Chemotherapy Protocols and Infusion Sequence

Iago Dillion Lima Cavalcanti

Chemotherapy Protocols and Infusion Sequence

Schedule Consideration in Cancer Treatment

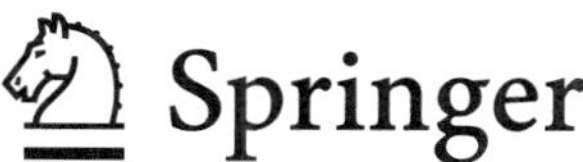 Springer

Iago Dillion Lima Cavalcanti
Federal University of Pernambuco
Recife, Pernambuco, Brazil

ISBN 978-3-031-10841-9   ISBN 978-3-031-10839-6   (eBook)
https://doi.org/10.1007/978-3-031-10839-6

This Springer imprint is published by the registered company Springer Nature Switzerland AG
The registered company address is: Gewerbestrasse 11, 6330 Cham, Switzerland

Preface

There are several types of cancer treatment modalities, such as surgery, radiotherapy, chemotherapy, immunotherapy, and targeted therapy, in which the choice of the best therapeutic option will depend on several factors such as type of tumor, stage of cancer, age, and clinical conditions of the patients. Due to the complexity of cancer, the association of therapeutic modalities has been shown to be effective, such as the application of chemotherapy and/or radiotherapy after surgical procedures or the association of chemotherapy that enhance the effects of radiotherapy.

The combination of anticancer drugs is also widely used, as they combine drugs that have different mechanisms of action, thereby enhancing the anticancer effect of the drugs. Although effective, the definition of chemotherapy protocols must be well planned to ensure maximum treatment efficacy and minimal toxic effects.

To define the best combination between chemotherapeutics, some parameters must be taken into account. Attention should be paid to the mechanisms of action and pharmacokinetic profile of each drug, diluent solutions and drug stability when infused concomitantly, as well as the drug's toxicity profiles, and the risks of dermatological toxicity due to vesicant, irritant, or not irritating characteristics. These characteristics are important as they provide safety and efficacy to the treatment.

Some studies highlight the importance of evaluating the order of infusion of the chemotherapy protocol due to possible pharmacodynamic and pharmacokinetic interactions, in which, depending on the infusion schedule, drugs may present antagonistic interactions with reduced therapeutic activity and increased toxicity, as well as depending on the order, they can present synergistic reactions with potentiation of therapeutic effects.

Therefore, this book tries to bring out the importance of combined chemotherapy in the treatment of cancer, highlighting the main parameters that must be considered when defining the infusion schedule of the protocols. In addition, I address the main solid cancers, such as breast, gastrointestinal, genitourinary, gynecological, head and neck cancers, among others, bringing the main protocols indicated for each type of cancer, with scientific studies of efficacy and data related to the infusion sequence.

Protocols were based on data made available in scientific articles, on the BC Cancer, University Hospital Southampton NHS Foundation websites, and in the book chemotherapy protocols 2017. The scarcity of articles that assess the infusion sequence of chemotherapy protocols reinforces the importance of this type of study to ensure maximum protocol effectiveness, as well as patient safety with the proposed therapy.

Recife, Pernambuco, Brazil   Iago Dillion Lima Cavalcanti 

Contents

Chapter 1
Polypharmacy in Cancer Therapy

1.1 Polypharmacy: Challenges in the Treatment of Chronic Diseases

Polypharmacy (Fig. 1.1) is defined as the routine and concomitant use of at least five medications (with or without a prescription) by a patient, being a common practice in older adult patients, especially people over 65 years of age [1, 2]. According to the study by Khezrian et al. [3], whose article traced the prevalence profile, determinants, and health outcomes related to polypharmacy. The authors observed that polypharmacy is related to the patient's age, being more common in the elderly, where it was estimated that by 2030, about 20% of people aged between 70 and 74 years can have a prescription for ten or more drugs, where the rate of polypharmacy is higher in the poorest population. According to Gu, Dillon, and Burt [4], the use of controlled medications increased from 6.3% to 10.7% when they compared the period 1999–2000 with the period 2007–2008, showing that more and more polypharmacy is present in therapy.

The increase in life expectancy has brought with it an increase in multimorbidity. Elderly patients with associated chronic diseases, such as diabetes mellitus, hypertension, cancer, cardiovascular and pulmonary diseases, among others, often need a combination of drugs to treat all their clinical conditions [5–9].

The presence of diseases in different organs makes patients look for different medical specialties, making each specialist act in the focus of the clinical condition and prescribe medications that can interact with other medications already in continuous use by the patient [10, 11]. In addition, the patient can also use over-the-counter medications, especially medications of natural origin that can interfere with their therapeutic follow-up [11–14]. Bui et al. [15] observed in their study, with patients with type 2 diabetes mellitus, that in addition to the drugs prescribed by physicians, 40.8% of the patients still used herbal and traditional drugs and food supplements.

I. D. Lima Cavalcanti, *Chemotherapy Protocols and Infusion Sequence*, https://doi.org/10.1007/978-3-031-10839-6_1

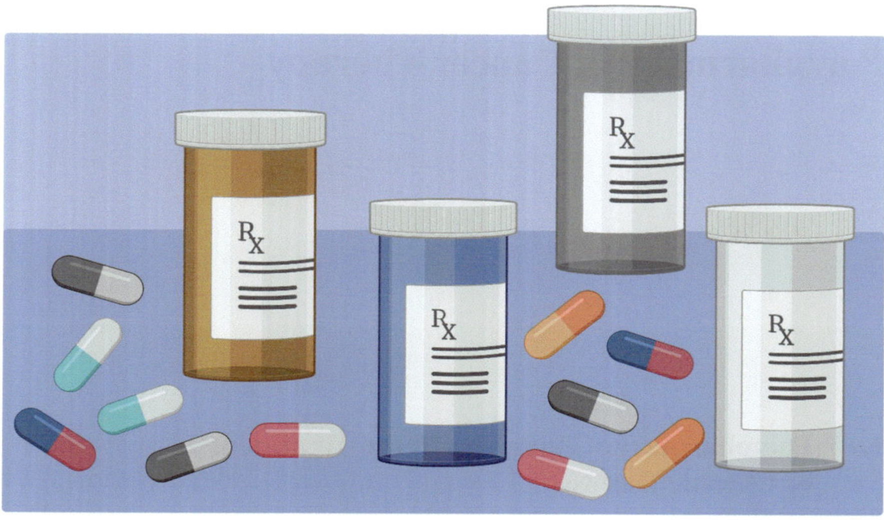

Fig. 1.1 Association of drugs as a therapeutic proposal. (Source: Created with BioRender.com)

Fig. 1.2 Diseases that are more related to the prevalence of polypharmacy. (Source: Marques et al. [16])

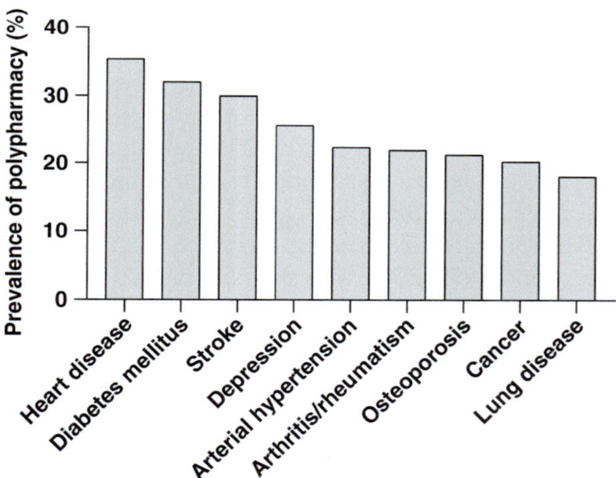

According to the study by Marques et al. [16], the prevalence of polypharmacy is more related to patients with heart disease with 35.3%, followed by diabetes mellitus with 32% (Fig. 1.2). Cancer patients also stand out in the study by Marques et al. [16] accounting for 20.3% of patients who use polypharmacy. This is a common practice in cancer treatment due to the complexity of the disease that requires the use of combined drugs, as well as the side effects of chemotherapy, thus requiring the use of drugs that reduce the side effects of chemotherapy [17, 18].

In many cases, polypharmacy is important, as it will allow all clinical conditions of the patient to receive adequate therapy. However, it is a practice that requires attention and multidisciplinary work, seeking integrative care, focused on reducing the risks of drug interactions and the effectiveness of combined therapy [19–21]. Table 1.1 presents studies that evaluated the use of polypharmacy in the treatment of diseases.

According to the study by Piccoliori et al. [22], 43% of patients had ≥5 diagnoses of chronic diseases and were the ones who used the most medications to treat their diseases (≥10 medications). Maxwell et al. [24] observed, in their cross-sectional study carried out in Canada, that multimorbidity is related to the increase in polypharmacy and is more prevalent in male patients. Pu et al. [28] report that in addition to greater age and multimorbidity, polypharmacy may also be associated with lower functional status and residence in a nursing home. The studies reported in Table 1.1 demonstrate the importance of assessing the need for polypharmacy and avoiding the development of undesirable drug interactions.

Table 1.1 Main findings of studies that evaluated polypharmacy for the treatment of diseases

Title article	Number of medicines	Diseases associated with polypharmacy	Conclusions	Reference
Epidemiology and associated factors of polypharmacy in older patients in primary care: a northern Italian cross-sectional study	≥8	Hypertension Arthrosis Type 2 diabetes mellitus Dyslipidemia Atrial fibrillation Coronary heart disease Osteoporosis Depression	Polypharmacy was associated with a number of chronic diseases that patients had and related to a decrease in the affective state and quality of life of patients	[22]
The phenomenon of polypharmacotherapy in polish geriatric population	6–10	Hypertension Diabetes Depression Dementia Ischemic heart disease Osteoporosis Heart failure Atrial fibrillation	Polypharmacy is related to the multimorbidity present in geriatric patients, which causes these patients to be treated by several specialist physicians, which contributes to the increase in the amount of medication that the patient has to use	[10]
Cardiovascular outcomes according to polypharmacy and drug adherence in patients with atrial fibrillation on long-term anticoagulation (from the RE-LY trial)	≥9	Hypertension Diabetes mellitus Coronary heart disease Heart failure	Polypharmacy and nonadherence to treatment in patients with atrial fibrillation may increase the risk of adverse cardiovascular and hemorrhagic events	[23]

(continued)

Table 1.1 (continued)

Title article	Number of medicines	Diseases associated with polypharmacy	Conclusions	Reference
Sex differences in multimorbidity and polypharmacy trends: A repeated cross-sectional study of older adults in Ontario, Canada	≥10	Acute myocardial infarction Asthma Cancer Cardiac arrhythmia Chronic coronary syndrome Chronic obstructive pulmonary disease Congestive heart failure Dementia Diabetes Hypertension Osteoarthritis	The prevalence of polypharmacy generally decreases among women, especially younger women with fewer chronic diseases, whereas polypharmacy increased at all ages and levels of multimorbidity among male patients	[24]
The effects of in-hospital deprescribing on potential prescribing omission in hospitalized elderly patients with polypharmacy	≥9	Hypertension Dyslipidemia Diabetes mellitus Asthma Dementia Ischemic stroke Ischemic heart disease Chronic kidney disease Heart failure Atrial fibrillation	The analysis of medication prescriptions allowed for a reduction in the number of medications for hospitalized elderly patients	[25]
Polypharmacy among people living with type 2 diabetes mellitus in rural communes in Vietnam	≥3.8	Type 2 diabetes mellitus	The number of medications increased according to the duration of type 2 diabetes mellitus, as well as the number of comorbidities	[15]

Table 1.1 (continued)

Title article	Number of medicines	Diseases associated with polypharmacy	Conclusions	Reference
The association of polypharmacy and high-risk drug classes with adverse health outcomes in the Scottish population with type 1 diabetes	≥5	Type 1 diabetes mellitus	The high number of prescription drugs are strong risk markers for the development of adverse health events, including acute complications of diabetes	[26]
The development of a scoring and ranking strategy for a patient-tailored adverse drug reaction prediction in polypharmacy	8	Cardiac failure Diabetes mellitus Hyperlipidemia	Tool capable of evaluating adverse drug reactions in polypharmacy therapies and may help in choosing the therapy and monitoring patient safety	[27]

Source: Research data

1.2   Scenario of Polypharmacy in Cancer Treatment

Polypharmacy has been a daily practice in cancer patients. Due to the narrow therapeutic window of antineoplastic chemotherapeutics, as well as the presence of other comorbidities in cancer patients, the combination of drugs in the therapeutic protocol of these patients becomes frequent [29]. With the complexity of cancer cells, many studies demonstrate that combination therapy has better results in tumor reduction when compared to monotherapy [17, 30]. The association of chemotherapeutic agents with different mechanisms of action (Fig. 1.3) allows a greater number of cancer cells to be reached, thus promoting a reduction in tumor mass and tumor regression [30, 31].

In addition, because cancer affects organs and compromises their functioning, it is common for cancer patients to use medication to relieve symptoms caused by tumor formation, where the pain is one of the main symptoms [8, 32, 33]. The use of drugs associated with chemotherapy can also be useful for reducing the toxicity of anticancer treatment [17, 34]. As well as the use of drugs whose objective is to reduce the toxicity of chemotherapy. The planning of the treatment protocol for cancer patients must be defined in a multi-professional way, to avoid serious drug interactions and reduce the quality of life of patients [35, 36].

Nieder et al. [37] studied the prevalence of polypharmacy in elderly patients ≥70 years old who received palliative radiotherapy and observed that 73% of the patients used five or more medications daily, with corticosteroids (59%) and analgesics opioids (55%) being the most used medications. Polypharmacy appears to be associated with symptom severity, as well as the pain medication used [37, 38].

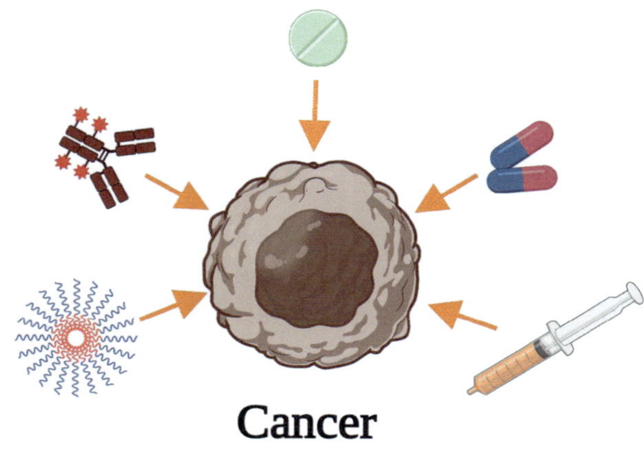

Fig. 1.3 Combination of different drugs with different mechanisms of action for the treatment of cancer. (Source: Created with BioRender.com)

In the study by Suzuki et al. [38], they observed that 70% of cancer patients used polypharmacy, where a part of the prescribed drugs was related to the symptoms presented by the patients, such as antiemetic drugs, analgesics, hypnotic sedatives, and laxatives, among others. After pharmaceutical evaluation of the prescription, at least one drug was recommended for suspension, being considered an unnecessary drug, reducing the use of antiemetics, gastrointestinal drugs, and hypnotic sedatives, thereby reducing or preventing adverse drug reactions [38, 39].

The presence of multimorbidity in cancer patients may be a factor that favors polypharmacy. According to the study by Keats et al. [40], 53% of adult cancer patients reported having multimorbidity, and 41% reported using ≥5 medications. Compared with a group that did not have cancer, the authors concluded that cancer appears to increase the risk of increased multimorbidity and polypharmacy, thereby increasing the health burden and the need for continuing education for the prevention of drug-related harm and focused interventions in reducing the prescription of unnecessary medications.

Alwhaibi et al. [41] also evaluated the association of comorbidities in cancer patients and the prevalence of polypharmacy. The authors observed that 79% of the patients used polypharmacy, being more prevalent in cancer patients with hypertension, diabetes, asthma, and anxiety. According to Nightingale, Skonecki, and Boparai [42], polypharmacy in elderly patients with cancer can induce adverse drug events, an increase in cases of falls, frailty, hospitalization, and postoperative complications and mortality.

1.3   Drug Interactions

The practice of polypharmacy, although important for the treatment of diseases such as diabetes, hypertension, and cancer, can present drug safety risks [7, 19, 43]. Polypharmacy is based on the prescription of drugs that will present different binding targets, seeking treatment efficacy or reducing resistance formation. This drug interaction may be beneficial, increasing the effectiveness of the therapy, or it may be unwanted, due to the development of adverse events [44]. Guthrie et al. [45] in a cross-sectional study in Scotland found that the greater the number of medications a patient uses, the greater the likelihood of potentially serious drug interactions. According to the study by Hoemme et al. [46], drug interactions influence in the overall survival of patients with breast cancer, in which patients without drug interactions had an overall survival of 34.9 months, while patients who had low- and high-risk drug interactions had an overall survival of 26.2 and 27 months, respectively.

Drug interaction is considered a form of adverse drug event, being identified as an avoidable cause of hospitalization related to drug use. One-third of cancer patients are prone to clinically relevant drug interactions, with around 2% of hospital admissions attributable to drug interactions in cancer patients [29, 47–49]. It is extremely important when defining the therapy that the patient will use, to assess the possible adverse reactions to which the treatment may be subject to develop and to assess the risk-benefit of the treatment [19, 50–53]. Given the complexity of drug interactions, polypharmacy is described as one of the greatest challenges of medical prescription [19, 54, 55].

1.3.1   Pharmacodynamic Interactions

Pharmacodynamic interactions refer to interactions related to the mechanism of action of drugs, where they directly influence the effects of each other and may potentiate the therapeutic effects of both drugs or reduce their effects [56–58]. Pharmacodynamic interactions may be desired when the potentiating effects are to be in the same direction as they were planned, and these synergistic effects are often aimed at in the treatment of infections or in pain therapy [57, 59]. When a drug blocks the effect of other drugs, they can be classified as antagonist drugs, which can be used in the desired way, when you want to reduce the exacerbated action of a particular drug, in cases of overdose and may be undesirable in the case of inhibiting the drug's action and reduce its therapeutic efficacy [56, 57, 60]. In Fig. 1.4 we observe the interaction of agonist and antagonist drugs that act on the same receptor.

Drugs can be classified according to their mechanism of action as nonspecific, with drugs that act independently of interaction with molecular targets, where their activities will depend on their physicochemical properties, such as solubility, oxi-reduction power, degree of ionization, and surface tension [56, 61]. On the other hand, specific drugs will interact with molecular targets, which can be enzymes, proteins, nucleic acids, and receptors [62, 63]. Figure 1.5 exemplifies the differences between nonspecific and specific drugs.

Antineoplastic therapy is based on the application of different drugs with different mechanisms of action that act together in the destruction of cancer cells. In this case, this type of interaction is desired, but also some interactions of antineoplastic

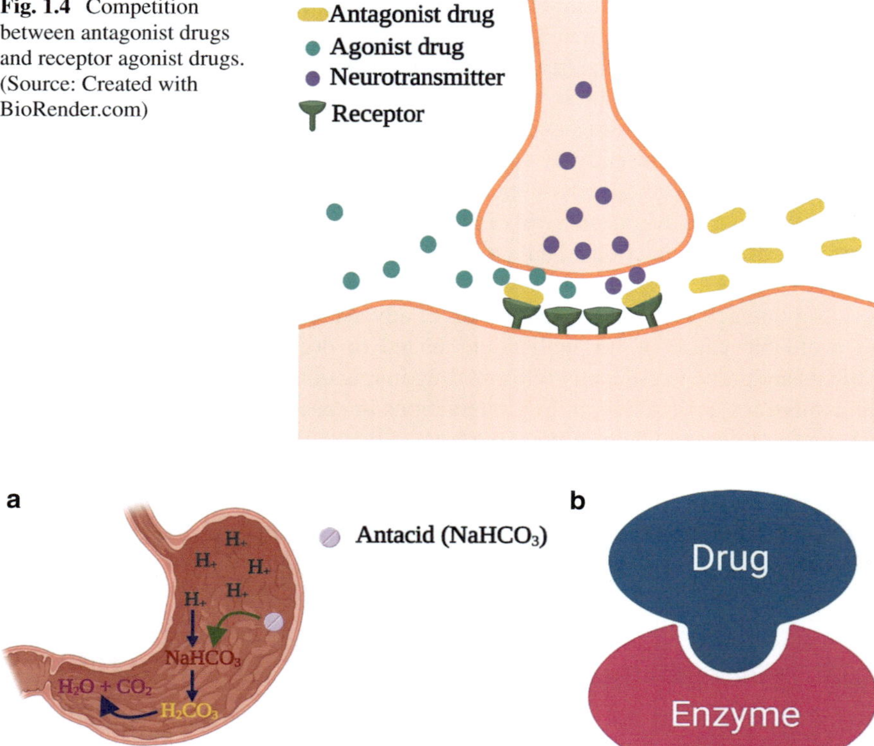

Fig. 1.4 Competition between antagonist drugs and receptor agonist drugs. (Source: Created with BioRender.com)

Fig. 1.5 Examples of mechanisms of action of nonspecific (**a**) and specific (**b**) drugs. (Source: Created with BioRender.com)

agents can potentiate their toxicity, which must be evaluated so as not to compromise the clinical status of the cancer patient [64–67].

Pharmacodynamic interactions can be classified as synergistic, when the effect of two drugs is greater than the sum of their individual effects; additive, when the effect of two drugs is just the sum of the effects of each; antagonist, when the effect of two drugs is less than the sum of their individual effects; and sequence-dependent effect, when the order of drug administration governs their effects [68–70].

An interaction widely used in cancer treatment is 5-fluorouracil (5-FU) with folinic acid (leucovorin). Leucovorin works by inhibiting the side effects of 5-FU and enhancing its anticancer efficacy [71]. Another interaction that may also be desired is methotrexate with leucovorin, as leucovorin may reduce the toxicity of methotrexate as well as reduce its effectiveness [72]. Figure 1.6 exemplifies the action of leucovorin on the mechanism of action of 5-FU and methotrexate.

Combination therapy for the treatment of cancer is based on pharmacodynamic interactions, synergistic, or additive, from a combination of drugs. With this in

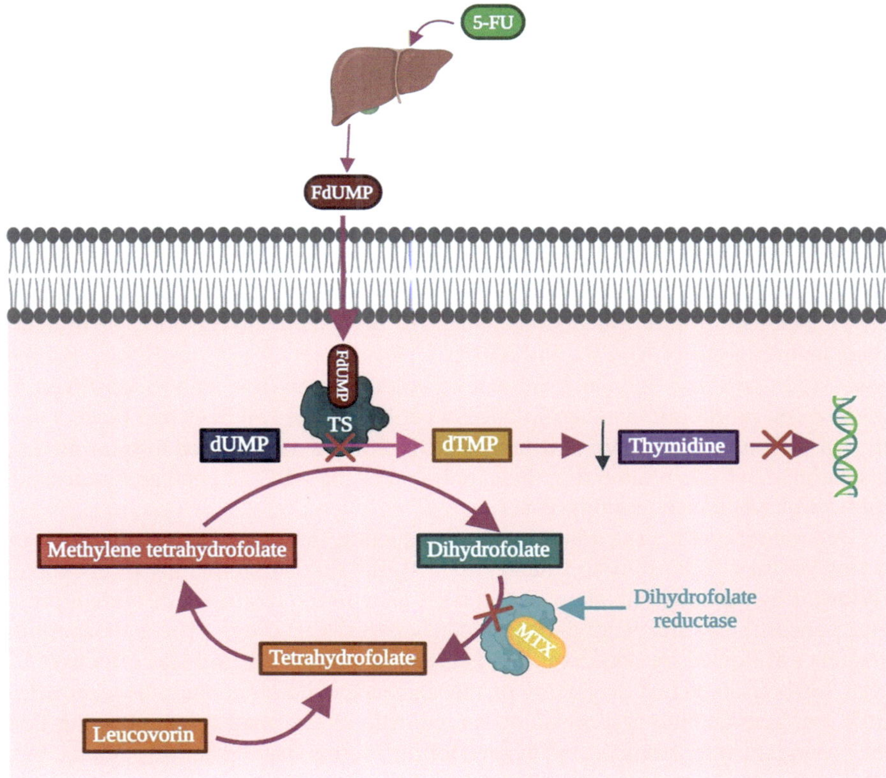

Fig. 1.6 Schematic of the interaction between 5-FU and leucovorin, where leucovorin will accelerate the thymidine synthesis process, thus facilitating the action of 5-FU in a step later with the inhibition of thymidylate synthase. We can also observe that methotrexate inhibits the formation of tetrahydrofolate, and when associated with leucovorin, because it is an analogue of tetrahydrofolate, it inhibits the action of methotrexate. *5-FU* 5-fluorouracil, *FdUMP* 5-fluoro-2′-deoxyuridine-5′-monophosphate, *dUMP* deoxyuridine monophosphate, *dTMP* deoxythymidine monophosphate, *TS* thymidylate synthase, *MTX* methotrexate. (Source: Created with BioRender.com)

mind, Milczarek, Pogorzelska, and Wiktorska [73] associated a natural compound derived from isothiocyanate and 5-FU in colon and prostate cancer cell lines. The authors observed synergistic effects between the substances, which seem to be more effective with more aggressive tumors, with the benefits observed in colon cancer cells of the HT-29 lineage.

Lam et al. [74] evaluated the interaction effects of herbal medicines such as Lingzhi and Yunzhi medicinal mushrooms with anticancer drugs. The authors observed that the antineoplastic agents most associated with mushrooms were cisplatin, 5-FU, mitomycin, tegafur, and paclitaxel, showing that the interactions increased the cytotoxic efficacy of the drugs, in addition to improving adverse effects and the quality of life of patients with cancer. Pawaskar et al. [75] evaluated the synergistic interactions between sorafenib and everolimus in pancreatic cancer xenografts noting that this interaction promoted a complete inhibition of tumor growth. Also in human pancreatic cancer cells, Ricciardi et al. [76] observed synergistic cytotoxic effects between sorafenib and gemcitabine, where sorafenib reduced the activation of c-Kit, extracellular signal-regulated kinases (ERK), and vascular endothelial growth factor receptor 2 (VEGFR2), while gemcitabine inhibited Akt phosphorylation.

Qian et al. [77] evaluated the effects of coix seed extract associated with gemcitabine in pancreatic cancer. The results of the study showed that coix seed extract greatly increased the effectiveness of gemcitabine with a tumor inhibition rate of $76.01 \pm 8.46\%$, where interactions appear to be related to regulation of protein-mediated drug efflux ABCB1 and ABCG2. Desidero et al. [78] also evaluated the association of drugs for the treatment of colon cancer. The authors observed in in vitro cell proliferation assays in different colon cancer cell lines that the association of the active metabolite of irinotecan (SN-38) when associated to sunitinib has a synergistic effect in inhibiting the expression of the ABCG2 gene and increasing intracellular of concentrations of SN-38.

Depending on the drug administration sequence, they may have different interaction profiles. According to Chen et al. [79], the sequential therapy of docetaxel followed by cabozantinib showed better efficacy in the treatment of human prostate cancer, showing synergistic effects between the drugs. The cabozantinib sequence followed by docetaxel had antagonistic effects, being less effective. Li et al. [80] observed that depending on the sequence of administration between erlotinib and gemcitabine synergistic or antagonistic effects may occur, showing that the synergistic interaction occurs when erlotinib is administered before gemcitabine, while the opposite occurs antagonism.

Also evaluating the interactions of combination therapy in the treatment of prostate cancer, Ben-Eltriki, Deb, and Guns [81] evaluated the use of calcitriol in combination therapy, bringing together several studies related to calcitriol in prostate cancer therapy. Calcitriol appears to increase the antiproliferative and cytotoxic effects of chemotherapy when combined with the antineoplastics mitoxantrone, docetaxel, and paclitaxel in vitro against cells of the PC3 lineage [82, 83]. This interaction of calcitriol with taxanes seems to be due to the action of calcitriol in reducing the expression of protein-1, and this protein is responsible for the mechanisms of resistance to multiple drugs [84].

Calcitriol has shown benefits in reducing cancer cell resistance mechanisms [81]. According to the study by Skowronski, Peehl, and Feldman [85], the combination of cetuximab with calcitriol suppresses the growth of hormone-resistant DU145 PCa cells, causing considerable interruption of the cell cycle in the G0/Gal phase and increased apoptosis.

Frances et al. [86] observed in clinical trials the synergistic effect of capecitabine associated with docetaxel in the treatment of metastatic breast cancer. Epidermal growth factor receptor (EGFR) inhibitor monoclonal antibodies also have pharmacodynamic interactions that can lead to the development of adverse reactions or increase antitumor activity. The combination of EGFR blockers combined with chemotherapy brings synergistic effects, thereby causing irreparable damage to cancer cells and may also reduce the resistance of tumor cells [87]. Other benefits of interactions are the association of curcumin that neutralizes the ototoxicity of cisplatin [88], and sulforaphane attenuates the cardiotoxicity of doxorubicin [89].

Despite the benefits of some pharmacodynamic interactions of anticancer treatment, others can cause serious adverse reactions [90]. Pritchard, McElwain, and Graham-Pole [91] observed that the association of high doses of melphalan with cyclophosphamide, vincristine, and doxorubicin can induce dangerous toxicity in the spinal cord and mucosa in children being treated for neuroblastoma.

Mouzon et al. [92] found in their cross-sectional study with anticancer agents a total of 41 potential interactions, of which 10 were considered more severe. As for the consequences of interactions, they increased the toxicity of drugs and led to a decrease in the effectiveness of the treatment. The authors emphasize that the drugs cisplatin, methotrexate, lapatinib, and fluorouracil were the ones that were most involved in drug interactions.

Some drugs may have additive interactions in increasing the risk of toxicity; examples are trastuzumab associated with doxorubicin, which increases the risk of cardiotoxicity and cisplatin when associated with nephrotoxic drugs such as aminoglycosides and rituximab induces renal toxicity [68, 93–96]. The use of vinorelbine associated with paclitaxel seems to induce the development of neuropathy [68, 97, 98].

1.3.2 Pharmacokinetic Interactions

Pharmacokinetic interactions are related to the route that the drug takes in the body and may occur during the processes of absorption, distribution, metabolization, or excretion of drugs. These interactions are identified when changes in pharmacokinetic parameters occur, such as changes in peak serum concentration, area under the curve, drug half-life, total amount of drug excreted, among others [99–101]. Figure 1.7 presents some mechanisms of pharmacokinetic interactions.

Pharmacokinetic interactions can reduce the effectiveness of a drug and increase its permanence in the body, with a consequent increase in its toxicity. Liu et al. [103] evaluated antipsychotic polypharmacy with clozapine and risperidone in in vitro and in vivo studies in healthy male Sprague-Dawley rats, with the aim of evaluating their interactions for the treatment of schizophrenia. The authors observed that clozapine inhibited the metabolism of risperidone in vivo and increased its concentration in plasma and brain, thereby causing brain exposure and possibly inducing toxic effects.

Some drugs can interact by reducing the absorption of a certain drug, an example is the interaction of proton pump inhibitors (rabeprazole, omeprazole, and esomeprazole) with tyrosine kinase inhibitors (erlotinib, lapatinib, nilotinib, imatinib, and axitinib). The proton pump inhibitors will cause changes in gastric pH and consequently inhibit the absorption of tyrosine kinase inhibitors [104, 105].

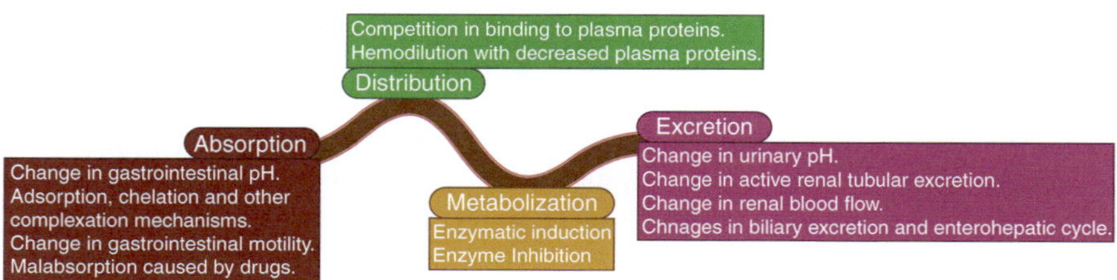

Fig. 1.7 Main mechanisms present in pharmacokinetic interactions. (Source: [100, 102]. Created with BioRender.com)

Another type of interaction is related to the distribution of drugs, to which some have a high binding with plasma proteins, requiring binding to be distributed to their site of action. Tyrosine kinase inhibitor drugs are highly protein-bound and may interact with other drugs that require this binding to plasma proteins, such as phenytoin and warfarin, which are highly protein-bound [104–107].

Gruzdeva, Khokhlov, and Ilyin [108] evaluated the drug interaction profile in patients with coronary heart disease using polypharmacy. The authors noted that drug interactions are more related to changes in the activity of cytochrome P450 isoenzymes, which is the most important biotransformation enzyme in drug metabolism [109].

Seeking to assess drug interactions in breast cancer patients, Fogli et al. [110] evaluated interactions of patients treated with CDK4/6 inhibitors (palbociclib, ribociclib, and abemacilib), where they could observe that the metabolic clearance of these inhibitors occurs mainly due to the metabolism in CYP3A4 in the liver. The interaction of these drugs can significantly change the pharmacokinetic profile of these inhibitors, which may influence their safety profile.

Another substance that is also metabolized by CYP3A4 is calcitriol [81]. This metabolization can cause interactions with drugs that are also metabolized by this enzyme, such as ketoconazole, tamoxifen, ritonavir, or clarithromycin, thereby causing a 60–100% inhibition of calcitriol inactivation by CYP3A4. Deb et al. [111] observed that calcitriol interacted with abiraterone mediated by CYP3A4 and inhibiting calcitriol inactivation in the liver and intestine and provided benefits in anticancer therapy of patients with prostate cancer.

Abiraterone inhibits enzymes important in the metabolism of several drugs, such as cytochrome P450-dependent enzymes, CYP2C8, and CYP2D6 in the liver; thus abiraterone can increase the plasma levels of drugs such as amitriptyline, oxycodone, risperidone, amiodarone, and carbamazepine. Due to the metabolism of enzalutamide by CYP2C8, abiraterone may also increase its plasma concentration. In addition, drugs that induce CYP2C8 can reduce the effectiveness of enzalutamide and should be avoided, as is the case with rifampicin [112].

Lipp and Miller [113] also evaluated the potential drug interactions of abiraterone and enzalutamide, used for the treatment of metastatic prostate cancer. The authors point out that because enzalutamide is a strong inducer of CYP3A4, it has the potential to decrease the plasma concentrations of several drugs. Concerning abiraterone, which is a strong inhibitor of CYP2D6, the situation is less worrying, as the metabolism mediated by CYP2D6 is much lower than with CYP3A4.

Regarding enzyme interactions, sorivudine is an inhibitor of dihydropyrimidine dehydrogenase, which is an important enzyme for 5-FU catabolism and responsible for 5-FU detoxification. With the inhibition of the enzyme by sorivudine, there is an increase in the levels of 5-FU, thereby increasing its toxicity, inducing the development of gastrointestinal disorders and bone marrow toxicity, as well as leading the patient to death [114–116].

Enzyme-inhibiting drugs can also reduce the effectiveness of a drug, for example, paroxetine can act by inhibiting the conversion of tamoxifen to endoxifen (active metabolite) due to targeted N-methylation of CYP3A4 and targeted hydroxylation of CYP2D6 [117, 118].

Another pharmacokinetic interaction profile is related to changes in drug excretion. An example of this type of interaction is methotrexate when combined with non-steroidal anti-inflammatory drugs (NSAIDs), which increase the exposure of plasma methotrexate, with a consequent decrease in the urinary flow rate [119]. The interaction of methotrexate with benzimidazoles may induce methotrexate toxicity, due to the increased serum concentration of its active metabolite 7-hydroxymethotrexate [120, 121].

1.4 Advantages in Drug Association

The use of polypharmacy, when properly applied, can help in the treatment of the patient, promoting the reduction of symptoms and the treatment of patients with multimorbidities [20, 122]. Cancer is a complex disease that can affect several organs, compromising their functioning, requiring a drug combination to improve the response in reducing cell proliferation of cancer cells, as well as to relieve symptoms [17, 123–125]. Furthermore, the cancer treatment itself can induce toxicity and compromise some organs, requiring the use of drugs to avoid the toxic effects of chemotherapy [8, 126–128]. Table 1.2 presents some advantages and disadvantages of polypharmacy.

Table 1.2 Main advantages and disadvantages of polypharmacy

Advantages	Disadvantages
Controlling chronic conditions or multiple comorbidities	Increased risk of drug interactions
Improve the quality of life of patients	Reduced quality of life due to treatment toxicity
Increased treatment effectiveness with synergism with therapeutic action of drugs	Reduced therapeutic effectiveness and increased toxicity
Increased disease control	Risk of nonadherence to treatment by the patient
Reduction of adverse events	Higher risk of medication errors

Source: [129, 130]

Seeking to develop a conjugate to multiple targets in cancer cells, Alam et al. [131] developed alkylphosphocholine-gefitinib conjugates, showing their benefits in inhibiting Akt phosphorylation and of EGFR tyrosine kinase, showing superior or comparable effects to erlotinib and miltefosine. Kim et al. [132] evaluated, in a phase 1 study, the combination of sorafenib and trametinib in patients with advanced hepatocellular cancer. The authors showed the safety in the association of these drugs in the treatment of hepatocellular cancer, although some patients had adverse reactions such as the elevation of aspartate aminotransferase (AST) in 37% of patients and hypertension in 24% of patients. But, on the other hand, the association led to 98.1% inhibition of phosphorylated ERK, which is an important pathway for cell proliferation.

Jiang et al. [133] evaluated the benefits of combined gemcitabine and sorafenib for the treatment of non-small cell lung cancer. In in vitro studies, the authors observed induction of cell cycle arrest and apoptosis of the A549 lineage cells. And in vivo studies showed a decrease in tumor mass in non-small cell lung cancer with the association of gemcitabine and sorafenib.

Combination therapy is more effective than monotherapy, but in some cases, combination chemotherapy can also increase the toxic profile of the therapy and lead to patient hospitalization and worsening of their clinical situation [134, 135]. Drug interactions are complex and require the action of a multidisciplinary team to provide comprehensive care to the patient and reduce drug-related problems [36, 136–138].

The use of premedication makes it possible to reduce the toxicity of chemotherapy. Groleau and Côte [139] evaluated the use of dexamethasone before pemetrexed-based chemotherapy, verifying that the use of dexamethasone allowed the reduction of skin toxicity due to treatment with pemetrexed. Saito et al. [140] evaluated the use of intravenous magnesium as a premedication to reduce cisplatin-induced nephrotoxicity, showing that magnesium had a protective effect. Kubo et al. [141] also used magnesium with a prophylactic effect on renal dysfunction in preoperative chemotherapy with the use of cisplatin in patients with esophageal cancer, thereby also showing the benefits of magnesium as a renal protector.

1.5   Risks of Polypharmacy

Polypharmacy, as important as it is for the treatment of patients, can have consequences in terms of reduced life expectancy, quality of life, frequency of readmissions, and financial costs [53, 122, 142–144]. These problems are related to the increase in adverse reactions to the treatment, which may be related to drug interactions present in the therapeutic protocol [18, 142, 145, 146]. Table 1.3 shows some studies that report adverse events due to drug interactions in patients undergoing polypharmacy.

According to the study by Millenaar et al. [23], patients with atrial fibrillation and who use polypharmacy should be advised when treatment adherence to avoid the development of adverse cardiovascular and hemorrhagic events that could lead to the patient's death. Pu et al. [28] observed in their study that the use of polypharmacy can induce signs of aspiration in the elderly, which can lead to swallowing disorders.

Hohn et al. [26] showed that polypharmacy in patients with type 1 diabetes can induce the development of reactions such as falls, hypoglycemia, and even the

Table 1.3 Main adverse events induced by drug interactions in patients using polypharmacy

Drugs in use	Most frequent adverse events	Reference
Antithrombotic/anticoagulant Antidepressants/antipsychotics Calcium carbonate Beta-blockers	Not reported	[22]
Antipsychotic	Gastrointestinal tract reactions Brain exposure	[103]
Antidepressants Diuretics Calcium channel blockers Beta blockers Antiepileptics Blood-glucose-lowering drugs Anticoagulant/antithrombotic	Falls Hypoglycemia Diabetic ketoacidosis	[26]
Antithrombotic ACE inhibitors Antiarrhythmic Diuretics Dihydropyridine calcium antagonists Beta blockers	Bradycardia Hypotension Thrombus formation	[108]
Valsartan Bisoprolol Bumetanide Digoxin Metformin Sitagliptin Gliclazide Simvastatin	Vomiting Renal failure Septic shock	[27]
Serotonin reuptake inhibitors Serotonin-noradrenalin reuptake inhibitors/ noradrenaline reuptake inhibitors Tricyclic antidepressants Gabapentinoids	Vascular risk factors	[147]
Opioid Antiepileptics Antipsychotics Beta blockers Diuretics Anxiolytic Antidepressant	Opioid overdose	[148]

(continued)

Table 1.3 (continued)

Drugs in use	Most frequent adverse events	Reference
Anthracyclines Fluoropyrimidines Platinum salts Antitubulins Anti-inflammatories Anticoagulants Antiplatelet Antihypertensives Corticosteroids	Decrease in renal creatinine clearance Myopathy Cardiovascular risk	[35]
Anthracyclines Fluoropyrimidines Platinum salts Antitubulins Antifolates Alkylators Tyrosine kinase inhibitors Monoclonal antibodies Non-steroidal antirheumatic drugs Low-dose aspirin Beta-blockers Opioids Proton pump inhibitors	Renal dysfunction Cardiac dysfunction Neurotoxicity Bradycardia Leucocytopenia Risk of bleeding Hypotension Hyperkalemia	[149]

Source: Research data

patient's death. Valeanu et al. [27] evaluated the effectiveness of a tool to prevent adverse reactions due to polypharmacy, evaluating the case of an 85-year-old patient who had three diseases and was using eight drugs, dying due to drug interactions.

Brett et al. [147] evaluated the use of psychotropic drugs in Australia in 2018, noting the use of polypharmacy. The authors observed that drug interactions with the use of serotonin reuptake inhibitors, serotonin-noradrenaline reuptake inhibitors, antidepressants, and gabapentinoids for the treatment of mental illness can bring serious cardiovascular problems. The study by Al-Qurain et al. [148] evaluated the risks of opioid interactions in elderly patients undergoing polypharmacy, where they observed that the interaction of opioids with antiepileptics may increase the risk of opioid overdose.

Some chemotherapy protocols for the treatment of cancer, despite showing greater efficacy, may be responsible for adverse reactions. Monteiro et al. [35] evaluated the main drug interactions in cancer patients, identifying serious interactions such as the association of paclitaxel with doxorubicin that can decrease renal clearance of creatinine induced by paclitaxel, also can lead to cardiovascular damage, as well as the interaction of cyclophosphamide with doxorubicin and aspirin with pemetrexed.

Hoemme et al. [149] highlight that the risk of drug interactions increases with the increase in the number of drugs in use, from 14% in patients with <4 drugs, 24% in patients with 4–7 drugs, 40% with 8–11 drugs, and 67% with >11 medications in use. The increase in the use of medication also seems to be related to the severity of the disease, being more frequent in patients with advanced cancer.

References

1. Almeida NA, Reiners AAO, Azevedo RCS, Silva AMC, Cardoso JDC, Souza LC. Prevalence of and factors associated with polypharmacy among elderly persons residents in the community. Revista Brasileira de Geriatria e Gerontologia. 2017;20(1):138–48. https://doi.org/10.1590/1981-22562017020.160086.
2. Halli-Tierney AD, Scarbrough C, Carroll D. Polypharmacy: evaluating risks and deprescribing. Am Fam Physician. 2019;100(1):32–8.
3. Khezrian M, McNeil CJ, Murray AD, Myint PK. An overview of prevalence, determinants and health outcomes of polypharmacy. Ther Adv Drug Saf. 2020;11:1–10. https://doi.org/10.1177/2042098620933741.
4. Gu Q, Dillon CF, Burt V. Prescription drug use continues to increase: U.S. prescription drug data for 2007-2008. NCHS Data Brief. 2010;(42):1–8.
5. Foscolou A, Chrysohoou C, Dimitriadis K, Masoura K, Vogiatzi G, Gkotzamanis V, Lazaros G, Tsioufis C, Stefanadis C. The association of healthy aging with multimorbidity IKARIA study. Nutrients. 2021;13:1386. https://doi.org/10.3390/nu13041386.
6. Nascimento RCRM, Álvares J, Guerra AA Jr, Gomes IC, Silveira MR, Costa EA, Leite SN, Costa KS, Soeiro OM, Guibu IA, Karnikowski MGO, Acurcio FA. Polifarmácia: uma realidade na atenção primária do Sistema Único de Saúde. Rev Saude Publica. 2017;51(Suppl 2):1S–12S. https://doi.org/10.11606/S1518-8787.2017051007136.
7. Nobili A, Garattini S, Mannucci PM. Multiple diseases and polypharmacy in the elderly: challenges for the internist of the third millennium. J Comorb. 2011;1:28–44. https://doi.org/10.15256/joc.2011.1.4.
8. Sarfati D, Koczwara B, Jackson C. The impact of comorbidity on cancer and its treatment. CA Cancer J Clin. 2016;66(4):337–50. https://doi.org/10.3322/caac.21342.
9. Vetrano DL, Roso-Llorach A, Fernández S, Guisado-Clavero M, Violán C, Onder G, Fratiglioni L, Calderón-Larrañaga A, Marengoni A. Twelve-year clinical trajectories of multimorbidity in a population of folder adults. Nat Commun. 2020;11:3223. https://doi.org/10.1038/s41467-020-16780-x.
10. Krenzel I, Rogalska A, Holecki T. The phenomenon of polypharmacotherapy in Polish geriatric population. Acta Poloniae Pharmaceutica Drug Res. 2021;78(1):129–34. https://doi.org/10.32383/appdr/131932.
11. Tonelli M, Wiebe N, Manns BJ, Klarenbach SW, James MT, Ravani P, Pannu N, Himmelfarb J, Hemmelgarn BR. Comparison of the complexity of patients seen by different medical subspecialists in a universal health care system. JAMA Netw Open. 2018;1(7):e184852. https://doi.org/10.1001/jamanetworkopen.2018.4852.
12. FitzGerald RJ. Medication errors: the importance of an accurate drug history. Br J Clin Pharmacol. 2009;67(6):671–5. https://doi.org/10.1111/j.1365-2125.2009.03424.x.
13. Jin J, Sklar GE, Oh VMS, Li SC. Factors affecting therapeutic compliance: a review from the patient's perspective. Ther Clin Risk Manag. 2008;4(1):269–86. https://doi.org/10.2147/tcrm.s1458.
14. Starfield B. The hidden inequity in health care. Int J Equity Health. 2011;10:15. https://doi.org/10.1186/1475-9276-10-15.
15. Bui DHT, Nguyen BX, Truong DC, Meyrowitsch DW, Søndergaard J, Gammeltoft T, Bygbjerg IC, Jannie N. Polypharmacy among people living with type 2 diabetes mellitus in rural communes in Vietnam. PLoS One. 2021;16(4):e0249849. https://doi.org/10.1371/journal.pone.0249849.

16. Marques PP, Assumpção D, Rezende R, Neri AL, Francisco PMSB. Polypharmacy in community-based older adults: results of the Fibra study. Revista Brasileira de Geriatria e Gerontologia. 2019;22(5):e190118. https://doi.org/10.1590/1981-22562019022.190118.

17. Mokhtari RB, Homayouni TS, Baluch N, Morgatskaya E, Kumar S, Das B, Yeger H. Combination therapy in combating cancer. Oncotarget. 2017;8(23):38022–43. https://doi.org/10.18632/oncotarget.16723.

18. Shrestha S, Shrestha S, Khanal S. Polypharmacy in elderly cancer patients: challenges and the way clinical pharmacists can contribute in resource-limited settings. Aging Med. 2019;2(1):42–9. https://doi.org/10.1002/agm2.12051.

19. Cadogan CA, Ryan C, Hughes CM. Appropriate polypharmacy and medicine safety: when many is not too many. Drug Saf. 2016;39:109–16. https://doi.org/10.1007/s40264-015-0378-5.

20. Rankin A, Cadogan CA, Patterson SM, Kerse N, Cardwell CR, Bradley MC, Ryan C, Hughes C. Interventions to improve the appropriate use of polypharmacy for older people. Cochrane Library. 2018;2018(9):CD008165. https://doi.org/10.1002/14651858.CD008165.pub4.

21. Saljoughian M. Polypharmacy and drug adherence in elderly patients. US Pharmacist. 2019;44(7):33–6.

22. Piccoliori G, Mahlknecht A, Sandri M, Valentini M, Vogele A, Schmid S, Deflorian F, Engl A, Sonnichsen A, Wiedermann C. Epidemiology and associated factors of polypharmacy in older patients in primary care: a northern Italian cross-sectional study. BMC Geriatr. 2021;21(1):197. https://doi.org/10.1186/s12877-021-02141-w.

23. Millenaar D, Schumacher H, Brueckmann M, Eikelboom JW, Ezekowitz M, Slawik J, Ewen S, Ukena C, Wallentin L, Connolly S, Yusuf S, Bohm M. Cardiovascular outcomes according to polypharmacy and drug adherence in patients with atrial fibrillation on long-term anticoagulation (from the RE-LY trial). Am J Cardiol. 2021;149:P27–35. https://doi.org/10.1016/j.amjcard.2021.03.024.

24. Maxwell CJ, Mondor L, Koné AJP, Hogan DB, Wodchis WP. Sex differences in multimorbidity and polypharmacy trends: a repeated cross-sectional study of older adults in Ontario, Canada. PLoS One. 2021;16(4):e0250567. https://doi.org/10.1371/journal.pone.0250567.

25. Kaminaga M, Komagamine J, Tatsumi S. The effects of in-hospital deprescribing on potential prescribing omission in hospitalized elderly patients with polypharmacy. Sci Rep. 2021;11:8898. https://doi.org/10.1038/s41598-021-88362-w.

26. Hohn A, Jeyam A, Caparrotta TM, McGurnaghan SJ, O'Reilly JE, Blackbourn LAK, McCrimmon RJ, Leese GP, McKnight JA, Kennon B, Lindsay RS, Sattar N, Wild SH, McKeigue PM, Colhoun HM. The association of polypharmacy and high-risk drug classes with adverse health outcomes in the Scottish population with type 1 diabetes. Diabetologia. 2021;64(6):1309–19. https://doi.org/10.1007/s00125-021-05394-7.

27. Valeanu A, Damian C, Marineci CD, Negres S. The development of a scoring and ranking strategy for a patient-tailored adverse drug reaction prediction in polypharmacy. Sci Rep. 2020;10:9552. https://doi.org/10.1038/s41598-020-66611-8.

28. Pu D, Wong MCH, Yiu EML, Chan KMK. Profiles of polypharmacy in older adults and medication associations with signs of aspiration. Expert Rev Clin Pharmacol. 2021;14(5):643–9. https://doi.org/10.1080/17512433.2021.1909474.

29. Riechelmann RP, Del Giglio A. Drug interactions in oncology: how common are they? Ann Oncol. 2009;20(12):1907–12. https://doi.org/10.1093/annonc/mdp369.

30. Falzone L, Salomone S, Libra M. Evolution of cancer pharmacological treatments at the turn of the third millennium. Front Pharmacol. 2018;9:1300. https://doi.org/10.3389/fphar.2018.01300.

31. Hernández AP, Juanes-Velasco P, Landeira-Viñuela A, Bareke H, Montalvillo E, Góngora R, Fuentes M. Restoring the immunity in the tumor microenvironment: insights into immunogenic cell death in onco-therapies. Cancers. 2021;13(11):2821. https://doi.org/10.3390/cancers13112821.

32. Nightingale G, Mohamed MR, Holmes HM, Sharma M, Ramsdale E, Lu-Yao G, Chapman A. Research priorities to address polypharmacy in older adults with cancer. J Geriat Oncol. 2021;12(6):964–70. https://doi.org/10.1016/j.jgo.2021.01.009.

33. Whitman A, Erdeljac P, Jones C, Pillarella N, Nightingale G. Managing polypharmacy in older adults with cancer across different healthcare settings. Drug Healthc Patient Saf. 2021;13:101–16. https://doi.org/10.2147/DHPS.S255893.

34. Zhang Z, Zhou L, Xie N, Nice EC, Zhang T, Cui Y, Huang C. Overcoming cancer therapeutic bottleneck by drug repurposing. Signal Transduct Target Ther. 2020;5:113. https://doi.org/10.1038/s41392-020-00213-8.

35. Monteiro CRA, Schoueri JHM, Cardial DT, Linhares LC, Turke KC, Steuer LV, Menezes LWA, Argani IL, Sette C, Cubero DIG, Giglio A. Evaluation of the systemic and therapeutic repercussions caused by drug interactions in oncology patients. Rev Assoc Med Bras. 2019;65(5):611–7. https://doi.org/10.1590/1806-9282.65.5.611.

36. Taberna M, Moncayo FG, Jané-Salas E, Antonio M, Arribas L, Vilajosana E, Torres EP, Mesía R. The multidisciplinary team (MDT) approach and quality of care. Front Oncol. 2020;10:85. https://doi.org/10.3389/fonc.2020.00085.

37. Nieder C, Mannasaker B, Pawinski A, Haukland E. Polypharmacy in older patients ≥70 years receiving palliative radiotherapy. Anticancer Res. 2017;37(2):795–9. https://doi.org/10.21873/anticanres.11379.

38. Suzuki S, Uchida M, Suga Y, Sugawara H, Kokubun H, Uesawa Y, Nakagawa T, Takase H. A Nationwide survey of community pharmacist contributions to polypharmacy in opioid-using and non-using cancer patients in Japan. Biol Pharm Bull. 2019;42(7):1164–71. https://doi.org/10.1248/bpb.b19-00043.

39. Uchida M, Suzuki S, Sugawara H, Suga Y, Kokubun H, Uesawa Y, Nakagawa T, Takase H. A Nationwide survey of hospital pharmacist interventions to improve polypharmacy for patients with cancer in palliative care in Japan. J Pharm Health Care and Sci. 2019;5:14. https://doi.org/10.1186/s40780-019-0143-5.

40. Keats MR, Cui Y, DeClercq V, Grandy SA, Sweeney E, Dummer TJB. Burden of multimorbidity and polypharmacy among cancer survivors: a population-based nested case-control study. Support Care Cancer. 2021;29(2):713–23. https://doi.org/10.1007/s00520-020-05529-3.

41. Alwhaibi M, AlRuthia Y, Alhawassi TM, Almalag H, Alsalloum H, Balkhi B. Polypharmacy and comorbidities among ambulatory cancer patients: a cross-sectional retrospective study. J Oncol Pharm Pract. 2020;26(5):1052–9. https://doi.org/10.1177/1078155219880255.

42. Nightingale G, Skonecki E, Boparai MK. The impact of polypharmacy on patient outcomes in older adults with cancer. Cancer J. 2017;23(4):211–8. https://doi.org/10.1097/PPO.0000000000000277.

43. Park JW, Roh JL, Lee SW, Kim SE, Choi SH, Nam SY, Kim SY. Effect of polypharmacy and potentially inappropriate medications on treatment and posttreatment courses in elderly patients with head and neck cancer. J Cancer Res Clin Oncol. 2016;142:1031–40. https://doi.org/10.1007/s00432-015-2108-x.

44. Liu X, Ye K, van Vlijmen HWT, Emmerich MTM, Ijzerman AP, van Westen GJP. DrugEx v2: de novo design of drug molecule by pareto-based multi-objective reinforcement learning in polypharmacology. ChemRxiv. 2021;1–34. https://doi.org/10.26434/chemrxiv.14474127.v2.

45. Guthrie B, Makubate B, Hernandez-Santiago V, Dreischulte T. The rising tide of polypharmacy and drug-drug interactions: population database analysis 1995-2010. BMC Med. 2015;13:74. https://doi.org/10.1186/s12916-015-0322-7.

46. Hoemme A, Barth H, Haschke M, Krahenbuhl S, Strasser F, Lehner C, von Kameke A, Walti T, Thurlimann B, Fruh M, Driessen C, Joerger M. Prognostic impact of polypharmacy and drug interactions in patients with advanced cancer. Cancer Chemother Pharmacol. 2019;83(4):763–74. https://doi.org/10.1007/s00280-019-03783-9.

47. Riechelmann RP, Zimmermann C, Chin SN, Wang L, O'Carroll A, Zarinehbaf S, Krzyzanowska MK. Potential drug interactions in cancer patients receiving supportive care exclusively. J Pain Symptom Manag. 2008;35(5):535–43. https://doi.org/10.1016/j.jpainsymman.2007.06.009.

48. Ussai S, Petelin R, Giordano A, Malinconico M, Cirillo D, Pentimalli F. A pilot study on the impacto f known drug-drug interactions in cancer patients. J Exp Clin Cancer Res. 2015;34(1):89. https://doi.org/10.1186/s13046-015-0201-2.

49. Yeoh TT, Tay XY, Si P, Chew L. Drug-related problems in elderly patients with cancer receiving outpatient chemotherapy. J Geriatr Oncol. 2015;6(4):280–7. https://doi.org/10.1016/j.jgo.2015.05.001.
50. Pretorius RW, Gataric G, Swedlund SK, Miller JR. Reducing the risk of adverse drug events in older adults. Am Fam Physician. 2013;85(5):331–6.
51. Lavan AH, Gallagher P. Predicting risk of adverse drug reactions in older adults. Therap Adv Drug Saf. 2016;7(1):11–22. https://doi.org/10.1177/2042098615615472.
52. Malki MA, Person ER. Drug-drug-gene interactions and adverse drug reactions. Pharmacogenomics J. 2020;20:355–66. https://doi.org/10.1038/s41397-019-0122-0.
53. Rodrigues MCS, Oliveira C. Drug-drug interactions and adverse drug reactions in polypharmacy among older adults: an integrative review. Rev Lat Am Enfermagem. 2016;24:e2800.
54. Masnoon N, Shakib S, Kallisch-Ellett L, Caughey GE. What is polypharmacy? A systematic review of definitions. BMC Geriatr. 2017;17:230. https://doi.org/10.1186/s12877-017-0621-2.
55. Medeiros-Souza P, Santos-Neto LL, Kusano LTE, Pereira MG. Diagnosis and control of polypharmacy in the elderly. Rev Saude Publica. 2007;41(6):1049–53. https://doi.org/10.1590/S0034-89102006005000050.
56. Brunton L, Chabner B, Knollman B. Goodman & Gilman's the pharmacological basis of therapeutics. 12th ed. New York: McGraw-Hill Professional; 2011. p. 2108.
57. Cascorbi I. Drug interactions – principles, examples and clinical consequences. Deutsch Arztebl Int. 2012;109(33–34):546–56. https://doi.org/10.3238/arztebl.2012.0546.
58. Snyder BD, Polasek TM, Doogue MP. Drug interactions: principles and practice. Aust Prescr. 2012;35(3):85–8. https://doi.org/10.18773/austprescr.2012.037.
59. Vakil V, Trappe W. Drug combinations: mathematical modeling and networking methods. Pharmaceutics. 2019;11(5):208. https://doi.org/10.3390/pharmaceutics11050208.
60. Negus SS. Some implications of receptor theory for in vivo assessment of agonists, antagonists and inverse agonists. Biochem Pharmacol. 2006;71(12):1663–70. https://doi.org/10.1016/j.bcp.2005.12.038.
61. Vinarov Z, Abrahamsson B, Artursson P, Batchelor H, Berben P, Bernkop-Schurch A, et al. Current challenges and future perspectives in oral absorption research: an opinion of the UNGAP network. Adv Drug Deliv Rev. 2021;171:289–331. https://doi.org/10.1016/j.addr.2021.02.001.
62. Feng Y, Wang Q, Wang T. Drug target protein-protein interaction networks: a systematic perspective. Biomed Res Int. 2017;2017:1289259. https://doi.org/10.1155/2017/1289259.
63. Santos R, Ursu O, Gaulton A, Bento AP, Donadi RS, Bologa CG, Karlsson A, Al-Lazikani B, Hersey A, Oprea TI, Overington JP. A comprehensive map of molecular drug targets. Nat Rev Drug Discov. 2017;16(1):19–34. https://doi.org/10.1038/nrd.2016.230.
64. Tocchetti CG, Cadeddu C, Lisi DD, Femminò S, Madonna R, Mele D, Monte I, Novo G, Penna C, Pepe A, Spallarossa P, Varricchi G, Zito C, Pagliaro P, Mercuro G. From molecular mechanisms to clinical management of antineoplastic drug-induced cardiovascular toxicity: a translational overview. Antioxid Redox Signal. 2019;30(8):2110–56. https://doi.org/10.1089/ars.2016.6930.
65. Silva AA, Carlotto J, Rotta I. Standardization of the infusion sequence of antineoplastic drugs used in the treatment of breast and colorectal cancers. Einstein. 2018;16(2):1–9. https://doi.org/10.1590/S1679-45082018RW4074.
66. Sak K. Chemotherapy and dietary phytochemical agents. Chemother Res Pract. 2012;2012:282570. https://doi.org/10.1155/2012/282570.
67. Trendowski M. Recent advances in the development of antineoplastic agents derived from natural products. Drugs. 2015;75:1993–2016. https://doi.org/10.1089/ars.2016.6930.
68. Scripture CD, Figg WD. Drug interactions in cancer therapy. Nat Rev Cancer. 2006;6(7):546–58. https://doi.org/10.1038/nrc1887.
69. Wicha SG, Chen C, Clewe O, Simonsson USH. A general pharmacodynamics interaction model identifies perpetrators and victims in drug interactions. Nat Commun. 2017;8:2129. https://doi.org/10.1038/s41467-017-01929-y.

70. Niu J, Straubinger RM, Mager DE. Pharmacodynamic drug-drug interactions. Clin Pharmacol Therapeut. 2019;105(6):1395–406. https://doi.org/10.1002/cpt.1434.

71. Thirion P, Michiels S, Pignon JP, Buyse M, Braud AC, Carlson RW, O'Connell M, Sargent P, Piedbois P. Modulation of fluorouracil by leucovorin in patients with advanced colorectal cancer: an updated meta-analysis. J Clin Oncol. 2004;22(18):3766–75. https://doi.org/10.1200/JCO.2004.03.104.

72. Madhyastha S, Prabhu LV, Saralaya V, Rai R. A comparison of vitamin a and leucovorin for the prevention of methotrexate-induced micronuclei production in rat bone marrow. Clinics. 2008;63(6):821–6. https://doi.org/10.1590/S1807-59322008000600019.

73. Milczarek M, Pogorzelska A, Wiktorska K. Synergistic interaction between 5-FU and an analog of sulforaphane—2-oxohexyl isothiocyanate—in an in vitro colon cancer mode. Molecules. 2021;26(10):3019. https://doi.org/10.3390/molecules26103019.

74. Lam CS, Cheng LP, Zhou LM, Cheung YT, Zuo Z. Herb-drug interactions between the medicinal mushrooms Lingzhi and Yunzhi and cytotoxic anticancer drugs: a systematic review. Chin Med. 2020;15:75. https://doi.org/10.1186/s13020-020-00356-4.

75. Pawaskar DK, Straubinger RM, Fetterly GJ, Hylander BH, Repasky EA, Ma WW, Jusko WJ. Synergistic interactions between sorafenib and everolimus in pancreatic cancer xenografts in mice. Cancer Chemother Pharmacol. 2013;71(5):1231–40. https://doi.org/10.1007/s00280-013-2117-x.

76. Ricciardi S, Mey V, Nannizzi S, Pasqualetti G, Crea F, Tacca MD, Danesi R. Synergistic cytotoxicity and molecular interaction on drug targets of sorafenib and gemcitabine in human pancreas cancer cells. Chemotherapy. 2010;56(4):303–12. https://doi.org/10.1159/000320031.

77. Qian Y, Xiong Y, Feng D, Wu Y, Zhang X, Chen L, Gu M. Coix seed extract enhances the anti-pancreatic cancer efficacy of gemcitabine through regulating ABCB1- and ABCG2-mediated drug efflux: a bioluminescent pharmacokinetic and pharmacodynamic study. Int J Mol Sci. 2019;20(21):5250. https://doi.org/10.3390/ijms20215250.

78. Desidero TD, Orlandi P, Fioravanti A, Alì G, Cremolini C, Loupakis F, Gentile D, Banchi M, Cucchiara F, Antoniotti C, Mais G, Fontanini G, Falcone A, Bocci G. Chemotherapeutic and antiangiogenic drugs beyond tumor progression in colon cancer: evaluation of the effects of switched schedules and related pharmacodynamics. Biochem Pharmacol. 2019;164:94–105. https://doi.org/10.1016/j.bcp.2019.04.001.

79. Chen W, Chen R, Li J, Fu Y, Yang L, Su H, Yao Y, Li L, Zhou T, Lu W. Pharmacokinetic/pharmacodynamic modeling of schedule-dependent interaction between docetaxel and cabozantinib in human prostate cancer xenograft models. J Pharmacol Exp Ther. 2018;364(1):13–25. https://doi.org/10.1124/jpet.117.243931.

80. Li M, Li H, Cheng X, Wang X, Li L, Zhou T, Lu W. Preclinical pharmacokinetic/pharmacodynamic models to predict schedule-dependent interaction between erlotinib and gemcitabine. Pharm Res. 2013;30(5):1400–8. https://doi.org/10.1007/s11095-013-0978-7.

81. Ben-Eltriki M, Deb S, Guns EST. Calcitriol in combination therapy for prostate cancer: pharmacokinetic and pharmacodynamics interactions. J Cancer. 2016;7(4):391–407. https://doi.org/10.7150/jca.13470.

82. Ahmed S, Johnson CS, Rueger RM, Trump DL. Calcitriol (1,25-dihydroxycholecalciferol) potentiates activity of mitoxantrone/dexamethasone in an androgen independent prostate cancer model. J Urol. 2002;168(2):756–61.

83. Hershberger PA, Yu WD, Modzelewski RA, Rueger RM, Johnson CS, Trump DL. Calcitriol (1,25-dihydroxycholecalciferol) enhances paclitaxel antitumor activity in vitro and in vivo and accelerates paclitaxel-induced apoptosis. Clin Cancer Res. 2001;7(4):1043–51.

84. Ting HJ, Hsu J, Bao BY, Lee YF. Docetaxel-induced growth inhibition and apoptosis in androgen independent prostate cancer cells are enhanced by 1alpha,25-dihydroxyvitamin D3. Cancer Lett. 2007;247(1):122–9. https://doi.org/10.1016/j.canlet.2006.03.025.

85. Skowronski RJ, Peehl DM, Feldman D. Vitamin D and prostate cancer: 1,25 dihydroxyvitamin D3 receptors and actions in human prostate cancer cell lines. Endocrinology. 1993;132(5):1952–60. https://doi.org/10.1210/endo.132.5.7682937.

86. Frances N, Claret L, Bruno R, Iliadis A. Tumor growth modeling from clinical trials reveals synergistic anticancer effect of the capecitabine and docetaxel combination in metastatic breast cancer. Cancer Chemother Pharmacol. 2011;68(6):1413–9. https://doi.org/10.1007/s00280-011-1628-6.

87. Visentin M, Biason P, Toffoli G. Drug interactions among the epidermal growth factor receptor inhibitors, other biologics and cytotoxic agents. Pharmacol Ther. 2010;128(1):82–90. https://doi.org/10.1016/j.pharmthera.2010.05.005.

88. Paciello F, Fetoni AR, Mezzogori D, Rolesi R, Pino AD, Paludetti G, Grassi C, Troiani D. The dual role of curcumin and ferulic acid in counteracting chemoresistance and cisplatin-induced ototoxicity. Sci Rep. 2020;10(1):1063. https://doi.org/10.1038/s41598-020-57965-0.

89. Bose C, Awasthi S, Sharma R, Benes H, Hauer-Jensen M, Boerma M, Singh SP. Sulforaphane potentiases anticâncer effects of doxorubicin and attenuates its cardiotoxicity in a breast cancer model. PLoS One. 2018;13(3):e0193918. https://doi.org/10.1371/journal.pone.0193918.

90. Rahaman ST, Pentakota R, Vasireddy P. An overview on various types of anticancer drugs and their drug-drug interactions: melphalan, 5-fluorouracil, and hydrazine. J Pharm Res. 2018;12(2):160–7.

91. Pritchard J, McElwain TJ, Graham-Pole J. High-dose melphalan with autologous marrow for treatment of advanced neuroblastoma. Br J Cancer. 1982;45(1):86–94. https://doi.org/10.1038/bjc.1982.11.

92. Mouzon A, Kerger J, D'Hondt L, Spinewine A. Potential interactions with anticancer agents: a cross-sectional study. Chemotherapy. 2013;59(2):85–92. https://doi.org/10.1159/000351133.

93. Małyszko J, Kozłowska K, Kozłowski L, Małyszko J. Nephrotoxicity of anticancer treatment. Nephrol Dialy Transpl. 2017;32(6):924–36. https://doi.org/10.1093/ndt/gfw338.

94. Onitilo AA, Engel JM, Stankowski RV. Cardiovascular toxicity associated with adjuvant trastuzumab therapy: prevalence, patient characteristics, and risk factors. Therapeut Adv Drug Saf. 2014;5(4):154–66. https://doi.org/10.1177/2042098614529603.

95. Herrmann J. Adverse cardiac effects of cancer therapies: cardiotoxicity and arrhythmia. Nat Rev Cardiol. 2020;17:474–502. https://doi.org/10.1038/s41569-020-0348-1.

96. Taguchi T, Nazneen A, Abid MR, Razzaque MS. Cisplatin-associated nephrotoxicity and pathological events. Contrib Nephrol. 2005;148:107–21. https://doi.org/10.1159/000086055.

97. Scalone S, Sorio R, Bortolussi R, Lombardi D, Mura NL, Veronesi A. Vinorelbine-induced acute reversible peripheral neuropathy in a patient with ovarian carcinoma pretreated with carboplatin and paclitaxel. Acta Oncol. 2004;43(2):209–11. https://doi.org/10.1080/02841860310020924.

98. Simão DAS, Murad M, Martins C, Fernandes VC, Captein KM, Teixeira AL. Chemotherapy-induced peripheral neuropathy: review for clinical practice. Revista Dor. 2015;16(3):215–20. https://doi.org/10.5935/1806-0013.20150043.

99. Shand DG, Mitchell JR, Oates JA. Pharmacokinetic drug interactions. In: Gillette JR, Mitchell JR, editors. Concepts in biochemical pharmacology. Handbuch der experimentellen pharmakologie/Handbook of Experimental Pharmacology 28/3. Berlin, Heidelberg: Springer; 1975. https://doi.org/10.1007/978-3-642-46314-3_11.

100. Mani S, Ghalib M, Chaudhary I, Goel S. Alterations of chemotherapeutic pharmacokinetic profiles by drug-drug interactions. Expert Opin Drug Metab Toxicol. 2009;5(2):109–30. https://doi.org/10.1517/17425250902753212.

101. Palleria C, Paolo AD, Giofrè C, Caglioti C, Leuzzi G, Siniscalchi A, Sarro GD, Gallelli L. Pharmacokinetic drug-drug interaction and their implication in clinical management. J Res Med Sci. 2013;18(7):601–10.

102. Hoefler R. Interações medicamentosas. Secretaria de Ciência, Tecnologia e Insumos Estratégicos/MS-FTN. 2005;1:1–4.

103. Liu X, Sun H, Zhang Y, Sun Y, Wang W, Xu L, Liu W. Clozapine affects the pharmacokinetics of risperidone and inhibits its metabolism and P-glycoprotein-mediated transport in vivo and in vitro: a safety attention to antipsychotic polypharmacy with clozapine and risperidone. Toxicol Appl Pharmacol. 2021;422:115560. https://doi.org/10.1016/j.taap.2021.115560.

104. Campen CJ, Vogel WH, Shah PJ. Managing drug interactions in cancer therapy: a guide for the advanced practitioner. J Adv Pract Oncol. 2017;8(6):609–20.

105. Zhao D, Chen J, Chu M, Long X, Wang J. Pharmacokinetic-based drug-drug interactions with anaplastic lymphoma kinase inhibitors: a review. Drug Des Devel Ther. 2020;14:1663–81. https://doi.org/10.2147/DDDT.S249098.

106. Bohnert T, Gan LS. Plasma protein binding: from discovery to development. J Pharm Sci. 2013;102(9):2953–94. https://doi.org/10.1002/jps.23614.

107. van Leeuwen RWF, van Gelder T, Mathijssen RHJ, Jansman FGA. Drug-drug interactions with tyrosine-kinase inhibitors: a clinical perspective. Lancet Oncol. 2014;15(8):E315–26. https://doi.org/10.1016/S1470-2045(13)70579-5.

108. Gruzdeva AA, Khokhlov AL, Ilyin MV. Risk management strategy for preventing the reduced treatment effectiveness from the position of drug interactions and polypharmacy. Res Res Pharmacol. 2020;6(4):85–92. https://doi.org/10.3897/rrpharmacology.6.60164.

109. Stepney R, Lichtman SM, Danesi R. Drug-drug interactions in older patients with cancer: a report from the 15th conference of the International Society of Geriatric Oncology, Prague, Czech Republic, November 2015. Ecancermedicalscience. 2016;10:611. https://doi.org/10.3332/ecancer.2016.611.

110. Fogli S, Re MD, Curigliano G, van Schaik RH, Lancellotti P, Danesi R. Drug-drug interactions in breast cancer patients treated with CDK4/6 inhibitors. Cancer Treat Rev. 2019;74:21–8. https://doi.org/10.1016/j.ctrv.2019.01.006.

111. Deb S, Chin MY, Adomat H, Guns EST. Abiraterone inhibits 1α,25-dihydroxyvitamin D3 metabolism by CYP3A4 in human liver and intestine in vitro. J Steroid Biochem Mol Biol. 2014;144(Pt A):50–8. https://doi.org/10.1016/j.jsbmb.2013.10.027.

112. Del Re M, Fogli S, Derosa L, Massari F, Souza PD, Crucitta S, Bracarda S, Santini D, Danesi R. The role of drug-drug interactions in prostate cancer treatment: focus on abiraterone acetate/prednisone and enzalutamide. Cancer Treat Rev. 2017;55:71–82. https://doi.org/10.1016/j.ctrv.2017.03.001.

113. Lipp HP, Miller K. Treatment of metastatic castration-resistant prostate cancer: drug interaction potentials of abiraterone acetate and enzalutamide. Urologe. 2016;55(6):766–71. https://doi.org/10.1007/s00120-016-0049-x.

114. Okuda H, Nishiyama T, Ogura K, Nagayama S, Ikeda K, Yamaguchi S, Nakamura Y, Kawaguchi K, Watabe T, Ogura Y. Lethal drug interactions of sorivudine, a new antiviral drug, with oral 5-fluorouracil prodrugs. Drug Metab Dispos. 1997;25(2):270–3.

115. Yan J, Tyring SK, McCrary MM, Lee PC, Haworth S, Raymond R, Olsen SJ, Diasio RB. The effect of sorivudine on dihydropyrimidine dehydrogenase activity in patients with acute herpes zoster. Clin Pharmacol Therapeut. 1997;61(5):563–73. https://doi.org/10.1016/S0009-9236(97)90136-3.

116. Diasio RB. Sorivudine and 5-fluorouracil; a clinically significant drug-drug interaction due to inhibition of dihydropyrimidine dehydrogenase. Br J Clin Pharmacol. 1998;46(1):1–4. https://doi.org/10.1046/j.1365-2125.1998.00050.x.

117. Stearns V, Johnson MD, Rae JM, Morocho A, Novielli A, Bhargava P, Hayes DF, Desta Z, Flockhart DA. Active tamoxifen metabolite plasma concentrations after coadministration of tamoxifen and the selective serotonin reuptake inhibitor paroxetine. J Natl Cancer Inst. 2003;95(23):1758–64. https://doi.org/10.1093/jnci/djg108.

118. Henry NL, Stearns V, Flockhart DA, Hayes DF, Riba M. Drug interactions and pharmacogenomics in the treatment of breast cancer and depression. Am J Psychiatry. 2008;165(10):1251–5. https://doi.org/10.1176/appi.ajp.2008.08040482.

119. Nozaki Y, Kusuhara H, Endou H, Sugiyama Y. Quantitative evaluation of the drug-drug interactions between methotrexate and nonsteroidal anti-inflammatory drugs in the renal uptake process based on the contribution of organic anion transporters and reduced folate carrier. J Pharmacol Exp Ther. 2004;309(1):226–34. https://doi.org/10.1124/jpet.103.061812.

120. Breedveld P, Zelcer N, Pluim D, Sonmezer O, Tibben MM, Beijnen JH, Schinkel AH, van Tellingen O, Borst P, Schellens JHM. Mechanism of the pharmacokinetic interaction between

methotrexate and benzimidazoles: potential role for breast cancer resistance protein in clinical drug-drug interactions. Cancer Res. 2004;64(16):5804–11. https://doi.org/10.1158/0008-5472.CAN-03-4062.

121. Joerger M, Huitema ADR, van den Bongard HJGD, Baas P, Schornagel JH, Schellens JHM, Beijnen JH. Determinants of the elimination of methotrexate and 7-hydroxy-methotrexate following high-dose infusional therapy to cancer patients. Br J Clin Pharmacol. 2006;62(1):71–80. https://doi.org/10.1111/j.1365-2125.2005.02513.x.

122. Molokhia M, Majeed A. Current and future perspectives on the management of polypharmacy. BMC Fam Pract. 2017;18:70. https://doi.org/10.1186/s12875-017-0642-0.

123. Florea AM, Busselberg D. Cisplatin as an anti-tumor drug: cellular mechanisms of activity, drug resistance and induced side effects. Cancers (Basel). 2011;3(1):1351–71. https://doi.org/10.3390/cancers3011351.

124. Wang X, Zhang H, Chen X. Drug resistance and combating drug resistance in cancer. Cancer Drug Resist. 2019;2:141–60. https://doi.org/10.20517/cdr.2019.10.

125. Henke E, Nandigama R, Ergun S. Extracellular matrix in the tumor microenvironment and its impact on cancer therapy. Front Mol Biosci. 2020;6:160. https://doi.org/10.3389/fmolb.2019.00160.v.

126. Olver I. Chemotherapy for elderly patients with advanced cancer: is it worth it? Aust Prescr. 2000;23:80–2. https://doi.org/10.18773/austprescr.2000.090.

127. Yeh ETH, Tong AT, Lenihan DJ, Yusuf SW, Swafford J, Champion C, Durand JB, Gibbs H, Zafarmand AA, Ewer MS. Cardiovascular complications of cancer therapy. Circulation. 2004;109:3122–31. https://doi.org/10.1161/01.CIR.0000133187.74800.B9.

128. Kroschinsky F, Stolzel F, von Bonin S, Beutel G, Kochanek M, Kiehl M, Schellongowski P. New drugs, new toxicities: severe side effects of modern targeted and immunotherapy of cancer and their management. Crit Care. 2017;21:89. https://doi.org/10.1186/s13054-017-1678-1.

129. Kaur G. Polypharmacy: the past, present and the future. J Adv Pharm Technol Res. 2013;4(4):224–5. https://doi.org/10.4103/2231-4040.121418.

130. Wojtczak D, Kasznicki J, Drzewoski J. Pros and cons of polypharmacy in elderly patients with diabetes. Clin Diabetol. 2017;6(1):34–8. https://doi.org/10.5603/DK.2017.0006.

131. Alam MM, Hassan AHE, Kwon YH, Lee HJ, Kim NY, Min KH, Lee SY, Kim DH, Lee YS. Design, synthesis and evaluation of alkylphosphocholine-gefitinib conjugates as multitarget anticancer agents. Arch Pharm Res. 2018;41(1):35–45. https://doi.org/10.1007/s12272-017-0977-z.

132. Kim R, Tan E, Wang E, Mahipal A, Chen DT, Cao B, Masawi F, Machado C, Yu J, Kim DW. A phase I trial of trametinib in combination with sorafenib in patients with advanced hepatocellular cancer. Oncologist. 2020;25(12):e1893–9. https://doi.org/10.1634/theoncologist.2020-0759.

133. Jiang S, Wang R, Zhang X, Wu F, Li S, Yuan Y. Combination treatment of gemcitabine and sorafenib exerts a synergistic inhibitory effect on non-small cell lung cancer in vitro and in vivo via the epithelial-to-mesenchymal transition process. Oncol Lett. 2020;20(1):346–56. https://doi.org/10.3892/ol.2020.11536.

134. Lordick F, Lorenzen S, Yamada Y, Ilson D. Optimal chemotherapy for advanced gastric cancer: is there a global consensus? Gastric Cancer. 2014;17:213–25. https://doi.org/10.1007/s10120-013-0297-z.

135. Miller KD, Nogueira L, Mariotto AB, Rowland JH, Yabroff R, Alfano CM, Jemal A, Kramer JL, Siegel RL. Cancer treatment and survivorship statistics, 2019. CA Cancer J Clin. 2019;69(5):363–85. https://doi.org/10.3322/caac.21565.

136. Davidsson M, Vibe OE, Ruths S, Blix HS. A multidisciplinary approach to improve drug therapy in nursing homes. J Multidiscip Healthc. 2011;4:9–13. https://doi.org/10.2147/JMDH.S15773.

137. Byrne A, Byrne S, Dalton K. A pharmacist's unique opportunity within a multidisciplinary team to reduce drug-related problems for older adults in an intermediate care setting. Res Soc Adm Pharm. 2021;18(4):2625–33. https://doi.org/10.1016/j.sapharm.2021.05.003.

138. Lenssen R, Heidenreich A, Schulz JB, Trautwein C, Fitzner C, Jaehde U, Eisert A. Analysis of drug-related problems in three departments of a German University hospital. Int J Clin Pharm. 2016;38:119–26. https://doi.org/10.1007/s11096-015-0213-1.

139. Groleau A, Côté J. Comparison between two premedication regimens of dexamethasone before a pemetrexed-based chemotherapy: a single-center experience study. J Oncol Pharm Pract. 2020;26(3):612–8. https://doi.org/10.1177/1078155219862040.

140. Saito Y, Kobayashi M, Yamada T, Kasashi K, Honma R, Takeuchi S, Shimizu Y, Kinoshita I, Dosaka-Akita H, Iseki K. Premedication with intravenous magnesium has a protective effect against cisplatin-induced nephrotoxicity. Support Care Cancer. 2017;25:481–7. https://doi.org/10.1007/s00520-016-3426-5.

141. Kubo Y, Miyata H, Sugimura K, Shinno N, Ushigome H, Yanagimoto Y, Takahashi Y, Yamamoto K, Nishimura J, Wada H, Takahashi H, Yasui M, Omori T, Ohue M, Yano M. Prophylactic effect of premedication with intravenous magnesium on renal dysfunction in preoperative cisplatin-based chemotherapy for esophageal cancer. Oncology. 2019;97:319–26. https://doi.org/10.1159/000501966.

142. Balducci L, Goetz-Parten D, Steinman MA. Polypharmacy and the management of the older cancer patient. Ann Oncol. 2013;24(Suppl 7):vii36–40. https://doi.org/10.1093/annonc/mdt266.

143. Błeszyńska E, Wierucki L, Zdrojewski T, Renke M. Pharmacological interactions in the elderly. Medicina (Kaunas). 2020;56(7):320. https://doi.org/10.3390/medicina56070320.

144. Domínguez-Alonso JA, Conde-Estévez D, Bosch D, Pi-Figueras M, Tusquets I. Breast cancer, placing drug interactions in the spotlight: is polypharmacy the cause of everything? Clin Transl Oncol. 2021;23(1):65–73. https://doi.org/10.1007/s12094-020-02386-8.

145. Triplitt C. Drug interactions of medications commonly used in diabetes. Diabet Spect. 2006;19(4):202–11. https://doi.org/10.2337/diaspect.19.4.202.

146. Zazzara MB, Palmer K, Vetrano DL, Carfi A, Graziano O. Adverse drug reactions in older adults: a narrative review of the literature. Eur Geriatr Med. 2021;12:463–73. https://doi.org/10.1007/s41999-021-00481-9.

147. Brett J, Pearson SA, Daniels B, Wylie CE, Buckley NA. A cross sectional study of psychotropic medicine use in Australia in 2018: a focus on polypharmacy. Br J Clin Pharmacol. 2021;87(3):1369–77. https://doi.org/10.1111/bcp.14527.

148. Al-Qurain AA, Gebremichael LG, Khan MS, Williams DB, Mackenzie L, Philips C, Russel P, Roberts MS, Wiese MD. Opioid prescribing and risk of drug-opioid interactions in older discharged patients with polypharmacy in Australia. Int J Clin Pharm. 2021;43:365–74. https://doi.org/10.1007/s11096-020-01191-1.

149. Hoemme A, Barth H, Haschke M, Krahenbuhl S, Strasser F, Lehner C, von Kameke A, Walti T, Thurlimann B, Fruh M, Driessen C, Joerger M. Prognostic impact of polypharmacy and drug interactions in patients with advanced cancer. Cancer Chemother Pharmacol. 2019;83:763–74. https://doi.org/10.1007/s00280-019-03783-9.

Chapter 2
Combined Therapy for the Treatment of Cancer

2.1 Anticancer Therapy

Antineoplastic chemotherapy is one of the modality of cancer treatment, which is based on the use of drugs seeking to destroy or slow down the growth of cancer cells [1–3]. Chemotherapy can be used for curative or palliative purposes, with the aim of prolonging life or reducing symptoms. This modality is one of the most used in cancer treatment and can be used alone or in association with other modality such as surgery and radiotherapy [4–6].

Chemotherapy is one of the most effective therapeutic approaches, which can alleviate painful symptoms, prolong life, and/or cure the disease. It has been used since ancient times and has been evolving every year with a reduction in its toxicity and successful therapeutic results [7–9]. However, the application of cytotoxic chemotherapy will not necessarily result in tumor regression in all cancer patients, due to the heterogeneity of the neoplasm, as well as the possibility of localization in different organs and tissues, so the chemotherapy response ends up being different for each type of tumor [9–12].

Neoplastic cells may have an invasive capacity, metastatic potential, higher growth rate, immunogenicity, and an intrinsic response to specific drugs [13, 14]. Therefore, patients with the same type of tumor, in the same region, with the same evolutionary stage, may present different responses to the same therapeutic regimen and may present favorable or unfavorable responses [3, 13, 15].

Some laboratory tests can help in the diagnosis of cancer as well as aid in the treatment, based on the analysis of tumor markers and the identification of overexpressed receptors on cancer cells [16, 17]. For example, in breast cancer, some patients may overexpress hormone receptors, and hormone therapy is indicated, or they may have overexpression of type 2 human epidermal growth factor receptors (HER2), which indicates the use of target therapy, with the use of monoclonal

I. D. Lima Cavalcanti, *Chemotherapy Protocols and Infusion Sequence*, https://doi.org/10.1007/978-3-031-10839-6_2

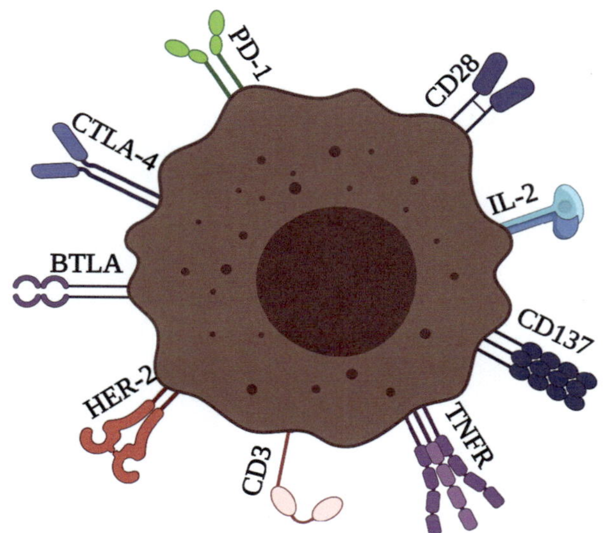

Fig. 2.1 Some receptors that may be overexpressed in cancer cells. *PD-1* programmed death 1 receptor, *CD28* cluster of differentiation 28, *IL-2* interleukin 2, *CD137* cluster of differentiation 137, *TNFR* tumor necrosis factor receptor, *CD3* cluster of differentiation 3, *HER-2* human epidermal growth factor receptor 2, *BTLA* B- and T-lymphocyte associated, *CTLA-4* cytotoxic T-lymphocyte-associated protein 4. Source: Created with BioRender.com

antibodies (trastuzumab and pertuzumab) [15, 18, 19]. In Fig. 2.1 some receptors that may be overexpressed in cancer cells are present.

With the discovery of overexpressed receptors, it was possible to develop targeted therapy directed at these overexpressed receptors in cancer cells [20–22]. Targeted therapy, unlike cytotoxic chemotherapy, is based on the application of drugs that will act exclusively or almost exclusively on specific molecules of cancer cells, thereby reducing toxicity in healthy cells and its side effects, which are common in cytotoxic chemotherapy [23–25].

The study of molecules overexpressed in cancer cells, in addition to aiding in the development of specific drugs, also allows the identification of mechanisms of resistance to antineoplastic agents [26–29]. The overexpression of drug-metabolizing enzymes in cancer cells causes the drugs to be converted quickly, and they can be inactivated and excreted more quickly, without showing their therapeutic action [30–33]. An example is the overexpression of glutathione, which inactivates antineoplastics due to its electrophilic properties [34, 35].

Given the complexity of cancer cells and due to the possibility of developing resistance to some antineoplastic drugs, combined therapy has been an ally, showing good results when compared to monotherapy for the treatment of cancer [36–39].

2.2 Combination Therapy in Cancer

Cytotoxic chemotherapy acts by inhibiting the cell proliferation of cancer cells during the process of cell division, being classified as alkylating agents, causing alterations in the DNA chains and preventing its replication, through the alkylation of nucleic acids [40]; antimetabolites, which act by inhibiting a metabolite, blocking the production of enzymes important to the process of cell division, and thereby interrupting nucleic acid synthesis [41–43]; cytotoxic antibiotics interfere with the synthesis of nucleic acids through intercalation processes, preventing the duplication and separation of DNA and RNA chains [42]; derived from natural products (vinca alkaloids and taxoids), they can act by inhibiting the formation of microtubules, promoting their rupture or making them nonfunctional, as well as acting by inhibiting topoisomerase, thereby interrupting DNA replication [44, 45]. Table 2.1 shows the classes of cytotoxic antineoplastic agents and examples of drugs belonging to each class.

Table 2.1 Classification of cytotoxic antineoplastic agents

Class	Function	Drugs	Reference
Alkylating agents	They bind to chemical groups such as phosphate, amino, sulfhydryl, and hydroxyl, which are commonly found in nucleic acids and other macromolecules, causing changes in DNA and RNA	Cyclophosphamide Nitrogen mustards Busulfan Nitrosoureas Dacarbazine Melphalan Chlorambucil Thiotepa	[46, 47]
Antimetabolites	They work by mimicking molecules needed for cell growth, causing cells to use these antimetabolites to inhibit DNA synthesis	5-Fluorouracil 6-Mercaptopurine Cytarabine Pentostatin Vidaza Decitabine Capecitabine Fludarabine Gemcitabine	[48–50]
Cytotoxic antibiotics	Drugs that have antibiotic activity as well as potent antitumor activity, being developed as anticancer agents	Bleomycin Dactinomycin Daunorubicin Doxorubicin Epirubicin Idarubicin Mitomycin C Mitoxantrone Plicamycin Valrubicin	[51, 52]
Taxoids	They promote the polymerization of tubulin and the formation of microtubules resistant to disassembly by physiological stimuli	Paclitaxel Docetaxel	[53–55]
Vinca alkaloids	It acts on tubulin, inhibiting the formation of microtubules and inhibiting the ability of cancer cells to divide	Vincristine Vinblastine Vinorelbine	[56–58]
Platinum composite	They form adducts with DNA, thereby preventing its synthesis and repair, inducing cell death	Cisplatin Carboplatin Oxaliplatin	[59–61]

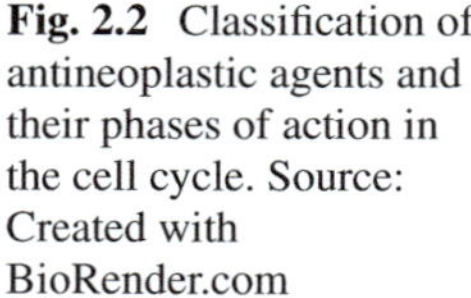

Fig. 2.2 Classification of antineoplastic agents and their phases of action in the cell cycle. Source: Created with BioRender.com

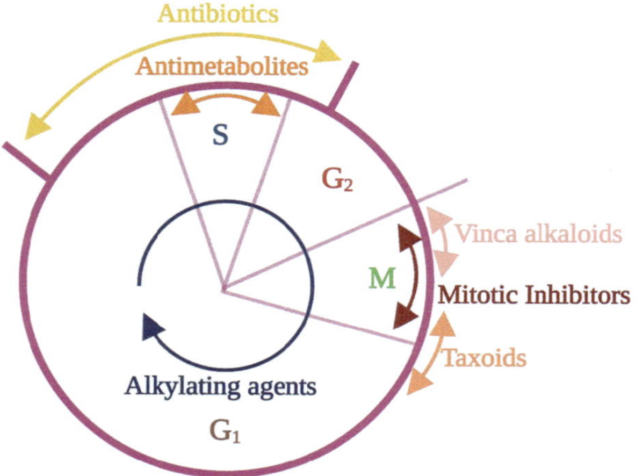

Cytotoxic drugs can act in different phases of the cell cycle, being classified as unspecific cycle and specific cycle, where specific cycle drugs can be further sub-classified in nonspecific or specific phase of the cell cycle [62, 63]. Drugs classified as unspecific phase can act in different phases of the cell cycle, such as alkylating agents, while phase-specific drugs will act in a phase of the cell cycle, such as anti-metabolites that act specifically on the S phase [47, 63, 64]. Figure 2.2 shows the phase of action of each class of antineoplastics.

Another class of drugs used for cancer treatment are biological agents, which stimulate natural defenses against neoplastic cells, and may act by blocking the cell cycle, inhibiting angiogenesis, in the rescue of apoptosis and the function of tumor suppressor genes or in the elimination of cells with mutated genes, acting selectively [9, 25, 65–67]. Among the drugs that are classified as biological agents, they include hematopoietic growth factors, interleukins, interferon, monoclonal antibodies, tyrosine kinase inhibitors, among others [68, 69]. Table 2.2 shows the classes of biological agents and their functions in cancer treatment.

Given the different options of drugs for the treatment of cancer with different mechanisms of action, the association of these drugs is interesting, as it will allow the blocking of the growth of cancer cells through different ways and be able to reduce the tumor mass, which may be more effective than monotherapy [3, 8, 92]. Therefore, combined therapy is widely used in cancer treatment, due to its advantages, with better response to cancer treatment, seeking to reduce the heterogeneity of tumor response [3, 93–95]. Combination therapy is more successful in metastatic cancer, where the guidelines to define the specific combination are as follows: the drugs must be effective when used alone, the associated drugs must have different mechanisms of action, and the degree of toxicity must not be higher than the admissible; thus, the drugs should not have the same toxicity profile [3, 96, 97].

Combination therapy also reduces the development of resistance in cancer cells by acting on different cellular mechanisms than cancer cells [98, 99]. Another advantage is that each drug can be used in its optimal concentration, avoiding its

Table 2.2 Main classes of biological agents, mechanism of action and drugs

Biological agents	Biological agent mechanism	Drugs	Reference
Granulocyte colony-stimulating factor (G-CSF) and granulocyte/macrophage colony-stimulating factor (GM-CSF)	They stimulate the proliferation of neutrophil line erythrocyte precursors, enhancing the function of neutrophils and macrophages	Filgrastim Pegfilgrastrim Sargromostim Recombinant human erythropoietin Darbepoetin alfa	[70, 71]
Interleukin	A group of cytokines that regulate immune cells by binding to receptors on the surface of lymphoid and hematopoietic cells, thereby interfering with the function and development of these cells	Interleukin 2 Interleukin 10 Interleukin 12 Interleukin 15 Interleukin 18	[72, 73]
Interferon	Responsible for NK cell activation, antiproliferative effects, angiogenesis inhibition, interaction with growth factors, oncogenes, and other cytokines	Octreotide Interferon alfa Bacillus Calmette-Guérin	[74–77]
Monoclonal antibodies	Immune system proteins produced in laboratories act on overexpressed receptors on cancer cells, but they can also act as immunotherapy helping to activate the immune system against cancer	Trastuzumab Rituximab Cetuximab Bevacizumab Ipilimumab Pertuzumab Pembrolizumab Tositumomab Blinatumomab	[78–80]
Tyrosine kinase inhibitors	They inhibit the enzyme tyrosine kinases that are responsible for activating proteins through signal transduction cascades	Imatinib Sorafenib Sunitinib Axitinib Erlotinib Gefitinib	[81, 82]
Anti-angiogenesis	They act by inhibiting the growth of new blood vessels, which may be due to the inhibition of vascular endothelial growth factor (VEGF) and leading to a reduction in the production of pro-angiogenic factors or through the endogenous regulation of angiogenesis-stimulating molecules	Bevacizumab Angiostatin Endostatin Thrombospondin Interferon-alpha	[9, 83–86]
CAR-T cells	It is based on the transfer of genes from a virus into the genetic material of T-lymphocyte cells, which then express the gene on their surface. The gene inserted into T lymphocytes will be able to recognize the tumor cell and fight the tumor	T lymphocytes obtained from patients and modified in the laboratory	[87–91]

intolerant side effects [100, 101]. Therapeutic combinations will depend on the type of tumor, its location, and whether they have overexpressed receptors [80, 102].

Multidrug therapy for the treatment of breast cancer is frequent; protocols such as doxorubicin associated with cyclophosphamide, epirubicin associated with cyclophosphamide and paclitaxel, docetaxel associated with carboplatin, and the association of paclitaxel with gemcitabine are some of the associations used [103, 104]. Bonadonna et al. [105] evaluated the use of the cyclophosphamide, methotrexate, and fluorouracil protocol in the treatment of adjuvant breast cancer, verifying that the association of these drugs reduced the risk of recurrence. Also evaluating the effectiveness of protocols for the treatment of breast cancer, Chan et al. [106] compared the association of gemcitabine plus docetaxel with capecitabine plus docetaxel, showing that the gemcitabine and docetaxel protocol had fewer adverse effects such as diarrhea, mucositis, and hand and foot syndrome, with fewer patients discontinuing treatment due to adverse events.

Marty et al. [107] evaluated the benefits of including trastuzumab in HER2-positive breast cancer therapy associated with docetaxel, showing that the combination increased overall survival to 31 months, overall response rate to 71%, duration of response to 12 months, time to disease progression of 12 months, and little additional toxicity compared to docetaxel monotherapy. Trastuzumab has shown benefits when combined with chemotherapy for the treatment of first-, second-, and third-line breast cancer [108].

The combination of anticancer drugs was also shown to be superior to monotherapy, in the study by Martin et al. [109], to the treatment of triple-negative breast cancer. In the study, the authors evaluated the efficacy of combining docetaxel with carboplatin, noting that the combination was more effective than doxorubicin monotherapy in treating triple-negative breast cancer. According to the study by Grem et al. [110], the combination of gemcitabine with 5-fluorodeoxyuridine was superior when compared to gemcitabine monotherapy. Patients had a lower toxicity profile with combination chemotherapy compared to gemcitabine monotherapy.

Seeking to assess the benefits of the combination of drugs in the treatment of refractory prostate cancer, Chiti et al. [111] associated vinorelbine with hormone therapy, resulting in a tumor response rate of 18%; 43% had stable PSA and 29% PSA progression. The authors identified that the use of oral vinorelbine proved to be safe.

Reni et al. [112] evaluated the combination of cisplatin, epirubicin, 5-fluorouracil, and gemcitabine in the treatment of advanced pancreatic cancer, proving to be a well-tolerated and safe protocol, with a response rate of 58%, mean duration of response of 8.5 months, and median survival of 11 months, achieving clinical benefit of 78% of the evaluable patients.

Braun et al. [113] evaluated the benefit of neoadjuvant polychemotherapy in the treatment of locally advanced rectal cancer. The authors compared patients who had received the chemotherapy protocol doxorubicin and fluorouracil followed by radical surgery with patients who had received surgery alone. The authors observed a reduction in the tumor vascular network of ~50–70%, as well as a better 5-year survival rate in patients who received neoadjuvant chemotherapy, thus demonstrating the benefits of combination therapy in the treatment of locally advanced rectal cancer.

2.2.1 Challenges in Combination Therapy

Not all combination therapies are as effective for a particular type of cancer. One of the great challenges is to choose appropriate associations that prove to be effective for the treatment of a given cancer. In addition to the combination, it is important to define the ideal concentration of each chemotherapy agent, meeting the patient's needs in terms of age, comorbidity, and pathological characteristics of the cancer. These values are important, as they will define the effectiveness of the chemotherapy treatment, in addition to reducing the toxicity profile [3, 114–117]. Fumet et al. [118] evaluated the safety of the gemcitabine, docetaxel, capecitabine, and cisplatin protocol as second-line therapy for the treatment of advanced pancreatic cancer after using the FOLFIRINOX protocol (oxaliplatin, irinotecan, leucovorin, and fluorouracil). The authors observed that the use of the protocol as a second line was not superior to the use of gemcitabine monotherapy; in addition it presented a grade 3 hematological toxicity profile, requiring dose adaptation.

Due to the difficulty of evaluating the efficacy and safety of a chemotherapy protocol for the treatment of cancer, Schlick et al. [119] observed new models for predicting the benefits and toxicity of treatment with the FOLFIRINOX protocol for the treatment of pancreatic cancer. The authors noted the importance of evaluating two new independent clinical and serum factors, which were the carcinoembryonic antigen (CEA) marker and the body mass index (BMI) that influenced the overall survival of patients, where high BMI negatively affected survival global.

Falcetta et al. [120] evaluated therapeutic regimens using paclitaxel, cisplatin, and bevacizumab for the treatment of ovarian cancer, noting that paclitaxel as monotherapy proved to be effective and that when associated with bevacizumab, there was an additional contribution. Bevacizumab promoted increased cell death in therapeutic regimens. However, the interaction of paclitaxel with cisplatin resulted in negative drug interactions, where cisplatin did not contribute to the efficacy of the regimen when the two drugs were administered on the same day.

Lopez and Banerji [115] highlight the challenges for combining drugs with targeted therapy, highlighting the importance of finding the best combinations due to the biological complexity of resistance mechanisms to targeted treatment, as well as the difficulties involved in combinations with respect to profiles of toxicity, pharmacokinetic interactions, and the correct time to use the combination.

Another challenge of combination therapy is related to treatment costs; according to the study by Latimer et al. [116], the combination of drugs that are under patent can result in an affordable challenge, in addition to delaying or denying the patient's access to treatment. This problem can be overcome by proving the cost-effectiveness of the therapy, concerning the clinical benefits of the therapy compared to monotherapy.

2.3   Toxicity of Combination Therapy for Cancer Treatment

One of the major problems of chemotherapy is its high toxicity, which often limits the therapeutic options and can contribute to the worsening of the clinical condition of cancer patients [7, 121, 122]. The drug association may have benefits by enhancing the therapeutic effect, destroying cancer cells by synergistic action, but it may also enhance the toxic effects of the drugs included in the protocol [3, 24, 123, 124].

Some chemotherapy protocols present toxicity to target organs due to the association of drugs that have similar toxicity profiles [9, 24, 125]. Breast cancer treatment protocols, for example, may be responsible for the development of cardiotoxicity, mainly due to the use of drugs from the anthracycline class (doxorubicin, epirubicin, among others) that are associated with a high degree of cardiotoxicity [126–129]. Another example is the protocols used for the treatment of colorectal cancer that have a high potential for hepatotoxicity [130–132], as well as the protocols used for ovarian cancer that are related to the development of nephrotoxicity [133–135]. The combination between docetaxel, cisplatin, and 5-fluorouracil, despite being efficient in the treatment of advanced gastric cancer, is a highly toxic regimen, which may be related to the development of febrile neutropenia, thrombocytopenia, nausea, and vomiting [136]. Likewise, the combination of gemcitabine and carboplatin in the treatment of lung cancer may be related to the development of neutropenia and thrombocytopenia [137].

2.3.1   Toxicity in the Treatment of Breast Cancer

Drugs used for breast cancer have significant toxicity that can be enhanced when they are in a combination regimen. Women undergoing chemotherapy usually report asthenia, myalgia, arthralgia, mucositis, abdominal pain, diarrhea, and neutropenia as adverse reactions, whose effects will depend on the class of chemotherapy used [138]. One of the most used classes in the treatment of breast cancer is anthracyclines, which can have irreversible side effects, such as cardiac toxicity and acute leukemia [109, 139, 140]. Another class of drugs widely used in the treatment of breast cancer is taxanes, which also have cardiotoxic effects [141, 142]. Therefore, Gianni, Salvatorelli, and Minotti [143] evaluated the cardiotoxicity of doxorubicin due to its synergistic use with taxanes and trastuzumab (monoclonal antibody used for the treatment of HER2-positive breast cancer), which is also cardiotoxic. The authors observed that there seems to be synergism in the cardiotoxicity of the drugs, despite their different toxicity mechanisms. Table 2.3 shows some studies that report the toxic effects of drugs used to treat breast cancer.

Table 2.3 Toxic effects of combinations used in the treatment of breast cancer

Drug	Interacting drug	Toxicity interactions	Reference
Doxorubicin	Paclitaxel	Paclitaxel stimulates the formation of anthracycline metabolites that play an important role in your heart failure mechanism. Increased area under the curve (AUC) and maximum concentration (C max) of doxorubicin and increased myelosuppression	[143, 144]
Doxorubicin	Trastuzumab	Trastuzumab interferes with heart-specific survival factors, helping the heart to resist stressors such as anthracyclines	[143]
Paclitaxel	Epirubicin	Increased myelosuppression	[145, 146]
Epirubicin	5-fluorouracil and cyclophosphamide	Interstitial pneumonitis Bilateral pleural effusions Pneumonitis	[147, 148]
Paclitaxel	Cyclophosphamide	Increased neutropenia and thrombocytopenia when paclitaxel is given before cyclophosphamide	[149, 150]

Petrelli et al. [151] evaluated, through a meta-analysis, the toxic effects of anthracyclines associated with taxanes for the treatment of breast cancer. The authors report that the association appears not to be related to an increased risk of cardiotoxicity, venous thromboembolic events, and leukemic risk, but increased mortality not related to breast cancer.

Paul et al. [152] evaluated the use of paclitaxel combined with 5-fluorouracil for the treatment of metastatic breast cancer. The authors observed that the patients who underwent treatment with the association presented as toxicity the development of mucositis, nausea/vomiting, paresthesia, alopecia, arthralgia/myalgia, and hypersensitivity reactions. In the case of patients who presented hypersensitivity, the protocol was suspended. With work similar to that of Paul et al. [152], Nicholson et al. [153] also evaluated the use of the association of paclitaxel, 5-fluorouracil, and leucovorin for the treatment of metastatic breast cancer, where patients presented as the toxicity of the treatment, neutropenia, arthralgia, and myalgia.

Loesch et al. [154] also evaluated the use of the protocol paclitaxel, 5-fluorouracil, and leucovorin for the treatment of metastatic breast cancer, noting that the main toxic effects of the treatment were leukopenia, neutropenia, sepsis, neuropathy, nausea/vomiting, diarrhea, and asthenia.

Berruti et al. [155] evaluated the toxicity of the combination of paclitaxel, vinorelbine, and 5-fluorouracil in the treatment of breast cancer. The authors observed that the dose-limiting toxicity was myelosuppression, with grade 3/4 leukopenia in 52.5% of the patients, in addition to non-hematological toxicities that included mucositis, diarrhea, skin, and cardiac toxicity. In 7.2% of patients, neurotoxicity was also identified.

2.3.2   Toxicity in the Treatment of Lung Cancer

Chemotherapy for the treatment of lung cancer can be performed with a single drug or can be used in combination with drugs. Despite its effectiveness, it can induce serious toxic events [156–158]. Cherif et al. [157] evaluated the toxicity profile of chemotherapy in advanced non-small-cell lung cancer. The authors observed that platinum-based protocols were the most used and that the main toxicities developed were hematological, gastrointestinal, and renal.

Fan et al. [159] in a phase II study evaluated the combination of gemcitabine and cisplatin in the treatment of advanced non-small-cell lung cancer; the authors noted that the combination can induce myelosuppression and gastrointestinal toxicity.

Some drugs used to treat lung cancer can also cause lung damage [148, 160]. This is the case of gefitinib, a drug used for the first-line treatment of advanced non-small-cell lung cancer. According to Niho et al. [161], treatment with gefitinib in patients with lung cancer can induce the development of grade 5 interstitial lung disease; in addition, the authors identified that this drug also induced liver toxicity (grade 2 or 3), rash (grade 1 or 2), and diarrhea (grade 1).

Erlotinib also appears to have pulmonary toxicity in the treatment of advanced non-small-cell lung cancer. Liu et al. [162] observed, through a case report, that the patient developed interstitial pneumonia after using erlotinib, with similar toxicity related to the use of gefitinib.

Chen et al. [163] also identified pulmonary toxicity in the association of ifosfamide and docetaxel for the treatment of non-small-cell lung cancer. In addition to pulmonary toxicity, through the induction of interstitial pneumonitis, the combination also induced myelosuppression, with the development of febrile neutropenia (grade 3 or 4) and anemia (grade 3). Table 2.4 shows some studies that observed pulmonary toxicity in drugs used to treat lung cancer.

Gemcitabine is a drug widely used for the treatment of cancer, indicated in the treatment of several solid tumors, such as pancreatic, ovarian, and non-small-cell lung cancer [159, 174, 175]. This drug has been linked to a pulmonary toxicity profile; Pavlakis et al. [160] reported fatal pulmonary toxicity after gemcitabine use, with patients presenting with respiratory distress syndrome and interstitial pneumonitis. Marruchella et al. [166] report diffuse alveolar damage induced by the use of gemcitabine during the treatment of non-small-cell lung cancer.

Methotrexate is also indicated for the treatment of lung cancer, and, like other antineoplastics, it induces the development of pulmonary toxicity [148]. Zimmerman et al. [170] evaluated the pulmonary toxicity profile of the combination of methotrexate, etoposide, and cyclophosphamide in the treatment of anaplastic small cell lung cancer. Methotrexate induces interstitial pneumonitis, and when associated with etoposide, it seems to enhance its toxicity because etoposide increases intracellular levels of methotrexate. In addition, etoposide also has a pulmonary toxicity profile, Gurjal et al. [172] report that the use of etoposide can induce subacute dyspnea and interstitial infiltrates. Dajczman et al. [171] show that pulmonary toxicity of etoposide can be fatal and can induce the development of pneumonitis, as well as methotrexate.

Table 2.4 Drugs used for the treatment of lung cancer that induces lung toxicity

Drugs	Pulmonary toxicity	Reference
Docetaxel plus ifosfamide	Interstitial pneumonitis	[163]
Gefitinib	Acute pneumonitis Diffuse alveolar damage Diffuse alveolar hemorrhage Pulmonary fibrosis	[148, 161]
Doxorubicin	Dyspnea Organizing pneumonia	[148, 164]
Gemcitabine	Dyspnea Bronchospasm Pulmonary edema Diffuse alveolar damage Alveolar hemorrhage	[165–168]
Erlotinib	Interstitial pneumonia	[162]
Methotrexate	Pneumonitis	[169]
Methotrexate, etoposide plus cyclophosphamide	Pneumonitis	[170]
Etoposide	Anaphylaxis Angioedema Chest discomfort Bronchospasm Pneumonitis Acute lung injury Diffuse alveolar damage Fibrin membrane formation Alveolar wall edema	[171–173]

2.3.3   Toxicity in the Treatment of Colorectal Cancer

Although antineoplastic chemotherapy has a good response for the treatment of colorectal cancer, the treatment can still induce severe toxicity [176, 177]. Chemotherapy-related toxicity for the treatment of colorectal cancer appears to be related to the development of neutropenia, thrombopenia, anemia, diarrhea, nausea/vomiting, mucositis, hand-foot syndrome, and peripheral neuropathy [178–180]. Chemotherapy treatment for colorectal cancer is mainly based on the association of drugs such as 5-fluorouracil, oxaliplatin, irinotecan, and leucovorin [176, 179, 181]. Cavalcanti et al. [131] reported the case of a patient who developed hepatotoxicity after treatment with a combination of oxaliplatin and irinotecan, with the appearance of liver nodules and worsening of the patient's clinical situation.

The use of 5-fluorouracil in the treatment of colorectal cancer, when administered as a bolus, results in hematological toxicity, such as neutropenia, and non-hematological toxicity, such as diarrhea and mucositis. When administered as an infusion, 5-fluorouracil can result in cases of hand-foot syndrome [182]. Irinotecan induces severe diarrhea and when combined with 5-fluorouracil results in high rates of severe diarrhea [183–185]. Goldberg et al. [186] and Saltz et al. [187] highlight that the association of 5-fluorouracil and irinotecan increases severe toxicity and treatment-related deaths.

The use of oxaliplatin is common in the treatment of colorectal cancer, but it has transient sensorineural toxicity, developing paresthesia due to cold sensitivity, and can also result in dose-dependent chronic peripheral sensory neuropathy [188]. Depending on the combination of drugs used, the toxicity profile changes; in the case of the combination 5-fluorouracil and leucovorin, there is a predominance in cases of vomiting, diarrhea, and neutropenia, while in the combination of oxaliplatin, leucovorin, and 5-fluorouracil, the prevalence is of cases of neutropenia, neurotoxicity, and diarrhea [182, 189]. Regarding the irinotecan, leucovorin, and 5-fluorouracil protocol, the prevalence is of cases of neutropenia, diarrhea, nausea, and vomiting, whereas the administration of capecitabine alone led to the development of diarrhea, neutropenia, nausea, and vomiting [182, 190, 191].

2.3.4 Toxicity in the Treatment of Prostate Cancer

Prostate cancer depends on hormones for its development, as cancer cells have hormone receptors, so their treatment is mainly based on the use of oral hormone therapy. Despite this, some chemotherapy protocols are effective for prostate cancer, but they are not free from toxic effects [192–196]. Behrens, Gulley, and Dahut [197] observed that the treatment of prostate cancer with docetaxel and thalidomide can induce pulmonary toxicity. Pulmonary toxicity of docetaxel and thalidomide can present from symptomatic effusions, dyspnea, interstitial lung disease, and pulmonary embolism [197].

Kellokumpu-Lehtinen et al. [198] evaluated toxicity in prostate cancer patients who had received docetaxel plus hormone after radical radiotherapy. After analyzing the results, the authors observed the induction of grade 3 or 4 adverse events, mainly due to bone marrow toxicity, such as neutropenia (72%), febrile neutropenia (24%), neutropenic infection (10%), and infection without neutropenia (4%). Some patients also presented anorexia, diarrhea, mucositis, nausea, pain, and fatigue, in addition to more severe toxicity such as pulmonary embolism and renal failure.

Terada et al. [199] evaluated the toxicity of cabazitaxel for the treatment of prostate cancer in Japanese patients. The authors observed that patients who used cabazitaxel presented neutropenia (45%), febrile neutropenia (25%), malaise (16%), nausea (14%), diarrhea (11%), thrombocytopenia (8%), and pneumonia (4%).

Scott et al. [200] evaluated the efficacy of treating advanced prostatic carcinoma with cyclophosphamide or 5-fluorouracil, where patients had minimal toxicity, with the development of leukopenia, nausea, and vomiting. Another drug tested for the treatment of prostate cancer was mitoxantrone. Tannock et al. [201] evaluated the use of mitoxantrone combined with prednisone for the treatment of prostate cancer, where despite being effective, it showed five episodes of cardiac toxicity.

Hudes et al. [202], in a phase II study, observed the use of estramustine and vinblastine in hormone-refractory prostate cancer, where they observed the development of leukopenia, anemia, nausea, vomiting, edema, fatigue, breast tenderness, paresthesias as treatment toxicity, cardiovascular toxicity, anorexia, indigestion, constipation, and leg cramps. In another phase II study, Hudes et al. [203] evaluated the association of paclitaxel plus estramustine in hormone-refractory metastatic prostate cancer, where the combination led to the development of mainly the toxic effects of nausea (33%), fluid retention (33%), and fatigue (24.2%).

The use of estramustine was also evaluated by Pienta et al. [204], this time associated with etoposide in the treatment of hormone-refractory prostate adenocarcinoma. The authors observed that this combination led to the development of toxicity such as alopecia (100%), leukopenia (57%), anemia (55%), edema (48%), and thrombocytopenia (36%), among others. Savarese et al. [205] evaluated the combination of docetaxel, estramustine, and hydrocortisone in hormone-refractory prostate cancer, with predominant toxicity being neutropenia (26%) and granulocytopenia (30%), in addition to milder reactions such as malaise/fatigue, peripheral edema, and hyperglycemia.

Sella et al. [206], in a phase II study, evaluated the use of ketoconazole combined with doxorubicin in patients with androgen-independent prostate cancer. The toxicity profile of this combination included stomatitis and acral erythema (29%), neutropenia (29%), and anal and urethral mucositis (13%), in addition to more severe reactions such as hypokalemia (39%) and adrenal insufficiency (63%).

2.3.5   Toxicity in the Treatment of Cervical Cancer

The main treatment modalities for cervical cancer are radiotherapy and chemotherapy, but their toxicity rates have been a concern, especially with the combination of the two modalities [7, 207–210]. Cisplatin is a widely used drug for the treatment of cervical cancer [211, 212]; with this in mind, Tan and Zahra [213] evaluated the combination of cisplatin with radiotherapy. Although the combination has benefits in improving patient survival, the association showed severe late toxicity, such as urinary and intestinal complications.

Tan et al. [214] evaluated the toxicity of chemoradiotherapy in the treatment of cervical cancer. The patients had received cisplatin associated with radiotherapy, where the observed toxicity of the treatment was diarrhea (80.6%), malaise (66.7%), and nausea (62.5%), in addition to hematological toxicity, anemia, thrombocytopenia, and neutropenia. Coronel et al. [215] evaluated the activity of oral cisplatin and vinorelbine as radiosensitizers for the treatment of cervical cancer, where the association of drugs with radiotherapy had grade 2 and 3 lymphopenias as the most frequent toxicity.

Wang et al. [216] evaluated the combination of cisplatin plus radiotherapy or cisplatin plus gemcitabine plus radiotherapy in the treatment of advanced cervical cancer. As for the toxicity profiles, the authors emphasize that the combination of cisplatin plus gemcitabine and radiotherapy led to the development of neutropenia and thrombocytopenia.

Kong et al. [217] evaluated the use of chemoradiation with weekly cisplatin compared to cisplatin plus monthly 5-fluorouracil. As for toxicity, the authors demonstrate that monthly chemoradiation had a higher toxicity profile, inducing anemia, leukopenia, thrombocytopenia, diarrhea, nausea, vomiting, and small bowel obstruction.

Araújo et al. [218] analyzed the toxicity of chemotherapy in cervical cancer. The authors observed that the most used chemotherapy protocols were cisplatin monotherapy, paclitaxel plus carboplatin, cisplatin plus paclitaxel, and carboplatin, cisplatin plus paclitaxel. As for the toxicity profile, the authors report that cisplatin is related to the development of leukopenia and that it increases the risks of thrombocytopenia in the protocols. The authors also noted that the combination of cisplatin and paclitaxel appears to increase the chances of developing nephrotoxicity and hepatotoxicity.

2.3.6 *Toxicity in the Treatment of Head and Neck Cancer*

Like cervical cancer, the treatment of head and neck cancer is based on the association of radiotherapy and chemotherapy modalities [219, 220]. The combination of the two modalities can lead to the development of systemic toxicities or local reactions, where mucositis is one of the main adverse reactions in the treatment of head and neck cancer [221–223].

Hu et al. [224] compared the treatment of head and neck cancer with the use of cisplatin versus cetuximab combined with radiotherapy. Side effects observed in both protocols showed that the effects of the combination of cisplatin and radiotherapy were more frequent than the combination of cetuximab and radiotherapy. Patients had cases of neutropenia, anemia, thrombocytopenia, mucositis, and radiation dermatitis, these being the most frequent reactions.

Albers et al. [225] studied the efficacy and toxicity of the combination of docetaxel, 5-fluorouracil, and cisplatin for the treatment of head and neck cancer. Among the adverse events of treatment, the most common were leucopenia (58%), anemia (51%), hepatotoxicity (53%), and nausea (27%). Posner et al. [226] compared the combination of cisplatin and 5-fluorouracil alone or with docetaxel in the treatment of head and neck cancer, showing that treatment with docetaxel plus cisplatin and 5-fluorouracil induced the development of febrile neutropenia and neutropenia, while patients who made use of the docetaxel and 5-fluorouracil protocol had their chemotherapy more frequently delayed due to the development of hematological adverse effects. Vermorken et al. [227] also compared the benefits of chemotherapy with cisplatin, 5-fluorouracil, and docetaxel in unresectable head and neck cancer, showing that this protocol induced the development of leukopenia and neutropenia, while the group receiving docetaxel and 5-fluorouracil had thrombocytopenia, nausea, vomiting, stomatitis, and hearing loss.

Qian et al. [228] evaluated the use of a combination taxane (docetaxel and paclitaxel), cisplatin, and 5-fluorouracil in the treatment of advanced head and neck cancer, showing that the toxicity of this protocol is related to cases of febrile neutropenia, alopecia, diarrhea, and leukopenia.

2.3.7 Toxicity in the Treatment of Lymphomas

Understanding the toxicity profiles of treatment for lymphomas is important; because of their chronic toxicity, many patients can achieve a cure and still later develop toxicity to the treatment [229, 230]. Two protocols widely used in the treatment of lymphomas are ABVD (doxorubicin, bleomycin, vinblastine, and dacarbazine) and R-CHOP (rituximab, cyclophosphamide, doxorubicin, vincristine, and prednisone), where both seem to induce cardiotoxicity, probably due to the presence of doxorubicin in the protocols [229, 231, 232].

Limat et al. [231] evaluated the incidence and risk factors of cardiotoxicity in the treatment of aggressive non-Hodgkin's lymphoma in patients using the CHOP/R--CHOP protocol. The authors confirmed the influence of the cardiotoxic effect of the R-CHOP protocol. Hershman et al. [233] demonstrate in their study that the administration of doxorubicin is a cardiac risk factor in elderly patients with diffuse B-cell non-Hodgkin's lymphoma, where the inclusion of doxorubicin in the treatment of these patients was associated with a 29% increase in the risk of congestive heart failure. Herbrecht et al. [234] compared the protocol containing pixantrone (R-CPOP) with the R-CHOP containing doxorubicin in the treatment of diffuse large B-cell lymphoma. Replacing doxorubicin with pixantrone reduced cardiotoxicity with a reduction in ejection fraction and troponin-T.

Swerdlow et al. [232] assessed the risk of mortality from myocardial infarction related to the treatment of Hodgkin's lymphoma. The risk of cardiotoxicity was increased in patients who were treated with radiotherapy, anthracyclines, or vincristine, being particularly high in patients who received doxorubicin, bleomycin, vinblastine, and dacarbazine. As for the chronic effect of cardiotoxicity, this was related to patients after 20 years or more who used it as the first treatment with radiotherapy and vincristine.

In addition to cardiotoxicity, the treatment of lymphomas can induce the development of other cancers. Hodgson [229] reports in his study that treatment for lymphomas can induce the development of breast, lung, and leukemia cancers. The use of alkylating agents (mechlorethamine and procarbazine) can induce the development of leukemia and lung cancer [235–237]. Van Leeuwen et al. [237] report that the cumulative dose of alkylating agents such as mechlorethamine and procarbazine increased the risk of developing leukemia in patients with Hodgkin's lymphoma eightfold.

References

1. Arruebo M, Vilaboa N, Sáez-Gutierrez B, Lambea J, Tres A, Valladares M, González-Fernández A. Assessment of the evolution of cancer treatment therapies. Cancer. 2011;3(3):3279–330. https://doi.org/10.3390/cancers3033279.
2. Abbas Z, Rehman S. An overview of cancer treatment modalities. London: Intechopen; 2018.

3. Mokhtari RB, Homayouni TS, Baluch N, Morgatskaya E, Kumar S, Das B, Yeger H. Combination therapy in combating cancer. Oncotarget. 2017;8(23):38022–43. https://doi.org/10.18632/oncotarget.16723.

4. Lutz ST, Jones J, Chow E. Role of radiation therapy in palliative care of the patient with cancer. J Clin Oncol. 2014;32(26):2913–9. https://doi.org/10.1200/JCO.2014.55.1143.

5. Roeland EJ, LeBlanc TW. Palliative chemotherapy: oxymoron or misunderstanding? BMC Palliat Care. 2016;15:33. https://doi.org/10.1186/s12904-016-0109-4.

6. Neugut AI, Prigerson HG. Curative, life-extending, and palliative chemotherapy: new outcomes need new names. Oncologist. 2017;22(8):883–5. https://doi.org/10.1634/theoncologist.2017-0041.

7. Harrington SE, Smith TJ. The role of chemotherapy at the end of life. When is enough, enough? JAMA. 2008;299(22):2667–78. https://doi.org/10.1001/jama.299.22.2667.

8. Falzone L, Salomone S, Libra M. Evolution of cancer pharmacological treatment at the turn of the third millennium. Front Pharmacol. 2018;9:1300. https://doi.org/10.3389/fphar.2018.01300.

9. Schirrmacher V. From chemotherapy to biological therapy: a review of novel concepts to reduce the side effects of systemic cancer treatment (review). Int J Oncol. 2019;54(2):407–19. https://doi.org/10.3892/ijo.2018.4661.

10. Gonzalez H, Hagerling C, Werb Z. Roles of the immune system in cancer: from tumor initiation to metastatic progression. Genes Dev. 2018;32(19-20):1267–84. https://doi.org/10.1101/gad.314617.118.

11. Sambi M, Bagheri L, Szewczuk MR. Current challenges in cancer immunotherapy: multimodal approaches to improve efficacy and patient response rates. J Oncol. 2019;2019:4508794. https://doi.org/10.1155/2019/4508794.

12. D'Alterio C, Scala S, Sozzi G, Roz L, Bertolini G. Paradoxical effects of chemotherapy on tumor relapse and metastasis promotion. Semin Cancer Biol. 2020;60:351–61. https://doi.org/10.1016/j.semcancer.2019.08.019.

13. Quail DF, Joyce JA. Microenvironmental regulation of tumor progression and metastasis. Nat Med. 2013;19(11):1423–37. https://doi.org/10.1038/nm.3394.

14. Welch DR, Hurst DR. Defining the hallmarks of metastasis. Cancer Res. 2019;79(12):3011–27. https://doi.org/10.1158/0008-5472.CAN-19-0458.

15. Harbeck N, Penault-Llorca F, Cortes J, Gnant M, Houssami N, Poortmans P, Ruddy K, Tsang J, Cardoso F. Breast cancer. Nat Rev Dis Primers. 2019;5:66. https://doi.org/10.1038/s41572-019-0111-2.

16. Hirata BKB, Oda JMM, Guembarovski RL, Ariza CB, Oliveira CEC, Watanabe MAE. Molecular markers for breast cancer: prediction on tumor behavior. Dis Markers. 2014;2014:513158. https://doi.org/10.1155/2014/513158.

17. Nagpal M, Singh S, Singh P, Chauhan P, Zaidi MA. Tumor markers: a diagnostic tool. Natl J Maxillofac Surg. 2016;7(1):17–20. https://doi.org/10.4103/0975-5950.196135.

18. Gutierrez C, Schiff R. HER 2: biology, detection, and clinical implications. Arch Pathol Lab Med. 2011;135(1):55–62. https://doi.org/10.1043/2010-0454-RAR.1.

19. Masoud V, Pagès G. Targeted therapies in breast cancer: new challenges to fight against resistance. World J Clin Oncol. 2017;8(2):120–34. https://doi.org/10.5306/wjco.v8.i2.120.

20. Al-Busairi W, Khajah M. The principles behind targeted therapy for cancer treatment. London: IntechOpen; 2019.

21. Rosenkranz AA, Slastnikova TA. Epidermal growth factor receptor: key to selective intracellular delivery. Biochemistry. 2020;85:967–93. https://doi.org/10.1134/S0006297920090011.

22. Worm DJ, Els-Heindl S, Beck-Sickinger AG. Targeting of peptide-binding receptors on cancer cells with peptide-drug conjugates. Pept Sci. 2020;112(3):e24171. https://doi.org/10.1002/pep2.24171.

23. Bailly C, Thuru X, Quesnel B. Combined cytotoxic chemotherapy and immunotherapy of cancer: modern times. NAR Cancer. 2020;2(1):1–20. https://doi.org/10.1093/narcan/zcaa002.

24. Senapati S, Mahanta AK, Kumar S, Maiti P. Controlled drug delivery vehicles for cancer treatment and their performance. Signal Transduct Target Ther. 2018;3:7. https://doi.org/10.1038/s41392-017-0004-3.

25. Zitvogel L, Apetoh L, Ghiringhelli F, Kroemer G. Immunological aspects of cancer chemotherapy. Nat Rev Immunol. 2008;8:59–73. https://doi.org/10.1038/nri2216.

26. Housman G, Byler S, Heerboth S, Lapinska K, Longacre M, Snyder N, Sarkar S. Drug resistance in cancer: an overview. Cancer. 2014;6(3):1769–92. https://doi.org/10.3390/cancers6031769.

27. Ramos P, Bentires-Alj M. Mechanism-based cancer therapy: resistance to therapy, therapy for resistance. Oncogene. 2015;34:3617–26. https://doi.org/10.1038/onc.2014.314.

28. Vaidya FU, Chhipa AS, Mishra V, Gupta VK, Rawat SG, Kumar A, Pathak C. Molecular and cellular paradigms of multidrug resistance in cancer. Cancer Rep. 2020;2020:e1291. https://doi.org/10.1002/cnr2.1291.

29. Bukowski K, Kciuk M, Kontek R. Mechanisms of multidrug resistance in cancer chemotherapy. Int J Mol Sci. 2020;21(9):3233. https://doi.org/10.3390/ijms21093233.

30. Ahmed S, Zhou Z, Zhou J, Chen SQ. Pharmacogenomics of drug metabolizing enzymes and transporters: relevance to precision medicine. Genomics Proteomics Bioinformatics. 2016;14(5):298–313. https://doi.org/10.1016/j.gpb.2016.03.008.

31. Kaur G, Gupta SK, Singh P, Ali V, Kumar V, Verma M. Drug-metabolizing enzymes: role in drug resistance in cancer. Clin Transl Oncol. 2020;22:1667–80. https://doi.org/10.1007/s12094-020-02325-7.

32. Tao G, Huang J, Moorthy B, Wang C, Hu M, Gao S, Ghose R. Role of drug metabolizing enzymes in chemotherapy-induced gastrointestinal toxicity and hepatotoxicity. Expert Opin Drug Metab Toxicol. 2020;16(11):1109–24. https://doi.org/10.1080/17425255.2020.1815705.

33. Pathania S, Bhatia R, Baldi A, Singh R, Rawal RK. Drug metabolizing enzymes and their inhibitors' role in cancer resistance. Biomed Pharmacother. 2018;105:53–65. https://doi.org/10.1016/j.biopha.2018.05.117.

34. Allocati N, Masulli M, Ilio CD, Federici L. Glutathione transferases: substrates, inhibitors and pro-drugs in cancer and neurodegenerative diseases. Oncogene. 2018;7(1):8. https://doi.org/10.1038/s41389-017-0025-3.

35. Singh RR, Reindl KM. Glutathione S-transferases in cancer. Antioxidants. 2021;10:701. https://doi.org/10.3390/antiox10050701.

36. Clara JA, Monge C, Yang Y, Takebe N. Targeting signalling pathways and the immune microenvironment of cancer stem cells – a clinical update. Nat Rev Clin Oncol. 2019;17:204–32. https://doi.org/10.1038/s41571-019-0293-2.

37. Pitt JM, Marabelle A, Eggermont A, Soria JC, Kroemer G, Zitvogel L. Targeting the tumor microenvironment: removing obstruction to anticancer immune responses and immunotherapy. Ann Oncol. 2016;27:1482–92. https://doi.org/10.1093/annonc/mdw168.

38. Harrison PT, Huang PH. Exploiting vulnerabilities in cancer signaling networks to combat targeted therapy resistance. Essays Biochem. 2018;62(4):583–93. https://doi.org/10.1042/EBC20180016.

39. Marshall HT, Djamgoz MB. Immuno-oncology: emerging targets and combination therapies. Front Oncol. 2018;8:315. https://doi.org/10.3389/fonc.2018.00315.

40. Kondo N, Takahashi A, Ono K, Ohnishi T. DNA damage induced by alkylating agents and repair pathways. J Nucl Acids. 2010;2010:543531. https://doi.org/10.4061/2010/543531.

41. Van Linden AA, Baturin D, Ford JB, Fosmire SP, Gardner L, Korch C, Reigan P, Porter CC. Inhibition of Wee1 sensitizes cancer cells to antimetabolite chemotherapeutics in vitro and in vivo, independent of p53 functionality. Mol Cancer Ther. 2013;12(12):2675–84. https://doi.org/10.1158/1535-7163.MCT-13-0424.

42. Weber GF. DNA damaging drugs. In: Molecular therapies of cancer. Cham: Springer; 2015. https://doi.org/10.1007/978-3-319-13278-5_2.

43. Mills CC, Kolb EA, Sampson VB. Development of chemotherapy with cell cycle inhibitors for adult and pediatric cancer therapy. Cancer Res. 2018;78(2):320–5. https://doi.org/10.1158/0008-5472.CAN-17-2782.

44. Khazir J, Riley DL, Pilcher LA, De-Maayer P, Mir BA. Anticancer agents from diverse natural sources. Nat Prod Commun. 2014;9(11):1655–69.

45. Minev BR. Cancer management in man: chemotherapy, biological therapy, hyperthermia and supporting measures. Cham: Springer; 2011.

46. Colvin M. Alkylating agents. In: Kufe DW, Pollock RE, Weichselbaum RR, et al., editors. Holland-Frei cancer medicine. 6th ed. Hamilton: BC Decker; 2003.

47. Weber GF. DNA damaging drugs. Mol Therap Cancer. 2014;2014:9–12. https://doi.org/10.1007/978-3-319-13278-5_2.

48. Wang LC, Okitsu Y, Zandi E. Tumor necrosis factor α-dependent drug resistance to purine and pyrimidine analogues in human colon tumor cells mediated through IKK. J Biol Chem. 2005;280(9):7634–44.

49. Parker WB. Enzymology of purine and pyrimidine antimetabolites used in the treatment of cancer. Chem Rev. 2009;109(7):2880–93. https://doi.org/10.1021/cr900028p.

50. Cheung-Ong K, Giaever G, Nislow C. DNA-damaging agents in cancer chemotherapy: serendipity and chemical biology. Chem Biol. 2013;20(5):648–59. https://doi.org/10.1016/j.chembiol.2013.04.007.

51. Bhattacharya B, Mukherjee S. Cancer therapy using antibiotics. J Cancer Ther. 2015;6:849–58. https://doi.org/10.4236/jct.2015.610093.

52. Quezada H, Martínez-Vázquez M, López-Jácome E, González-Pedrajo B, Andrade A, Fernández-Presas AM, Tovar-García A, García-Contreras R. Repurposed anti-cancer drugs: the future for anti-infective therapy? Expert Rev Anti-Infect Ther. 2020;18(7):609–12. https://doi.org/10.1080/14787210.2020.1752665.

53. Schrijvers D, Vermorken JB. Role of toxoids in head and neck cancer. Oncologist. 2000;5(3):199–208. https://doi.org/10.1634/theoncologist.5-3-199.

54. Abal M, Andreu JM, Barasoain I. Taxanes: microtubule and centrosome targets, and cell cycle dependent mechanisms of action. Curr Cancer Drug Targets. 2003;3:193–203. https://doi.org/10.2174/1568009033481967.

55. Orr GA, Verdier-Pinard P, McDaid H, Horwitz SB. Mechanisms of taxol resistance to microtubules. Oncogene. 2003;22(47):7280–95. https://doi.org/10.1038/sj.onc.1206934.

56. Bates D, Eastman A. Microtubule destabilizing agents: far more than just antimitotic anticancer drugs. Br J Clin Pharmacol. 2017;83(2):255–68. https://doi.org/10.1111/bcp.13126.

57. Chagas CM, Alisaraie L. Metabolites of vinca alkaloid vinblastine: tubulin binding and activation of nausea-associated receptors. ACS Omega. 2019;4(6):9784–99. https://doi.org/10.1021/acsomega.9b00652.

58. Krause W. Resistance to anti-tubulin agents: from vinca alkaloids to epothilones. Cancer Drug Resist. 2019;2:82–106.

59. Kruger K, Thomale J, Stojanovic N, Osmak M, Henninger C, Bormann S, Fritz G. Platinum-induced kidney damage: unraveling the DNA damage response (DDR) of renal tubular epithelial and glomerular endothelial cells following platinum injury. Biochim Biophys Acta. 2015;1853(3):685–98. https://doi.org/10.1016/j.bbamcr.2014.12.033.

60. Rocha CRR, Silva MM, Quinet A, Cabral-Neto JB, Menck CFM. DNA repair pathways and cisplatin resistance: an intimate relationship. Clinics. 2018;73(1):e478. https://doi.org/10.6061/clinics/2018/e478s.

61. Wenmaekers S, Viergever BJ, Kumar G, Kranenburg O, Black PC, Daugaard M, Meijer RP. A potential role for HUWE1 in modulating cisplatin sensitivity. Cell. 2021;10(5):1262. https://doi.org/10.3390/cells10051262.

62. Silva AA, Carlotto J, Rotta I. Standardization of the infusion sequence of antineoplastic drugs used in the treatment of breast and colorectal cancers. Einstein. 2018;16(2):1–9. https://doi.org/10.1590/S1679-45082018RW4074.

63. Cavalcanti IDL, Soares JCS. Conventional cancer treatment. In: Advances in cancer treatment. Cham: Springer; 2021. https://doi.org/10.1007/978-3-030-68334-4_4.
64. Konstantinov SM, Berger MR. Alkylating agents. In: Offermann S, Rosenthal W, editors. Encyclopedia of molecular pharmacology. Berlin: Springer; 2008. https://doi.org/10.1007/978-3-540-38918-7_178.
65. Wang Z, Sun Y. Targeting p53 for novel anticancer therapy. Transl Oncol. 2010;3(1):1–12. https://doi.org/10.1593/tlo.09250.
66. Farkona S, Diamandis EP, Blasutig IM. Cancer immunotherapy: the beginning of the end of cancer? BMC Med. 2016;14:73. https://doi.org/10.1186/s12916-016-0623-5.
67. Mantovani F, Collavin L, Del Sal G. Mutant p53 as a guardian of the cancer cell. Cell Death Differ. 2019;26:199–212. https://doi.org/10.1038/s41418-018-0246-9.
68. Bisht M, Bist SS, Dhasmana DC. Biological response modifiers: current use and future prospects in cancer therapy. Indian J Cancer. 2010;47(4):443–51. https://doi.org/10.4103/0019-509X.73559.
69. Corraliza-Gorjón I, Somovilla-Crespo B, Santamaria S, Garcia-Sanz JÁ, Kremer L. New strategies using antibody combinations to increase cancer treatment effectiveness. Front Immunol. 2017;8:1804. https://doi.org/10.3389/fimmu.2017.01804.
70. Bociek RG, Armitage JO. Hematopoietic growth factors. CA Cancer J Clin. 1996;46(3):165–84. https://doi.org/10.3322/canjclin.46.3.165.
71. Mehta HM, Malandra M, Corey SJ. G-CSF and GM-CSF in neutropenia. J Immunol. 2015;195(4):1341–9. https://doi.org/10.4049/jimmunol.1500861.
72. Wigley P, Kaiser P. Avian cytokines in health and disease. Braz J Poultry Sci. 2003;5(1):1–14. https://doi.org/10.1590/S1516-635X2003000100001.
73. Briukhovetska D, Dorr J, Endres S, Libby P, Dinarello CA, Kobold S (2021) Interleukins in cancer: from biology to therapy. Nat Rev Cancer. https://doi.org/10.1038/s41568-021-00363-z.
74. Janson EMT, Ahlstrom H, Andersson T, Oberg KE. Octreotide and interferon alfa: a new combination for the treatment of malignant carcinoid tumours. Eur J Cancer. 1992;28(10):1647–50. https://doi.org/10.1016/0959-8049(92)90060-F.
75. Dinney CPN, Fisher MB, Navai N, C'Donnell MA, Cutler D, Abraham A, Young S, Hutchins B, Caceres M, Kishnani N, Sode G, Cullen C, Zhang G, Grossman HB, Kamat AM, Gonzales M, Kincaid M, Ainslie N, Maneval DC, Wszolek MF, Benedict WF. Phase I trial of intravesical recombinant adenovirus mediated interferon-α2b formulated in Syn3 for Bacillus Calmette-Guérin failures in nonmuscle invasive bladder cancer. J Urol. 2013;190(3):850–6. https://doi.org/10.1016/j.juro.2013.03.030.
76. Medrano RFV, Hunger A, Mendonça AS, Barbuto JAM, Strauss BE. Immunomodulatory and antitumor effects of type I interferons and their application in cancer therapy. Oncotarget. 2017;8(41):71249–84. https://doi.org/10.18632/oncotarget.19531.
77. Castro F, Cardoso AP, Gonçalves RM, Serre K, Oliveira MJ. Interferon-gamma at the crossroads of tumor immune surveillance or evasion. Front Immunol. 2018;9:847. https://doi.org/10.3389/fimmu.2018.00847.
78. Weiner LM, Dhodapkar MV, Ferrone S. Monoclonal antibodies for cancer immunotherapy. Lancet. 2009;373(9668):1033–40. https://doi.org/10.1016/S0140-6736(09)60251-8.
79. Waldman AD, Fritz JM, Lenardo MJ. A guide to cancer immunotherapy: from T cell basic science to clinical practice. Nat Rev Immunol. 2020;20:651–68. https://doi.org/10.1038/s41577-020-0306-5.
80. Zahavi D, Weiner L. Monoclonal antibodies in cancer therapy. Antibodies. 2020;9(3):34. https://doi.org/10.3390/antib9030034.
81. Paul MK, Mukhopadhyay AK. Tyrosine kinase – role and significance in cancer. Int J Med Sci. 2004;1(2):101–15. https://doi.org/10.7150/ijms.1.101.
82. Metibemu DS, Akinloye OA, Akamo AJ, Ojo DA, Okeowo OT, Omotuyi IO. Exploring receptor tyrosine kinases-inhibitors in cancer treatment. Egyp J Med Hum Genet. 2019;20:35. https://doi.org/10.1186/s43042-019-0035-0.

83. Indraccolo S. Interferon-alpha as angiogenesis inhibitor: learning from tumor models. Autoimmunity. 2010;43(3):244–7. https://doi.org/10.3109/08916930903510963.

84. Niu G, Chen X. Vascular endothelial growth factor as an anti-angiogenic target for cancer therapy. Curr Drug Targets. 2010;11(8):1000–17.

85. Yoo SY, Kwon SM. Angiogenesis and its therapeutic opportunities. Mediat Inflamm. 2013;2013:127170. https://doi.org/10.1155/2013/127170.

86. Haibe Y, Kreidieh M, Hajj HE, Khalifeh I, Mukherji D, Temraz S, Shamseddine A. Resistance mechanisms to anti-angiogenic therapies in cancer. Front Oncol. 2020;10:221. https://doi.org/10.3389/fonc.2020.00221.

87. Sharpe M, Mount N. Genetically modified T cells in cancer therapy: opportunities and challenges. Dis Model Mech. 2015;8(4):337–50. https://doi.org/10.1242/dmm.018036.

88. Li H, Zhao Y. Increasing the safety and efficacy of chimeric antigen receptor T cell therapy. Protein Cell. 2017;8:573–89. https://doi.org/10.1007/s13238-017-0411-9.

89. Zhao L, Cao YJ. Engineered T cell therapy for cancer in the clinic. Front Immunol. 2019;10:2250. https://doi.org/10.3389/fimmu.2019.02250.

90. Rafiq S, Hackett CS, Brentjens RJ. Engineering strategies to overcome the current roadblocks in CAR T cell therapy. Nat Rev Clin Oncol. 2020;17:147–67. https://doi.org/10.1038/s41571-019-0297-y.

91. Tian Y, Li Y, Shao Y, Zhang Y. Gene modification strategies for next-generation CAR T cells against solid cancers. J Hematol Oncol. 2020;13:54. https://doi.org/10.1186/s13045-020-00890-6.

92. Fung MKL, Chan GCF. Drug-induced amino acid deprivation as strategy for cancer therapy. J Hematol Oncol. 2017;10:144. https://doi.org/10.1186/s13045-017-0509-9.

93. Palmer AC, Sorger PK. Combination cancer therapy can confer benefit via patient-to-patient variability without drug additivity or synergy. Cell. 2017;171(7):1678–91. https://doi.org/10.1016/j.cell.2017.11.009.

94. Cajal SR, Sesé M, Capdevila C, Aasen T, Mattos-Arruda LD, Diaz-Cano SJ, Hernández-Losa J, Castellví J. Clinical implications of intratumor heterogeneity: challenges and opportunities. J Mol Med. 2020;98:161–77. https://doi.org/10.1007/s00109-020-01874-2.

95. Huang A, Yang XR, Chung WY, Dennison AR, Zhou J. Targeted therapy for hepatocellular carcinoma. Signal Transduct Target Ther. 2020;5:146. https://doi.org/10.1038/s41392-020-00264-x.

96. Baba AI, Câtoi C. Principles of anticancer therapy. In: Comparative oncology. Bucharest: The Publishing House of the Romanian Academy; 2007.

97. Anderson RL, Balasas T, Callaghan J, Coombes RC, Evans J, Hall JA, Kinrade S, Jones D, Jones PS, Jones R, Marshall JF, Panico MB, Shaw JA, Steeg PS, Sullivan M, Tong W, Westwell AD, Ritchie JWA. A framework for the development of effective anti-metastatic agents. Nat Rev Clin Oncol. 2019;16:185–204. https://doi.org/10.1038/s41571-018-0134-8.

98. Delou JMA, Souza ASO, Souza LCM, Borges HL. Highlights in resistance mechanism pathways for combination therapy. Cell. 2019;8(9):1013. https://doi.org/10.3390/cells8091013.

99. Henke E, Nandigama R, Ergun S. Extracellular matrix in the tumor microenvironment and its impact on cancer therapy. Front Mol Biosci. 2020;6:160. https://doi.org/10.3389/fmolb.2019.00160.

100. Hu Q, Sun W, Wang C, Gu Z. Recent advances of cocktail chemotherapy by combination drug delivery systems. Adv Drug Deliv Rev. 2016;98:19–34. https://doi.org/10.1016/j.addr.2015.10.022.

101. Malyutina A, Majumder MM, Wang W, Pessia A, Hecjman CA, Tang J. Drug combination sensitivity scoring facilitates the discovery of synergistic and efficacious drug combinations in cancer. PLoS Comput Biol. 2019;15(5):e1006752. https://doi.org/10.1371/journal.pcbi.1006752.

102. Levitzki A, Klein S. My journey from tyrosine phosphorylation inhibitors to targeted immune therapy as strategies to combat cancer. Proc Natl Acad Sci. 2019;116(24):11579–86. https://doi.org/10.1073/pnas.1816012116.

103. Conte FM, Sgnaolin V, Sgnaolin V. Neutropenia associated with the treatment of breast cancer: integrative literature review. Rev Bras Cancerol. 2019;65(3):11307. https://doi.org/10.32635/2176-9745.RBC.2019v65n3.307.

104. Fisusi FA, Akala EO. Drug combinations in breast cancer therapy. Pharm Nanotechnol. 2019;7(3):3–23. https://doi.org/10.2174/2211738507666190122111224.

105. Bonadonna G, Brusamolino E, Valagussa P, Rossi A, Brugnatelli L, Brambilla C, De Lena M, Tancini G, Bajetta E, Musumeci R, Veronesi U. Combination chemotherapy as an adjuvant treatment in operable breast cancer. N Engl J Med. 1976;294(8):405–10. https://doi.org/10.1056/NEJM197602192940801.

106. Chan S, Romieu G, Huober J, Delozier T, Tubiana-Hulin M, Schneeweiss A, Lluch A, Llmbart A, Bois A, Kreienberg R, Mayordomo JI, Antón A, Harrison M, Jones A, Carrasco E, Vaury AT, Frimodt-Moller B, Fumoleau P. Phase III study of gemcitabine plus docetaxel compared with capecitabine plus docetaxel for anthracycline-pretreated patients with metastatic breast cancer. J Clin Oncol. 2009;27(11):1753–60. https://doi.org/10.1200/JCO.2007.15.8485.

107. Marty M, Cognetti F, Maraninchi D, Snyder R, Mauriac L, Tubiana-Hulin M, Chan S, Grimes D, Antón A, Lluch A, Kennedy J, O'Byrne K, Conte P, Green M, Ward C, Mayne K, Extra JM. Randomized phase II trial of the efficacy and safety of trastuzumab combined with docetaxel in patients with human epidermal growth factor receptor 2-positive metastatic breast cancer administered as first-line treatment: the M77001 study group. J Clin Oncol. 2005;23(19):4265–74. https://doi.org/10.1200/JCO.2005.04.173.

108. Li H, Shao B, Yan Y, Guohong C, Liu X, Wang J, Liang X. Efficacy and safety of trastuzumab combined with chemotherapy for first-line treatment and beyond progression of HER2-overexpressing advanced breast cancer. Chin J Cancer Res. 2016;28(3):330–8. https://doi.org/10.21147/j.issn.1000-9604.2016 03.07.

109. Martin M, Ramos-Medina R, Bernat R, García-Saenz JÁ, Monte-Millan M, Alvarez E, Cebollero M, Moreno F, Gonzalez-Haba E, Bueno O, Romero P, Massarrah T, Echavarria I, Jerez Y, Herrero B, Rincon P, Palomero MI, Marquez-Rodas I, Lizarraga S, Asensio F, Lopez-Tarruella S. Activity of docetaxel, carboplatin, and doxorubicin in patient-derived triple-negative breast cancer xenografts. Sci Rep. 2021;11:7064. https://doi.org/10.1038/s41598-021-85962-4.

110. Grem JL, Quinn MG, Keith B, Monahan BP, Hamilton JM, Xu Y, Harold N, Nguyen D, Takimoto CH, Rowedder A, Pang J, Morrison G, Chen A. A phase I and pharmacologic study of weekly gemcitabine in combination with infusional 5-fluorodeoxyuridine and oral calcium leucovorin. Chem Fac Publ. 2003;167:487–96. https://doi.org/10.1007/s00280-003-0698-5.

111. Chiti F, Silva FMC, Canelas A, Gonçalves P, Gomes JM. Phase II study of oral vinorelbine plus hormone therapy in hormone-refractory prostate cancer. J Clin Oncol. 2008;26(15):16075. https://doi.org/10.1200/jco.2008.26.15_suppl.16075.

112. Reni M, Passoni P, Panucci MG, Nicoletti R, Galli L, Balzano G, Zerbi A, Di Carlo V, Villa E. Definitive results of a phase II trial of cisplatin, epirubicin, continuous-infusion fluorouracil, and gemcitabine in stage IV pancreatic adenocarcinoma. J Clin Oncol. 2016;19(10):2679–86. https://doi.org/10.1200/JCO.2001.19.10.2679.

113. Braun EM, Kikot VA, Ugrinov OG, Lishchishina EM. Neoadjuvant intra-arterial polychemotherapy of locally advanced rectal cancer. Eur J Surg Oncol. 1997;23(3):P228–32. https://doi.org/10.1016/S0748-7983(97)92412-4.

114. LoRusso PM, Canetta R, Wagner JÁ, Balogh EP, Nass SJ, Boerner SA, Hohneker J. Accelerating cancer therapy development: the importance of combination strategies and collaboration. Summary of an institute of medicine workshop. Clin Cancer Res. 2012;18(22):6101–9. https://doi.org/10.1158/1078-0432.CCR-12-2455.

115. Lopez JS, Banerji U. Combine and conquer: challenges for targeted therapy combinations in early phase trials. Nat Rev Clin Oncol. 2017;14(1):57–66. https://doi.org/10.1038/nrclinonc.2016.96.

116. Latimer NR, Pollard D, Towse A, Henshall C, Sansom L, Ward RL, Bruce A, Deakin C. Challenges in valuing and paying for combination regimens in oncology: reporting

the perspectives of a multi-stakeholder, international workshop. BMC Health Serv Res. 2021;21:412. https://doi.org/10.1186/s12913-021-06425-0.

117. Shalom-Sharabi I, Lavie O, Samuels N, Keinan-Boker L, Lev E, Ben-Arye E. Can complementary medicine increase adherence to chemotherapy dosing protocol? A controlled study in an integrative oncology setting. J Cancer Res Clin Oncol. 2017;143(12):2535–43. https://doi.org/10.1007/s00432-017-2509-0.

118. Fumet JD, Vincent J, Bengrine L, Hennequin A, Granconato L, Palmier R, Ghiringhelli F. Safety and efficacy of gemcitabine, docetaxel, capecitabine, cisplatin as second-line therapy for advanced pancreatic cancer after FOLFIRINOX. Anticancer Res. 2020;40(7):4011–5. https://doi.org/10.21873/anticanres.14395.

119. Schlick K, Magnes T, Ratzinger L, Jaud B, Weiss L, Melchardt T, Greil R, Egle A. Novel models for prediction of benefit and toxicity with FOLFIRINOX treatment of pancreatic cancer using clinically available parameters. PLoS One. 2018;13(11):e0206688. https://doi.org/10.1371/journal.pone.0206688.

120. Falcetta F, Bizzaro F, D'Agostini E, Bani MR, Giavazzi R, Ubezio P. Modeling cytostatic and cytotoxic responses to new treatment regimens for ovarian cancer. Cancer Res. 2017;77(23):6759–69. https://doi.org/10.1158/0008-5472.CAN-17-1099.

121. Senkova AV, Mironova NL, Patutina AO, Ageeva TA, Zenkova MA. The toxic effects of polychemotherapy onto the liver are accelerated by the upregulated MDR of lymphosarcoma. Int Sch Res Not. 2012;2012:721612. https://doi.org/10.5402/2012/721612.

122. Cameron AC, Touyz RM, Lang NN. Vascular complications of cancer chemotherapy. Can J Cardiol. 2016;32(7):852–62. https://doi.org/10.1016/j.cjca.2015.12.023.

123. Huang CY, Ju DT, Chang CF, Reddy PM, Velmurugan BK. A review on the effects of current chemotherapy drugs and natural agents in treating non-small cell lung cancer. Biomedicine. 2017;7(4):23. https://doi.org/10.1051/bmdcn/2017070423.

124. Wang X, Zhang H, Chen X. Drug resistance and combating drug resistance in cancer. Cancer Drug Resist. 2019;2:141–60. https://doi.org/10.20517/cdr.2019.10.

125. Torrisi JM, Schwartz LH, Gollub MJ, Ginsberg MS, Bosl GJ, Hrick H. CT findings of chemotherapy-induced toxicity: what radiologists need to know about the clinical and radiologic manifestations of chemotherapy toxicity. Radiology. 2011;258(1):41–56.

126. Adão R, Keulenaer G, Leite-Moreira A, Brás-Silva C. Cardiotoxicity associated with cancer therapy: pathophysiology and prevention. Rev Port Cardiol. 2013;32(5):395–409. https://doi.org/10.1016/j.repce.2012.11.019.

127. Barbosa RR, Bourguignon TB, Torres LD, Arruda LS, Jacques TM, Serpa RG, Calil AO, Barbosa LFM. Anthracycline-associated cardiotoxicity in adults: systematic review on the cardioprotective role of beta-blockers. Rev Assoc Med Bras. 2018;64(8):745–54. https://doi.org/10.1590/1806-9282.64.08.745.

128. Cai F, Luis MAF, Lin X, Wang M, Cai L, Cen C, Biskup E. Anthracycline-induced cardiotoxicity in the chemotherapy treatment of breast cancer: preventive strategies and treatment. Mol Clin Oncol. 2019;11(1):15–23. https://doi.org/10.3892/mco.2019.1854.

129. Sobczuk P, Czerwinska M, Kleibert M, Cudnoch-Jedrzejewska A. Anthracycline-induced cardiotoxicity and renin-angiotensin-aldosterone system-from molecular mechanisms to therapeutic applications. Heart Fail Rev. 2020;27(1):295–319. https://doi.org/10.1007/s10741-020-09977-1.

130. Tannapfel A, Reinacher-Schick A. Chemotherapy associated hepatotoxicity in the treatment of advanced colorectal cancer (CRC). Z Gastroenterol. 2008;46(5):435–40. https://doi.org/10.1055/s-2008-1027151.

131. Cavalcanti IDL, Costa DT, Silva ATA, Peres AL, Coimbra CGO. Importance of pharmacist in oxaliplatin hepatotoxicity associated with inadequate nutritional diet: case report. Curr Nutr Food Sci. 2020;16(5):839–44. https://doi.org/10.2174/1573401316666200120110632.

132. Gangi A, Lu SC. Chemotherapy-associated liver injury in colorectal cancer. Ther Adv Gastroenterol. 2020;13:1756284820924194. https://doi.org/10.1177/1756284820924194.

133. Perse M, Veceric-Haler Z. Cisplatin-induced rodent model of kidney injury: characteristics and challenges. Biomed Res Int. 2018;2018:1462802. https://doi.org/10.1155/2018/1462802.

134. Santos MLC, Brito BB, Silva FAF, Botelho ACS, Melo FF. Nephrotoxicity in cancer treatment: an overview. World J Clin Oncol. 2020;11(4):190–204. https://doi.org/10.5306/wjco.v11.i4.190.

135. Miyoshi T, Uoi M, Omura F, Tsumagari K, Maesaki S, Yokota C. Induced nephrotoxicity: a multicenter retrospective study. Oncology. 2021;99:105–13. https://doi.org/10.1159/000510384.

136. Unek IT, Akman T, Oztop I, Unal OU, Salman T, Yilmaz U. Bimonthly regimen of high-dose leucovorin, infusional 5-fluorouracil, docetaxel, and cisplatin (modified DCF) in advanced gastric adenocarcinoma. Gastric Cancer. 2013;16(3):428–34. https://doi.org/10.1007/s10120-012-0206-x.

137. Xu N, Shen P, Zhang XC, Yu LF, Bao HY, Shi GM, Huang S, Chen J, Mou HB, Fang WJ. Phase II trial of a 2-h infusion of gemcitabine plus carboplatin as first-line chemotherapy for advanced non-small-cell lung cancer. Cancer Chemother Pharmacol. 2007;59(1):1–7. https://doi.org/10.1007/s00280-006-0237-2.

138. Paula DP, Costa VIB, Jorge RV, Nobre FF. Impact of protocol change on individual factors related to course of adverse reactions to chemotherapy for breast cancer. Support Care Cancer. 2020;28(1):395–403. https://doi.org/10.1007/s00520-019-04841-x.

139. Azim HA, Azambuja E, Colozza M, Bines J, Piccart MJ. Long-term toxic effects of adjuvant chemotherapy in breast cancer. Ann Oncol. 2011;22(9):1939–47. https://doi.org/10.1093/annonc/mdq683.

140. Volkova M, Russel R. Anthracycline cardiotoxicity: prevalence, pathogenesis and treatment. Curr Cardiol Rev. 2011;7(4):214–20. https://doi.org/10.2174/157340311799960645.

141. Peroukides S, Alexopoulos A, Kalofonos H, Papadaki H. Cardiovascular effects of treatment with taxanes. J Cardiovasc Med. 2012;13(5):319–24. https://doi.org/10.2459/JCM.0b013e3283529060.

142. Florescu M, Mihalcea D, Enescu AO, Radu E, Chirca A, Acasandrei AM, Magda LS, Rimbas RC, Cirstoiu C, Vinereanu D. Eur Heart J. 2011;34(1):541. https://doi.org/10.1093/eurheartj/eht309.P3006.

143. Gianni L, Salvatorelli E, Minotti G. Anthracycline cardiotoxicity in breast cancer patients: synergism with trastuzumab and taxanes. Cardiovasc Toxicol. 2007;7:67–71. https://doi.org/10.1007/s12012-007-0013-5.

144. Baker AF, Dorr RT. Drug interactions with the taxanes: clinical implications. Cancer Treat Rev. 2001;27(4):221–33. https://doi.org/10.1053/ctrv.2001.0228.

145. Esposito M, Venturini M, Vannozzi MO, Tolino G, Lunardi G, Garrone O, Angiolini C, Viale M, Bergaglio M, Del Mastro L, Rosso R. Comparative effects of paclitaxel and docetaxel on the metabolism and pharmacokinetics of epirubicin in breast cancer patients. J Clin Oncol. 1999;17(4):1132. https://doi.org/10.1200/JCO.1999.17.4.1132.

146. Venturini M, Lunardi G, Del Mastro L, Vannozzi MO, Tolino G, Numico G, Viale M, Pastrone I, Angiolini C, Bertelli G, Straneo M, Rosso R, Eposito M. Sequence effect of epirubicin and paclitaxel treatment on pharmacokinetics and toxicity. J Clin Oncol. 2000;18(10):2116–25. https://doi.org/10.1200/JCO.2000.18.10.2116.

147. Dang CT, D'Andrea GM, Moynahan ME, Dickler MN, Seidman AD, Fornier M, Robson ME, Theodoulou M, Lake D, Currie VE, Hurria A, Panageas KS, Norton L, Hudis CA. Phase II study of feasibility of dose-dense FEC followed by alternating weekly taxanes in high-risk, four or more node-positive breast cancer. Clin Cancer Res. 2004;10(17):5754–61. https://doi.org/10.1158/1078-0432.CCR-04-0634.

148. Vahid B, Marik PE. Pulmonary complications of novel antineoplastic agents for solid tumors. Chest J. 2008;133(2):528–38. https://doi.org/10.1378/chest.07-0851.

149. Kennedy MJ, Zahurak ML, Donehower RC, Noe DA, Sartorius S, Chen TL, Bowling K, Rowinsky EK. Phase I and pharmacologic study of sequences of paclitaxel and cyclophosphamide supported by granulocyte colony-stimulating factor in women with previously

treated metastatic breast cancer. J Clin Oncol. 1996;14(3):783–91. https://doi.org/10.1200/JCO.1996.14.3.783.
150. Tolcher AW, Cowan KH, Noone MH, Denicoff AM, Kohler DR, Goldspiel BR, Barnes CS, McCabe M, Gossard MR, Zujewski J, O'Shaughnessy JA. Phase I study of paclitaxel in combination with cyclophosphamide and granulocyte colony-stimulating factor in metastatic breast cancer patients. J Clin Oncol. 1996;14(1):95–102. https://doi.org/10.1200/JCO.1996.14.1.95.
151. Petrelli F, Borgonovo K, Cabiddu M, Lonati V, Barni S. Mortality, leukemic risk, and cardiovascular toxicity of adjuvant anthracycline and taxane chemotherapy in breast cancer: a meta-analysis. Breast Cancer Res Treat. 2012;135:335–46. https://doi.org/10.1007/s10549-012-2121-6.
152. Paul DM, Garrett AM, Meshad M, DeVore RD, Porter LL, Johnson DH. Paclitaxel and 5-fluorouracil in metastatic breast cancer: the US experience. Semin Oncol. 1996;23(1):48–52.
153. Nicholson BP, Paul DM, Hande KR, Shyr Y, Meshad M, Cohen A, Johnson DH. Paclitaxel, 5-fluorouracil, and leucovorin (TFL) in the treatment of metastatic breast cancer. Clin Breast Cancer. 2000;1(2):136–43. https://doi.org/10.3816/CBC.2000.n.012.
154. Loesch DM, Asmar L, Canfield VA, Parker GA, Hynes HE, Ellis PG, Ferri WA Jr, Robert NJ. A phase II trial of weekly paclitaxel, 5fluorouracil, and leucovorin as first-line treatment for metastatic breast cancer. Breast Cancer Res Treat. 2003;77:115–23.
155. Berruti A, Bitossi R, Gorzegno G, Bottini A, Generali D, Milani M, Katsaros D, Rigault de la Longrais IA, Bellino R, Donadio M, Ardine M, Bertetto O, Danese S, Sarobba MG, Farris A, Lorusso V, Dogliotti L. Paclitaxel, vinorelbine and 5-fluorouracil in breast câncer patients pretreated with adjuvant anthracyclines. Br J Cancer. 2005;92:634–8.
156. Steward WP, Dunlop DJ. New drugs in the treatment of non-small cell lung cancer. Ann Oncol. 1995;6(1):49–54.
157. Cherif H, Bacha S, Habibech S, Racil H, Cheikhrouhou S, Chaouech N, Chabbou A, Megdiche ML. Chemotherapy toxicity in advanced non-small cell lung cancer and its impact on survival. Eur Respir J. 2016;48:4841. https://doi.org/10.1183/13993003.congress-2016.PA4841.
158. Lee SH. Chemotherapy for lung cancer in the era of personalized medicine. Tuberc Respir Dis. 2019;82(3):179–89. https://doi.org/10.4046/trd.2018.0068.
159. Fan Y, Lin NM, Ma SL, Luo LH, Fang L, Huang ZY, Yu HF, Wu FQ. Phase II trial of gemcitabine plus cisplatin in patients with advanced non-small cell lung cancer. Acta Pharmacol Sin. 2010;31:746–52. https://doi.org/10.1038/aps.2010.50.
160. Ryu JH. Chemotherapy-induced pulmonary toxicity in lung cancer patients. J Thorac Oncol. 2010;5(9):1313–4. https://doi.org/10.1097/JTO.0b013e3181e9dbb9.
161. Niho S, Kubota K, Goto K, Yoh K, Ohmatsu H, Kakinuma R, Saijo N, Nishiwaki Y. First-line single agent treatment with gefitinib in patients with advanced non-small-cell lung cancer: a phase II study. J Clin Oncol. 2006;24(1):64–9. https://doi.org/10.1200/JCO.2005.02.5825.
162. Liu V, White DA, Zakowski MF, Travis W, Kris MG, Ginsberg MS, Miller VA, Azzoli CG. Pulmonary toxicity associated with erlotinib. Chest J. 2007;132(3):1042–4. https://doi.org/10.1378/chest.07-0050.
163. Chen YM, Shih JF, Lee CS, Chen MC, Lin WC, Tsai CM, Perng RP. Phase II study of docetaxel and ifosfamide combination chemotherapy in non-small-cell lung cancer patients failing previous chemotherapy with or without paclitaxel. Lung Cancer. 2003;39(2):209–14. https://doi.org/10.1016/s0169-5002(02)00445-2.
164. Skubitz KM, Skubitz AP. Mechanism of transient dyspnea induced by pegylated-liposomal doxorubicin (Doxil). Anti-Cancer Drugs. 1998;9(1):45–50. https://doi.org/10.1097/00001813-199801000-00005.
165. Pavlakis N, Bell DR, Millward MJ, Levi JA. Fatal pulmonary toxicity resulting from treatment with gemcitabine. Cancer. 1997;80(2):286–91.
166. Marruchella A, Fiorenzano G, Merizzi A, Rossi G, Chiodera PL. Diffuse alveolar damage in a patient treated with gemcitabine. Eur Respir J. 1998;11(2):504–6. https://doi.org/10.1183/09031936.98.11020504.

167. Roychowdhury DF, Cassidy CA, Peterson P, Arning M. A report on serious pulmonary toxicity associated with gemcitabine-based therapy. Investig New Drugs. 2002;20(3):311–5. https://doi.org/10.1023/a:1016214032272.
168. Barlési F, Villani P, Doddoli C, Gimenez C, Kleisbauer JP. Gemcitabine-induced severe pulmonar toxicity. Fundam Clin Pharmacol. 2004;18(1):85–91. https://doi.org/10.1046/j.0767-3981.2003.00206.x.
169. Saravanan V, Kelly CA. Reducing the risk of methotrexate pneumonitis in rheumatoid arthritis. Rheumatology. 2004;43(2):143–7. https://doi.org/10.1093/rheumatology/keg466.
170. Zimmerman MS, Ruckdeschel JC, Hussain M. Chemotherapy-induced interstitial pneumonitis during treatment of small cell anaplastic lung cancer. J Clin Oncol. 1984;2(5):396–405. https://doi.org/10.1200/JCO.1984.2.5.396.
171. Dajczman E, Srolovitz H, Kreisman H, Frank H. Fatal pulmonary toxicity following oral etoposide therapy. Lung Cancer. 1995;12(1):81–6. https://doi.org/10.1016/0169-5002(94)00410-o.
172. Gurjal A, An T, Valdivieso M, Kalemkerian GP. Etoposide-induced pulmonary toxicity. Lung Cancer. 1999;26(2):109–12. https://doi.org/10.1016/s0169-5002(99)00081-1.
173. Siderov J, Prasad P, De Boer R, Desai J. Safe administration of etoposide phosphate after hypersensitivity reaction to intravenous etoposide. Br J Cancer. 2002;86(1):12–3. https://doi.org/10.1038/sj.bjc.6600003.
174. Toschi L, Finocchiaro G, Bartolini S, Gioia V, Cappuzzo F. Role of gemcitabine in cancer therapy. Future Oncol. 2005;1(1):7–17. https://doi.org/10.1517/14796694.1.1.7.
175. Ciccolini J, Serdjebi C, Peters GJ, Giovanneti E. Pharmacokinetics and pharmacogenetics of Gemcitabine as a mainstay in adult and pediatric oncology: an EORTC-PAMM perspective. Cancer Chemother Pharmacol. 2016;78:1–12. https://doi.org/10.1007/s00280-016-3003-0.
176. Mohelnikova-Duchonova B, Melichar B, Soucek P. FOLFOX/FOLFIRI pharmacogenetics: the call for a personalized approach in colorectal cancer therapy. World J Gastroenterol. 2014;20(30):10316–30. https://doi.org/10.3748/wjg.v20.i30.10316.
177. Xie YH, Chen YX, Fang JY. Comprehensive review of targeted therapy for colorectal cancer. Signal Transduct Target Ther. 2020;5:22. https://doi.org/10.1038/s41392-020-0116-z.
178. Eng C. Toxic effects and their management: daily clinical challenges in the treatment of colorectal cancer. Nat Rev Clin Oncol. 2009;6:207–18. https://doi.org/10.1038/nrclinonc.2009.16.
179. Tong L, Ahn C, Symanski E, Lai D, Du XL. Effects of newly developed chemotherapy regimens, comorbidities, chemotherapy-related toxicities on the changing patterns of the leading causes of death in elderly patients with colorectal cancer. Ann Oncol. 2014;25(6):1234–42. https://doi.org/10.1093/annonc/mdu131.
180. Aoullay Z, Slaoui M, Razine R, Er-Raki A, Meddah B, Cherrah Y. Therapeutic characteristics, chemotherapy-related toxicities and survivorship in colorectal cancer patients. Ethiop J Health Sci. 2020;30(1):65–74. https://doi.org/10.4314/ejhs.v30i1.9.
181. Grivicich I, Mans DRA, Peters GJ, Schwartsmann G. Irinotecan and oxaliplatin: an overview of the novel chemotherapeutic options for the treatment of advanced colorectal cancer. Braz J Med Biol Res. 2001;34(9):1087–103. https://doi.org/10.1590/S0100-879X2001000900001.
182. Braun MS, Seymour MT. Balancing the efficacy and toxicity of chemotherapy in colorectal cancer. Therap Adv Med Oncol. 2011;3(1):43–52. https://doi.org/10.1177/1758834010388342.
183. Cunningham D, Pyrhonen S, James RD, Punt CJ, Hickish TF, Heikkila R, Johannesen TB, Starkhammar H, Topham CA, Awad L, Jacques C, Herait P. Randomised trial of irinotecan plus supportive care versus supportive care alone after fluorouracil failure for patients with metastatic colorectal cancer. Lancet. 1998;352(9138):1413–8. https://doi.org/10.1016/S0140-6736(98)02309-5.
184. Ledermann JA, Leonard P, Seymour M. Recommendation for caution with irinotecan fluorouracil, and leucovorin for colorectal cancer. N Engl J Med. 2001;345(2):145–6.
185. Sargent DJ, Niedzwiecki D, O'Connell MJ, Schilsky RL. Recommendation for caution with irinotecan, fluorouracil, and leucovorin for colorectal cancer. N Engl J Med. 2001;345(2):144–5. https://doi.org/10.1056/NEJM200107123450213.

186. Goldberg RM, Sargent DJ, Morton RF, Fuchs CS, Ramanathan RK, Williamson SK, Findlay BP, Pitot HC, Alberts SR. A randomized controlled trial of fluorouracil plus leucovorin, irinotecan, and oxaliplatin combinations in patients with previously untreated metastatic colorectal cancer. J Clin Oncol. 2004;22(1):23–30. https://doi.org/10.1200/JCO.2004.09.046.

187. Saltz LB, Niedzwiecki D, Hollis D, Goldberg RM, Hantel A, Thomas JP, Fields ALA, Mayer RJ. Irinotecan fluorouracil plus leucovorin is not superior to fluorouracil plus leucovorin alone as adjuvant treatment for stage III colon cancer: results of CALGB 89803. J Clin Oncol. 2007;25(23):3456–61. https://doi.org/10.1200/JCO.2007.11.2144.

188. Grothey A. Clinical management of oxaliplatin-associated neurotoxicity. Clin Colorectal Cancer. 2005;5(1):38–46. https://doi.org/10.3816/ccc.2005.s.006.

189. Gramont A, Figer A, Seymour M, Homerin M, Hmissi A, Cassidy J, Boni C, Cortes-Funes H, Cervantes A, Freyer G, Papamichael D, Le Bail N, Louvet C, Hendler D, Braud F, Wilson C, Morvan F, Bonetti A. Leucovorin and fluorouracil with or without oxaliplatin as first-line treatment in advanced colorectal cancer. J Clin Oncol. 2000;18(16):2938–47. https://doi.org/10.1200/JCO.2000.18.16.2938.

190. Cassidy J, Twelves C, Van Cutsem E, Hoff P, Bajetta E, Boyer M, Bugat R, Burger U, Garin A, Graeven U, McKendric J, Maroun J, Marshall J, Osterwalder B, Pérez-Manga G, Rosso R, Rougier P, Schilsky RL. First-line oral capecitabine therapy in metastatic colorectal cancer: a favorable safety profile compared with intravenous 5-fluorouracil/leucovorin. Ann Oncol. 2002;13(4):566–75. https://doi.org/10.1093/annonc/mdf089.

191. Tournigand C, André T, Achille E, Lledo G, Flesh M, Mery-Mignard D, Quinaux E, Couteau C, Buyse M, Ganem G, Landi B, Colin P, Louvet C, Gramont A. FOLFIRI followed by FOLFOX6 or the reverse sequence in advanced colorectal cancer: a randomized GERCOR study. J Clin Oncol. 2004;22(2):229–37. https://doi.org/10.1200/JCO.2004.05.113.

192. Eisenberger MA, Simon R, O'Dwyer PJ, Wittes RE, Friedman MA. A reevaluation of non-hormonal cytotoxic chemotherapy in the treatment of prostatic carcinoma. J Clin Oncol. 1985;3(6):827–41. https://doi.org/10.1200/JCO.1985.3.6.827.

193. Beer TM, Bubalo JS. Complications of chemotherapy for prostate cancer. Semin Urol Oncol. 2001;19(3):222–30.

194. Denmeade SR, Isaacs JT. A history of prostate cancer treatment. Nat Rev Cancer. 2002;2(5):389–96. https://doi.org/10.1038/nrc801.

195. Sciarra A, Cardi A, Salvatori G, D'Eramo G, Mariotti G, Silverio FD. Which patients with prostate cancer are actually candidates for hormone therapy? Int Braz J Urol. 2004;30(6):455–65. https://doi.org/10.1590/S1677-55382004000600002.

196. Kaliks RA, Giglio AD. Management of advanced prostate cancer. Rev Assoc Med Bras. 2008;54(2):178–82. https://doi.org/10.1590/S0104-42302008000200025.

197. Behrens RJ, Gulley JL, Dahut WL. Pulmonary toxicity during prostate cancer treatment with docetaxel and thalidomide. Am J Ther. 2003;10(3):228–32. https://doi.org/10.1097/00045391-200305000-00011.

198. Kellokumpu-Lehtinen PL, Hjalm-Eriksson M, Thellenberg-Karlsson C, Astrom L, Franzen L, Marttila T, Seke M, Taalikka M, Ginman C. Toxicity in patients receiving adjuvant docetaxel + hormonal treatment after radical radiotherapy for intermediate or high-risk prostate cancer: a preplanned safety report of the SPCG-13 trial. Prostate Cancer Prostatic Dis. 2012;15:303–7. https://doi.org/10.1038/pcan.2012.13.

199. Terada N, Kamoto T, Tsukino H, Mukai S, Akamatsu S, Inoue T, Ogawa O, Narita S, Habuchi T, Yamashita S, Mitsuzuka K, Arai Y, Kandori S, Kojima T, Nishiyama H, Kawamura Y, Shimizu Y, Terachi T, Sugi M, Kinoshita H, Matsuda T, Yamada Y, Yamamoto S, Hirama H, Sugimoto M, Kakehi Y, Sakurai T, Tsuchiya N. The efficacy and toxicity of cabazitaxel for treatment of docetaxel-resistant prostate cancer correlating with the initial doses in Japanese patients. BMC Cancer. 2019;19:156. https://doi.org/10.1186/s12885-019-5342-9.

200. Scott WW, Johnson DE, Schimidt JE, Gibbons RP, Prout GR, Joiner JR, Saroff J, Murphy GP. Chemotherapy of advanced prostatic carcinoma with cyclophosphamide or

5-fluorouracil: results of first national randomized study. J Urol. 1975;114(6):909–11. https://doi.org/10.1016/s0022-5347(17)67172-6.

201. Tannock IF, Osoba D, Stockler MR, Ernst DS, Neville AJ, Moore MJ, Armitage GR, Wilson JJ, Venner PM, Coppin CM, Murphy KC. Chemotherapy with mitoxantrone plus prednisone or prednisone alone for symptomatic hormone-resistant prostate cancer: a Canadian randomized trial with palliative end points. J Clin Oncol. 1996;14(6):1756–64. https://doi.org/10.1200/JCO.1996.14.6.1756.

202. Hudes GR, Greenberg R, Krigel RL, Fox S, Scher R, Litwin S, Watts P, Speicher L, Tew K, Comis R. Phase II study of estramustine and vinblastine, two microtubule inhibitors, in hormone-refractory prostate cancer. J Clin Oncol. 1992;10(11):1754–61. https://doi.org/10.1200/JCO.1992.10.11.1754.

203. Hudes GR, Nathan F, Khater C, Haas N, Cornfield M, Giantonio B, Greenberg R, Gomella L, Litwin S, Ross E, Roethke S, McAleer C. Phase II trial of 96-hour paclitaxel plus oral estramustine phosphate in metastatic hormone-refractory prostate cancer. J Clin Oncol. 1997;15(9):3156–63. https://doi.org/10.1200/JCO.1997.15.9.3156.

204. Pienta KJ, Redman B, Hussain M, Cummings G, Esper PS, Appel C, Flaherty LE. Phase II evaluation of oral estramustine and oral etoposide in hormone-refractory adenocarcinoma of the prostate. J Clin Oncol. 1994;12(10):2005–12. https://doi.org/10.1200/JCO.1994.12.10.2005.

205. Savarese DM, Halabi S, Hars V, Akerley WL, Taplin ME, Godley PA, Hussain A, Small EJ, Vogelzang NJ. Phase II study of docetaxel, estramustine, and low-dose hydrocortisone in men with hormone-refractory prostate cancer: a final report of CALGB 9780. Cancer and Leukemia Group B. J Clin Oncol. 2001;19(9):2509–16. https://doi.org/10.1200/JCO.2001.19.9.2509.

206. Sella A, Kilbourn R, Amato R, Bui C, Zukiwski AA, Ellerhorst J, Logothetis CJ. Phase II study of ketoconazole combined with weekly doxorubicin in patients with androgen-independent prostate cancer. J Clin Oncol. 1994;12(4):683–8. https://doi.org/10.1200/JCO.1994.12.4.683.

207. Jones B. Toxicity after cervical cancer treatment using radiotherapy and chemotherapy. Clin Oncol J. 2009;21(1):56–63. https://doi.org/10.1016/j.clon.2008.10.009.

208. Zuliani AC, Cunha MO, Esteves SCB, Teixeira JC. Brachytherapy for stage IIIB squamous cell carcinoma of the uterine cervix: survival and toxicity. Rev Assoc Med Bras. 2010;56(1):37–40. https://doi.org/10.1590/S0104-42302010000100013.

209. Chen HHW, Kuo MT. Improving radiotherapy in cancer treatment: promises and challenges. Oncotarget. 2017;8(37):62742–58. https://doi.org/10.18632/oncotarget.18409.

210. Fu ZZ, Li K, Peng Y, Zheng Y, Cao LY, Zhang YJ, Sun YM. Efficacy and toxicity of different concurrent chemoradiotherapy regimens in the treatment of advanced cervical cancer: a network meta-analysis. Medicine. 2017;96(2):e5853. https://doi.org/10.1097/MD.0000000000005853.

211. Dasari S, Tchounwou PB. Cisplatin in cancer therapy: molecular mechanisms of action. Eur J Pharmacol. 2014;740:364–78. https://doi.org/10.1016/j.ejphar.2014.07.025.

212. Ghosh S. Cisplatin: the first metal based anticancer drug. Bioorg Chem. 2019;88:102925. https://doi.org/10.1016/j.bioorg.2019.102925.

213. Tan LT, Zahra M. Long-term survival and late toxicity after chemoradiotherapy for cervical cancer – the Addenbrooke's experience. Clin Oncol. 2008;20(5):358–64. https://doi.org/10.1016/j.clon.2008.03.001.

214. Tan LT, Russell S, Burgess L. Acute toxicity of chemo-radiotherapy for cervical cancer: the Addenbrooke's experience. Clin Oncol J. 2004;16(4):255–60. https://doi.org/10.1016/j.clon.2003.12.004.

215. Coronel JA, Cetina LC, Cantú D, Cerezo O, Hernández CS, Rivera L, Chacón AP, Duenas-Gonzalez A. A randomized comparison of cisplatin and oral vinorelbine as radiosensitizers in aged or comorbid locally advanced cervical cancer patients. Int J Gynecol Cancer. 2013;23(5):884–9. https://doi.org/10.1097/IGC.0b013e3182915c69.

216. Wang CC, Chou HH, Yang LY, Lin H, Liou WS, Tseng CW, Liu FY, Liou JD, Huang KG, Huang HJ, Huang EY, Chen CH, Chang TC, Chang CJ, Hong JH, Lai CH. A randomized trial comparing concurrent chemoradiotherapy with single-agent cisplatin versus cisplatin plus gemcitabine in patients with advanced cervical cancer: An Asian Gynecologic Oncology Group study. Gynecol Oncol. 2015;137(3):462–7. https://doi.org/10.1016/j.ygyno.2015.03.046.
217. Kong TW, Chang SJ, Paek J, Yoo SC, Yoon JH, Chang KH, Chun M, Ryu HS. Comparison of concurrent chemoradiation therapy with weekly cisplatin versus monthly fluorouracil plus cisplatin in FIGO stage IIB-IVA cervical cancer. J Gynecol Oncol. 2012;23(4):235–41. https://doi.org/10.3802/jgo.2012.23.4.235.
218. Araújo DFB, Cavalcanti IDL, Larrazabal-Hadj-Idris BR, Peres AL. Hematological and biochemical toxicity analysis of chemotherapy in women diagnosed with cervical cancer. J Bras Patol Med Lab. 2020;56:1–6. https://doi.org/10.5935/1676-2444.20200038.
219. Cognetti DM, Weber RS, Lai SY. Head and neck cancer: an evolving treatment paradigm. Cancer. 2008;113(7):1911–32. https://doi.org/10.1002/cncr.23654.
220. Yeh SA. Radiotherapy for head and neck cancer. Semin Plast Surg. 2010;24(2):127–36. https://doi.org/10.1055/s-0030-1255330.
221. Trotti A. Toxicity in head and neck cancer: a review of trends and issues. Int J Radiat Oncol Biol Phys. 2000;47(1):1–12. https://doi.org/10.1016/s0360-3016(99)00558-1.
222. Biswal BM. Current trends in the management of oral mucositis related to cancer treatment. Malays J Med Sci. 2008;15(3):4–13.
223. Corrêa DS, Oliveira TFL, Santos PSS. Management of oral adverse effects related to cetuximab plus radiotherapy. J Oral Diagn. 2017;2:e20170003. https://doi.org/10.5935/2525-5711.20170003.
224. Hu MH, Wang LW, Lu HJ, Chu PY, Tai SK, Lee TL, Chen MH, Yang MH, Chang PMH. Cisplatin-based chemotherapy versus cetuximab in concurrent chemoradiotherapy for locally advanced head and neck cancer treatment. Biomed Res Int. 2014;2014:904341. https://doi.org/10.1155/2014/904341.
225. Albers AE, Grabow R, Qian X, Jumah MD, Holfmann VM, Krannich A, Pecher G. Efficacy and toxicity of docetaxel combination chemotherapy for advanced squamous cell cancer of the head and neck. Mol Clin Oncol. 2017;7(1):151–7. https://doi.org/10.3892/mco.2017.1281.
226. Posner MR, Hershock DM, Blajman CR, Mickiewicz E, Winquist E, Gorbounova V, Tjulandin S, Shin DM, Cullen K, Ervin TJ, Murphy BA, Raez LE, Cohen RB, Spaulding M, Tishler RB, Roth B, Viroglio RC, Venkatesan V, Romanov I, Agarwala S, Harter KW, Dugan M, Cmelak A, Markoe AM, Read PW, Read PW, Steinbrenner L, Colevas AD, Norris CM, Haddad RI. Cisplatin and fluorouracil alone or with docetaxel in head and neck cancer. N Engl J Med. 2007;357(17):1705–15. https://doi.org/10.1056/NEJMoa070956.
227. Vermorken JB, Remenar E, van Herpen C, Gorlia T, Mesia R, Degardin M, Stewart JS, Jelic S, Betka J, Preiss JH, van den Weyngaert D, Awada A, Cupissol D, Kienzer HR, Rey A, Desaunois I, Bernier J, Lefebvre JL. Cisplatin, fluorouracil, and docetaxel in unresectable head and neck cancer. N Engl J Med. 2007;357(17):1695–704. https://doi.org/10.1056/NEJMoa071028.
228. Qian X, Ma C, Hoffmann TK, Kaufmann AM, Albers AE. Taxane-cisplatin-fluorouracil as induction chemotherapy for advanced head and neck cancer: a meta-analysis of the 5-year efficacy and safety. Springerplus. 2015;4:208. https://doi.org/10.1186/s40064-015-0988-5.
229. Hodgson DC. Long-term toxicity of chemotherapy and radiotherapy in lymphoma survivors: optimizing treatment for individual patients. Clin Adv Hematol Oncol. 2015;13(2):103–12.
230. Shanbhag S, Ambinder R. Hodgkin lymphoma: a review and update on recent progress. CA Cancer J Clin. 2018;68(2):116–32. https://doi.org/10.3322/caac.21438.
231. Limat S, Daguindau E, Cahn JY, Nerich V, Brion A, Perrin S, Woronoff-Lemsi MC, Deconinck E. Incidence and risk-factors of CHOP/R-CHOP-related cardiotoxicity in patients with aggressive non-Hodgkin's lymphoma. J Clin Pharm Ther. 2014;39(2):168–74. https://doi.org/10.1111/jcpt.12124.

232. Swerdlow AJ, Higgins CD, Smith P, Cunningham D, Hancock BW, Horwich A, Hoskin PJ, Lister A, Radford JA, Rohatiner AZS, Linch DC. Myocardial infarction mortality risk after treatment for Hodgkin disease: a collaborative British cohort study. J Natl Cancer Inst. 2007;99(3):206–14. https://doi.org/10.1093/jnci/djk029.
233. Hershman DL, McBride RB, Eisenberger A, Tsai WY, Grann VR, Jacobson JS. Doxorubicin, cardiac risk factors, and cardiac toxicity in elderly patients with diffuse B-cell non-Hodgkin's lymphoma. J Clin Oncol. 2008;26(19):3159–65. https://doi.org/10.1200/JCO.2007.14.1242.
234. Herbrecht R, Cernohous P, Engert A, Le Gouill S, Macdonald D, Machida C, Myint H, Saleh A, Singer J, Wilhelm M, van der Jagt R. Comparison of pixantrone-based regimen (CPOP-R) with doxorubicin-based therapy (CHOP-R) for treatment of diffuse large B-cell lymphoma. Ann Oncol. 2013;24(10):2618–23. https://doi.org/10.1093/annonc/mdt289.
235. Swerdlow AJ, Schoemaker MJ, Allerton R, Horwich A, Barber JA, Cunningham D, Lister TA, Rohatiner AZ, Vaughan Hudson G, Williams MV, Linch DC. Lung cancer after Hodgkin's disease: a nested case-control study of the relation to treatment. J Clin Oncol. 2001;19(6):1610–8. https://doi.org/10.1200/JCO.2001.19.6.1610.
236. Travis LB, Gospodarowicz M, Curtis RE, Clarke EA, Andersson M, Glimelius B, Joensuu T, Lynch CF, van Leeuwen FE, Holowaty E, Storm H, Glimelius I, Pukkala E, Stovall M, Fraumeni JF Jr, Boice JD Jr, Gilbert E. Lung cancer following chemotherapy and radiotherapy for Hodgkin's disease. J Natl Cancer Inst. 2002;94(3):182–92. https://doi.org/10.1093/jnci/94.3.182.
237. Van Leeuwen FE, Chorus AM, van den Belt-Dusebout AW, Hagenbeek A, Noyon R, van Kerkhoff EH, Pinedo HM, Somers R. Leukemia risk following Hodgkin's disease: relation to cumulative dose of alkylating agents, treatment with teniposide combinations, number of episodes of chemotherapy, and bone marrow damage. J Clin Oncol. 1994;12(5):1063–73. https://doi.org/10.1200/JCO.1994.12.5.1063.

Chapter 3
Importance of the Infusion Order in the Treatment of Cancer

3.1 Drug Infusion Therapy

Infusion therapy is defined as medication or fluids which are administered through a needle or catheter. It is a form of drug administration that often cannot be administered orally [1, 2]. In infusion therapy, drugs are usually given intravenously, but they can also be given epidurally, intramuscularly, or subcutaneously [3–5]. Figure 3.1 shows some drug administration routes.

Some drugs are not stable when administered orally and may lose their effectiveness due to exposure to the digestive system. Thus, some drugs have to be administered by another route, which is usually the route of choice is intravenous [4, 6, 7]. The intravenous route has the advantage of quickly obtaining effects, as the drug will not need to be absorbed, as it is already inserted into the bloodstream. Some classes of drugs administered by infusion include antibiotics, antiemetics, antifungals, antivirals, and chemotherapeutics, among others [7–9].

An advantage of infusion therapy over oncology is the possibility of administering large volumes in slow infusion, allowing controlled drug dosage, as well as allowing the administration of irritating substances [4, 10]. Many of the anticancer agents are given by infusion, allowing the drug to be delivered directly into the bloodstream. As this is generally a therapy that combines several drugs, administration by infusion also allows the patient to receive the medication in the same access, without having to obtain another venous access [11, 12].

I. D. Lima Cavalcanti, *Chemotherapy Protocols and Infusion Sequence*, https://doi.org/10.1007/978-3-031-10839-6_3

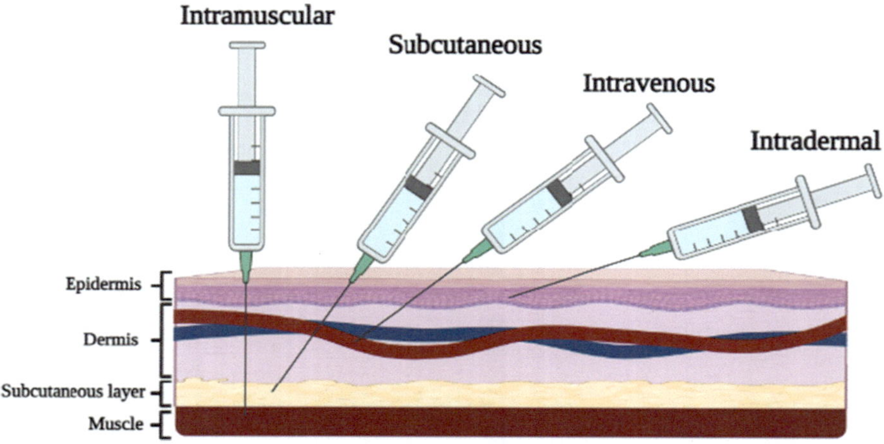

Fig. 3.1 Drug administration routes. Source: Created with BioRender.com

3.1.1   Types of Infusion According to Administration Time

Drug infusion can be classified according to the time of drug administration (Fig. 3.2). Bolus infusion is related to the application of the drug directly into the patient's bloodstream in less than or equal to 1 min. The administration in bolus allows a rapid increase in the concentration of the drug in the blood, and it can be carried out intravenously, intramuscularly, subcutaneously, or intrarectally [13–16].

Some classes of chemotherapy drugs that are commonly administered in bolus, according to the study by Lokich and Anderson [14], and include antimetabolites, alkylating agents, plant alkaloids, platinum analogues, and cytotoxic antibiotics. The authors noted that the administration of antimetabolites generally decreases the dose intensity and the maximum tolerated dose, except for 5-fluorouracil. Carlson and Sikic [17] point out that bolus administration can induce chemotherapy toxicity compared to continuous infusion and may reduce bleomycin pulmonary toxicity, doxorubicin cardiac toxicity, and 5-fluorouracil myelosuppression.

Another form of infusion is rapid infusion, which is related to administering the drug for 1–30 min [13, 18, 19]. Some drugs are administered in rapid infusion because they are well tolerated and are safe during infusion [20]. Sehn et al. [21] evaluated the administration of rituximab by rapid infusion in combination with chemotherapy, where the authors observed that the rapid infusion of rituximab did not increase its toxicity, being safe during its administration. Zhao et al. [22] also evaluated the safety and efficacy of rapid infusion of rituximab combined with chemotherapy in patients with non-Hodgkin's lymphoma, showing the safety of rapid administration without increased infusion reactions, with overall survival rates of 93.1% and progression-free survival of 81.1% in 3 years.

Segeren et al. [23] evaluated the administration of vincristine, doxorubicin, and dexamethasone in rapid infusion in the treatment of multiple myeloma. The authors

Types of Intravenous Infusion	Infusion time
Bolus infusion	Less than or equal to 1 minute
Rapid infusion	1 to 30 minutes
Continuous infusion	Greater than 60 minutes

Fig. 3.2 Main types of intravenous infusion used in antineoplastic chemotherapy. Source [13]

observed that administration of the protocol by rapid infusion promoted a partial response in 86% of patients and a complete response in 5%, with a response rate of 67%. Furthermore, developed toxicity was acceptable, with mild neurotoxicity in 18% and fever or infections in 27% of patients.

Despite the tolerable toxic profile, presented by Segeren et al. [23] regarding the rapid infusion of chemotherapeutic agents, in some cases, the rapid infusion of a certain antineoplastic agent can increase its toxic profile. Shapira et al. [24] compared rapid infusion with continuous infusion of doxorubicin. The authors observed that the slow infusion of doxorubicin for 6 h reduced the cardiotoxicity of this drug. Continuous infusion of various antineoplastics such as bleomycin, cytosine arabinoside, and doxorubicin appears to show an apparent improvement in the therapeutic index [25–27].

Poorter et al. [28] evaluated the administration of 5-fluorouracil and fluorodeoxyuridine by continuous infusion, showing it to be feasible, but the results of response rate and survival, from the survey carried out by the authors, were disappointing. In another study, Kollmannsberger et al. [29] evaluated the administration of 5-fluorouracil by continuous infusion combined with paclitaxel, cisplatin, and folinic acid. The results were positive, showing that the continuous infusion of these antineoplastics seemed to be highly active in the treatment of advanced gastric cancer, with acceptable general toxicity, allowing its use in the palliative setting, and it can also be indicated for neoadjuvant or adjuvant treatment.

Georgiadis et al. [30] showed the benefits of continuous 96-h paclitaxel infusion combined with cisplatin in the treatment of advanced lung cancer. The results showed a median time to progression of 5 months and median survival duration of 10 months, being a well-tolerated and active protocol in patients with lung cancer.

Ortega et al. [31] compared the cisplatin, vincristine, and 5-fluorouracil protocol with the cisplatin and doxorubicin protocol in continuous infusion in the treatment of pediatric hepatoblastoma. The authors observed that both protocols were similar, with excellent results achieved in stage I and II patients, as well as for subsets of stage III patients.

Fabrício et al. [15] evaluated the use of the cisplatin, 5-fluorouracil, and leucovorin protocol in the treatment of advanced head and neck and esophageal carcinomas. 5-Fluorouracil and leucovorin were administered by bolus infusion, while cisplatin was by continuous infusion over 90 min. The results showed an overall response rate of 36%, mean overall survival of 6 months, and progression-free survival of 3 months, in addition to the protocol presenting tolerable toxicity and a favorable impact on the quality of life.

3.2   Dilution of Drugs and Their Stability

Some drugs to be administered intravenously need to be reconstituted because they are in powder form [32–35]. Reconstitution consists of returning the drug to its original liquid form, requiring the addition of diluents such as sterile water, 0.9% sodium chloride, or 5% glucose, following the manufacturer's instructions, as the proper choice of diluent may interfere in drug stability, where some are incompatible with a particular diluent [34–36]. In Table 3.1, we include the main anticancer agents that need to be reconstituted, as well as their diluents and their stability.

After reconstitution, for the drug to be administered intravenously, it is necessary to dilute it in serum bags [33, 52]. The dilution aims to change the concentration of the drug that is already in liquid form, which can be a solution, suspension, or

Table 3.1 Anticancer drugs that need to be reconstituted, their diluents, and their stability after reconstitution

Drug	Diluent	Stability	Reference
Brentuximab vedotin	Water for injection	24 h at a temperature of 2–8 °C	[37]
Bleomycin	0.9% sodium chloride	24 h at a temperature between 2 and 8 °C and 12 h at room temperature	[38]
Cisplatin	Water for injection	20 h at room temperature	[39]
Cyclophosphamide	Water for injection or 0.9% sodium chloride	Up to 6 days at a temperature of 2–8 °C and 24 h at room temperature	[40]
Dacarbazine	Water for injection	36 h at a temperature between 2 and 8 °C and 8 h at room temperature	[41]
Doxorubicin	Water for injection	15 days at a temperature between 2 and 8 °C and 7 days at room temperature	[42]
Epirubicin	Water for injection	24 h at a temperature between 2 to 8 °C	[43]
Fludarabine	Water for injection	8 h at room temperature	[44]
Ganciclovir	Water for injection	12 h at room temperature	[45]
Gemcitabine	0.9% sodium chloride	24 h at room temperature	[46]
Ifosfamide	Water for injection or bacteriostatic water	24 h at a temperature between 2 and 8 °C	[47]
Mitomycin	Water for injection	14 days at a temperature between 2 and 8 °C and 7 days at room temperature	[48]
Oxaliplatin	Water for injection or 5% dextrose	24–48 h at a temperature between 2 and 8 °C	[49]
Trastuzumab	Water for injection	48 h at room temperature	[50]
Trastuzumab emtansine	Water for injection	48 h at a temperature between 2 and 8 °C	[51]

Source: Research data

reconstituted powder. The diluents used can be saline (0.9% sodium chloride), glucose (5% glucose), and ringer lactate, among others [33, 53, 54]. Table 3.2 shows some anticancer agents and their main diluents.

Some anticancer drugs may be incompatible with a particular diluent, being one of the critical points in the manipulation of chemotherapy, which may impair their activity, as well as prevent the exact dosage of the drug and influence the formulation's appearance. It is important to know the incompatibility of the drug to design solutions that help cancer therapy, such as the replacement of the diluent [12, 73–75].

Table 3.2 Main anticancer agents and their diluents

Drug	Dosage forms	Diluent	Reference
Brentuximab vedotin	50 mg	0.9% sodium chloride, 5% dextrose, and lactated ringer	[37]
Bevacizumab	100 mg/4 mL or 400 mg/10 mL	0.9% sodium chloride	[55]
Bleomycin	15 units	0.9% sodium chloride	[38]
Calcium folinate	10 mg/mL or 20 mg/mL	0.9% sodium chloride or 5% dextrose	[56]
Carboplatin	50 mg/5 mL 150 mg/15 mL 450 mg/45 mL 600 mg/60 mL	5% dextrose	[57]
Cetuximab	2 mg/mL	0.9% sodium chloride	[58]
Cyclophosphamide	200 mg or 1000 mg	5% dextrose or 5% dextrose and 0.9% sodium chloride	[40]
Cisplatin	1 mg/mL	0.9% sodium chloride	[59]
Dacarbazine	600 mg	0.9% sodium chloride or 5% dextrose	[41]
Docetaxel	20 mg/2 mL 80 mg/8 mL 160 mg/16 mL	0.9% sodium chloride or 5% dextrose	[60]
Doxorubicin	10 mg, 20 mg or 50 mg	0.9% sodium chloride or 5% dextrose	[42]
Epirubicin	50 mg/25 mL 200 mg/100 mL	0.9% sodium chloride or 5% dextrose	[43]
Etoposide	100 mg/5 mL	0.9% sodium chloride or 5% dextrose	[61]
Fludarabine	50 mg	0.9% sodium chloride or 5% dextrose	[44]
Fluorouracil	2.5g/50 mL	0.9% sodium chloride or 5% dextrose	[62]
Gemcitabine	200 mg or 1 g	0.9% sodium chloride	[46]
Ifosfamide	1 g or 3 g	0.9% sodium chloride, 5% dextrose, and lactated ringer	[47]
Ipilimumab	50 mg/10 mL 200 mg/40 mL	0.9% sodium chloride or 5% dextrose	[63]
Irinotecan	40 mg/2 mL 100 mg/5 mL 300 mg/15 mL	5% dextrose (preferred) or 0.9% sodium chloride	[64]

(continued)

Table 3.2 (continued)

Drug	Dosage forms	Diluent	Reference
Mesna	100 mg/mL	0.9% sodium chloride, 5% dextrose, lactated ringer or 5% dextrose, and 0.9% sodium chloride	[65]
Methotrexate	50 mg/2 mL 100 mg/4 mL 200 mg/8 mL 250 mg/10 mL 1 g/40 mL	0.9% sodium chloride or 5% dextrose	[66]
Mitomycin	5 mg	0.9% sodium chloride or 5% dextrose	[48]
Oxaliplatin	50 mg or 100 mg	5% dextrose	[49]
Paclitaxel	30 mg/5 mL 100 mg/16.7 mL 300 mg/50 mL	0.9% sodium chloride, 5% dextrose or 5% dextrose, and 0.9% sodium chloride	[67]
Rituximab	100 mg/10 mL 500 mg/50 mL	0.9% sodium chloride or 5% dextrose	[68]
Tocilizumab	20 mg/mL	0.9% sodium chloride	[69]
Trastuzumab	440 mg	0.9% sodium chloride	[50]
Trastuzumab emtansine	100 mg or 160 mg	0.9% sodium chloride	[51]
Vinblastine	1 mg/mL	0.9% sodium chloride	[70]
Vincristine	1 mg/1 mL 2 mg/2 mL	0.9% sodium chloride	[71]
Vinorelbine	10 mg/1 mL 50 mg/5 mL	0.9% sodium chloride, 5% dextrose, lactated ringer, or 5% dextrose and 0.9% sodium chloride	[72]

Source: Research data

The incompatibility can induce the reduction of the drug's activity or inactivation, as well as can induce the formation of a new compound with toxic activity. In addition, organoleptic changes and precipitation formation may occur. These problems related to incompatibility must be evaluated mainly between drugs that will be administered in the same infusion bag or the same access route [12, 76–78].

A classic example of incompatibility in oncology is related to oxaliplatin. Oxaliplatin is a platinum compound used in the treatment of colorectal cancer in combination with other drugs such as irinotecan and 5-fluorouracil [79–81]. This drug is incompatible in sodium chloride solution, inducing its precipitation and degradation with the formation of oxalate, so it should be indicated that oxaliplatin is diluted in glucose serum and that all drugs present in the protocol are diluted in glycosylated serum to avoid its conversion [82–84]. Jerremalm et al. [82] evaluated the cytotoxicity of the complex obtained after oxaliplatin degradation in the presence of chloride. The results showed that the monochloro monooxalate complex did not show the same cytotoxic effect as oxaliplatin, highlighting that this degradation can reduce the drug's efficacy.

Li and Koda [85] verified the stability of irinotecan after reconstitution in a phosphate buffer solution (pH 4.0, 6.0, and 7.4), 5% dextrose, and 0.9% sodium chloride. The authors managed to relate the rate of degradation of irinotecan according to temperature and pH, showing that the extent of hydrolysis of this drug increases with pH, converting it into its carboxylate form, being reversible. Thus, among the vehicles, reconstitution with 5% dextrose is more suitable, as it can maintain the stability of the drug before administration.

Another study also proposes the evaluation of the stability of irinotecan, this time administered concomitantly with 5-fluorouracil. Tan and Hu [86] observed that simultaneous infusions of irinotecan diluted in 0.9% sodium chloride and 5-fluorouracil in the same intravenous route can induce drug precipitation and color change to yellow, indicating possible drug degradation.

Another drug that undergoes degradation in the presence of sodium chloride is carboplatin, where, through a hydrolysis process, it can be converted into cisplatin [87, 88]. Myers et al. [89] performed a stability study of carboplatin diluted in 0.9% sodium chloride. The authors noted that carboplatin appears to be stable for 24 h at room temperature or 3 days under refrigeration.

3.3 Risks of Chemotherapy Infusion

During the intravenous administration of anticancer chemotherapy, it is important to check the venous permeability, flow, and reflux with saline solution and assess the conditions of the insertion site [90, 91]. The professional nurse responsible for administering these medications must be aware of the risks to which the patient may be exposed, such as cases of infection, extravasation, phlebitis, and falls [92–94].

The professional nurse may also be exposed due to the characteristics of the antineoplastic agent that can form aerosols and induce the development of acute or chronic adverse reactions, which will depend on the concentration of drug to which the professional was exposed [95, 96].

All professionals working in the chemotherapy sector must know the risks that anticancer drugs can induce after occupational exposure and know what biosafety procedures are necessary to protect these professionals [97, 98]. Antineoplastics, as they are highly cytotoxic, can cause cell damage in normal cells and thus induce toxic effects, which will depend on the route of exposure to which the patient was exposed, which may be through contact with the skin and mucous membranes, as well as through inhalation of aerosols [99–101]. Table 3.3 shows some acute and chronic side effects that professionals exposed to chemotherapy may experience.

As for biosafety care to reduce the risk of exposure to antineoplastic drugs, it is recommended that the professional nurse during drug administration use personal protective equipment, which includes waterproof aprons, latex gloves, activated charcoal masks, among others, during administration of antineoplastics. In

Table 3.3 Acute and chronic side effects after exposure of professionals to antineoplastic agents

Acute effects	Chronic effects
Allergic reactions	Infertility
Irritation eye	Miscarriages
Nausea	Stillbirths
Vomiting	Ectopic pregnancy
Syncope	Fetal birth defects
Diarrhea	Cancer
Constipation	Menstrual dysfunctions
Cough	Mutagenicity
Headache	

Source: [95, 96]

addition, the nurse needs to assess the patient's venous access, to avoid cases of extravasation of antineoplastic agents [96, 102–104].

3.3.1   Drug Extravasation

The term extravasation is used in cases where a drug-infused intravenously, which is a vesicant or irritant, leaks into the extravascular space [105–107]. Extravasation is different from the term infiltration, as infiltration occurs with medications that are neither vesicant nor irritant [102, 108]. Early signs of extravasation include persistent pain, burning, swelling, and whitening or erythema in the area where the drug was infused [106, 108].

Because some drugs have vesicant and irritating characteristics, they cause tissue damage and may cause necrosis, blister formation, and ulceration [102, 108]. There is no exact incidence of extravasation cases, but it is estimated that it occurs in 0.1 to 6% during the administration of vesicant and antineoplastic drugs [102, 104, 105, 109].

Risk factors that contribute to cases of extravasation include the quality of the infusion equipment used, which allows venous access to the patient for infusion of the medication [93, 108, 110, 111]. Factors may also be patient-related, such as predisposition to infiltrating lesions [106]. In addition, the pharmacological characteristics of the drug can favor its extravasation, such as pH, osmolality, vasoactivity, and cytotoxicity of the infusate; an example is drugs that irritate the veins, inducing an inflammatory response of the endothelial cells, thus allowing the drug to leak of the vein [108, 110].

Many anticancer drugs have a vesicant and/or irritant characteristic, and the fact that many are used in combination for the treatment of cancer can be infused in the same access route, and this can lead to compromise of the patient's vein and increase the probability of extravasation [102, 106, 112].

3.3.1.1 Irritating Antineoplastics

Antineoplastic drugs can be classified according to their potential for local dermatological toxicity into irritants, vesicants, and non-vesicants [108, 113]. Irritating drugs cause a local inflammatory response inducing phlebitis, with pain, heat, and erythema, with rare cases in the development of necrosis or ulcerations [110, 114–116]. When the extravasation of these drugs occurs, they cause a burning sensation on the skin, and when in large concentrations, it can cause ulceration in soft tissue. Inflammation-induced by the extravasation of irritating drugs is usually self-limiting and is not related to long-term sequelae [106, 115, 117, 118]. Some irritating antineoplastic drugs are listed in Table 3.4.

The clinical manifestations observed in patients who have suffered from extravasation of irritating drugs include discomfort or burning sensation, redness, edema, heat, and local hyperalgesia. The presence of edema at the drug infusion site may be an indication of extravasation, with local hypersensitivity reactions or vasospasm and phlebitis (Fig. 3.3). Another common manifestation is hyperpigmentation and cutaneous sclerosis in the venous path [110, 120, 121].

Table 3.4 Anticancer drugs that are irritating

Therapeutic class	Drugs
Alkylating agents	Busulfan Carmustine Cyclophosphamide Dacarbazine Ifosfamide Melphalan Thiotepa
Antimetabolites	Cladribine 5-Fluorouracil Gemcitabine
Cytotoxic antibiotics	Daunorubicin (liposomal) Doxorubicin (liposomal) Streptozocin
Platinum compounds	Carboplatin Cisplatin Oxaliplatin
Vegetable derivatives	Docetaxel Etoposide Irinotecan Teniposide Topotecan
Others	Trastuzumab Mitoxantrone

Source: [115, 119, 120]

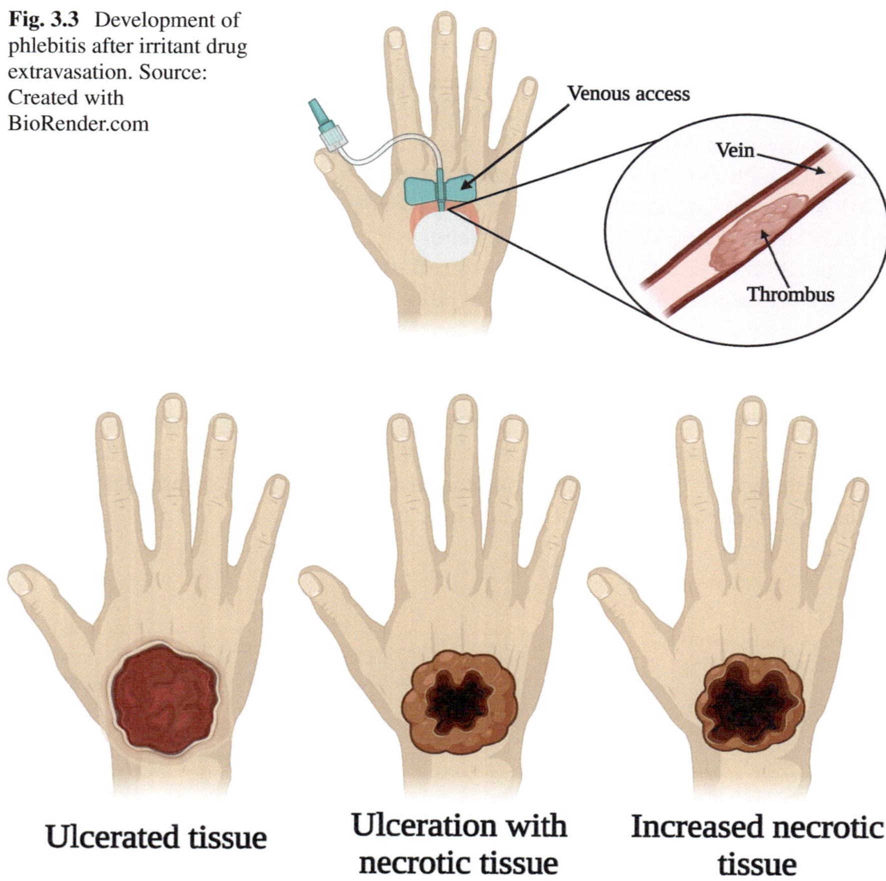

Fig. 3.3 Development of phlebitis after irritant drug extravasation. Source: Created with BioRender.com

Fig. 3.4 Degrees of tissue damage after extravasation of the vesicant drug. Source: Created with BioRender.com

3.3.1.2 Vesicant Antineoplastics

Vesicant drugs, unlike irritants, when they overflow cause progressive damage to the underlying tissue, inducing the formation of vesicles and ulcerations, leading to tissue destruction. They can also injure tendons, bones, ligaments, and nerves, leading to functional impairment and severe limitations [102, 106, 122–124]. Figure 3.4 shows tissue damage caused after the extravasation of vesicant drugs.

Vesicant drugs can be classified into DNA-binders, to which they will bind to tissue nucleic acids and induce the formation of free radicals, thereby inhibiting protein synthesis and leading to progressive tissue destruction, causing the lesion to become present deeper, more extensive, and painful, where the drug is retained in the tissue for a long time (up to 28 days), increasing the lesion [102, 108, 119, 125]. Vesicant drugs that do not bind to DNA, bind to healthy tissue cells and are more easily metabolized and neutralized, where the lesion is usually localized, with

Table 3.5 Vesicant antineoplastic drugs

Therapeutic class	DNA binding drugs	DNA nonbinding drugs
Alkylating agents	Bendamustine Mechlorethamine	–
Cytotoxic antibiotics	Daunorubicin Doxorubicin Epirubicin Idarubicin Dactinomycin Mitomycin Mitoxantrone	–
Platinum compounds	Cisplatin	–
Vegetable derivatives	–	Vinblastine Vincristine Vindesine Vinorelbine Paclitaxel Docetaxel Cabazitaxel
Others	Amsacrine Trabectedin	–

Source: [115, 119, 120]

Table 3.6 Non-vesicant antineoplastic drugs

Therapeutic class	Drugs
Alkylating agents	Cyclophosphamide
Antimetabolites	Cytarabine Fludarabine Gemcitabine Methotrexate Raltitrexed
Cytotoxic antibiotics	Bleomycin
Vegetable derivatives	Cabazitaxel Paclitaxel Albumin
Others	Aldesleukin Asparaginase Bortezomib Interferon Pemetrexed Arsenic trioxide Monoclonal antibodies

Source: [119]

moderate pain, improving over time [102, 108, 119]. Table 3.5 shows some anticancer drugs that are vesicants.

Non-vesicant drugs, unlike other classes, if extravasated, will rarely produce acute reactions or tissue necrosis. They are inert or neutral compounds that do not cause inflammation and ulceration, but tend to cause pain at the injection site, around and along the vein [102, 106]. In Table 3.6 we highlight the non-vesicant antineoplastics.

3.4 Concept and Importance of Infusion Order

Defining the order of infusion of the drug allows for planning the therapeutic regimens and thus optimizing the effect of chemotherapy [126, 127]. The sequence of administration of chemotherapeutic agents is important because it can avoid drug interaction due to possible incompatibilities regarding the dilution in serum of 5% dextrose or 0.9% sodium chloride. Another point that can also be avoided, depending on the order of drug infusion, is the protocol's toxicity profile, as it can also reduce the risk of extravasation due to the dermatological toxicity of each drug inserted in the protocol [128–130].

The infusion sequence of antineoplastic agents can directly impact the patient's response to treatment, as well as their safety and toxicological profile [127, 131]. Drug interactions can contribute to the therapeutic effect of a given drug as well as delay or inactivate its pharmacological activity [127, 132]. A classic example is the interaction of leucovorin with 5-fluorouracil, where leucovorin when administered before 5-fluorouracil potentiates the therapeutic effect of 5-fluorouracil [133, 134]. On the other hand, when we combine calcium folinate with methotrexate, calcium folinate inhibits the cytotoxic effect of methotrexate, thereby reducing its therapeutic effectiveness [135–137].

When defining a therapeutic protocol, it is important to carry out a study of possible drug interactions that allows choosing the best order of drug administration during therapy, as the inappropriate infusion order can compromise the treatment of the patient with cancer. The knowledge of possible drug interactions is important in optimizing the dose of the antineoplastic agent in combination therapy [138–141].

When a specific cycle drug is administered before an unspecific cycle drug, it is believed that maximization of the effects on cells at a high rate of cell division will occur [127, 142]. Another important point is when administering vesicant drugs first, as over time vascular integrity decreases, and it is more advantageous to administer vesicant drugs when the vein is more stable to avoid vascular disruption and drug extravasation [104, 127, 143].

3.4.1 Factors That May Influence in the Order of Infusion of Antineoplastic Agents

Most therapeutic protocols for the treatment of cancer are based on the combination of anticancer drugs, with different mechanisms of action, but when combined, they potentiate the anticancer effect, being cytotoxic to a greater number of cells compared to monotherapy [144–146]. A chemotherapy protocol can present the association of two or more drugs, which will be administered in sequence on the same day [73, 147, 148].

Antineoplastic drugs will present drug interactions with synergistic or summative effects, regarding their therapeutic effect, as well as potentiating toxic effects

Table 3.7 Factors that influence the order of infusion of anticancer drugs

Factors	Influence	Reference
Incompatibility of drug with diluent	When they come into contact with diluents with which they are incompatible, some drugs can precipitate and cause undesirable symptoms	[152, 153]
Vesicant or irritant drugs	Vesicant and irritant drugs tend to be harmful to the vascular wall and can compromise blood vessels, and they should be administered as a priority at the beginning of therapy to reduce the risk of extravasation	[102, 105, 106]
Drug interactions	Drug interactions can contribute to increasing the therapeutic effect of the drug, as well as contributing to reducing its effectiveness and increasing the toxicity of the treatment	[132, 154–156]
Infusion time	Infusion time can be a factor that determines the sequence of medication in therapy, and medications compatible with each other can be administered concurrently to reduce the patient's length of stay in the facility	[157, 158]

[149, 150]. The sequence of administration of antineoplastic agents can influence the drug's mechanism of action, contributing to drug interactions that will favor the drug's effect or reduce its effectiveness and increase its toxicity [127, 131, 151].

Therefore, it is essential to plan the sequence of administration of antineoplastic agents for a better therapeutic response to the applied protocol. The study of the pharmacokinetic and pharmacodynamic profiles of each antineoplastic agent can provide evidence of drug interactions that may favor therapy and define the best order of infusion of antineoplastic agents [127, 131]. In Table 3.7 are some important factors that must be evaluated before defining the order of infusion of antineoplastic agents.

The order of infusion of antineoplastic agents, when well studied and planned, favors cancer treatment, increasing the therapeutic response and benefiting the patient by promoting a better quality of life [159, 160]. Stanford, Zondor, and Jumper [154] found in their study that interactions related to the infusion sequence were related to toxicity, pharmacokinetics, and efficacy. The authors emphasize that the inadequate sequence can lead to increased toxicity, decreased efficacy, and pharmacokinetic differences. These results presented by Stanford et al. [154] only reinforce the importance of planning the sequence of antineoplastic agents in cancer treatment.

References

1. Fox LM. Remington: the science and practice of pharmacy. Am J Pharm Educ. 2006;70(3):3.
2. Scales K. Intravenous therapy: a guide to good practice. Br J Nurs. 2008;17(8):4–12.
3. Lavery I, Ingram P. Safe practice in intravenous medicines administration. Nurs Stand. 2008;22(46):44–8.
4. Jin JF, Zhu LL, Chen M, Xu HM, Wang HF, Feng XQ, Zhu XP, Zhou Q. The optimal choice of medication administration route regarding intravenous, intramuscular, and subcutaneous injection. Patient Prefer Adherence. 2015;9:923–42. https://doi.org/10.2147/PPA.S87271.

5. Lister S, Hofland J, Grafton H, Wilson C. The Royal Marsden manual of clinical nursing procedures. Hoboken: Wiley; 2021.

6. Homayun B, Lin X, Choi HJ. Challenges and recent progress in oral drug delivery systems for biopharmaceuticals. Pharmaceutics. 2019;11(3):129. https://doi.org/10.3390/pharmaceutics11030129.

7. Le J. Drug administration. MSD manual consumer version. New Jersey, USA, 2020. Available https://www.msdmanuals.com/home/drugs/administration-and-kinetics-of-drugs/drug-administration. Access July 9, 2021.

8. Shimizu S. Routes of administration. In: Hedrich H, editor. The laboratory mouse (handbook of experimental animals). Cambridge: Academic; 2004.

9. Gale RP. Management of adverse effects of cancer therapy. MSD manual professional version. New Jersey, USA, 2020. Available https://www.msdmanuals.com/professional/hematology-and-oncology/principles-of-cancer-therapy/management-of-adverse-effects-of-cancer-therapy. Access July 9, 2021.

10. Diehl KH, Hull R, Morton D, Pfister R, von Rabemampianina Y, Smith D, Vidal JM, van de Vorstenbosch C. A good practice guide to the administration of substances and removal of blood, including routes and volumes. J Appl Toxicol. 2001;21:15–23.

11. Lewis HL, Bloomston M. Hepatic artery infusional chemotherapy. Surg Clin N Am. 2016;96(2):341–55. https://doi.org/10.1016/j.suc.2015.11.002.

12. Marsilio NR, Silva D, Bueno D. Drug incompatibilities in the adult intensive care unit of a university hospital. Rev Bras Terapia Intens. 2016;28(2):147–53. https://doi.org/10.5935/0103-507X.20160029.

13. Boehm AB, Salomão D, Lemes PM. Manual de Diluição de Medicamentos Injetáveis. Joinville: Pronto Atendimento e Unidade de Pronto Atendimento. Secretaria da Saúde; 2018.

14. Lokich J, Anderson N. Dose intensity for bolus versus infusion chemotherapy administration: review of the literature for 27 anti-neoplastic agents. Ann Oncol. 1997;8(1):15–25. https://doi.org/10.1023/A:1008243806415.

15. Fabrício VDC, Amado F, Del Giglio A. Low-cost outpatient chemotherapy regimen of cisplatin, 5-fluorouracil and leucovorin for advanced head and neck and esophageal carcinomas. Sao Paulo Med J. 2008;126(1):63–6.

16. Ahmed TA. Pharmacokinetics of drugs following IV bolus, IV infusion, and oral administration. London: IntechOpen; 2015.

17. Carlson RW, Sikic BI. Continuous infusion or bolus injection in cancer chemotherapy. Ann Intern Med. 1983;99(6):823–33. https://doi.org/10.7326/0003-4819-99-6-823.

18. Zahrani AA, Ibrahim N, Eid AA. Rapid infusion rituximab changing practice for patient care. J Oncol Pharm Pract. 2009;15(3):183–6. https://doi.org/10.1177/1078155208100527.

19. Matsuba CST, Ciosak SI, Serpa LF, Poltronieri M, Oliseski MS. Terapia Nutricional: Administração e Monitoramento. In: Sociedade Brasileira Nutrição Parenteral e Enteral. Associação Brasileira de Nutrologia. Diretrizes Brasileiras para Terapia Nutricional Enteral e Parenteral. São Paulo: Associação Médica Brasileira; 2011.

20. Atmar J. Review of the safety and feasibility of rapid infusion of rituximab. J Oncol Pract. 2010;6(2):91–3. https://doi.org/10.1200/JOP.200001.

21. Sehn LH, Donaldson J, Filewich A, Fitzgerald C, Gill KK, Runzer N, Searle B, Souliere S, Spinelli JJ, Sutherland J, Connors JM. Rapid infusion rituximab in combination with corticosteroid-containing chemotherapy or as maintenance therapy is well tolerated and can safely be delivered in the community setting. Blood. 2007;109:4117–73. https://doi.org/10.1182/blood-2006-11-059469.

22. Zhao W, Gao Y, Bai B, Cai QC, Wang XX, Cai QQ, Huang HQ. Safety and efficacy of non-initial rapid infusion of rituximab plus chemotherapy in Chinese patients with CD20+ non-Hodgkin's lymphoma. Expert Opin Drug Saf. 2015;14(1):21–9. https://doi.org/10.1517/14740338.2015.988138.

23. Segeren CM, Sonneveld P, van der Holt B, Baars JW, Biesma DH, Cornellissen JJ, Croockewit AJ, Dekker AW, Fibbe WE, Lowenberg B, van Marwijk KM, van Oers MH, Richel DJ,

Schouten HC, Vellenga E, Verhoef GE, Wijermans PW, Wittebol S, Lokhorst HM. Vincristine, doxorubicin and dexamethasone (VAD) administered as rapid intravenous infusion for first-line treatment in untreated multiple myeloma. Br J Haematol. 1999;105(1):127–30.

24. Shapira J, Gotfried M, Lishner M, Ravid M. Reduced cardiotoxicity of doxorubicin by a 6-hour infusion regimen. A prospective randomized evaluation. Cancer. 1990;65(4):870–3.

25. Vogelzang NJ. Continuous infusion chemotherapy: a critical review. J Clin Oncol. 1984;2(11):1289–304. https://doi.org/10.1200/JCO.1984.2.11.1289.

26. Rosenthal CJ, Rotman M. Clinical applications of continuous infusion chemotherapy and concomitant radiation therapy. Boston: Springer; 1986. https://doi.org/10.1007/978-1-4613-2197-2.

27. Nanninga AG, Vries EGE, Willemse PHB, Oosterhuis BE, Sleijfer DT, Hoekstra HJ, Mulder NH. Continuous infusion of chemotherapy on an outpatient basis via a totally implanted venous access port. Eur J Cancer Clin Oncol. 1991;27(2):147–9. https://doi.org/10.1016/0277-5379(91)90474-R.

28. Poorter RL, Bakker PJM, Veenhof CHN. Continuous infusion of chemotherapy: focus on 5-fluorouracil and fluorodeoxyuridine. Pharm World Sci. 1998;20:45–59. https://doi.org/10.1023/A:1008605600414.

29. Kollmannsberger C, Quietzsch D, Haag C, Lingenfelser T, Schroeder M, Hartmann JT, Baronius W, Hempel V, Clemens M. Kanz L, Bokemeyer C. A phase II study of paclitaxel, weekly, 24-hour continuous infusion 5-fluorouracil, folinic acid and cisplatin in patients with advanced gastric cancer. Br J Cancer. 2000;83:458–62. https://doi.org/10.1054/bjoc.2000.1295.

30. Georgiadis MS, Schuler BS, Brown JE, Kieffer LV, Steinberg SM, Wilson WH, Takimoto CH, Kelley MJ, Johnson BE. Paclitaxel by 96-hour continuous infusion in combination with cisplatin: a phase I trial in patients with advanced lung cancer. J Clin Oncol. 1997;15(2):735–43. https://doi.org/10.1200/JCO.1997.15.2.735.

31. Ortega JA, Douglass EC, Feusner JH, Reynolds M, Quinn JJ, Haas MJFE, King DR, Liu-Mares W, Sensel MG, Krailo MD. Randomized comparison of cisplatin/vincristine/fluorouracil and cisplatin/continuous infusion doxorubicin for treatment of pediatric hepatoblastoma: a report from the Children's Cancer Group and the Pediatric Oncology Group. J Clin Oncol. 2000;18(14):2665–75. https://doi.org/10.1200/JCO.2000.18.14.2665.

32. European Commission. Enterprise and industry directorate-general. A guideline on summary of product characteristics. Brussels: European Commission; 2009.

33. ISMP – Institute for Safe Medication Practices. Safe practice guidelines for adult iv push medications. A compilation of safe practices from the ISMP adult IV push medication safety summit, Horsham, Pennsylvania, 2015.

34. Tritak-Elmiger A, Edd RN, Daingerfield M. Brown and Mulholland's drug calculations e-book: process and problems for clinical practice. St. Louis: Elsevier; 2019.

35. Brown M, Mulholland JL. Drug calculations-e-book: ratio and proportion problems for clinical practice. St. Louis: Elsevier; 2016.

36. Benizri F, Bonan B, Ferrio AL, Brandely ML, Castagné V, Théou-Anton N, Verlinde-Carvalho M, Havard L. Stability of antineoplastic agents in use for home-based intravenous chemotherapy. Pharm World Sci. 2008;31(1):1–13. https://doi.org/10.1007/s11096-008-9270-z.

37. ADCETRIS® (brentuximab vedotin): injection. Seattle Genetics Inc., Bothell, 2014. Available https://www.accessdata.fda.gov/drugsatfda_docs/label/2014/125388_s056s078lbl.pdf. Accessed July 14, 2021.

38. BLENOXANE® (bleomycin sulfate): injection. Nippon Kayaku Co., Ltd. Tokyo, 2010. Available https://www.accessdata fda.gov/drugsatfda_docs/label/2010/050443s036lbl.pdf. Accessed July 14, 2021.

39. Cisplatin: injection. WG Critical Care, LLC. Paramus, 2019. Available https://www.accessdata.fda.gov/drugsatfda_docs/label/2019/018057s089lbl.pdf. Accessed July 14, 2021.

40. Cyclophosphamide: Injection. Baxter Healthcare Corporation. Deerfield, 2012. Available https://www.accessdata.fda.gov/drugsatfda_docs/label/2012/012142s109lbl.pdf. Accessed July 14, 2021.

41. Dacarbazine: Injection. Pfizer Canada ULC, Kirkland, 2019. Available https://www.pfizer.ca/sites/default/files/201902/Dacarbazine_PM_E_221511_25Jan2019.pdf. Accessed July 14, 2021.
42. ADRIAMYCIN (Doxorubicin): injection. Bedford Laboratories, Bedford, 2012. Available https://www.accessdata.fda.gov/drugsatfda_docs/label/2012/062921s022lbl.pdf. Accessed July 14, 2021.
43. ELLENCE® (epirubicin hydrochloride): injection. Pharmacia & Upjohn Ca., New York, 2014. Available https://www.accessdata.fda.gov/drugsatfda_docs/label/2014/050778s021lbl.pdf. Accessed July 14, 2021.
44. Fludara® (fludarabine phosphate): injection. Bayer HealthCare Pharmaceuticals Inc., Wayne, 2008. Available https://www.accessdata.fda.gov/drugsatfda_docs/label/2009/020038s032lbl.pdf. Accessed July 14, 2021.
45. GANCICLOVIR: injection. Exela Pharma Sciences, Lenoir, 2017. Available https://www.accessdata.fda.gov/drugsatfda_docs/label/2017/209347lbl.pdf. Accessed July 14, 2021.
46. GEMZAR (gemcitabine): injection. Lilly USA, LLC., Indianapolis, 2014. Available https://www.accessdata.fda.gov/drugsatfda_docs/label/2014/020509s077lbl.pdf. Accessed July 14, 2021.
47. IFEX (ifosfamide): injection. Baxter Healthcare Corporation, Deerfield, 2012. Available https://www.accessdata.fda.gov/drugsatfda_docs/label/2012/019763s017lbl.pdf. Accessed July 14, 2021.
48. Mitozytrex™ (mitomycin): injection. SuperGen, Inc., Dublin, 2002. Available https://www.accessdata.fda.gov/drugsatfda_docs/label/2002/50763_Mitozytrex_lbl.pdf. Accessed July 14, 2021.
49. ELOXATIN (oxaliplatin): injection. Sanofi-avenis U.S. LLC., Bridgewater, 2011. Available https://www.accessdata.fda.gov/drugsatfda_docs/label/2011/021759s012lbl.pdf. Accessed July 14, 2021.
50. HERCEPTIN® (trastuzumab): injection. Genentech, Inc., South San Francisco, 2010. Available https://www.accessdata.fda.gov/drugsatfda_docs/label/2010/103792s5250lbl.pdf. Accessed July 14, 2021.
51. KADCYLA™ (ado-trastuzumab emtansine): injection. Genentech, Inc., South San Francisco, 2013. Available https://www.accessdata.fda.gov/drugsatfda_docs/label/2013/125427lbl.pdf. Accessed July 14, 2021.
52. Doyle GR, McCutcheon JA. Clinical procedures for safer patient care. BC open textbook. Victoria: BCcampus; 2015.
53. Kim SH, Heeb RM, Kramer I. Physicochemical stability of reconstituted decitabine (Dacogen®) solutions and ready-to-administer infusion bags when stored refrigerated or frozen. Pharm Technol Hosp Pharm. 2017;2(4):145–57. https://doi.org/10.1515/pthp-2017-0025.
54. Rudloff E, Hopper K. Crystalloid and colloid compositions and their impact. Front Vet Sci. 2021;8:639848. https://doi.org/10.3389/fvets.2021.639848.
55. AVASTIN® (bevacizumab): solution. Genentech, Inc., South San Francisco, 2009. Available https://www.accessdata.fda.gov/drugsatfda_docs/label/2009/125085s0169lbl.pdf. Accessed July 14, 2021.
56. LEUCOVORIN CALCIUM: injection. Ben Venue Laboratories, Inc., Bedford, 2011. Available https://www.accessdata.fda.gov/drugsatfda_docs/label/2012/040347s010lbl.pdf. Access July 14, 2021.
57. PARAPLATIN® (carboplatin): injection. Bristol-Myers Squibb Company, Princeton, 2010. Available https://www.accessdata.fda.gov/drugsatfda_docs/label/2010/020452s005lbl.pdf. Accessed July 14, 2021.
58. ERBITUX® (cetuximab): injection. Eli Lilly and Company, Indianapolis, 2019. Available https://www.accessdata.fda.gov/drugsatfda_docs/label/2019/125084s273lbl.pdf. Access July 14, 2021.
59. CISplatin: injection. WG Critical Care, LLC., Paramus, 2015. Available https://www.accessdata.fda.gov/drugsatfda_docs/label/2015/018057s083lbl.pdf. Accessed July 14, 2021.

60. Docetaxel: solution. EBEWE Pharma Ges.m.b.H. Unterach, 2012. Available https://www.accessdata.fda.gov/drugsatfda_docs/label/2012/201525s002lbl.pdf. Accessed July 14, 2021.

61. ETOPOPHOS® (etoposide phosphate): injection. Baxter Healthcare Corporation, Deerfield, 2017. Available https://www.accessdata.fda.gov/drugsatfda_docs/label/2017/020457s016lbl.pdf. Accessed July 14, 2021.

62. Fluorouracil: Injection. Spectrum Pharmaceuticals, Inc., Irvine, 2016. Available https://www.accessdata.fda.gov/drugsatfda_docs/label/2016/012209s040lbl.pdf. Accessed July 14, 2021.

63. YERVOY® (ipilimumab): injection. Bristol-Myers Squibb Company, Princeton, 2015. Available https://www.accessdata.fda.gov/drugsatfda_docs/label/2015/125377s073lbl.pdf. Accessed July 14, 2021.

64. CAMPTOSAR® (irinotecan): injection. Pharmacia & Upjohn Co. Division of Pfizer Inc., New York, 2014. Available https://www.accessdata.fda.gov/drugsatfda_docs/label/2014/020571s048lbl.pdf. Accessed July 14, 2021.

65. MESNEX (mesna): Injection. Baxter Healthcare Corporation, Deerfield, 2014. Available https://www.accessdata.fda.gov/drugsatfda_docs/label/2014/019884s013lbl.pdf. Accessed July 14, 2021.

66. Methotrexate: injection. Division of Pfizer Inc., New York, 2012. Available https://cdn.pfizer.com/pfizercom/products/uspi_methotrexate.pdf. Accessed July 14, 2021.

67. TAXOL® (paclitaxel): injection. Bristol-Myers Squibb Company, Princeton, 2011. Available https://www.accessdata.fda.gov/drugsatfda_docs/label/2011/020262s049lbl.pdf. Accessed July 14, 2021.

68. Rituxan (rituximab): injection. Genentech Inc., South San Francisco, 2010. Available https://www.accessdata.fda.gov/drugsatfda_docs/label/2010/103705s5311lbl.pdf. Accessed July 14, 2021.

69. ACTEMRA® (tocilizumab): injection. Genentech, Inc., South San Francisco, 2013. Available https://www.accessdata.fda.gov/drugsatfda_docs/label/2013/125276s092lbl.pdf. Accessed July 14, 2021.

70. VinBLAStine sulfate: injection. Bedford Laboratories, Bedford, 2012. Available https://docs.boehringer-ingelheim.com/Prescribing%20Information/PIs/Ben%20Venue_Bedford%20Labs/55390-091-10%20VIN%2010MG/5539009110. Accessed July 14, 2021.

71. VinCRIStine sulfate: injection. Hospira, Inc., Lake Forest, 2013. Available https://www.accessdata.fda.gov/drugsatfda_docs/label/2014/071484s042lbl.pdf. Accessed July 14, 2021.

72. NAVELBINE® (vinorelbine): injection. Pierre Fabre Médicament, Boulogne, 2020. Available https://www.accessdata.fda.gov/drugsatfda_docs/label/2020/020388s037lbl.pdf. Accessed July 14, 2021.

73. Neuss MN, Gilmore TR, Belderson KM, Billett AL, Conti-Kalchik T, Harvey BE, Hendricks C, LeFebvre KB, Mangu PB, McNiff K, Olsen M, Schulmeister L, Gehr AV, Polovich M. 2016 Updated American Society of Clinical Oncology/Oncology Nursing Society Chemotherapy Administration. Oncol Nurs Forum. 2017;44(1):1–13. https://doi.org/10.1200/JOP.2016.017905.

74. Aguiar KS, Santos JM, Cambrussi MC, Picolotto S, Carneiro MB. Patient safety and the value of pharmaceutical intervention in a cancer hospital. Einstein. 2018;16(1):1–7. https://doi.org/10.1590/S1679-45082018AO4122.

75. Lee Y, Fong SY, Shon J, Zhang SL, Brooks R, Lahens NF, Chen D, Dang CV, Field JM, Sehgal A. Time-of-day specificity of anticancer drugs may be mediated by circadian regulation of the cell cycle. Sci Adv. 2021;7(7):2645. https://doi.org/10.1126/sciadv.abd2645.

76. Miranda TMM, Ferraresi AA. Compatibility: drugs and parenteral nutrition. Einstein. 2016;14(1):52–5. https://doi.org/10.1590/S1679-45082016AO3440.

77. Paes GO, Moreira SO, Moreira MB, Martins TG. Drug incompatibility in the ICU: review of implications in nursing practice. Rev Eletrôn Enfermagem. 2017;19:1–12. https://doi.org/10.5216/ree.v19.38718.

78. Patel P. Preformulation studies: an integral part of formulation design. London: IntechOpen; 2019.

79. Lévi F, Metzger G, Massari C, Milano G. Oxaliplatin, pharmacokinetics and chronopharmacological aspects. Clin Pharmacokinet. 2000;38(1):1–21. https://doi.org/10.2165/00003088-200038010-00001.
80. Cavalcanti IDL, Costa DT, Silva ATA, Peres AL, Coimbra CGO. Importance of pharmacist in oxaliplatin hepatotoxicity associated with inadequate nutritional diet: case report. Curr Nutr Food Sci. 2020;16:839–44. https://doi.org/10.2165/00003088-200038010-00001.
81. Wen F, Tang R, Sang Y, Li M, Hu Q, Du Z, Zhou Y, Zhang P, He X, Li Q. Which is false: oxaliplatin or fluoropyrimidine? An analysis of patients with KRAS wild-type metastatic colorectal cancer treated with first-line epidermal growth factor receptor monoclonal antibody. Cancer Sci. 2013;104(10):1330–8. https://doi.org/10.1111/cas.12224.
82. Jerremalm E, Hedeland M, Wallin I, Bondesson U, Ehrsson H. Oxaliplatin degradation in the presence of chloride: identification and cytotoxicity of the monochloro monooxalato complex. Pharm Res. 2004;21(5):891–4. https://doi.org/10.1023/b:pham.0000026444.67883.83.
83. Eto S, Yamamoto K, Shimazu K, Sugiura T, Baba K, Sato A, Goromaru T, Hagiwara Y, Hara K, Shinohara Y, Takahashi K. Formation of oxalate in oxaliplatin injection diluted with infusion solutions. Gan To Kagaku Ryoho. 2014;41(1):71–5.
84. Mehta AM, Van den Hoven JM, Rosing H, Hillebrand MJX, Nuijen B, Huitema ADR, Beijnen JH, Verwaal VJ. Stability of oxaliplatin in chloride-containing carrier solutions used in hyperthermic intraperitoneal chemotherapy. Int J Pharm. 2015;479(1):23–7. https://doi.org/10.1016/j.ijpharm.2014.12.025.
85. Li WY, Koda RT. Stability of irinotecan hydrochloride in aqueous solutions. Am J Health Syst Pharm. 2002;59(6):539–44. https://doi.org/10.1093/ajhp/59.6.539.
86. Tan X, Hu J. Incompatibility between irinotecan and fluorouracil injections. Am J Health Syst Pharm. 2016;73(11):755. https://doi.org/10.2146/ajhp150664.
87. Allsopp MA, Sewell GJ, Rowland CG, Riley CM, Schowen RL. The degradation of carboplatin in aqueous solutions containing chloride or other selected nucleophiles. Int J Pharm. 1991;69(3):197–210. https://doi.org/10.1016/0378-5173(91)90362-R.
88. Benaji B, Dine T, Luyckx M, Brunet C, Goudaliez F, Mallevais ML, Cazin M, Gressier B, Cazin JC. Stability and compatibility of cisplatin and carboplatin with PVC infusion bags. J Clin Pharm Ther. 1994;19(2):95–100. https://doi.org/10.1111/j.1365-2710.1994.tb01118.x.
89. Myers AL, Zhang YP, Kawedia JD, Trinh VA, Tran H, Smith JA, Kramer MA. Stability study of carboplatin infusion solutions in 0.9% sodium chloride in polyvinyl chloride bags. J Oncol Pharm Pract. 2014;1(1):1–6. https://doi.org/10.1177/1078155214546016.
90. Cabrera VF, Suguimoto JCP, Dini AP, Cornélio ME, Lima MHM. Maintenance of central venous access devices permeability in cancer patients. Rev Enferm. 2019;27:e39230. https://doi.org/10.12957/reuerj.2019.39230.
91. Olsen M, LeFebvre K, Brassil K. Chemotherapy and immunotherapy guidelines and recommendations for practice. 1st ed. Pittsburgh: Oncology Nursing Society; 2019.
92. Martinho RFS, Rodrigues AB. Occurrence of phlebitis in patients on intravenous amiodarone. Einstein. 2008;6(4):459–62.
93. Gomes ACR, Silva CAG, Gamarra CJ, Faria JCO, Avelar AFM, Rodrigues EC. Assessment of phlebitis, infiltration and extravasation events in neonates submitted to intravenous therapy. Escola Anna Nery. 2011;15(3):472–9. https://doi.org/10.1590/S1414-81452011000300005.
94. Kim M, Seomun GA. Errors in high-risk intravenous injections administered by nurses: the causes according to healthcare professionals. Health Sci J. 2014;8(2):249–61.
95. Rocha FLR, Marziale MHP, Robazzi MLCC. Perigos potenciais a que estão expostos os trabalhadores de enfermagem na manipulação de quimioterápicos antineoplásicos: conhece-los para preveni-los. Rev Lat Am Enfermagem. 2004;12(3):511–7. https://doi.org/10.1590/S0104-11692004000300009.
96. Ferreira AR, Ferreira EB, Campos MCT, Reis PED, Vasques CI. Medidas de biossegurança na administração de quimioterapia antineoplásica: conhecimento dos enfermeiros. Rev Bras Cancerol. 2016;62(2):137–45.
97. Kwon P. Guide to handling cytotoxic drugs and related waste. Qld Nurse. 1997;16(4):22.

98. Polovich M. Safe handling of hazardous drugs. Online J Issues Nurs. 2004;9(3):6.
99. Conklin KA. Chemotherapy-associated oxidative stress: impact on chemotherapeutic effectiveness. Integr Cancer Ther. 2004;3(4):294–300.
100. Xelegati R, Robazzi MLCC, Marziale MHP, Haas VJ. Chemical occupational risks identified by nurses in a hospital environment. Rev Lat Am Enfermagem. 2006;14(2):214–9. https://doi.org/10.1590/S0104-11692006000200010.
101. Connor TH, Lawson CC, Polovich M, McDiarmid MA. Reproductive health risks associated with occupational exposures to antineoplastic drugs in health care settings: a review of the evidence. J Occup Environ Med. 2014;56(9):901–10. https://doi.org/10.1097/JOM.0000000000000249.
102. Boschi R, Rostagno E. Extravasation of antineoplastic agents: prevention and treatments. Pediat Rep. 2012;4(3):e28. https://doi.org/10.4081/pr.2012.e28.
103. Cavalcanti IDL, Santos RJ, Cordeiro RP. Evolução conceitual da biossegurança na manipulação de antineoplásicos. Electron J Pharm. 2016;13(1):6–17. https://doi.org/10.5216/ref.v13i1.31435.
104. Souza NR, Bushatsky M, Figueiredo EG, Melo JTS, Freire DA, Santos ICRV. Oncological emergency: the work of nurses in the extravasation of antineoplastic chemotherapeutic drugs. Escola Anna Nery. 2017;21(1):e20170009. https://doi.org/10.5935/1414-8145.20170009.
105. Cassagnol M, McBride A. Management of chemotherapy extravasations. US Pharm. 2009;34(9):3–11.
106. Al-Benna S, O'Boyle C, Holley J. Extravasation injuries in adults. ISRN Dermatol. 2013;2013:856541. https://doi.org/10.1155/2013/856541.
107. Park HJ, Kim KH, Lee HJ, Jeong EC, Kim KW, Suh DI. Compartment syndrome due to extravasation of peripheral parenteral nutrition: extravasation injury of parenteral nutrition. Korean J Pediatr. 2015;58(11):454–8. https://doi.org/10.3345/kjp.2015.58.11.454.
108. Kreidieh FY, Moukadem HA, El Saghir NS. Overview, prevention and management of chemotherapy extravasation. World J Clin Oncol. 2016;7(1):87–97. https://doi.org/10.5306/wjco.v7.i1.87.
109. Sakaida E, Sekine I, Iwasawa S, Kurimoto R, Uehara T, Ooka Y, Akanuma N, Tada Y, Imai C, Oku T, Takiguchi Y. Incidence, risk factors and treatment outcomes of extravasation of cytotoxic agents in an outpatient chemotherapy clinic. Jpn J Clin Oncol. 2014;44(2):168–71. https://doi.org/10.1093/jjco/hyt186.
110. Reynolds PM, MacLaren R, Mueller SW, Fish DN, Kiser TH. Management of extravasation injuries: a focused evaluation of noncytotoxic medications. Pharmacotherapy. 2014;34(6):617–32. https://doi.org/10.1002/phar.1396.
111. Kim JT, Park JY, Lee HJ, Cheon YJ. Guidelines for the management of extravasation. J Educ Eval Health Professions. 2020;17:21. https://doi.org/10.3352/jeehp.2020.17.21.
112. Martins EZ, Friedrich N, Gozzo TO, Prado MAS, Almeida AM. Complications in the venous network of women with breast cancer during chemotherapy treatment. Acta Paulista Enfermagem. 2010;23(4):552–6.
113. Fidalgo JAP, Fabregat LG, Cervantes A, Margulies A, Vidall C, Roila F. Management of chemotherapy extravasation: ESMO-EONS clinical practice guidelines. Ann Oncol. 2012;23(7):167–73. https://doi.org/10.1093/annonc/mds294.
114. Duque FLV, Chagas CAA. Intramuscular accident with drug injection in the deltoid muscle: local and distant lesions, review of 32 cases. J Vasc Bras. 2009;8(3):238–46. https://doi.org/10.1590/S1677-54492009000300009.
115. Roberto AFV. Lesões de extravasamento de terapêutica intravenosa com propriedades vesicantes. Lisboa: Universidade de Lisboa; 2014.
116. Goulart CB. Effectiveness of topical interventions to prevent or treat phlebitis-related to intravenous therapy: a systematic review and meta-analysis. Brasília: Universidade de Brasília; 2019.
117. Ener RA, Meglathery SB, Styler M. Extravasation of systemic hemato-oncological therapies. Ann Oncol. 2004;15(6):858–62. https://doi.org/10.1093/annonc/mdh214.

118. Schneider F, Pedrolo E. Extravasamento de drogas antineoplásicas: avaliação do conhecimento da equipe de enfermagem. REME Rev Mineira Enferm. 2011;15(4):522–9.
119. Gama CS, Nobre SMPC, Neusquen LPDG. Extravasamento de medicamentos antineoplásicos. São Paulo: Eurofarma; 2016.
120. Criado PR, Moure ERD, Sanches Júnior JA, Brandt HRC, Pereira GLS. Adverse mucocutaneous reactions related to chemotherapeutic agents – part II. An Bras Dermatol. 2010;85(5):591–608. https://doi.org/10.1590/S0365-05962010000500002.
121. Hecker JF. Failure of intravenous infusions from extravasation and phlebitis. Anaesth Intensive Care. 1989;17(4):433–9. https://doi.org/10.1177/0310057X8901700406.
122. Adami NP, Baptista AR, Fonseca SM, Paiva DRS. Extravasamento de drogas antineoplásicas – notificação e cuidados prestados. Rev Bras Cancerol. 2001;47(2):143–51.
123. Thakur JS, Chauhan CGS, Diwana VK, Chauhan DC, Thakur A. Extravasational side effects of cytotoxic drugs: a preventable catastrophe. Indian J Plast Surg. 2008;41(2):145–50.
124. Barbee MS, Owonikoko TK, Harvey RD. Taxanes: vesicants, irritants, or just irritating? Therap Adv Med Oncol. 2014;6(1):16–20. https://doi.org/10.1177/1758834013510546.
125. Wengstrom Y. Managing anthracycline extravasations and protecting tissue. Eur Oncol. 2009;5(1):14–6. https://doi.org/10.17925/EOH.2009.05.1.14.
126. Mulkerin DL, Bergsbaken JJ, Fischer JA, Mulkerin MJ, Bohler AM, Mably MS. Multidisciplinary optimization of oral chemotherapy delivery at the University of Wisconsin Carbone Cancer Center. J Oncol Pract. 2016;12(10):e912–23. https://doi.org/10.1200/JOP.2016.013748.
127. Silva AA, Carlotto J, Rotta I. Standardization of the infusion sequence of antineoplastic drugs used in the treatment of breast and colorectal cancers. Einstein. 2018;16(2):1–9. https://doi.org/10.1590/S1679-45082018RW4074.
128. FDA – Food and Drug Administration. Guidance for industry. Dosage and administration section of labeling for human prescription drug and biological products—content and format. Washington: US Department of Health and Human Services; 2011.
129. Goldspiel B, Hoffman JM, Griffith NL, Goodin S, DeChristoforo R, Montello M, Chase JL, Bartel S, Patel JT. ASHP guidelines on preventing medication errors with chemotherapy and biotherapy. Am J Health Syst Pharm. 2015;72(8):e6–e35.
130. Senapati S, Mahanta AK, Kumar S, Maiti P. Controlled drug delivery vehicles for cancer treatment and their performance. Signal Transduct Target Ther. 2018;3:7. https://doi.org/10.1038/s41392-017-0004-3.
131. Mendonça AB, Pereira ER, Magnago C, Barreto BMF, Goes TRP, Silva RM. Sequencing of antineoplastic drug administration: contributions to evidence-based oncology nursing practice. Rev Eletrôn Enfermagem. 2018;20:20–51. https://doi.org/10.5216/ree.v20.52232.
132. Palleria C, Paolo AD, Giofrè C, Caglioti C, Leuzzi G, Siniscalchi A, Sarro GD, Gallelli L. Pharmacokinetic drug-drug interaction and their implication in clinical management. J Res Med Sci. 2013;18(7):601–10.
133. Smith R, Wickerham DL, Wieand HS, Colangelo L, Mamounas EP. UFT plus calcium folinate vs 5-FU plus calcium folinate in colon cancer. Oncology. 1999;13(7):44–7.
134. Saif MW, Makrilia N, Syrigos K. CoFactor: folate requirement for optimization of 5-fluouracil activity in anticancer chemotherapy. J Oncol. 2010;2010:934359. https://doi.org/10.1155/2010/934359.
135. Boarman DM, Baram J, Allegra CJ. Mechanism of leucovorin reversal of methotrexate cytotoxicity in human MCF-7 breast cancer cells. Biochem Pharmacol. 1990;40(12):2651–60. https://doi.org/10.1016/0006-2952(90)90583-7.
136. Ortiz Z, Shea B, Almazor MS, Moher D, Wells G, Tugwell P. Folic acid and folinic acid for reducing side effects in patients receiving methotrexate for rheumatoid arthritis. Cochrane Libr. 2000;2:CD000951. https://doi.org/10.1002/14651858.CD000951.
137. Madhyastha S, Prabhu LV, Saralaya V, Rai R. A comparison of vitamin A and leucovorin for the prevention of methotrexate-induced micronuclei production in rat bone marrow. Clinics. 2008;63(6):821–6. https://doi.org/10.1590/S1807-59322008000600019.

138. Scripture CD, Figg WD. Drug interactions in cancer therapy. Nat Rev Cancer. 2006;6:546–58. https://doi.org/10.1038/nrc1887.
139. Ma CSJ. Role of pharmacists in optimizing the use of anticancer drugs in the clinical setting. Integr Pharm Res Pract. 2014;2014(3):11–24. https://doi.org/10.2147/IPRP.S40428.
140. Reinert CA, Ribas MR, Zimmermann PR. Drug interactions between antineoplastic and antidepressant agents: analysis of patients seen at an oncology clinic at a general hospital. Trends Psychiatry Psychother. 2015;37(2):87–93. https://doi.org/10.1590/2237-6089-2015-0003.
141. van As JW, van den Berg H, van Dalen EC. Different infusion durations for preventing platinum-induced hearing loss in children with cancer. Cochrane Libr. 2018;2018(7):CD010885. https://doi.org/10.1002/14651858.CD010885.pub4.
142. Rodrigues R. Ordem de infusão de medicamentos antineoplásicos – Sistematização de informações para auxiliar a discussão e criação de protocolos assistenciais. São Paulo: Atheneu; 2015.
143. How C, Brown J. Extravasation of cytotoxic chemotherapy from peripheral veins. Eur J Oncol Nurs. 1998;2(1):51–8. https://doi.org/10.1016/S1462-3889(98)81261-1.
144. Mokhtari RB, Homayouni TS, Baluch N, Morgatskaya E, Kumar S, Das B, Yeger H. Combination therapy in combating cancer. Oncotarget. 2017;8(23):38022–43. https://doi.org/10.18632/oncotarget.16723.
145. Falzone L, Salomone S, Libra M. Evolution of cancer pharmacological treatments at the turn of the third millennium. Front Pharmacol. 2018;9:1300. https://doi.org/10.3389/fphar.2018.01300.
146. Jardim DL, Gagliato DDM, Nikanjam M, Barkauskas DA, Kurzrock R. Efficacy and safety of anticancer drug combinations: a meta-analysis of randomized trials with a focus on immunotherapeutics and gene-targeted compounds. OncoImmunology. 2020;9(1):e1710052. https://doi.org/10.1080/2162402X.2019.1710052.
147. Dear RF, McGeechan K, Jenkins MC, Barratt A, Tattersall MHN, Wilcken N. Combination versus sequential single agent chemotherapy for metastatic breast cancer. Cochrane Libr. 2013;2013(12):CD008792. https://doi.org/10.1002/14651858.CD008792.pub2.
148. Morales ASR, Joy JK, Zbona DM. Administration sequence for multi-agent oncolytic regimens. J Oncol Pharm Pract. 2020;26(4):933–42. https://doi.org/10.1177/1078155219895070.
149. Voll ML, Yap KD, Terpstra WE, Crul M. Potential drug-drug interactions between anti-cancer agents and community pharmacy dispensed drugs. Pharm World Sci. 2010;32(5):575–80. https://doi.org/10.1007/s11096-010-9410-0.
150. Roell KR, Reif DM, Motsinger-Reif AA. An introduction to terminology and methodology of chemical synergy – perspectives from across disciplines. Front Pharmacol. 2017;8:158. https://doi.org/10.3389/fphar.2017.00158.
151. Stout NL, Wagner SS. Antineoplastic therapy side effects and polypharmacy in older adults with cancer. Topic Geriatr Rehabil. 2019;35(1):15–30. https://doi.org/10.1097/TGR.0000000000000212.
152. Bentley J, Heard K, Collins G, Chung C. Mixing medicines: how to ensure patient safety. Pharm J. 2015;294:7859. https://doi.org/10.1211/PJ.2015.20068289.
153. Murney P. To mix or not to mix – compatibilities of parenteral drug solutions. Aust Prescr. 2008;31(4):98–101. https://doi.org/10.18773/austprescr.2008.057.
154. Stanford BL, Zondor SD, Jumper CA. Chemotherapy administration sequences – review of the literature & administration recommendations. J Clin Oncol. 2005;23(16):6121. https://doi.org/10.1200/jco.2005.23.16_suppl.6121.
155. Cascorbi I. Drug interactions – principles, examples and clinical consequences. Dtsch Arzteblatt Int. 2012;109(33-34):546–56. https://doi.org/10.3238/arztebl.2012.0546.
156. Snyder BD, Polasek TM, Doogue MP. Drug interactions: principles and practice. Aust Prescr. 2012;35(3):85–8. https://doi.org/10.18773/austprescr.2012.037.
157. Jin J, Sklar GE, Oh VMS, Li SC. Factors affecting therapeutic compliance: a review from the patient's perspective. Ther Clin Risk Manag. 2008;4(1):269–86. https://doi.org/10.2147/tcrm.s1458.

158. Tariq RA, Vashisht R, Sinha A, Scherback Y. Medication dispensing errors and prevention. Treasure Island: StatPearls Publishing; 2021.
159. Oncology Working Party. Guideline on the clinical evaluation of anticancer medicinal products. Amsterdam: European Medicines Agency; 2021.
160. Minami H, Kiyota N, Kimbara S, Ando Y, Shimokata T, Ohtsu A, Fuse N, Kuboki Y, Shimizu T, Yamamoto N, Nishio K, Kawakami Y, Nihira SI, Sase K, Nonaka T, Takahashi H, Komori Y, Kiyohara K. Guidelines for clinical evaluation of anti-cancer drugs. Cancer Sci. 2021;112(7):2563–77. https://doi.org/10.1111/cas.14967.

Chapter 4
Chemotherapeutic Protocols for the Treatment of Breast Cancer

4.1 Breast Cancer: Epidemiology

Breast cancer is characterized by abnormal cells that multiply in a disorderly fashion, arising from cells lining (epithelium) in the ducts or lobes of the glandular tissue of the breast (Fig. 4.1) [1, 2]. There are a variety of types of breast cancer, where depending on the type, cancer can grow fast or slow [3, 4]. Despite being a tumor closely related to women, this cancer can also affect men, with an incidence of 1% concerning the total number of cases of the disease [5, 6].

It is cancer that has the highest incidence in women worldwide, where according to data from the World Health Organization (WHO) [7], 2.3 million women were diagnosed with breast cancer and 685,000 deaths worldwide. Figure 4.2 shows the incidence and mortality estimates for breast cancer in 2040. Some factors can increase the risk of developing breast cancer, such as age, obesity, family history, radiation exposure, excessive use of alcohol and tobacco, and postmenopausal hormone therapy, among others, but they are not determining factors since half of the women who develop breast cancer do not have any risk factors [6, 8].

Among the types of breast cancer, according to cell type, ductal is more prevalent, present in 85% of cases, and lobular in 15% [7]. Regarding the spectrum of abnormalities in the lobules and ducts, including hyperplasia, atypical hyperplasia, carcinoma in situ, and invasive carcinoma, infiltrating ductal carcinoma is the most common, representing 80–90% of all cases [9, 10]. Regarding the immunohisto-chemical classification of breast cancer, the most prevalent, according to the studies by Acheampong et al. [11] and Pandit et al. [12], was luminal A, followed by luminal B and human epidermal growth factor receptor type 2 (HER2) positive and triple-negative.

I. D. Lima Cavalcanti, *Chemotherapy Protocols and Infusion Sequence*,
https://doi.org/10.1007/978-3-031-10839-6_4

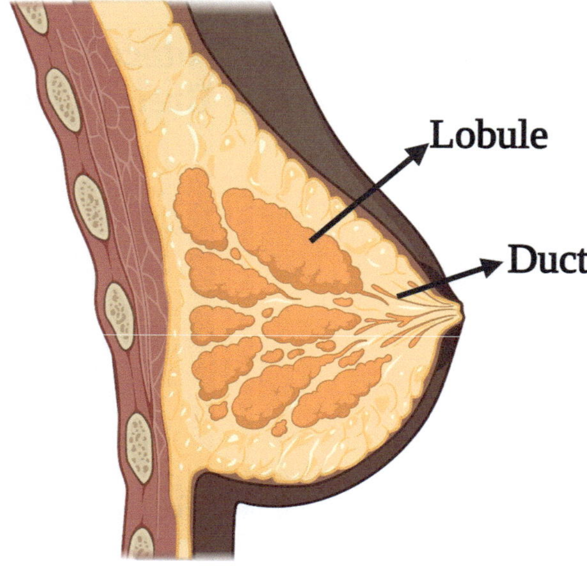

Fig. 4.1 Glandular tissue of the breast. Source: Created with BioRender.com

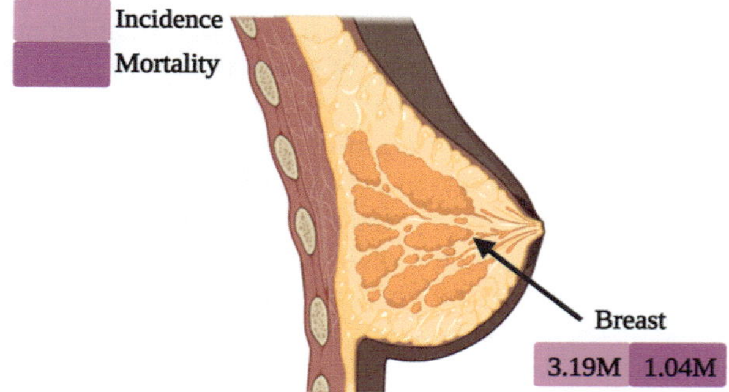

Fig. 4.2 Estimate of breast cancer incidence and mortality for the year 2040. Source: Created with BioRender.com. and data were extracted from [7]

4.2 Pathophysiology of Breast Cancer

DNA damage and genetic mutations are some of the factors that can contribute to the development of breast cancer. Exposure to estrogen can induce DNA damage, as well as familial inheritance of mutations in tumor suppressor genes such as *BRCA1*, *BRCA2*, and p53 that contribute to an increased risk of breast cancer [13–16].

Breast cancer can be classified as invasive or noninvasive, where noninvasive is classified as lobular carcinoma in situ and ductal carcinoma in situ [17, 18]. Lobular carcinoma in situ conforms to the contour of the normal lobule with expanded and filled acini, while ductal carcinoma in situ is more heterogeneous and can be classified as papillary, cribriform, solid, and comedo [18–20]. The papillary and cribriform types are lesions, generally low-grade, and may take longer to develop into invasive cancer, whereas the solid and comedo types are usually high-grade and if not treated can turn into invasive cancer [2, 20, 21].

Concerning invasive cancer, it can be classified as invasive lobular or invasive ductal cancer [22–24]. Invasive lobular carcinoma tends to permeate the breast in a single file, while invasive ductal carcinoma tends to grow as a cohesive mass, being easier to be detected by mammography and by palpating a smaller discrete lump in the breast than in lobular cancers [20, 23, 25].

After its local development, breast cancer can spread through regional lymph nodes and/or the bloodstream, affecting organs such as the lungs, liver, bones, brain, and skin (Fig. 4.3), where most cutaneous metastases occur in the region of breast surgery [26, 27].

There are other types of breast cancer that affect other types of breast cells, being less common cancers. Paget's disease initially occurs in the breast ducts and spreads to the skin of the nipple and areola, with a prevalence of 1–3% of breast cancer cases [2, 28–30]. Another type is angiosarcoma, which represents 1% of breast cancer cases, in which cancer starts in the cells lining blood or lymphatic vessels, and may involve the breast tissue or the skin of the breast [2, 31]. There is also a phylloid tumor, which develops in breast stromal cells, most of which are benign, but about a quarter are malignant [2]. Papillary carcinoma is also rare, accounting for less than 3% of all breast cancer cases, presenting as finger-like projections, where cancer cells are very small in size and form micropapillary cells [2, 32, 33].

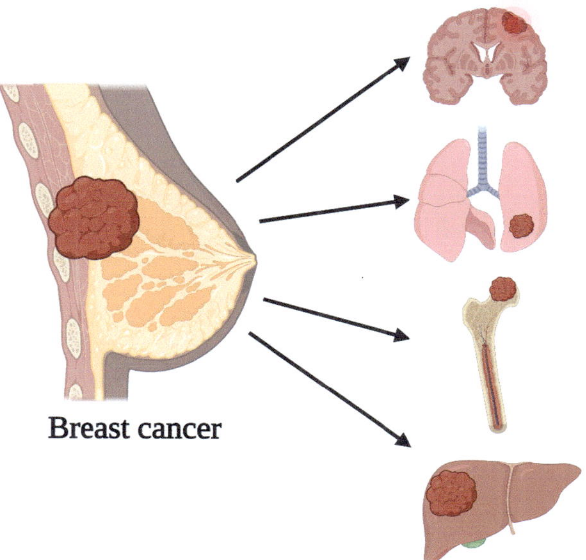

Fig. 4.3 Breast cancer with metastasis to the brain, lung, bone, and liver. Source: Created with BioRender.com

4.3 Molecular Subtypes of Breast Cancer

With the introduction of immunohistochemistry, it was possible to differentiate the molecular subtypes of breast cancer. Immunohistochemistry allows the detection of specific antigens and tissue immunophenotyping, allowing confirmation of the diagnosis, as well as the prognostic evaluation of the patient, as well as helping to choose the best therapeutic option for breast cancer [34–36]. Molecular subtypes of breast cancer include hormone receptors and other types of proteins involved or not involved in each cancer [37, 38]. Table 4.1 presents the breast cancer subtypes and their differences concerning the data obtained in immunohistochemistry.

Luminal type A cancer is the most common, generally slow-growing than other types of breast cancer, being popularly called hormone-positive due to the expression of positive hormone receptors for estrogen and progesterone [39, 42]. In addition, luminal A cancers have HER2-negative receptors; this receptor plays an important role in cell growth and repair; when a patient has a normal amount of HER2 protein, she will have HER2-negative breast cancer [43, 44].

Concerning luminal B cancers, they tend to grow faster than luminal A, being considered more aggressive, which are also positive for hormone receptors, as well as for a higher than normal amount of HER2; thus, they are hormone receptors and HER2 positive [37, 45]. As for triple-negative cancers, cells do not overexpress estrogen, progesterone, or HER2 receptors, being a more invasive cancer, starting in the breast ducts. Finally, the HER2-positive subtypes are cancers in which there is an overexpression of the HER2 receptor and hormone receptors are negative [46–48].

Table 4.1 Molecular subtypes of breast cancer according to immunohistochemistry

	ER	PR	HER2	ki67	ck 5/6	Aggressiveness
Luminal type A	+++	+	−	<15 or <20%	−	+
Luminal type B	++/+++	+/−	+/−	>15 or >20%	−	++/+++
HER2	−	−	+	>20%	−	+++
Basal-like	−	−	−	>20%	+	+++
Triple-negative	−	−	−	>20%	+/-	+++

ER estrogen receptor, *PR* progesterone receptor, *HER2* human epidermal growth factor receptor type 2, *ck5/6* cytokeratins 5 and 6, + low, ++ medium, +++ high
Source: [39–41]

4.4   Breast Cancer Treatment Modalities

There are several treatment modalities for breast cancer including surgery, radiation therapy, hormone therapy, chemotherapy, and targeted therapy. The choice of therapeutic modality will depend on the stage of the disease, as well as on the presence of receptors on the surface of cancer cells [49–51]. In the case of surgery, it can be of conservation, when the tumor is in situ or after neoadjuvant therapy to reduce tumor volume. Cancer cells that remain after surgery can be destroyed after radiation to reduce the risk of cancer recurrence [51–54].

The choice of hormone therapy is related to tumors that have hormone-positive receptors, whereas targeted therapy with trastuzumab or pertuzumab will depend on HER2 receptor overexpression [55–58]. In the case of patients with triple-negative cancer, the use of systemic chemotherapy is more indicated, as well as surgery and radiotherapy, as this type of cancer does not have specific receptors, making the use of hormone therapy and/or targeted therapy unfeasible [59, 60].

4.5   Adjuvant Chemotherapy

Adjuvant therapy occurs when the drug is administered after a surgical procedure to destroy cancer cells remaining from the surgical procedure or disseminated that cannot be visualized by imaging exams [50, 61, 62]. It is also considered adjuvant therapy when the administration is performed after radiotherapy treatment, being less common [63, 64].

Adjuvant therapy can consist of the administration of chemotherapy, hormone therapy, radiotherapy, immunotherapy, or targeted therapy, the choice of which will depend on the type of tumor and its stage [49, 65, 66]. The indication for adjuvant therapy will depend on the possibility of the patient presenting some microscopic focus of cancer cells, which is estimated based on the clinical presentation and the characteristics of the tumor [65, 67]. Below, we will discuss some protocols [68–70] used for the adjuvant treatment of breast cancer and their infusion sequence indications.

4.5.1   AC Protocol (Doxorubicin and Cyclophosphamide)

The AC protocol is based on the association of the drugs doxorubicin and cyclophosphamide, being one of the most used protocols in the treatment of breast cancer [71–73]. Doxorubicin is a cytotoxic antibiotic that belongs to the anthracycline class, being a drug with a vesicant characteristic [74, 75]. Doxorubicin is part of the group of nonspecific cycle drugs and has cardiotoxicity as limiting toxicity, which is dose-dependent and, when identified, is a factor for suspending the use of doxorubicin [76–79].

On the other hand, cyclophosphamide is a nitrogen mustard that acts through alkylation, being part of the class of alkylating agents, with an irritating characteristic [80–82]. Cyclophosphamide is not specific to the cell cycle phase, needing to be metabolized to its active form, which is capable of inhibiting protein synthesis through the crosslinking of DNA and RNA [82–84]. Regarding toxic effects, the greatest concern is with bladder and gonadal toxicity; in addition, it can cause cardiotoxicity, pulmonary toxicity, hepatic veno-occlusive disease, and secondary neoplasms [82, 85–87].

As for interactions, doxorubicin may have its metabolism increased when associated with cyclophosphamide. According to the study by Dodion et al. [88] when cyclophosphamide is administered before doxorubicin, there is an inhibition of the reduction of 7-deoxydoxorubicin aglycone to 7-deoxydoxorubicinol aglycone by microsomes. Doxorubicin and cyclophosphamide can alter the activities of a variety of drug-metabolizing enzymes through multiple mechanisms which are still unknown in humans [88, 89].

Elkiran et al. [89] evaluated the activity of enzymes responsible for drug metabolism after treatment with doxorubicin and cyclophosphamide, observing an increase in CYP1A2 activity by 20% and a decrease in CYP2C9 activity by 315% in 3 weeks after the administration of these drugs. Therefore, the safest order of administration for the AC protocol would be to start with doxorubicin, as it is a vesicant agent, thus reducing the risk of extravasation and avoiding the inhibition of its metabolism by the action of cyclophosphamide (Fig. 4.4) [90–92].

With the interaction between doxorubicin and cyclophosphamide in enzymes responsible for drug metabolism, it can delay drug excretion and increase the toxic profile [93–95]. Cyclophosphamide is a prodrug that needs to be metabolized in its activated form to have its pharmacological action and has been associated with the development of hemorrhagic cystitis [82, 96, 97]. Some studies report that the association between cyclophosphamide and doxorubicin increases the risk of developing hemorrhagic cystitis; another event that can also be increased is related to cardiotoxicity [95, 96, 98–100]. It is extremely important that when prescribing the AC protocol, doctors, nurses, and pharmacists monitor the possible toxic effects of the protocol.

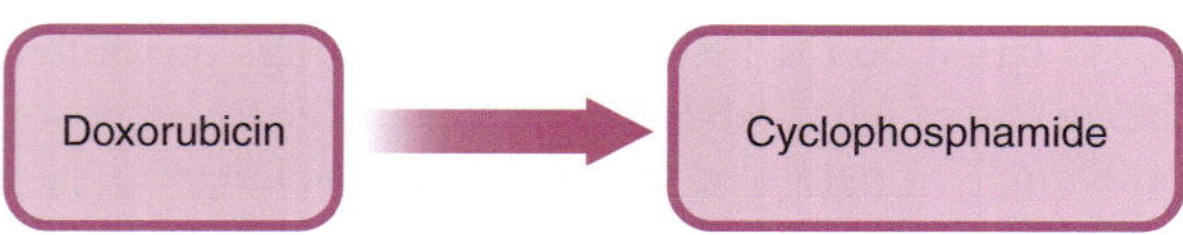

Fig. 4.4 AC protocol infusion sequence

4.5.2 ACT, T-AC, or AC-T Protocol (Doxorubicin, Cyclophosphamide, and Paclitaxel)

The ACT or AC-T protocol is similar to the AC protocol, where the difference is in the inclusion of paclitaxel that can be administered on the same day as doxorubicin and cyclophosphamide (ACT) or the AC-T protocol, where doxorubicin and cyclophosphamide are started, being generally applied for four cycles for 2 or 3 weeks, and after completion paclitaxel (AC-T) is started (Fig. 4.5). The scheme can also be inverted, where the physician chooses to start paclitaxel alone first and after the end of the cycles, AC (T-AC) is started (Fig. 4.6) [101, 102].

Paclitaxel is a natural product of the taxane class, which acts specifically in the M phase of the cell cycle, inhibiting the formation of microtubules, preventing their depolymerization, which is necessary for cell replication, thereby blocking cell division [103, 104]. As for dermatological toxicity, paclitaxel has an irritating characteristic [105]. Like doxorubicin and cyclophosphamide, paclitaxel is also metabolized by the cytochrome P450 enzyme, in addition to having high levels of plasma protein binding [92, 106].

Combining paclitaxel with cyclophosphamide may increase paclitaxel metabolism. According to the study by Martínez et al. [107], paclitaxel is metabolized by CYP3A4, forming its main metabolite 3'-p-hydroxypaclitaxel in colorectal cancer, thereby giving cancer cells the ability to inactivate paclitaxel. However, cyclophosphamide is metabolized by the enzyme CYP3A4 in its active form, and, when interacting with this enzyme, it can increase the metabolism of paclitaxel in the liver by the enzyme CYP2C8 [107, 108]. According to the study by Kaledin et al. [109], the association of cyclophosphamide with paclitaxel can add its antitumor effects in some tumors.

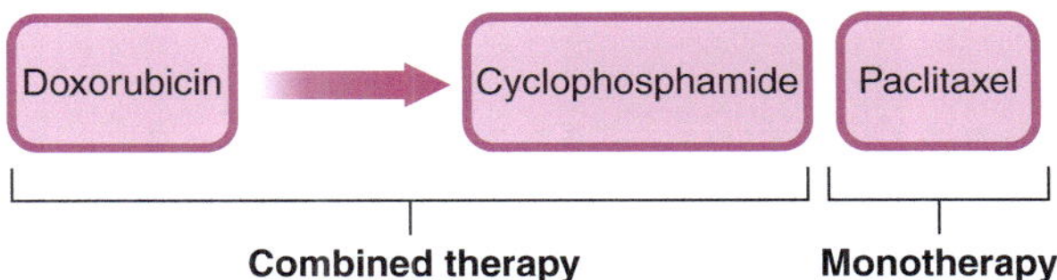

Fig. 4.5 AC-T protocol. Initially, doxorubicin and cyclophosphamide (AC) are administered, and after completion of the AC cycles, paclitaxel (T) is administered alone

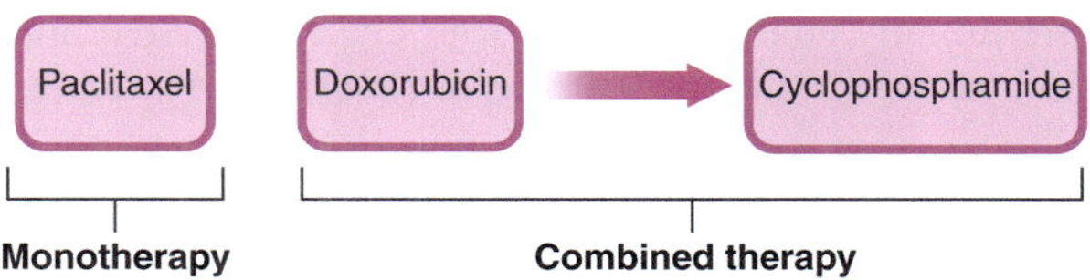

Fig. 4.6 T-AC protocol. Paclitaxel (T) is initially administered, and after completion of the cycles, doxorubicin and cyclophosphamide (AC) are administered in combination therapy

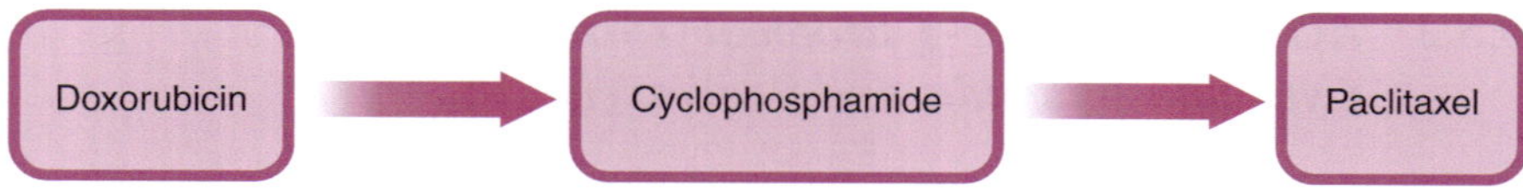

Fig. 4.7 Infusion sequence of the ACT protocol

Paclitaxel can be metabolized by the liver through the enzyme CYP2C8 to form the 6α-hydroxypaclitaxel metabolite, while metabolism through the enzyme CYP3A4 forms two smaller metabolites, 3-p-hydroxypaclitaxel and 6α,3′-p-dihydroxypaclitaxel [106, 110, 111]. As mentioned in the study by Martínez et al. [107], the inhibition of the activity of the enzyme CYP3A4 induces a decrease in the formation of the metabolite 3-p-hydroxypaclitaxel. In the case of doxorubicin, it induces a reduction in the main metabolite of paclitaxel, which is 6α-hydroxypaclitaxel, in human liver microsomes [112]. According to Perez [113], the association of doxorubicin with paclitaxel can induce congestive heart failure, where paclitaxel seems to decrease doxorubicin clearance by approximately 30% when the two drugs are administered in close succession.

Colombo et al. [114] demonstrated in their study that when paclitaxel is administered together with doxorubicin, it modifies the distribution and metabolism, thereby increasing the levels of doxorubicin in tissues, including the heart, thus increasing the cardiotoxicity of doxorubicin. Thus, although cyclophosphamide has a pharmacokinetic interaction with paclitaxel, its interaction with doxorubicin is more severe; therefore, it is preferable that cyclophosphamide be administered between doxorubicin and paclitaxel [101, 102, 113, 115]. Due to the vesicant characteristic of doxorubicin, it is preferable that it be administered first; therefore, the most suitable infusion sequence for the ACT protocol would be first doxorubicin followed by cyclophosphamide and finally paclitaxel, as shown in Fig. 4.7.

4.5.3 ACTT Protocol (Doxorubicin, Cyclophosphamide, Paclitaxel, and Trastuzumab)

The ACTT protocol is a protocol that combines doxorubicin, cyclophosphamide, paclitaxel, and trastuzumab, being used in the treatment of breast cancer in patients who have a positive HER2 receptor [116, 117]. Generally, doxorubicin and cyclophosphamide are initially administered for four cycles at 21-day intervals, following the infusion order of the AC protocol (Sect. 4.5.1), while paclitaxel is administered after the four cycles of the AC protocol, associated with trastuzumab [117, 118].

Trastuzumab is a monoclonal antibody that acts directly on cells that overexpress the HER2 receptor, so it is indicated only for patients who have positive HER2 immunohistochemistry [119, 120]. As for dermatological toxicity, it presents a non-vesicating characteristic [121]. As it is a monoclonal antibody, it can be immunogenic and should be administered as an infusion for 90 min to reduce

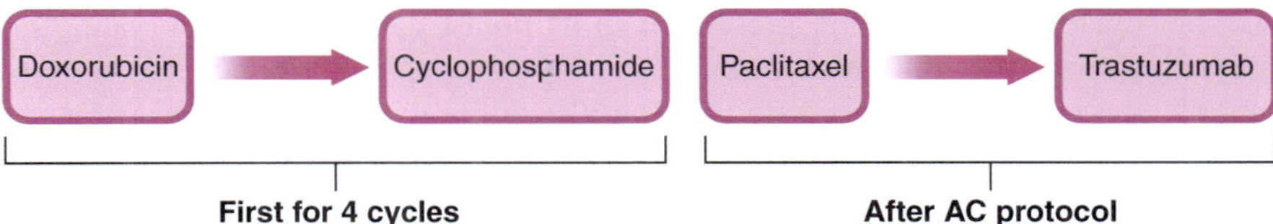

Fig. 4.8 ACTT protocol infusion sequence when trastuzumab is administered for the first time

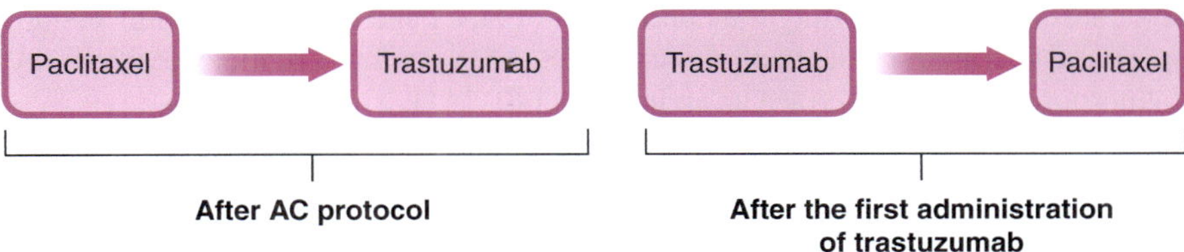

Fig. 4.9 Change in the order of trastuzumab infusion after the first administration of trastuzumab

damage if the patient presents immunogenicity during the infusion of the drug [122, 123].

The interaction of trastuzumab with paclitaxel seems to favor the antitumor action of both drugs [124, 125]. According to Diéras et al. [126], the combination of trastuzumab and paclitaxel showed additive and synergistic interactions, with an increase in the response rate of 41% when compared to monotherapy with paclitaxel (17%), also proving to be a well-tolerated regimen. Paclitaxel can increase the activity of trastuzumab, where in some cases it may be interesting to readjust the doses to avoid possible side effects due to the use of trastuzumab, such as cardiotoxicity, which when present is indicated to discontinue the use of trastuzumab [127, 128].

Given the information mentioned above, trastuzumab is a monoclonal antibody and can induce immunogenicity in some patients. The ideal would be to administer the trastuzumab last, after administration of paclitaxel, in case the patient is using it for the first time, with infusion in 90 min. In the case he develops an immunogenic reaction, it does not compromise the entire protocol (Fig. 4.8) [129, 130].

After the patient uses trastuzumab for the first time and has not developed an immunogenic reaction, trastuzumab can be administered initially (Fig. 4.9), with infusion within 30 min, as it is a specific cycle drug, allowing trastuzumab to act on cells with overexpression of HER2 and leaving other cancer cells susceptible to the action of paclitaxel [129, 130].

4.5.4   CMF Protocol (Cyclophosphamide, Methotrexate, and 5-Fluorouracil)

The CMF protocol is another protocol of choice for the treatment of adjuvant breast cancer, which is based on the combination of antineoplastic agents cyclophosphamide, methotrexate, and 5-fluorouracil [131–134]. As we saw in the previous section, cyclophosphamide is present in most breast cancer protocols, being an alkylating agent [82, 101]. Methotrexate and 5-fluorouracil are drugs of the antimetabolite class, where methotrexate is an antifolate drug with a structure similar to folic acid and acts by inhibiting the enzyme dihydrofolate-reductase, acting specifically in the S phase of cell division [135, 136]. As for dermatological toxicity, methotrexate is classified as a non-vesicating agent [137].

Regarding 5-fluorouracil, it, like methotrexate, is an antimetabolite agent, but it is a pyrimidine analog that acts by inhibiting the enzyme thymidylate synthetase and consequently preventing the duplication of DNA and cancer cells, thus being a specific S-phase drug-like methotrexate [138, 139]. As for dermatological toxicity, 5-fluorouracil is characterized as an irritant [140, 141].

Regarding drug interactions, according to Tattersall et al. [142], the combination of methotrexate and 5-fluorouracil reduces the efficacy of 5-fluorouracil, because methotrexate induces the accumulation of cellular deoxyuridylic acid, while 5-fluorouracil reduces the blockage of purine biosynthesis caused by methotrexate, thus being able to reverse the toxicity of methotrexate and also reduce its effectiveness. Despite these findings, the sequential administration of these drugs does not seem to induce these interactions. According to Benz et al. [143] and Pronzato et al. [144], sequential administration of methotrexate and 5-fluorouracil may result in synergistic antitumor activity. Sasaki [145] explains that the sequence-dependent synergism between these drugs may be related to the incorporation of 5-fluorouracil into RNA or due to more sustained inhibition of DNA synthesis by the two drugs.

According to Berne et al. [146], the administration of methotrexate followed by 5-fluorouracil induced an increase in the persistence of the active metabolite of 5-fluorouracil, 5-fluoro-2'-deoxyuridylate, which may be the mechanism of synergism of the drugs, but in relation to inhibition of thymidylate synthetase, they had antagonistic effects, being less effective in inhibiting this enzyme.

5-Fluorouracil also interacts with cyclophosphamide, where both compete for binding with plasma proteins, which can interfere with the distribution of these drugs in the body, delaying the therapeutic effect and even inducing toxicity [93, 147, 148]. As for methotrexate and cyclophosphamide, Bruijn et al. [149] reports that cyclophosphamide decreased the concentration-time curve of methotrexate. Given the data available so far, the infusion sequence that has been used in practice in the CMF protocol is 5-fluorouracil followed by methotrexate and cyclophosphamide (Fig. 4.10) [150].

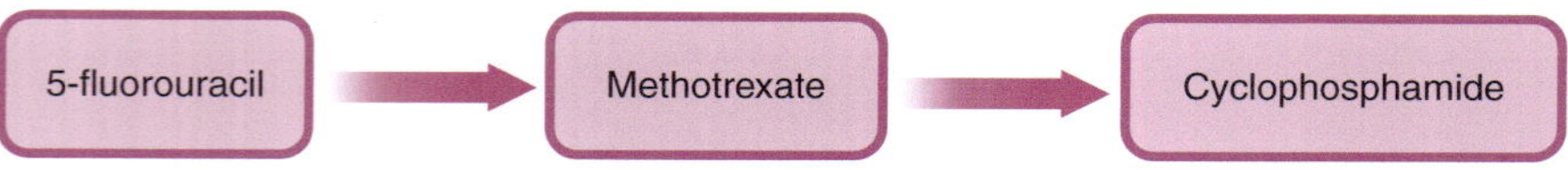

Fig. 4.10 Infusion sequence of the CMF protocol

4.5.5   *FAC Protocol (5-Fluorouracil, Doxorubicin, and Cyclophosphamide)*

The FAC protocol combined the drugs 5-fluorouracil, doxorubicin, and cyclophosphamide in the treatment of adjuvant breast cancer [151, 152]. Buzdar et al. [151] evaluated the efficacy of the FAC protocol as an adjuvant treatment in patients with stage II or III breast cancer. The results showed an estimated 10-year disease-free survival of 58 and 36% for stage II and III cancers, respectively. The combination has been shown to be effective in improving the disease and overall survival.

Martin et al. [153] compared the effectiveness of the FAC protocol followed or not by weekly paclitaxel in the treatment of breast cancer, as adjuvant therapy. Both regimens had similar results, but the inclusion of weekly paclitaxel was related to a small improvement in disease-free survival as well as controllable toxicity. Martin et al. [153] highlight the cases of cardiotoxicity, where seven patients in the study who received FAC died due to cardiovascular disease.

Tecza et al. [154] reported in their study that adverse events may be related to the interaction of the FAC protocol with polygenic inheritance and clinical risk factors. The identification of genes and their polymorphisms can be an alternative for the early intervention of possible adverse events, since some genes may be involved in the transport of drugs, their metabolism and DNA recognition, and repair and control of the cell cycle.

According to Pereira-Oliveira et al. [155], the cardiotoxicity of the FAC protocol is mainly related to the presence of doxorubicin, which is increasingly cardiotoxic. When comparing the cardiotoxicity of drugs alone and when combined, the authors observed that the cardiotoxicity profile of the FAC protocol was similar to that presented by doxorubicin alone. According to Volkova and Russell [77], the combination of doxorubicin with cyclophosphamide may increase the risk of cardiotoxicity, as cyclophosphamide also presents cardiotoxicity. Because of this possible increase in cardiotoxicity, perhaps an infusion order starting with doxorubicin followed by 5-fluorouracil and cyclophosphamide is more appropriate to reduce cardiotoxicity (Fig. 4.11).

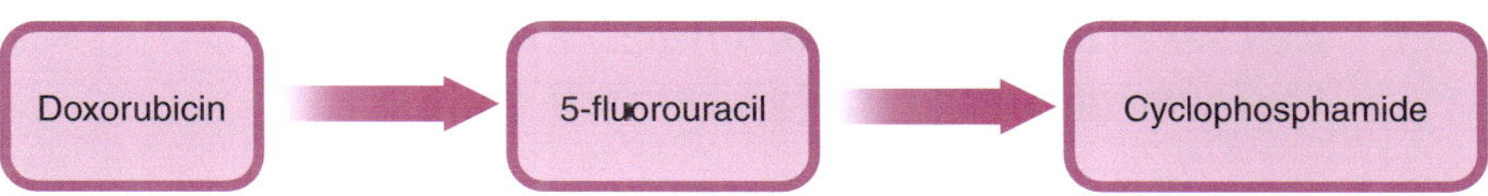

Fig. 4.11   FAC protocol infusion sequence

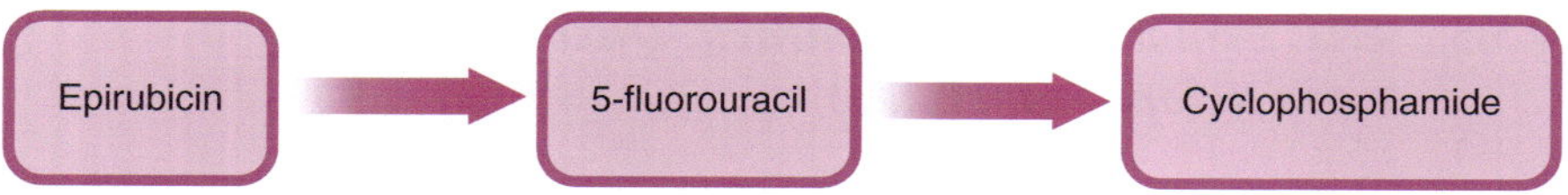

Fig. 4.12 FEC protocol infusion sequence

4.5.6 FEC Protocol (5-Fluorouracil, Epirubicin, and Cyclophosphamide)

Another protocol used in the adjuvant treatment of breast cancer is the FEC, which is based on a combination of the antineoplastic drugs 5-fluorouracil, epirubicin, and cyclophosphamide [156–158]. Epirubicin, like doxorubicin, is a cytotoxic antibiotic of the anthracycline class, acting specifically in the S phase of cell division, inhibiting DNA and RNA synthesis. It is a drug with dermatological toxicity with a vesicant characteristic [159, 160].

The limiting toxicity of epirubicin is cardiotoxicity; however, there are no reports that associated with cyclophosphamide, which also has cardiac toxicity, can increase the cardiotoxicity of the epirubicin [76, 79, 161–164]. The FEC protocol has shown a good therapeutic response in early breast cancer, as evidenced in the study by von Heideman et al. [158] who highlighted the benefits of the combination of epirubicin, 5-fluorouracil, and cyclophosphamide in primary cell cultures, showing synergistic and additive effects in cells extracted from breast cancer patients.

Burnell et al. [165] observe the benefits of the FEC protocol compared to other protocols, such as the AC-T, showing superior recurrence-free survival in the group that received the FEC. Regarding the toxicity profile, the most frequent ones are nausea and vomiting, stomatitis, and leukopenia [166]. As they do not have serious interactions that limit the use of the protocol, we can establish the infusion sequence according to the risk of extravasation and dermatological toxicity, starting the protocol with epirubicin, which is a vesicant; followed by 5-fluorouracil, which is irritating; and finally, cyclophosphamide which is non-vesicant (Fig. 4.12) [167, 168].

4.5.7 FEC-D Protocol (5-Fluorouracil, Epirubicin, Cyclophosphamide, and Docetaxel)

The FEC-D protocol is similar to the FEC protocol with the addition of docetaxel [169]. Docetaxel is a plant derivative of the taxane class, as well as paclitaxel, which acts specifically in the M phase of the cell cycle, inhibiting the formation of microtubules. As for dermatological toxicity, docetaxel has an irritating characteristic [170–173].

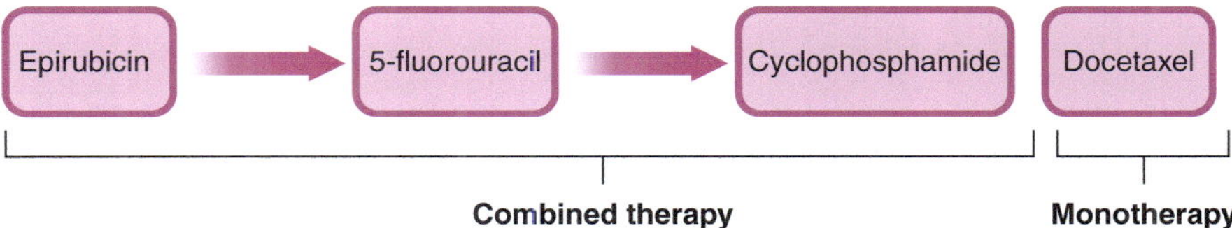

Fig. 4.13 FEC-D protocol infusion sequence

Ceruti et al. [174] evaluated the interaction of the combination between docetaxel and epirubicin, showing that a transient drug interaction occurs when docetaxel is infused for 1 hour after administration of epirubicin, leading to a transient increase in plasma epirubicin due to the maximum concentration of docetaxel. However, when administered during 10 min of infusion, there was no evidence of this interaction. Trying to verify an appropriate infusion sequence between epirubicin and docetaxel, Lunardi et al. [175] observed that regardless of the sequence chosen, it did not affect the pharmacokinetic profile of the drugs, nor the hematological and non-hematological toxicity profile.

Joensuu et al. [176] evaluated the effectiveness of the FEC protocol with the addition of docetaxel in the adjuvant treatment of breast cancer showing that docetaxel improved long-term disease-free survival. Martin et al. [177] also looked at the benefits of combining docetaxel with epirubicin and cyclophosphamide in early node-positive breast cancer. The administration regimen of the FEC-D protocol is generally based on the application of the FEC for three cycles with 21-day intervals, and after completion, the administration of docetaxel is started for three cycles with 21-day intervals. Thus, the order of infusion is similar to FEC, as the addition of docetaxel is only after completion of FEC (Fig. 4.13) [178].

4.5.8   FEC-DT Protocol (5-Fluorouracil, Epirubicin, Cyclophosphamide, Docetaxel, and Trastuzumab)

The FEC-DT protocol is based on the administration of the FEC protocol for three cycles at intervals of 21 days, and after completion, the administration of the DT starts [179]. The FEC infusion sequence remains in the order discussed in Sect. 4.5.5. Because it features the monoclonal antibody trastuzumab, this protocol is indicated for patients with HER2-positive breast cancer [92, 180]. The combination of trastuzumab with docetaxel had benefits in increasing the time to progression and response rate to breast cancer treatment [181]. According to Pegram et al. [127], the combination of trastuzumab with docetaxel causes a synergistic interaction.

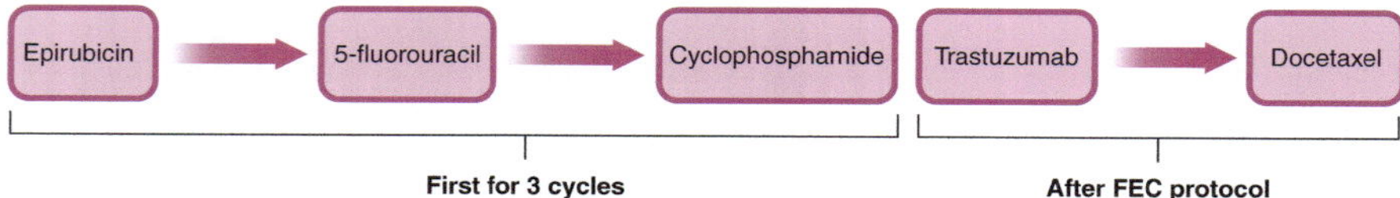

Fig. 4.14 FEC-DT protocol infusion sequence

Regarding the toxicity profile of the DT combination, there is an increase in adverse events characteristic of docetaxel, which include febrile neutropenia, neutropenia, and anemia, but the hematological toxicity profile was within manageable limits [181–183]. Non-hematological toxicity included diarrhea, fatigue, nausea and vomiting, neuropathy, dyspepsia, pruritus, thrombosis, and hyperglycemia, among others, remaining within reasonable occurrence rates [181, 182]. Regarding the cardiotoxicity of trastuzumab, studies are not conclusive that the combination with docetaxel may increase the cardiac toxicity of trastuzumab in the development of congestive heart failure [184–186].

The DT combination infusion sequence is preferred to start with trastuzumab as it is a target-directed drug followed by docetaxel (Fig. 4.14) [56, 116, 187]. However, it is important to know if the patient presents immunogenicity to trastuzumab, in which the first time of administration, it is chosen, for safety, to administer trastuzumab last [188, 189].

4.5.9   DAC (Docetaxel, Doxorubicin, and Cyclophosphamide) and DC (Docetaxel and Cyclophosphamide) Protocols

Another protocol widely used in the treatment of adjuvant breast cancer is DAC, which is a protocol similar to the ACT (Sect. 4.5.2), differing only in the replacement of paclitaxel by docetaxel, where both are from the same therapeutic class and have similar pharmacological profiles. The combination of these three drugs seems to bring important results for the treatment of breast cancer not only as an adjuvant treatment but also in advanced and metastatic cancer [190–193].

Nabholtz et al. [190] evidenced the benefits of the DAC protocol in their phase II study in patients with metastatic breast cancer, showing that the combination resulted in a response rate of 80%, and regarding toxicity, grade 4 neutropenia, febrile neutropenia, and grades 3 to 4 infection were observed, but cardiac toxicity was rare, with only one case of reversible congestive heart failure.

Bear et al. [194] evaluated the benefits of including docetaxel in the AC protocol in terms of the response rate to breast cancer and disease-free survival, with

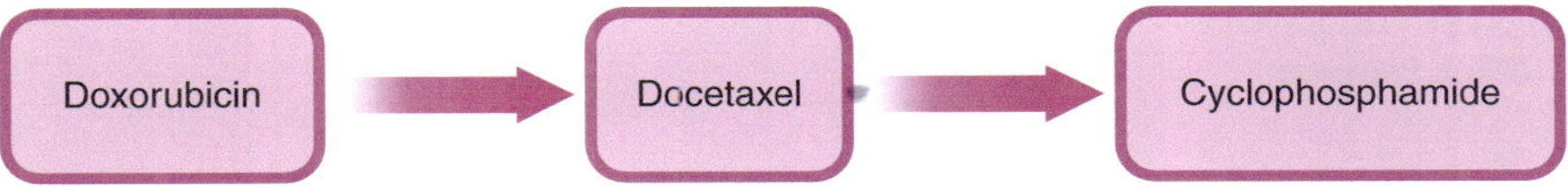

Fig. 4.15 Infusion sequence of the DAC protocol

preoperative or postoperative administration of docetaxel failing to identify significant improvement in disease-free survival, but observed a decrease in the incidence of local recurrences.

Older studies, such as the one by Colombo et al. [114], suggested the concern in combining docetaxel with doxorubicin, believing that the combination could increase the cardiotoxic effects of doxorubicin, but clinical studies such as those by Nabholtz et al. [190], Baltali et al. [195], and Bear et al. [194] show rare cases of cardiotoxicity. Zeng et al. [196] observed the interactions of docetaxel and doxorubicin in vitro, according to the sequence of administration, showing that doxorubicin, when administered before docetaxel, seems to interfere with mitotic arrest and cell death induced by docetaxel, with antagonistic effects. When docetaxel is given first, they did not observe an antagonistic effect, indicating that the combination is schedule-dependent and sequential exposure to docetaxel followed by doxorubicin would be the ideal regimen.

Itoh et al. [197], on the other hand, in their study with patients with advanced breast cancer, did not observe significant differences in the pharmacokinetic parameters related to the infusion sequence of doxorubicin and docetaxel, but with regard to toxicity. Administration of docetaxel followed by doxorubicin had a longer duration of grade 4 neutropenia than when doxorubicin was administered first. The authors recommend administering doxorubicin first followed by docetaxel. Given these data, perhaps the DAC protocol sequence with doxorubicin is interesting due to its vesicant characteristic, followed by docetaxel and cyclophosphamide (Fig. 4.15) [198].

Regarding the interactions between docetaxel and cyclophosphamide, it is related to metabolism, where cyclophosphamide needs to be metabolized to its active form in cytochrome P450, and docetaxel is also oxidized by cytochrome P450 enzymes, mainly by the enzyme CYP3A4 in the liver [199, 200]. It is believed that docetaxel can inhibit the biotransformation of cyclophosphamide, due to the study by Ando et al. [201] who suggested that docetaxel could inhibit the biotransformation of the prodrug ifosfamide, which is an analog of cyclophosphamide. However, the identified studies do not have clear evidence for an order of administration of these drugs. Because docetaxel is a cycle-specific drug, in addition to having an irritating characteristic, starting the DC protocol with docetaxel could bring greater benefit to the treatment (Fig. 4.16) [92, 202].

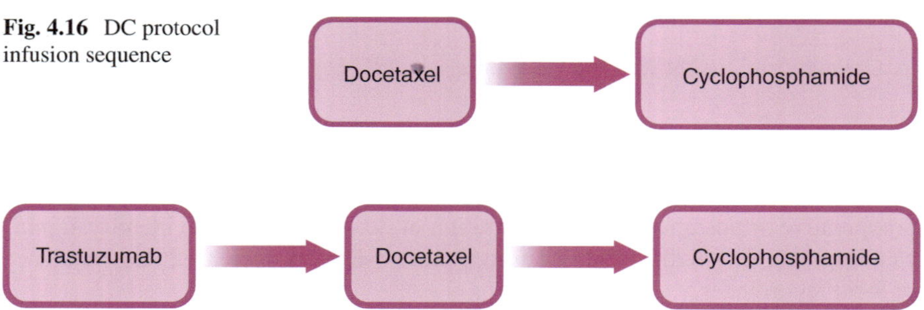

Fig. 4.16 DC protocol infusion sequence

Fig. 4.17 TDC protocol infusion sequence

4.5.10 *TDC Protocol (Trastuzumab, Docetaxel, and Cyclophosphamide)*

The TDC protocol is based on a combination of trastuzumab, docetaxel, and cyclophosphamide. As we saw in Sect. 4.5.7, it is believed that docetaxel can interact with cyclophosphamide inhibiting its biotransformation and therefore interfering with its activity, but there are no studies that prove this interaction. Given the specificity of the cell cycle, the option is to start with the target-specific agent, trastuzumab, which will act on cells with overexpression of the HER2 receptor, followed by docetaxel, which is a specific cycle drug, and cyclophosphamide (Fig. 4.17) [92, 202].

4.5.11 *DCARBT Protocol (Docetaxel, Carboplatin, and Trastuzumab)*

The DCARBT protocol combines docetaxel with carboplatin and trastuzumab, being a protocol also indicated for the adjuvant treatment of breast cancer in patients with HER-2 receptor overexpression [203–205]. Carboplatin is an antineoplastic in the class of platinum compounds that acts as an alkylating agent thereby inhibiting DNA synthesis [206]. It is a nonspecific cycle drug, which binds to plasma proteins and is rapidly excreted by the kidneys, thus presenting reduced renal and gastrointestinal toxicity, but with myelosuppressive toxicity [206, 207].

Eppler et al. [203] evaluated possible pharmacokinetic interactions between trastuzumab and carboplatin in the DCARBT protocol in the treatment of patients with HER2-positive metastatic inoperable solid tumors. The authors observed that the blood concentration of carboplatin remained independent of the presence or absence of trastuzumab, suggesting that there are no pharmacokinetic-type interactions between the drugs.

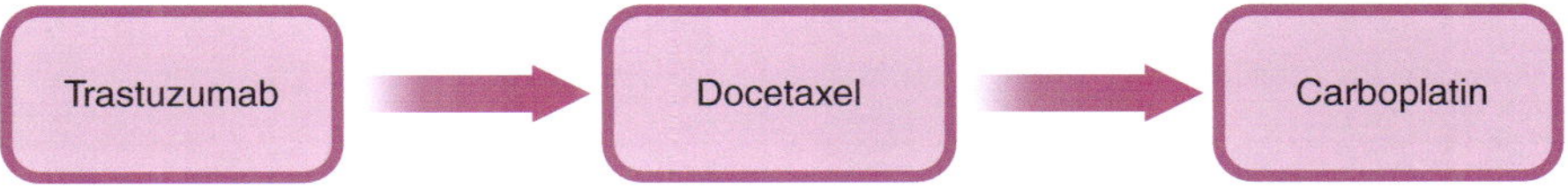

Fig. 4.18 Infusion sequence of the DCARBT protocol

Xu et al. [208] evaluated the possible cardiac toxicity of the combination of trastuzumab with carboplatin and docetaxel, noting that the combination did not prolong the QT interval of the electrocardiogram, and similarly to Eppler et al. [203], no pharmacokinetic interactions between drugs were observed either, thus evidencing the safety profile of this protocol.

According to the study by Wu and Xiong [205], the combination of trastuzumab, docetaxel, and carboplatin has high efficacy in the treatment of HER2-positive breast cancer, safety, and disease-free survival, and 5-year overall survival, in addition to a good effect on inflammation recovery, immune response, and oxidative stress. There are no reports of serious toxicity due to drug interactions in this protocol; therefore, the infusion sequence could start with the monoclonal antibody trastuzumab, as it is a target-specific drug, followed by docetaxel, which is a specific cycle drug, and finally carboplatin, which it is a nonspecific cycle drug (Fig. 4.18) [209].

4.6 Chemotherapy in Locally Advanced Breast Cancer

Locally advanced breast cancer is defined as patients with stage III disease and stage II patients with lymph node invasion, as well as patients with metastases limited to the ipsilateral supraclavicular lymph nodes (stage IV) [210–213]. The goal of treating locally advanced breast cancer is to achieve control of locoregional disease and the eradication of occult systemic metastases, so it requires a multimodal treatment including combinatorial chemotherapy, surgery, and radiotherapy [65, 214, 215].

The oncologist may indicate neoadjuvant chemotherapy, which precedes surgery, in order to reduce the size of tumors that are initially unresectable and become candidates for surgery [216–218]. After chemotherapy and surgery, it is important that patients receive radiotherapy to the breast or chest wall and draining lymphatic vessels. In addition, patients with hormone receptors should receive hormone therapy, and patients with HER2-positive receptors should receive treatment with target-directed therapy [6, 219–223].

Some protocols that were mentioned in the previous section (Sect. 4.5) can also be used in the treatment of locally advanced breast cancer, such as the DAC and ACT protocols [102, 191, 224, 225]. In the following sections, we discuss some chemotherapy protocols and their infusion sequences in the treatment of locally advanced breast cancer.

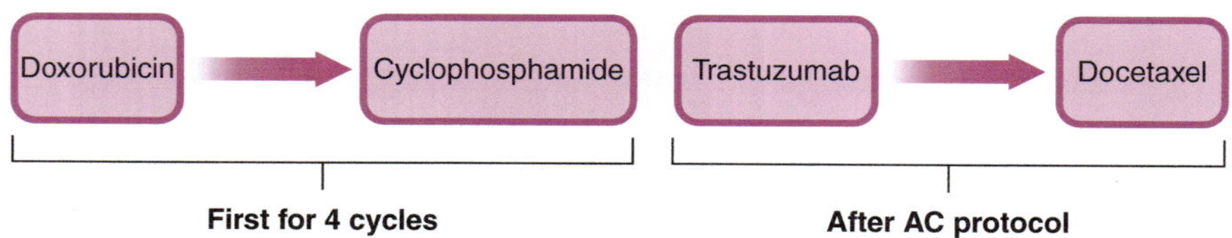

Fig. 4.19 AC-DT protocol infusion sequence

4.6.1   AC-DT Protocol (Doxorubicin, Cyclophosphamide, Docetaxel, and Trastuzumab)

The AC-DT protocol is a derivation of the DAC protocol (Sect. 4.5.7) with the inclusion of trastuzumab, indicated for patients with HER2-positive breast cancer. As there is the inclusion of trastuzumab, which is a drug that targets cells with HER2 overexpression, this monoclonal antibody has cardiotoxicity, as well as doxorubicin, which can increase the risk of developing cardiotoxicity if administered in combination [226–228]. Therefore, the ideal is to start the administration of the AC protocol, as we saw in Sect. 4.5.1, starting with doxorubicin, which is a vesicant, followed by cyclophosphamide for four cycles with intervals of 21 days [229].

In the fifth cycle, the AC protocol is interrupted to start the DT protocol, which is based on the combination of trastuzumab and docetaxel. The ideal is to start the protocol with the monoclonal antibody because it is target-directed, reinforcing that in the first cycle, the ideal is to end with trastuzumab in the case of patients who do not know if they will develop immunogenicity, as a form of safety [229, 230]. Figure 4.19 shows the order of infusion of drugs present in the AC-DT protocol.

4.6.2   CT-AC Protocol (Carboplatin, Paclitaxel, Doxorubicin, and Cyclophosphamide)

The CT-AC protocol is also divided into two phases, in which, in the first, the patient uses the drugs carboplatin and paclitaxel in combination for four cycles with 21-day intervals, and at the end, the AC protocol starts [231]. The combination of carboplatin and paclitaxel appears to demonstrate additive cytotoxic effect; furthermore paclitaxel also appears to reduce the risk of thrombocytopenia caused by carboplatin. However, the association of carboplatin with paclitaxel seems to increase myelosuppression [232, 233]. The combination can also increase the risks of neurotoxicity, from the induction of nerve damage, being a side effect of both drugs and can induce the development of weakness, numbness, pain, burning, or tingling in the hands, feet, or limbs [234–237].

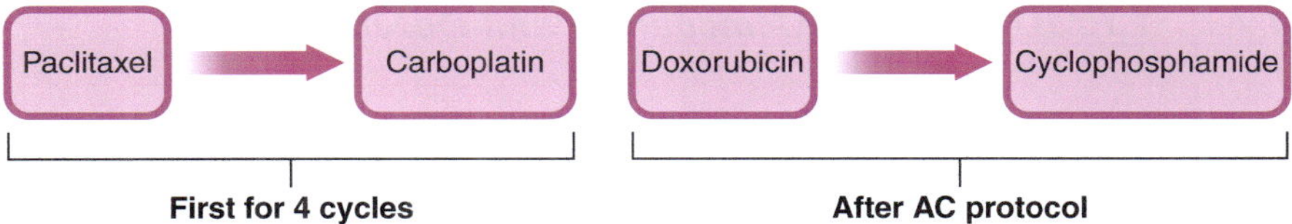

Fig. 4.20 CT-AC protocol infusion sequence

Despite the hematological toxicity and neurotoxicity of the combination, Pentheroudakis et al. [238] evaluated the effectiveness of the combination of paclitaxel and carboplatin in the treatment of advanced breast cancer, showing that the combination exhibits schedule-dependent synergistic effects of the combination with paclitaxel being administered first followed by carboplatin.

More recently, Yu et al. [239] demonstrated the efficacy of the combination of carboplatin and paclitaxel in the adjuvant treatment of operable triple-negative breast cancer, with improvements in the 5-year disease-free survival rate when compared to the combination of cyclophosphamide, epirubicin and 5-fluororuracil followed by docetaxel. Given this information and the information covered in Sect. 4.5.1, which talks about the AC protocol, Fig. 4.20 shows the infusion sequence for the CT-AC protocol [90–92, 238, 240].

4.7   Chemotherapy in Advanced Breast Cancer

Advanced or metastatic breast cancer is considered the latest stage of breast cancer, where the tumor has spread to other organs such as bones, lungs, brain, and liver, among other organs [6, 241–243]. There is currently no cure for advanced breast cancer, but there are many treatments available, which aim to prolong life and preserve the quality of life, seeking to relieve symptoms [244, 245].

Therapeutic modalities are diverse and may include chemotherapy, hormone therapy, radiotherapy, targeted therapy, and surgery [6, 65, 246]. Chemotherapy is usually based on monotherapy, and the antineoplastic drugs docetaxel, capecitabine, paclitaxel, abraxane, doxorubicin, gemcitabine, and high-dose methotrexate with leucovorin and vinorelbine can be administered as monotherapy, in addition to specific drugs for the therapy of hormonal positive breast cancer, such as anastrozole, tamoxifen, palbociclib, ribociclib, and fulvestrant, among others [247–250].

Some combination therapies used in other stages of breast cancer may also be indicated in the treatment of advanced breast cancer; examples are the AC and CMF protocols [101, 133, 251]. Some drugs that are not commonly used in the treatment of early and locally advanced breast cancer are included in protocols for the treatment of advanced breast cancer, such as gemcitabine and cisplatin [252–256]. In the following sections, we will address the main protocols used in advanced breast cancer and their infusion sequences.

4.7.1 GEMD Protocol (Gemcitabine and Docetaxel)

The GEMD protocol is a combination of the antineoplastic agents gemcitabine and docetaxel [257, 258]. Gemcitabine is a deoxycytidine nucleoside analogue that is incorporated into DNA during its replication, causing changes in DNA synthesis [259–262]. Gemcitabine is part of the class of antimetabolites, being cycle specific, acting in the S phase of the cell cycle, and its dermatological toxicity is characterized by being an irritant [262–264].

Many studies have shown the benefits of the combination of gemcitabine and docetaxel in the treatment of advanced breast cancer because they have different mechanisms of action, as well as partially nonoverlapping toxicity profiles and good activities as single agents [258, 265, 266]. Seidman [258] highlights in his study that the combination of gemcitabine and docetaxel in metastatic breast cancer produced a response rate of 36% to 79% in patients who received mainly second-line treatment, with a response rate greater than 50% in most of the studies that the author evaluated. As for the toxicity profile, Seidman [258] reports neutropenia as the primary combination-related toxicity.

Chan et al. [266] compared in a phase III study the effects of gemcitabine plus docetaxel with capecitabine plus docetaxel in patients with metastatic breast cancer who were pretreated with anthracycline, showing that there was no difference between the protocols in free survival data progression, overall response rate, and overall survival, as well as hematologic toxicity data. However, the results of non-hematological toxicity were significantly higher in patients who received capecitabine combined with docetaxel, with diarrhea, mucositis, and hand and foot syndrome, suggesting that the use of gemcitabine combined with docetaxel is a better option.

The combination of gemcitabine with docetaxel appears to have synergistic cytotoxicity when gemcitabine is administered before docetaxel. The GEMD protocol is based on the combination of drugs on day 1, and from day 2 to day 8, gemcitabine is administered alone [92, 267–270].

Alexopoulos et al. [257] evaluated the use of the combination of gemcitabine and docetaxel in patients with metastatic breast cancer after failure of treatment with docetaxel monotherapy, showing that the combination led to a high overall response rate and could be related to a synergistic action. In this study, the authors administered docetaxel before gemcitabine on day 8 of gemcitabine administration. Given the data from the study by Alexopoulos et al. [257], the introduction of the protocol with the infusion of docetaxel may bring benefits for the therapy of metastatic breast cancer (Fig. 4.21).

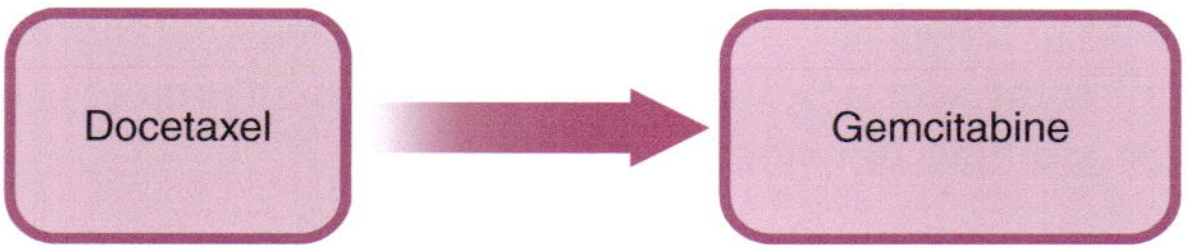

Fig. 4.21 GEMD protocol infusion sequence

4.7.2 GEMP Protocol (Gemcitabine and Cisplatin)

The combination of gemcitabine and cisplatin in the GEMP protocol has also been used for the treatment of advanced breast cancer [253, 271]. Cisplatin is part of the class of drugs composed of platinum, being one of the most used drugs in the treatment of cancer, where its activity is based on DNA alkylation and is also part of the class of alkylating agents [272–274]. Cisplatin is not cell cycle specific and may have a vesicant or irritant character depending on the extravasated dose [275–277].

Heinemann [252] highlights that the combination of gemcitabine, and cisplatin proved to be effective in the first-line treatment of breast cancer, with a response rate of 80% and an average response rate of 43%, with moderate toxicity that could induce thrombocytopenia and neutropenia. Zhang et al. [278] also demonstrate the benefits of the combination in the treatment of triple-negative metastatic breast cancer, with significant activity and a favorable safety profile. The results showed a progression-free survival of 7.2 months, overall survival of 19.1 months, and an overall response rate of 62.5%. Toxicity was also similar to that observed by Heinemann [252], with pictures of neutropenia, thrombocytopenia, anemia, and nausea and vomiting.

In a randomized phase III study, Hu et al. [279] highlight the benefits of the GEMP protocol compared to the combination of paclitaxel and gemcitabine for the first-line treatment of triple-negative metastatic breast cancer. According to Koshy et al. [253], the benefits of the GEMP protocol seem to be related to the treatment of triple-negative metastatic breast cancer with better results than when compared to the treatment of non-triple-negative breast cancer.

The combination of gemcitabine with cisplatin can be used as a rescue regimen for the treatment of breast cancer patients who have failed the use of anthracyclines and/or taxanes [280]. The results of the study by Chitapanarux et al. [280] showed an overall response rate of 51%, with a mean time to disease progression of 8.1 months and a mean response time of 4 weeks, with a toxicity profile similar to other studies with cases of thrombocytopenia and neutropenia.

According to Peters et al. [281], the interactions between cisplatin and gemcitabine in in vitro studies seem to be synergistic, while in in vivo studies, it seems to show at least additive effect, where the synergism will depend on the infusion schedule. Bergman et al. [282] believe that the synergistic effect between these drugs appears to be the result of the incorporation of the metabolite of gemcitabine into the DNA and/or the formation of a cisplatin adduct with the DNA.

Seeking to define the best schedule for the GEMP protocol, Kroep et al. [283] evaluated the administration of gemcitabine 4 h before cisplatin, cisplatin 4 h before gemcitabine, gemcitabine 24 h before cisplatin, and cisplatin 24 h before gemcitabine. The authors noted that myelosuppression was the main toxicity, where leukopenia was schedule dependent, where when gemcitabine is given before cisplatin, it appears to be less toxic. The infusion sequence, starting for gemcitabine, appears to be the most suitable, as gemcitabine is a specific cycle drug and can reduce the toxicity profile of the protocol (Fig. 4.22).

Fig. 4.22 GEMP protocol infusion sequence

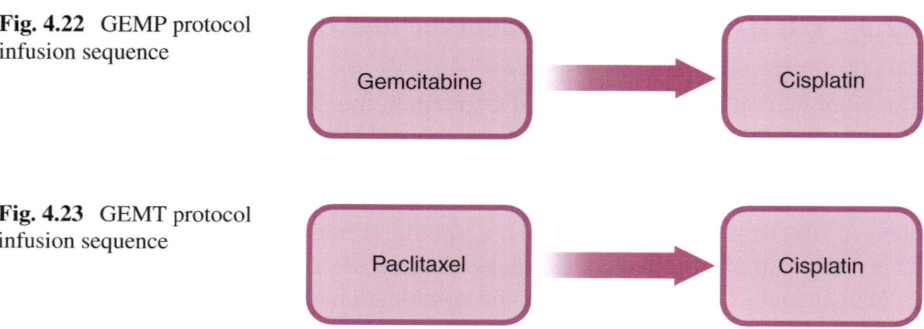

Fig. 4.23 GEMT protocol infusion sequence

4.7.3 GEMT Protocol (Gemcitabine and Paclitaxel)

The use of the GEMT protocol, a combination of gemcitabine and paclitaxel, may also be indicated for the treatment of advanced breast cancer [284–287]. The combination of drugs seems to have synergistic activity against metastatic breast cancer, in which the study by Colomer [284] reports that the use of the GEMT protocol as the first line presents a response rate higher than 71% compared to the use of the protocol in patients who had received previous chemotherapy, with a response rate of 46%. As for the toxicity profile, according to the study by Colomer [284], it has been low, with cases of rare neutropenia or non-hematological toxicity.

Allouache et al. [288], in a phase II study, observed the effectiveness of the GEMT protocol in recurrent or metastatic breast cancer, with tolerable toxicity as first-line therapy. The results showed a response rate of 40%, with a median duration of response of 12 months, the median time to progression of 7.2 months, and median survival of 25.7 months. As for the toxicity profile, cases of neutropenia, leukopenia, and alopecia were observed.

Albain et al. [289] highlight the importance of including gemcitabine combined with paclitaxel in the treatment of metastatic breast cancer in patients who had been previously treated with an anthracycline. The authors demonstrate that the inclusion of gemcitabine may be a reasonable choice, with increased median survival and manageable toxicity.

Rau et al. [286] also evaluated the efficacy of combined treatment with gemcitabine and paclitaxel in advanced breast cancer with the administration of paclitaxel before gemcitabine. The protocol was effective and safe with an overall response rate of 56%, median progression-free survival of 7.4 months and median overall survival of 19 months. Demiray et al. [290] also used in their study paclitaxel followed by gemcitabine in the treatment of metastatic breast cancer, proving to be an effective protocol with a controllable toxicity profile. Ahead of the studies, the infusion sequence starting with paclitaxel seems to bring benefits to patients with advanced breast cancer (Fig. 4.23).

4.7.4   PTRAD Protocol (Pertuzumab, Trastuzumab, and Docetaxel)

Another protocol indicated for the treatment of advanced HER2-positive breast cancer is PTRAD, which is based on a combination of the drugs pertuzumab, trastuzumab, and docetaxel [291–294]. Pertuzumab, like trastuzumab, is a monoclonal antibody that acts on cells that overexpress the HER2 receptor, acting on the extracellular domain of dimerization (subdomain II), thereby blocking HER2-dependent ligand heterodimerization with other members of the HER family, like HER1, HER3, and HER4, unlike trastuzumab which will act on the HER2 receptor subdomain IV (Fig. 4.24) [295, 296]. As it is a monoclonal antibody, it can also be immunogenic, and care must be taken during its administration, and it has a non-vesicating characteristic [56, 297, 298].

The combination of pertuzumab with trastuzumab has synergistic activity, where trastuzumab is preferentially active against tumors driven by HER2 homodimers, while pertuzumab prevents HER2 ligand-induced dimerization with HER3 and inhibits the activation of downstream cell signaling pathways, thereby preventing tumor growth [56]. According to the study by Swain et al. [291], the addition of pertuzumab in the treatment of HER2-positive metastatic breast cancer improved median overall survival to 56.5 months, with a median duration of response of 7.7 months, and median progression-free survival improved by 6.3 months.

The combination of pertuzumab, trastuzumab, and docetaxel significantly improved the response rate, from 39.3% to 21.8% with the inclusion of pertuzumab,

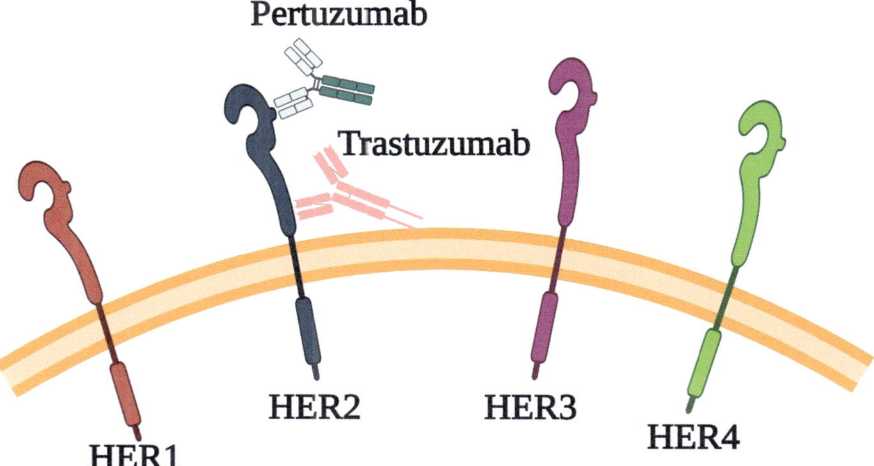

Fig. 4.24 Pertuzumab and trastuzumab double blockade at the HER2 receptor. Source: Created with BioRender.com

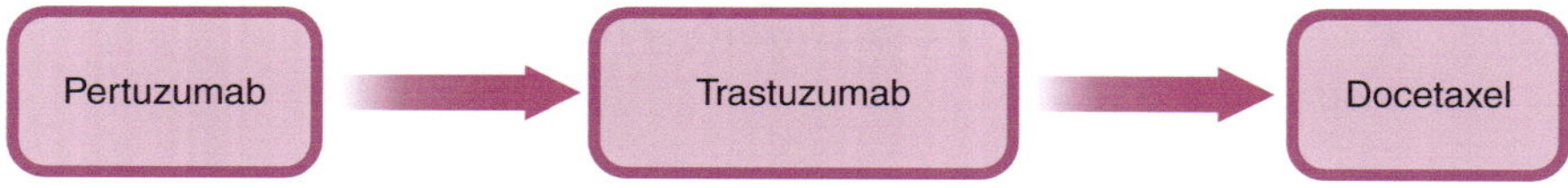

Fig. 4.25 PTRAD protocol infusion sequence

against early or locally advanced HER2-positive breast cancer. The most frequent adverse event was neutropenia [292].

In a phase III study, Swain et al. [293] observed similar results to other studies with a median overall survival of 57.1 months, an overall survival rate of 8 years, and the most common adverse event was neutropenia. This time, the authors observed the occurrence of one case of congestive heart failure and symptomatic left ventricular systolic dysfunction. Despite this, the results were promising, showing that this combination increased the overall 8-year survival rate with the double blockade of pertuzumab and trastuzumab.

Positive results were also presented in the study by Ramagopalan et al. [294], demonstrating data on overall survival of 48.6 months. As for the infusion sequence of the PTRAD protocol, the ideal is to start with target-directed therapy, starting with pertuzumab followed by trastuzumab to induce a double blockade of the HER2 receptor and finally docetaxel infusion (Fig. 4.25) [292, 299].

4.7.5 PTRAT Protocol (Pertuzumab, Trastuzumab, and Paclitaxel)

The PTRAT protocol is similar to the PTRAD protocol, differing only in the substitution of docetaxel for paclitaxel in the treatment of advanced HER2-positive breast cancer [300–302]. Smyth et al. [303] evaluated the use of weekly paclitaxel combined with trastuzumab and pertuzumab in metastatic breast cancer with HER2 overexpression. The authors noted that the combination led to the overall survival of 44 months, with a progression-free survival of 6 months being 86%, well-tolerated, and could be an alternative to therapy using docetaxel.

Wang et al. [301] also evaluated the use of weekly paclitaxel with trastuzumab and pertuzumab in patients with metastatic breast cancer with HER2-positive receptors, with a 5-year follow-up. The results showed that the protocol's efficacy was maintained for almost 5 years, providing a median progression-free survival of 24.2 months, but overall survival was not achieved. As for the toxicity profile, Gupta et al. [304] found that patients with HER2-positive breast cancer who received a neoadjuvant regimen had neutropenia, diarrhea, neuropathy, and a drop in left ventricular ejection fraction (LVEF) of more than 10%. Despite the toxicity profile that is acceptable compared to other protocols, the patients in the study had a complete pathological response of 41.6%. The infusion order of the PTRAT protocol can be

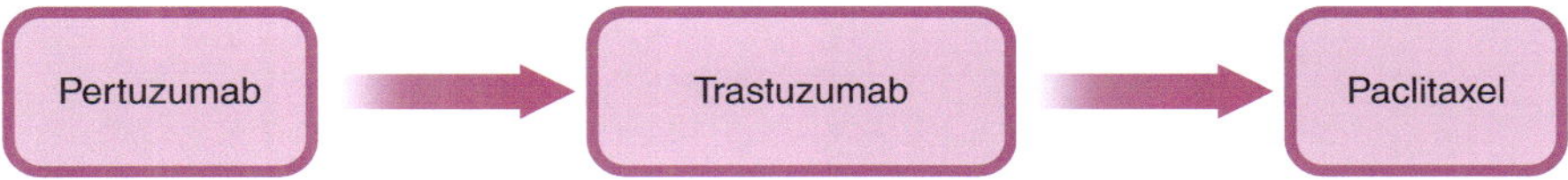

Fig. 4.26 PTRAT protocol infusion sequence

similar to the PTRAD protocol (Sect. 4.7.5) substituting docetaxel for paclitaxel (Fig. 4.26) [300, 301, 305].

4.7.6   TRVIN Protocol (Trastuzumab and Vinorelbine)

The combination of trastuzumab and vinorelbine may be an alternative for the treatment of advanced breast cancer [306, 307]. Vinorelbine is a plant derivative that belongs to the class of vinca alkaloids and is indicated for the treatment of various cancers. This drug is specific for the M phase of the cell cycle, as well as drugs from the taxane class, and it works by inhibiting the formation of microtubules. As for dermatological toxicity, vinorelbine is classified as a vesicant drug.

Suzuki et al. [306] evaluated the efficacy of the combination of vinorelbine and trastuzumab, showing that the combination led to a response rate of 42%, with manageable adverse events that included neutropenia, vasculitis, generalized fatigue, anemia, and thrombocytopenia. Burstein et al. [308] evaluated the combination in the treatment of metastatic breast cancer with HER2 overexpression as a first-line protocol. The authors noted that the TRVIN protocol achieved an overall response rate of 68% as the toxicity, two patients had cardiotoxicity above grade 1, and one patient had symptomatic heart failure. Despite this, the protocol proved to be effective and well-tolerated, requiring LVEF follow-up.

Stravodimou et al. [309] evaluated the contribution of vinorelbine when combined with trastuzumab in the treatment of metastatic breast cancer. The combination proved to be highly effective concerning overall survival and time to progression. Chan et al. [310] evaluated the efficacy and safety of the combination as first-line therapy for HER2-positive metastatic breast cancer, noting an overall response rate of 62.9%, meantime to the response of 8.4 weeks, the median duration of response of 17.5 months, and progression-free survival of 9.9 months. As for the toxicity profile, it was similar to those presented in the other studies with cases of neutropenia, febrile neutropenia, and one case of symptomatic cardiac dysfunction that led to the interruption of the protocol.

Burstein et al. [311] evaluated the response rate and toxicity profile with a weekly infusion of trastuzumab followed by vinorelbine in HER2-positive advanced breast cancer. The authors observed a response rate of 84% in patients who re-initiated the combination as first-line therapy, with a tolerable toxicity profile with neutropenia as the only grade 4 toxicity and grade 2 cardiotoxicity in three patients. The infusion

Fig. 4.27 TRVIN protocol infusion sequence

sequence starting with trastuzumab appears to have benefits for the treatment of advanced breast cancer (Fig. 4.27).

References

1. Hassiotou F, Geddes D. Anatomy of the human mammary gland: current status of knowledge. Clin Anat. 2012;26(1):29–48.
2. Feng Y, Spezia M, Huang S, Yuan C, Zeng Z, Zhang L, Ji X, Liu W, Huang B, Luo W, Liu B, Lei Y, Du S, Vuppalapatu A, Luu HH, Haydon RC, He TC, Ren G. Breast cancer development and progression: risk factors, cancer stem cells, signaling pathways, genomics, and molecular pathogenesis. Genes Dis. 2018;5(2):77–106. https://doi.org/10.1016/j.gendis.2018.05.001.
3. Kopans DB, Rafferty E, Georgian-Smith D, Yeh E, D'Alessandro H, Moore R, Hughes K, Halpern E. A simple model of breast carcinoma growth may provide explanations for observations of apparently complex phenomena. Cancer. 2003;97(12):2951–9. https://doi.org/10.1002/cncr.11434.
4. Alaidy Z, Mohamed A, Euhus D. Breast cancer progression when definitive surgery is delayed. Breast J. 2021;27(4):307–13. https://doi.org/10.1111/tbj.14177.
5. Yalaza M, Inan A, Bozer M. Male breast cancer. J Breast Health. 2016;12(1):1–8. https://doi.org/10.5152/tjbh.2015.2711.
6. Harbeck N, Penault-Llorca F, Cortes J, Gnant M, Houssami N, Poortmans P, Ruddy K, Tsang J, Cardoso F. Breast cancer. Nat Rev Dis Primers. 2019;5:66. https://doi.org/10.1038/s41572-019-0111-2.
7. WHO – World Health Organization. Estimated number of incident cases from 2018 to 2040. International Agency for Research on Cancer. 2020. Available https://gco.iarc.fr/tomorrow/graphic-isotype?type=0&type_sex=0&mode=population&sex=0&populations=900&cancers=36&age_group=value&apc_male=0&apc_female=0&single_unit=100000&print=0. Accessed Aug 5, 2021.
8. Olver IN. Prevention of breast cancer. Med J Aust. 2016;205(10):475–9. https://doi.org/10.5694/mja16.01007.
9. American Cancer Society. Breast cancer facts & figures 2019-2020. Atlanta: American Cancer Society, Inc.; 2019.
10. INCA – Instituto Nacional de Câncer. Controle do Câncer de Mama: Conceito e Magnitude, 2021. Available https://www.inca.gov.br/controle-do-cancer-de-mama/conceito-e-magnitude. Accessed July 24, 2021.
11. Acheampong T, Kehm RD, Terry MB, Argov EL, Tehranifar P. Incidence trends of breast cancer molecular subtypes by age and race/ethnicity in the US from 2010 to 2016. JAMA Netw Open. 2020;3(8):e2013226. https://doi.org/10.1001/jamanetworkopen.2020.13226.
12. Pandit P, Patil R, Palwe V, Gandhe S, Patil R, Nagarkar R. Prevalence of molecular subtypes of breast cancer: a single institutional experience of 2062 patients. Eur J Breast Health. 2020;16(1):39–43. https://doi.org/10.5152/ejbh.2019.4997.
13. Martin AM, Weber BL. Genetic and hormonal risk factors in breast cancer. JNCI. 2000;92(14):1126–35. https://doi.org/10.1093/jnci/92.14.1126.

14. Davis JD, Lin SY. DNA damage and breast cancer. World J Clin Oncol. 2011;2(9):329–38. https://doi.org/10.5306/wjco.v2.i9.329.
15. Shiovitz S, Korde LA. Genetics of breast cancer: a topic in evolution. Ann Oncol. 2015;26(7):1291–9. https://doi.org/10.1093/annonc/mdv022.
16. Petrucelli N, Daly MB, Pal T. *BRCA1*- and *BRCA2*-associated hereditary breast and ovarian cancer. In: GeneReviews. Seattle: University of Washington Seattle; 2016.
17. Sinn HP, Kreipe H. A brief overview of the WHO classification of breast tumors, 4th edition, focusing on issues and updates from the 3rd edition. Breast Care. 2013;8:149–54. https://doi.org/10.1159/000350774.
18. Makki J. Diversity of breast carcinoma: histological subtypes and clinical relevance. Clin Med Insights Pathol. 2015;8:23–31. https://doi.org/10.4137/CPath.S31563.
19. Boghaert E, Radisky DC, Nelson CM. Lattice-based model of ductal carcinoma *in situ* suggests rules for breast cancer progression to an invasive state. PLoS Comput Biol. 2014;10(12):e1003997. https://doi.org/10.1371/journal.pcbi.1003997.
20. Alkabban FM, Ferguson T. Breast cancer. Treasure Island: StatPearls Publishing; 2020.
21. Bane A. Ductal carcinoma *in situ*: what the pathologist needs to know and why. Int J Breast Cancer. 2013;2013:914053. https://doi.org/10.1155/2013/914053.
22. Dossus L, Benusiglio PR. Lobular breast cancer: incidence and genetic and non-genetic risk factors. Breast Cancer Res. 2015;17:37. https://doi.org/10.1186/s13058-015-0546-7.
23. Du T, Levine KM, Tasdemir N, Lee AV, Vignali DAA, Houten BV, Tseng GC, Oesterreich S. Invasive lobular and ductal breast carcinoma differ in immune response, protein translation efficiency and metabolism. Sci Rep. 2018;8:7205. https://doi.org/10.1038/s41598-018-25357-0.
24. Barroso-Sousa R, Metzger-Filho O. Differences between invasive lobular and invasive ductal carcinoma of the breast: results and therapeutic implications. Therap Adv Med Oncol. 2016;8(4):261–6. https://doi.org/10.1177/1758834016644156.
25. Kohler HF, Maciel MS, Collins JD, Rozenowicz RL, Netto MM. A multivariate analysis on prognostic factors for lobular carcinoma of the breast. Sao Paulo Med J. 2010;128(3):125–9. https://doi.org/10.1590/S1516-31802010000300004.
26. Bittencourt MJS, Carvalho AH, Nascimento BAM, Freitas LKM, Parijós AM. Cutaneous metastasis of a breast cancer diagnosed 13 years before. An Bras Dermatol. 2015;90(3):S134–7. https://doi.org/10.1590/abd1806-4841.20153842.
27. Al-Mahmood S, Sapiezynski J, Garbuzenko OB, Minko T. Metastatic and triple-negative breast cancer: challenges and treatment options. Drug Deliv Transl Res. 2018;8(5):1483–507. https://doi.org/10.1007/s13346-018-0551-3.
28. Karakas C. Paget's disease of the breast. J Carcinog. 2011;10:31. https://doi.org/10.4103/1477-3163.90676.
29. Lim HS, Jeong SJ, Lee JS, Park MH, Kim JW, Shin SS, Park JG, Kang HK. Paget disease of the breast: mammographic, US, and MR imaging findings with pathologic correlation. RadioGraphics. 2011;31:1973–87. https://doi.org/10.1148/rg.317115070.
30. Lopes Filho LL, Lopes IMRS, Lopes LRS, Enokihara MMSS, Michalany AO, Matsunaga N. Mammary and extramammary Paget's disease. An Bras Dermatol. 2015;90(2):225–31. https://doi.org/10.1590/abd1806-4841.20153189.
31. Cabral ANF, Rocha RH, Amaral ACV, Medeiros KB, Nogueira PSE, Diniz LM. Cutaneous angiosarcoma: report of three different and typical cases admitted in a unique dermatology clinic. An Bras Dermatol. 2017;92(2):235–8. https://doi.org/10.1590/abd1806-4841.20175326.
32. Trovisco V, Soares P, Preto A, Castro P, Máximo V, Sobrinho-Simões M. Molecular genetics of papillary thyroid carcinoma: great expectations. Arq Bras Endocrinol Metabol. 2007;51(5):643–53. https://doi.org/10.1590/S0004-27302007000500002.
33. Pal SK, Lau SK, Kruper L, Nwoye U, Garberoglio C, Gupta RK, Paz B, Vora L, Guzman E, Artinyan A, Somlo G. Papillary carcinoma of the breast: an overview. Breast Cancer Res Treat. 2010;122(3):637–45. https://doi.org/10.1007/s10549-010-0961-5.

34. Hawes D, Shi SR, Dabbs DJ, Taylor CR, Cote RJ. Immunohistochemistry. In: Modern surgical pathology. Amsterdam: Elsevier; 2009. p. 48–70. https://doi.org/10.1016/B978-1-4160-3966-2.00016-3.
35. Blows FM, Driver KE, Schmidt MK, Broeks A, van Leeuwen FE, Wesseling J, Cheang MC, Gelmon K, Nielsen TO, Blomqvist C, Heikkila P, Heikkinen T, Nevanlinna H, Pharoah PD. Subtyping of breast cancer by immunohistochemistry to investigate a relationship between subtype and short and long term survival: a collaborative analysis of data for 10,159 cases from 12 studies. PLoS Med. 2010;7(5):e1000279. https://doi.org/10.1371/journal.pmed.1000279.
36. Ramos EAS, Silva CT, Manica GCM, Pereira IT, Klassen LMB, Ribeiro SEM, Cavalli IJ, Braun-Prado K, Lima RS, Urban CA, Costa FF, Noronha L, Klassen G. Worse prognosis in breast cancer patients can be predicted by immunohistochemical analysis of positive MMP-2 and negative estrogen and progesterone receptors. Rev Assoc Med Bras. 2016;62(8):774–81. https://doi.org/10.1590/1806-9282.62.08.774.
37. Fragomeni SM, Sciallis A, Jeruss JS. Molecular subtypes and local-regional controlo f breast cancer. Surg Oncol Clin N Am. 2018;27(1):95–120. https://doi.org/10.1016/j.soc.2017.08.005.
38. Nascimento RG, Otoni KM. Histological and molecular classification of breast cancer: what do we know? Mastology. 2020;30:e20200024. https://doi.org/10.29289/25945394202020200024.
39. Cirqueira MB, Moreira MAR, Soares LR, Freitas-Júnior R. Subtipos moleculares do cancer de mama. Femina. 2011;39(10):499–503.
40. Barros ACSD, Leite KRM. Classificação molecular dos carcinomas de mama: uma visão contemporânea. Rev Bras Mastol. 2015;25(4):146–55. https://doi.org/10.5327/Z201500040006RBM.
41. Santos DMV, Silva LG, Pardi PC, Santos GAA, Segura MEA, Xavier JS. Breast carcinoma: molecular classification using immunohistochemistry. Saúde Coletiva. 2020;10(58):3863–74. https://doi.org/10.36489/saudecoletiva.2020v10i58p3863-3874.
42. Inic Z, Zegarac M, Inic M, Markovic I, Kozomara Z, Djurisic I, Inic I, Pupic G, Jancic S. Difference between luminal A and luminal B Subtypes according to Ki-67, tumor size, and progesterone receptor negativity providing prognostic information. Clin Med Insights Oncol. 2014;8:107–11. https://doi.org/10.4137/CMO.S18006.
43. Anderson DH. Chapter 1 – luminal A breast cancer resistance mechanisms and emerging treatments. In: Biological mechanisms and the advancing approaches to overcoming cancer drug resistance, vol. 12. Amsterdam: Elsevier; 2021. p. 1–22. https://doi.org/10.1016/B978-0-12-821310-0.00010-3.
44. Horvath E. Molecular subtypes of breast cancer – what beast imaging radiologists need to know. Rev Chil Radiol. 2021;27(1):17–26.
45. Dai X, Li T, Bai Z, Yang Y, Liu X, Zhan J, Shi B. Breast cancer intrinsic subtypes classification, clinical use and future trends. Am J Cancer Res. 2015;5(10):2929–43.
46. Anders C, Carey LA. Understanding and treating triple-negative breast cancer. Oncology. 2008;22(11):1233–43.
47. Yao H, He G, Yan S, Chen C, Song L, Rosol TJ, Deng X. Triple-negative breast cancer: is there a treatment on the horizon. Oncotarget. 2017;8(1):1913–24. https://doi.org/10.18632/oncotarget.12284.
48. Yin L, Duan JJ, Bian XW, Yu SC. Triple-negative breast cancer molecular subtyping and treatment progress. Breast Cancer Res. 2020;22:61. https://doi.org/10.1186/s13058-020-01296-5.
49. Abbas Z, Rehman S. Na overview of cancer treatment modalities. London: IntechOpen; 2018.
50. Arruebo M, Vilaboa N, Sáez-Gutierrez B, Lambea J, Tres A, Valladares M, González-Fernández A. Assessment of the evolution of cancer treatment therapies. Cancer. 2011;3(30):3279–330. https://doi.org/10.3390/cancers3033279.
51. Nounou M, ElAmrawy F, Ahmed N, Abdelraouf K, Goda S, Syed-Sha-Qhattal H. Breast cancer: conventional diagnosis and treatment modalities and recent patents and technologies. Breast Cancer Basic Clin Res. 2015;9(2):17–34. https://doi.org/10.4137/BCBCR.S29420.

52. Teshome M, Hunt KK. Neoadjuvant therapy in the treatment of breast cancer. Surg Oncol Clin N Am. 2014;23(3):505–23. https://doi.org/10.1016/j.soc.2014.03.006.

53. Magri KD, Bin FC, Formiga FB, Manzione TS, Gomes CMCN, Candelári PAP, Ortiz JÁ, Klug WA, Neto JM, Capelhuchnik P. Impact of neoadjuvant therapy in downstaging of lower rectal adenocarcinoma and the role of pelvic magnetic resonance in staging. Rev Col Bras Cir. 2016;43(2):102–9. https://doi.org/10.1590/0100-69912016002006.

54. Heil J, Kuerer HM, Pfob A, Rauch G, Sinn HP, Golatta M, Liefers GJ. Eliminating the breast cancer surgery paradigm after neoadjuvant systemic therapy: current evidence and future challenges. Ann Oncol. 2020;31(1):61–71. https://doi.org/10.1016/j.annonc.2019.10.012.

55. Prat A, Baselga J. The role of hormonal therapy in the management of hormonal-receptor-positive breast cancer with co-expression of HER2. Nat Rev Clin Oncol. 2008;5(9):531–42. https://doi.org/10.1038/ncponc1179.

56. Richard S, Selle F, Lotz JP, Khalil A, Gligorov J, Soares DG. Pertuzumab and trastuzumab: the rationale way to synergy. An Acad Bras Cienc. 2016;88(1):565–77. https://doi.org/10.1590/0001-3765201620150178.

57. Masoud V, Pagès G. Targeted therapies in breast cancer: new challenges to fight against resistance. World J Clin Oncol. 2017;8(2):120–34. https://doi.org/10.5306/wjco.v8.i2.120.

58. Wang J, Xu B. Targeted therapeutic options and future perspectives for HER2-positive breast cancer. Signal Transduct Target Ther. 2019;4:34. https://doi.org/10.1038/s41392-019-0069-2.

59. Collignon J, Lousberg L, Schroeder H, Jerusalem G. Triple-negative breast cancer: treatment challenges and solutions. Breast Cancer Targets Ther. 2016;8:93–107. https://doi.org/10.2147/BCTT.S69488.

60. Waks A, Winer EP. Breast cancer treatment: a review. JAMA. 2019;321(3):288–300. https://doi.org/10.1001/jama.2018.19323.

61. Chew HK. Adjuvant therapy for breast cancer. West J Med. 2001;174(4):284–7. https://doi.org/10.1136/ewjm.174.4.284.

62. Graham LJ, Shupe MP, Schneble EJ, Flynt FL, Clemenshaw MN, Kirkpatrick AD, Gallagher C, Nissan A, Henry L, Stojadinovic A, Peoples GE, Shumway NM. Current approaches and challenges in monitoring treatment responses in breast cancer. J Cancer. 2014;5(1):58–68. https://doi.org/10.7150/jca.7047.

63. Nazário ACP, Facina G, Filassi JR. Breast cancer: news in diagnosis and treatment. Rev Assoc Med Bras. 2015;61(6):543–52. https://doi.org/10.1590/1806-9282.61.06.543.

64. Chen JLY, Huang YS, Huang CY, Hsu CY, Lan KH, Cheng WF, Kuo SH. Impact of adjuvant radiotherapy on the survival of women with optimally resected stage III endometrial cancer in the era of modern radiotherapy: a retrospective study. Radiat Oncol. 2020;15:72. https://doi.org/10.1186/s13014-020-01523-5.

65. Moo TA, Sanford R, Dang C, Morrow M. Overview of breast cancer therapy. PET Clin. 2018;13(3):339–54. https://doi.org/10.1016/j.cpet.2018.02.006.

66. Miller KD, Nogueira L, Mariotto AB, Rowland JH, Yabroff R, Alfano CM, Jemal A, Kramer JL, Siegel RL. Cancer treatment and survivorship statistics. CA Cancer J Clin. 2019;69(5):363–85. https://doi.org/10.3322/caac.21565.

67. Riggio AI, Varley KE, Welm AL. The lingering mysteries of metastatic recurrence in breast cancer. Br J Cancer. 2021;124:13–26. https://doi.org/10.1038/s41416-020-01161-4.

68. Kuehr T, Thaler J, Woell E. Chemotherapy protocols 2017: current protocols and "targeted therapies". Klinikum Wels-Grieskirchen and Caritas Christi URGET NOS, Austria, 2017. www.chemoprotocols.eu.

69. BC Cancer. Supportive care protocols. BC Cancer, British Columbia, 2021. Available http://www.bccancer.bc.ca/health-professionals/clinical-resources/chemotherapy-protocols/supportive-care. Accessed July 2, 2021.

70. NHS. Chemotherapy protocols. NHS, University Hospital Southampton, NHS Foundation Trust, England, 2021. Available https://www.uhs.nhs.uk/HealthProfessionals/Chemotherapy-protocols/Chemotherapy-protocols.aspx. Accessed July 2, 2021.

71. Jones RL, Walsh G, Ashley S, Chua S, Agarwal R, O'Brien M, Johnston S, Smith IE. A randomised pilot Phase II study of doxorubicin and cyclophosphamide (AC) or epirubicin

and cyclophosphamide (EC) given 2 weekly with pegfilgrastim (accelerated) vs 3 weekly (standard) for women with early breast cancer. Br J Cancer. 2009;100(2):305–10. https://doi.org/10.1038/sj.bjc.6604862.

72. Clavarezza M, Mustacchi G, Gardini AC, Mastro LD, Matteis AD, Riccardi F, Adamo V, Aitini E, Amoroso D, Marchetti P, Gori S, Carrozza F, Maiello E, Giotta F, Dondi D, Venturini M. Biological characterization and selection criteria of adjuvant chemotherapy for early breast cancer: experience from the Italian observational NEMESI study. BMC Cancer. 2012;12:216. https://doi.org/10.1186/1471-2407-12-216.

73. Denduluri N, Chavez-MacGregor M, Telli ML, Eisen A, Graff SL, Hassett MJ, Holloway JN, Hurria A, King TA, Lyman GH, Partridge AH, Somerfield MR, Trudeau ME, Wolff AC, Giordano SH. Selection of optimal adjuvant chemotherapy and targeted therapy for early breast cancer: ASCO clinical practice guideline focused update. J Clin Oncol. 2018;36(23):2433–43. https://doi.org/10.1200/JCO.2018.78.8604.

74. Aubel-Sadron G, Londos-Gagliardi D. Daunorubicin and doxorubicin, anthracycline antibiotics, a physicochemical and biological review. Biochimie. 1984;66(5):333–52. https://doi.org/10.1016/0300-9084(84)90018-x.

75. Curtit E, Chaigneau L, Pauchot J, Nguyen T, Nerich V, Bazan F, Thiery-Vuillemin A, Demarchi M, Pivot X, Villanueva C. Extravasation of liposomal doxorubicin induces irritant reaction without vesicant injury. Anticancer Res. 2012;32(4):1481–3.

76. Floyd JD, Nguyen DT, Lobins RL, Bashir Q, Doll DC, Perry MC. Cardiotoxicity of cancer therapy. J Clin Oncol. 2005;23(30):7685–96. https://doi.org/10.1200/JCO.2005.08.789.

77. Volkova M, Russell R. Anthracycline cardiotoxicity: prevalence, pathogenesis and treatment. Curr Cardiol Rev. 2011;7(4):214–20. https://doi.org/10.2174/157340311799960645.

78. Bansal N, Adams MJ, Ganatra S, Colan SD, Aggarwal S, Steiner R, Amdani S, Lipshultz ER, Lipshultz SE. Cardio-Oncology. 2019;5:18. https://doi.org/10.1186/s40959-019-0054-5.

79. Cardinale D, Lacopo F, Cipolla CM. Cardiotoxicity of anthracyclines. Front Cardiovasc Med. 2020;7:26. https://doi.org/10.3389/fcvm.2020.00026.

80. Chen Y, Jia Y, Song W, Zhang L. Therapeutic potential of nitrogen mustard based hybrid molecules. Front Pharmacol. 2018;9:1453. https://doi.org/10.3389/fphar.2018.01453.

81. Lehmann F, Wennerberg J. Evolution of nitrogen-based alkylating anticancer agents. PRO. 2021;9:377. https://doi.org/10.3390/pr9020377.

82. Ogino MH, Tadi P. Cyclophosphamide. Treasure Island: StatPearls Publishing; 2021.

83. Zitvogel L, Apetoh L, Ghiringhelli F, Kroemer G. Immunological aspects of cancer chemotherapy. Nat Rev Immunol. 2008;8:59–73. https://doi.org/10.1038/nri2216.

84. Weber G. DNA damaging drugs. In: Molecular therapies of cancer. Cham: Springer; 2015. https://doi.org/10.1007/978-3-319-13278-5_2.

85. Jonge ME, Huitema ADR, Beijnen JH, Rodenhuis S. High exposures to bioactivated cyclophosphamide are related to the occurrence of veno-occlusive disease of the liver following high-dose chemotherapy. Br J Cancer. 2006;94:1226–30. https://doi.org/10.1038/sj.bjc.6603097.

86. Torrisi JM, Schwartz LH, Gollub MJ, Ginsberg MS, Bosl GJ, Hricak H. CT findings of chemotherapy-induced toxicity: what radiologists need to know about the clinical and radiologic manifestations of chemotherapy toxicity. Radiology. 2011;258(1):41–56. https://doi.org/10.1148/radiol.10092129.

87. Ponticelli C, Escoli R, Moroni G. Does cyclophosphamide still play a role in glomerular diseases? Autoimmun Rev. 2018;17(10):1022–7. https://doi.org/10.1016/j.autrev.2018.04.007.

88. Dodion P, Akman SR, Tamburini JM, Riggs CE Jr, Colvin OM, Bachur NR. Interactions between cyclophosphamide and doxorubicin metabolism in rats. II. Effect of cyclophosphamide on the aldoketoreductase system. J Pharmacol Exp Ther. 1986;237(1):271–4.

89. Elkiran T, Harputluoglu H, Yasar U, Babaoglu MO, Dincel AK, Altundag K, Ozisik Y, Guler N, Bozkurt A. Differential alteration of drug-metabolizing enzyme activities after cyclophosphamide/Adriamycin administration in breast cancer patients. Methods Find Exp Clin Pharmacol. 2007;29(1):27–32. https://doi.org/10.1358/mf.2007.29.1.1074690.

90. How C, Brown J. Extravasation of cytotoxic chemotherapy from peripheral veins. Eur J Oncol Nurs. 1998;2(1):51–8. https://doi.org/10.1016/S1462-3889(98)81261-1.

91. Rodrigues R. Ordem de infusão de medicamentos antineoplásicos – sistematização de informações para auxiliar a discussão e criação de protocolos assistenciais. São Paulo: Atheneu; 2015.

92. Silva AA, Carlotto J, Rotta I. Standardization of the infusion sequence of antineoplastic drugs used in the treatment of breast and colorectal cancers. Einstein. 2018;16(2):1–9. https://doi.org/10.1590/S1679-45082018RW4074.

93. van Leeuwen RWF, Swart EL, Boven E, Boom FA, Schuitenmaker MG, Hugtenburg JG. Potential drug interactions in cancer therapy: a prevalence study using an advanced screening method. Ann Oncol. 2011;22(10):2334–41. https://doi.org/10.1093/annonc/mdq761.

94. Tacar O, Sriamornsak P, Dass CR. Doxorubicin: an update on anticancer molecular action, toxicity and novel drug delivery systems. J Pharm Pharmacol. 2012;65(2):157–70. https://doi.org/10.1111/j.2042-7158.2012.01567.x.

95. Monteiro CRA, Schoueri JHM, Cardial DT, Linhares LC, Turke KC, Steuer LV, Menezes LWA, Argani IL, Sette C, Cubero DIG, Giglio A. Evaluation of the systemic and therapeutic repercussions caused by drug interactions in oncology patients. Rev Assoc Med Bras. 2019;65(5):611–7. https://doi.org/10.1590/1806-9282.65.5.611.

96. Ershler WB, Gilchrist KW, Citrin DL. Adriamycin enhancement of cyclophosphamide-induced bladder injury. J Urol. 1980;123(1):121–2. https://doi.org/10.1016/s0022-5347(17)55813-9.

97. Teles KA, Medeiros-Souza P, Lima FAC, Araújo BG, Lima RAC. Cyclophosphamide administration routine in autoimune rheumatic diseases: a review. Rev Bras Reumatol. 2017;57(6):596–604. https://doi.org/10.1016/j.rbre.2016.09.008.

98. Broder H, Gottlieb RA, Lepor NE. Chemotherapy and cardiotoxicity. Rev Cardiovasc Med. 2013;9(2):75–83.

99. Atalay F, Gulmez O, Ugurlu AO. Cardiotoxicity following cyclophosphamide therapy: a case report. J Med Case Rep. 2014;8:252. https://doi.org/10.1186/1752-1947-8-252.

100. Lobo RED, Bahia BPG, Silva GEA, Cruz LN, Sarges ES, Prete ACL, Carneiro TX, Ribeiro CHMA. Interação medicamentosa em pacientes com câncer: revisão integrativa da literatura. Braz J Dev. 2021;7(3):32289–303. https://doi.org/10.34117/bjdv7n3-784.

101. Anampa J, Makower D, Sparano JÁ. Progress in adjuvant chemotherapy for breast cancer: an overview. BMC Med. 2015;13:195. https://doi.org/10.1186/s12916-015-0439-8.

102. Mamounas EP, Bryant J, Lembersky B, Fehrenbacher L, Sedlacek SM, Fisher B, Wickerham DL, Yothers G, Soran A, Wolmark N. Paclitaxel after doxorubicin plus cyclophosphamide as adjuvant chemotherapy for node-positive breast cancer: results from NSABP B-28. J Clin Oncol. 2005;23(16):3686–96. https://doi.org/10.1200/JCO.2005.10.517.

103. Abal M, Andreu JM, Barasoain I. Taxanes: microtubule and centrosome targets, and cell cycle dependent mechanisms of action. Curr Cancer Drug Targets. 2003;3:193–203. https://doi.org/10.2174/1568009033481967.

104. Mukhtar E, Adhami VM, Mukhtar H. Targeting microtubules by natural agents for cancer therapy. Mol Cancer Ther. 2014;13(2):275–84. https://doi.org/10.1158/1535-7163.MCT-13-0791.

105. Criado PR, Brandt HRC, Moure ERD, Pereira GLS, Júnior JAS. Adverse mucocutaneous reactions related to chemotherapeutic agents: part II. An Bras Dermatol. 2010;85(5):591–608. https://doi.org/10.1590/S0365-05962010000500002.

106. Rodriguez-Antona C, Ingelman-Sundberg M. Cytochrome P450 pharmacogenetics and cancer. Oncogene. 2006;25:1679–91. https://doi.org/10.1038/sj.onc.1209377.

107. Martínez C, García-Martín E, Pizarro RM, García-Gamito FJ, Agúndez JAG. Expression of paclitaxel-inactivating CYP3A activity in human colorectal cancer: implications for drug therapy. Br J Cancer. 2002;87(6):681–6. https://doi.org/10.1038/sj.bjc.6600494.

108. Yang L, Yan C, Zhang F, Jiang B, Gao S, Liang Y, Huang L, Chen W. Effects of ketoconazole on cyclophosphamide metabolism: evaluation of CYP3A4 inhibition effect using the in vitro and in vivo models. Exp Anim. 2018;67(1):71–82. https://doi.org/10.1538/expanim.17-0048.

109. Kaledin VI, Nikolin VP, Popova NA, Pyshnaya IA, Bogdanova LA, Morozkova TS. Effect of paclitaxel on antitumor activity of cyclophosphamide: study on two transplanted tumors in mice. Bull Exp Biol Med. 2015;160(1):81–3. https://doi.org/10.1007/s10517-015-3103-6.

110. Desai PB, Duan JZ, Zhu YW, Kouzi S. Human liver microsomal metabolism of paclitaxel and drug interactions. Eur J Drug Metab Pharmacokinet. 1998;23(3):417–24. https://doi.org/10.1007/BF03192303.

111. Daily EB, Aquilante CL. Cytochrome P450 2C8 pharmacogenetics: a review of clinical studies. Pharmacogenomics. 2009;10(9):1489–510. https://doi.org/10.2217/pgs.09.82.

112. Bun SS, Ciccolini J, Bun H, Aubert C, Catalin EJ. Drug interactions of paclitaxel metabolism in human liver microsomes. J Chemother. 2013;15(3):266–74. https://doi.org/10.1179/joc.2003.15.3.266.

113. Perez EA. Doxorubicin and paclitaxel in the treatment of advanced breast cancer: efficacy and cardiac considerations. Cancer Investig. 2001;19(2):155–64. https://doi.org/10.1081/cnv-100000150.

114. Colombo T, Parisi I, Zucchetti M, Sessa C, Goldhirsch A, D'Incalci M. Pharmacokinetic interactions of paclitaxel, docetaxel and their vehicles with doxorubicin. Ann Oncol. 1999;10(4):391–5. https://doi.org/10.1023/a:1008309916974.

115. Henderson IC, Berry DA, Demetri GD, Cirrincione CT, Goldstein LJ, Ingle SMJN, Cooper MR, Hayes DF, Tkaczuk KH, Fleming G, Holland JF, Duggan DB, Carpenter JT, Frei E, Schilsky RL, Wood WC, Muss HB, Norton L. Improved outcomes from adding sequential paclitaxel but not from escalating doxorubicin dose in an adjuvant chemotherapy regimen for patients with node-positive primary breast cancer. J Clin Oncol. 2003;21(6):976–83. https://doi.org/10.1200/JCO.2003.02.063.

116. Slamon D, Eiermann W, Robert N, Pienkowski T, Martin M, Press M, Mackey J, Glaspy J, Chan A, Pawlicki M, Pinter T, Valero V, Liu MC, Sauter G, von Minckwitz G, Visco F, Bee V, Buyse M, Bendahmane B, Tabah-Fisch I, Lindsay MA, Riva A, Crown J. Adjuvant trastuzumab in HER2-positive breast cancer. N Engl J Med. 2011;365(14):1273–83. https://doi.org/10.1056/NEJMoa0910383.

117. NCT00004067. Doxorubicin and cyclophosphamide plus paclitaxel with or withour trastuzumab in treating women with node-positive breast cancer that overexpresses HER2. Clinical Trials. 2021. Available https://clinicaltrials.gov/ct2/show/study/NCT00004067. Accessed Aug 1, 2021.

118. Gelmon K. BC cancer protocol summary for neoadjuvant or adjuvant therapy for breast cancer using DOXOrubicin and cyclophosphamide followed by PACLitaxel and trastuzumab. BC Cancer, British Columbia. 2021. Available http://www.bccancer.bc.ca/chemotherapy-protocols-site/Documents/Breast/BRAJACTT_Protocol.pdf. Accessed Aug 1, 2021.

119. Spector NL, Blackwell KL. Understanding the mechanisms behind trastuzumab therapy for human epidermal growth factor receptor 2–positive breast cancer. J Clin Oncol. 2009;27(34):5838–47. https://doi.org/10.1200/JCO.2009.22.1507.

120. Gajria D, Chandarlapaty S. HER2-amplified breast cancer: mechanisms of trastuzumab resistance and novel targeted therapies. Expert Rev Anticancer Ther. 2011;11(2):263–75. https://doi.org/10.1586/era.10.226.

121. Tewari-Singh N, Agarwal R. Mustard vesicating agent-induced toxicity in the skin tissue and silibinin as a potential countermeasure. Ann N Y Acad Sci. 2016;1374(1):184–92. https://doi.org/10.1111/nyas.13099.

122. Guan M, Zhou YP, Sun JL, Chen SC. Adverse events of monoclonal antibodies used for cancer therapy. Biomed Res Int. 2015;2015:428169. https://doi.org/10.1155/2015/428169.

123. Jarvi NL, Balu-Iyer SV. Immunogenicity challenges associated with subcutaneous delivery of therapeutic proteins. BioDrugs. 2021;35:125–46. https://doi.org/10.1007/s40259-020-00465-4.

124. Griguolo G, Pascual T, Dieci MV, Guarneri V, Prat A. Interaction of host immunity with HER2-targeted treatment and tumor heterogeneity in HER2-positive breast cancer. J Immunother Cancer. 2019;7:90. https://doi.org/10.1186/s40425-019-0548-6.

125. Shu S, Tamashita-Kashima Y, Yanagisawa M, Nakanishi H, Kodera Y, Harada N, Yoshimura Y. Trastuzumab in combination with paclitaxel enhances antitumor activity by promoting apoptosis in human epidermal growth factor receptor 2-positive trastuzumab-resistant gastric cancer xenograft models. Anti-Cancer Drugs. 2020;31(3):241–50. https://doi.org/10.1097/CAD.0000000000000853.

126. Diéras V, Beuzeboc P, Laurence V, Pierga JY, Pouillart P. Interaction between herceptin and taxanes. Oncology. 2001;61(2):43–9. https://doi.org/10.1159/000055401.

127. Pegram MD, Lopez A, Konecny G, Slamon DJ. Trastuzumab and chemotherapeutics: drug interactions and synergies. Semin Oncol. 2000;27(6):21–5.

128. Merlin JL, Barberi-Heyob M, Bachmann N. In vitro comparative evaluation of trastuzumab (Herceptin®) combined with paclitaxel (Taxol®) or docetaxel (Taxotere®) in HER2-expressing human breast cancer cell lines. Ann Oncol. 2002;13(11):1743–8. https://doi.org/10.1093/annonc/mdf263.

129. Seidman AD, Fornier MN, Esteva FJ, Tan L, Kaptain S, Bach A, Panageas KS, Arroyo C, Valero V, Currie V, Gilewski T, Theodoulou M, Moynahan ME, Moasser M, Sklarin N, Dickler M, D'Andrea G, Cristofanilli M, Rivera E, Hortobagyi GN, Norton L, Hudis CA. Weekly trastuzumab and paclitaxel therapy for metastatic breast cancer with analysis of efficacy by HER2 immunophenotype and gene amplification. J Clin Oncol. 2001;19(10):2587–95. https://doi.org/10.1200/JCO.2001.19.10.2587.

130. Hasmann. Chapter 9 – targeting HER2 by monoclonal antibodies for cancer therapy. In: Introduction to biological and small molecule drug research and development. Amsterdam: Elsevier; 2013. p. 283–305. https://doi.org/10.1016/B978-0-12-397176-0.00009-1.

131. Tormey DC, Gray R, Gilchrist K, Grage T, Carbone PP, Wolter J, Woll JE, Cummings FJ. Adjuvant chemohormonal therapy with cyclophosphamide, methotrexate, 5-fluorouracil, and prednisone (CMFP) or CMFP plus tamoxifen compared with CMF for premenopausal breast cancer patients. An Eastern Cooperative Oncology Group trial. Cancer. 1990;65(2):200–6.

132. Bonadonna G, Valagussa P, Moliterni A, Zambetti M, Brambilla C. Adjuvant cyclophosphamide, methotrexate, and fluorouracil in node-positive breast cancer – the results of 20 years of follow-up. N Engl J Med. 1995;332:901–6. https://doi.org/10.1056/NEJM199504063321401.

133. Fujii T, Du FL, Xiao L, Kogawa T, Barcenas CH, Alvarez RH, Valero V, Shen Y, Ueno NT. Effectiveness of an adjuvant chemotherapy regimen for early-stage breast cancer: a systematic review and network meta-analysis. JAMA Oncol. 2015;1(9):1311–8. https://doi.org/10.1001/jamaoncol.2015.3062.

134. NCT00615901. Dose dense adjuvant CMG (cyclophosphamide, methotrexate, fluorouracil) at 14 and 10-11 day intervals for women with early stage breast cancer. Clinical Trials. 2017. Available https://clinicaltrials.gov/c:2/show/NCT00615901. Accessed Aug 2, 2021.

135. McGuire JJ. Anticancer antifolates: current status and future directions. Curr Pharm Des. 2003;9(31):2593–613. https://doi.org/10.2174/1381612033453712.

136. Kozminski P, Halik PK, Chesori R, Gniazdowska E. Overview of dual-acting drug methotrexate in different neurological diseases, autoimmune pathologies and cancers. Int J Mol Sci. 2020;21(10):3483. https://doi.org/10.3390/ijms21103483.

137. Souza CFD, Suarez OMZ, Silva TFM, Gorenstein ACLA, Quintella LP, Avelleira JCR. Ulcerations due to methotrexate toxicity in a psoriasis patient. An Bras Dermatol. 2016;91(3):375–7. https://doi.org/10.1590/abd1806-4841.20163960.

138. Mellor HR, Callaghan R. Resistance to chemotherapy in cancer: a complex and integrated cellular response. Pharmacology. 2008;81:275–300. https://doi.org/10.1159/000115967.

139. Zhang N, Yin Y, Xu SJ, Chen WS. 5-fluorouracil: mechanisms of resistance and reversal strategies. Molecules. 2008;13(8):1551–69. https://doi.org/10.3390/molecules13081551.

140. Hussain A, Samad A, Ramzan M, Ahsan MN, Rehman ZU, Ahmad FJ. Elastic liposome-based gel for topical delivery of 5-fluorouracil: in vitro and in vivo investigation. Drug Deliv. 2016;23(4):1115–29. https://doi.org/10.3109/10717544.2014.976891.

141. Lacouture ME, Sibaud V, Gerber PA, van den Hurk C, Fernández-Peñas P, Santini D, Jahn F, Jordan K. Prevention and management of dermatological toxicities related to anticancer agents: ESMO clinical practice guidelines. Ann Oncol. 2020;32(2):157–70. https://doi.org/10.1016/j.annonc.2020.11.005.

142. Tattersall MHN, Jackson RC, Connors TA, Harrap KR. Combination chemotherapy: the interaction of methotrexate and 5-fluorouracil. Eur J Cancer. 1973;9(10):733–9. https://doi.org/10.1016/0014-2964(73)90064-9.

143. Benz C, DeGregorio M, Saks S, Sambol N, Holleran W, Ignoffo R, Lewis B, Cadman E. Sequential infusions of methotrexate and 5-fluorouracil in advanced cancer: pharmacology, toxicity, and response. Cancer Res. 1985;45:3354–8.

144. Pronzato P, Amoroso D, Ardizzoni A, Bertelli G, Canobbio L, Conte PF, Cusimano MP, Fusco V, Gulisano M, Lionetto R, Repetto L, Rosso R. Sequential administration of cyclophosphamide, methotrexate, 5-fluorouracil, and folinic acid as salvage treatment in metastatic breast cancer. Am J Clin Oncol. 1987;10(5):404–6. https://doi.org/10.1097/00000421-198710000-00007.

145. Sasaki T. Sequential methotrexate and 5-fluorouracil. Gan To Kagaku Ryoho. 1996;23(14):1907–10.

146. Berne MHO, Gustavsson BG, Almersjo O, Spears PC, Frosing R. Sequential methotrexate/5-FU: FdUMP formation and TS inhibition in a transplantable rodent colon adenocarcinoma. Cancer Chemother Pharmacol. 1986;16:237–42. https://doi.org/10.1007/BF00293984.

147. Henriksson R, Grankvist K. Interactions between anticancer drugs and other clinically used pharmaceuticals: a review. Acta Oncol. 1989;28(4):451–62. https://doi.org/10.3109/02841868909092250.

148. Thoppil AA, Choudhary S, Kishore N. Competitive binding of anticancer drugs 5-fluorouracil and cyclophosphamide with serum albumin: calorimetric insights. Biochim Biophys Acta. 2016;1860(5):917–29. https://doi.org/10.1016/j.bbagen.2016.01.026.

149. Bruijn EA, Driessen O, Leeflang P, van den Bosch N, van Strijen E, Slee PH, Hermans J. Pharmacokinetic interactions of cyclophosphamide and 5-fluorouracil with methotrexate in an animal model. Cancer Treat Rev. 1986;70(10):1159–65.

150. NHS. Chemotherapy protocol. Breast cancer. Cyclophosphamide-fluorouracil-methotrexate (CMF). NHS, University Hospital Southampton, NHS Foundation Trust, England, 2020. Available https://www.uhs.nhs.uk/Media/SUHTExtranet/Services/Chemotherapy-SOPs/Breastcancer/CyclophosphamideFluorouracilMethotrexateCMF-IV.pdf. Accessed Aug 4, 2021.

151. Buzdar AU, Kau SW, Smith TL, Hortobagyi GN. Ten-year results of FAC adjuvant chemotherapy trial in breast cancer. Am J Clin Oncol. 1989;12(2):123–8. https://doi.org/10.1097/00000421-198904000-00007.

152. Rivera E, Holmes FA, Buzdar AU, Asmar L, Kau SW, Fraschini G, Walters R, Theriault RL, Hortobagyi GN. Fluorouracil, doxorubicin, and cyclophosphamide followed by tamoxifen as adjuvant treatment for patients with stage IV breast cancer with no evidence of disease. Breast J. 2002;8(1):2–9. https://doi.org/10.1046/j.1524-4741.2002.08002.x.

153. Martín M, Ruiz A, Borrego MR, Barnadas A, González S, Calvo L, Vila MM, Antón A, Rodríguez-Lescure A, Seguí-Palmer MA, Muñoz-Mateu M, Ribugent JD, López-Veja JM, Jara C, Espinosa E, Fernández CM, Andrés R, Ribelles N, Plazaola A, Sánchez-Rovira P, Bofill JS, Crespo C, Carabantes FJ, Servitja S, Chacón JI, Rodríguez CA, Hernando B, Álvarez I, Carrasco E, Lluch A. Fluorouracil, doxorubicin, and cyclophosphamide (FAC) versus FAC followed by weekly paclitaxel as adjuvant therapy for high-risk, node-negative breast cancer: results from the GEICAM/2003-02 study. J Clin Oncol. 2013;31(20):2593–9. https://doi.org/10.1200/JCO.2012.46.9841.

154. Tecza K, Pamula-Pilat J, Lanuszewska J, Butkiewicz D, Grzybowska E. Pharmacogenetics of toxicity of 5-fluorouracil, doxorubicin and cyclophosphamide chemotherapy in breast cancer patients. Oncotarget. 2018;9:9114–36. https://doi.org/10.18632/oncotarget.24148.

155. Pereira-Oliveira M, Reis-Mendes A, Carvalho F, Remião F, Bastos ML, Costa VM. Doxorubicin is key for the cardiotoxicity of FAC (5-fluorouracil + adriamycin + cyclo-

phosphamide) combination in differentiated H9c2 cells. Biomol Ther. 2019;9(1):21. https://doi.org/10.3390/biom9010021.

156. Bergh J, Wiklind T, Erikstein B, Lidbrink E, Lindman H, Malmstrom P, Kellokumpu-Lehtinen P, Bengtsson NO, Soderlund G, Anker G, Wist E, Ottosson S, Salminen E, Ljungman P, Holte H, Nilsson J, Blomqvist C, Wilking N. Tailored fluorouracil, epirubicin, and cyclophosphamide compared with marrow-supported high-dose chemotherapy as adjuvant treatment for high-risk breast cancer: a randomised trial. Scandinavian Breast Group 9401 study. Lancet. 2000;356(9239):1384–91. https://doi.org/10.1016/s0140-6736(00)02841-5.

157. Pacini P, Rinaldini M, Algeri R, Guarneri A, Tucci E, Barsanti G, Neri B, Bastiani P, Marzano S, Fallai C. FEC (5-fluorouracil, epidoxorubicin and cyclophosphamide) versus EM (epidoxorubicin and mitomycin-C) with or without lonidamine as first-line treatment for advanced breast cancer. A multicentric randomised study. Final results. Eur J Cancer. 2000;36(8):966–75. https://doi.org/10.1016/s0959-8049(00)00068-x.

158. von Heideman A, Sandstrom M, Csoka K, Tholander B, Larsson R, Bergh J, Nygren P. Evaluation of drug interactions in the established FEC regimen in primary cultures of tumour cells from patients. Ann Oncol. 2000;11(10):1301–7. https://doi.org/10.1023/a:1008332816407.

159. Cersosimo RJ, Hong WK. Epirubicin: a review of the pharmacology, clinical activity, and adverse effects of an Adriamycin analogue. J Clin Oncol. 1986;4(3):425–39. https://doi.org/10.1200/JCO.1986.4.3.425.

160. Tsukagoshi S. Epirubicin (4′-epi-adriamycin). Gan To Kagaku Ryoho. 1990;17(1):151–9.

161. Fumoleau P, Roché H, Kerbrat P, Bonneterre J, Romestaing P, Fargeot P, Namer M, Monnier A, Montcuquet P, Goudier MJ, Luporsi E. Long-term cardiac toxicity after adjuvant epirubicin-based chemotherapy in early breast cancer: French adjuvant study group results. Ann Oncol. 2006;17(1):85–92. https://doi.org/10.1093/annonc/mdj034.

162. Saad ED, Facina G, Gebrim LH. Epirrubicina no tratamento do câncer de mama. Rev Bras Cancerol. 2006;53(1):47–53.

163. Ryberg M, Nielsen D, Cortese G, Nielsen G, Skovsgaard T, Andersen PK. New insight into epirubicin cardiac toxicity: competing risks analysis of 1097 breast cancer patients. JNCI. 2008;100(15):1058–67. https //doi.org/10.1093/jnci/djn206.

164. van Boxtel W, Bulten BF, Mavinkurve-Groothuis AMC, Bellersen L, Mandigers CMPW, Joosten LAB, Kapusta L, Geus-Oei LF, van Laarhoven HWM. New biomarkers for early detection of cardiotoxicity after treatment with docetaxel, doxorubicin and cyclophosphamide. Biomarkers. 2015;20(2):143–8. https://doi.org/10.3109/1354750X.2015.1040839.

165. Burnell M, Levine MN, Chapman JAW, Bramwell V, Gelmon K, Walley B, Vandenberg T, Chalchal H, Albain KS, Perez EA, Rugo H, Pritchard K, O'Brien P, Shepherd LE. Cyclophosphamide, epirubicin, and fluorouracil versus dose-dense epirubicin and cyclophosphamide followed by paclitaxel versus doxorubicin and cyclophosphamide followed by paclitaxel in node-positive or high-risk node-negative breast cancer. J Clin Oncol. 2010;28(1):77–82. https://doi.org/10.1200/JCO.2009.22.1077.

166. Mastro LD, Levaggi A, Michelotti A, Cavazzini G, Adami F, Scotto T, Piras M, Danese S, Garrone O, Durando A, Accortanzo V, Bighin C, Miglietta L, Pastorino S, Pronzato P, Castiglione F, Landucci E, Conte P, Bruzzi P. 5-Fluorouracil, epirubicin and cyclophosphamide versus epirubicin and paclitaxel in node-positive early breast cancer: a phase-III randomized GONO-MIG5 trial. Breast Cancer Res Treat. 2016;155:117–26. https://doi.org/10.1007/s10549-015-3655-1.

167. Cupertino A, Marcondes MA, Gatti RM. Estudo retrospectivo das reações adversas e interações medicamentosas na quimioterapia no tratamento do câncer de mama: relato de caso. Rev Bras Ciên Saúde. 2008;6(17):26–36. https://doi.org/10.13037/rbcs.vol6n17.356.

168. Pérez Fidalgo JA, Fabregat LG, Cervantes A, Margulies A, Vidall C, Roila F. Management of chemotherapy extravasation: ESMO-EONS clinical practice guidelines. Ann Oncol. 2012;23(7):167–73. https://doi.org/10.1093/annonc/mds294.

169. Miguel I, Winckler P, Sousa M, Cardoso C, Moreira A, Brito M. Febrile neutropenia in FEC-D regimen for early stage breast cancer: is there a place for G-CSF primary prophylaxis? Breast Dis. 2015;35(3):167–71. https://doi.org/10.3233/BD-150411.

170. Dumontet C, Jordan MA. Microtubule-binding agents: a dynamic field of cancer therapeutics. Nat Rev Drug Discov. 2010;9(10):790–803. https://doi.org/10.1038/nrd3253.

171. Weaver BA. How taxol/paclitaxel kills cancer cells. Mol Biol Cell. 2014;25(18):2677–81. https://doi.org/10.1091/mbc.E14-04-0916.

172. Maloney SM, Hoover CA, Morejon-Lasso LV, Prosperi JR. Mechanisms of taxane resistance. Cancer. 2020;12:3323. https://doi.org/10.3390/cancers12113323.

173. Skubnik J, Pavlicková V, Ruml T, Rimpelová S. Current perspectives on taxanes: focus on their bioactivity, delivery and combination therapy. Plan Theory. 2021;10(3):569. https://doi.org/10.3390/plants10030569.

174. Ceruti M, Tagini V, Recalenda V, Arpicco S, Cattel L, Airoldi M, Bumma C. Docetaxel in combination with epirubicin in metastatic breast cancer: pharmacokinetic interactions. Farmaco. 1999;54(11-12):733–9. https://doi.org/10.1016/s0014-827x(99)00092-0.

175. Lunardi G, Venturini M, Vannozzi MO, Tolino G, Del Mastro L, Bighin C, Schettini G, Esposito M. Influence of alternate sequences of epirubicin and docetaxel on the pharmacokinetic behavior of both drugs in advanced breast cancer. Ann Oncol. 2002;13(2):280–5. https://doi.org/10.1093/annonc/mdf016.

176. Joensuu H, Bono P, Kataja V, Alanko T, Kokko R, Asola R, Utriainen T, Turpeenniemi-Hujanen T, Jyrkkio S, Moykkynen K, Helle L, Ingalsuo S, Pajunen M, Huusko M, Salminen T, Auvinen P, Leinonen H, Leinonen M, Isola J, Kellokumpu-Lehtinen PL. Fluorouracil, epirubicin, and cyclophosphamide with either docetaxel or vinorelbine, with or without trastuzumab, as adjuvant treatments of breast cancer: final results of the FinHer trial. J Clin Oncol. 2009;27(34):5685–92. https://doi.org/10.1200/JCO.2008.21.4577.

177. Martín M, Simón AR, Borrego MR, Ribelles N, Rodríguez-Lescure A, Muñoz-Mateu M, Vila MM, Barnadas A, Ramos M, Berron SDB, Jara C, Calvo L, Martínez-Jáñez N, Fernández CM, Rodríguez CA, Dueñas EM, Andrés R, Plazaola A, Haba-Rodríguez J, López-Veja JM, Adrover E, Ballesteros AI, Santaballa A, Sánchez-Rovira P, Baena-Cañada JM, Casas M, Cámara MC, Carrasco EM, Lluch A. Epirubicin plus cyclophosphamide followed by docetaxel versus epirubicin plus docetaxel followed by capecitabine as adjuvant therapy for node-positive early breast cancer: results from the GEICAM/2003-10 study. J Clin Oncol. 2015;33(32):3788–95. https://doi.org/10.1200/JCO.2015.61.9510.

178. Chia S. BC cancer protocol summary for neoadjuvant or adjuvant therapy for breast cancer using fluorouracil, epirubicin, cyclophosphamide and DOCEtaxel. BC Cancer, British Columbia, 2021. Available http://www.bccancer.bc.ca/chemotherapy-protocols-site/Documents/Breast/BRAJFECD_Protocol.pdf. Accessed Aug 3, 2021.

179. Chia S. BC cancer protocol summary for neoadjuvant or adjuvant therapy for breast cancer using fluorouracil, epirubicin and cyclophosphamide followed by DOCEtaxel and trastuzumab. BC Cancer, British Columbia, 2021. Available http://www.bccancer.bc.ca/chemotherapy-protocols-site/Documents/Breast/BRAJFECDT_Protocol.pdf. Accessed Aug 4, 2021.

180. Tedesco KL, Thor AD, Johnson DH, Shyr Y, Blum KA, Goldstein LJ, Gradishar WJ, Nicholson BP, Merkel DE, Murrey D, Edgerton S, Sledge GW Jr. Docetaxel combined with trastuzumab is an active regimen in HER-2 3+ overexpressing and fluorescent in situ hybridization–positive metastatic breast cancer: a multi-institutional phase II trial. J Clin Oncol. 2004;22(6):1071–7. https://doi.org/10.1200/JCO.2004.10.046.

181. Demonty G. Docetaxel plus trastuzumab as treatment for Her-2 positive metastatic breast cancer: review of the existing evidence. Womens Health. 2007;3(5):523–8. https://doi.org/10.2217/17455057.3.5.523.

182. Swain SM, Im YH, Im SA, Chan V, Miles D, Knott A, Clark E, Ross G, Baselga J. Safety profile of pertuzumab with trastuzumab and docetaxel in patients from Asia with human epidermal growth factor receptor 2-positive metastatic breast cancer: results from the phase III Trial CLEOPATRA. Oncologist. 2014;19(7):693–701. https://doi.org/10.1634/theoncologist.2014-0033.

183. Hirata T, Ozaki S, Tabata M, Iwamoto T, Hinotsu S, Hamada A, Motoki T, Nogami T, Shien T, Taira N, Matsuoka J, Doihara H. A multicenter study of docetaxel at a dose of 100 mg/m^2 in Japanese patients with advanced or recurrent breast cancer. Intern Med. 2021;60(8):1183–90. https://doi.org/10.2169/internalmedicine.5089-20.

184. Marty M, Cognetti F, Maraninchi D, Snyder R, Mauriac L, Tubiana-Hulin M, Chan S, Grimes D, Antón A, Lluch A, Kennedy J, O'Byrne K, Conte P, Green M, Ward C, Mayne K, Extra JM. Randomized phase II trial of the efficacy and safety of trastuzumab combined with docetaxel in patients with human epidermal growth factor receptor 2-positive metastatic breast cancer administered as first-line treatment: the M77001 study group. J Clin Oncol. 2005;23(19):4265–74. https://doi.org/10.1200/JCO.2005.04.173.

185. Forbes JF, Pienkowski T, Valero V, Eiermann W, von Minckwitz G, Martin M, Smylie M, Crown MJ, Noel N, Pegram M. BCIRG 007: randomized phase III trial of trastuzumab plus docetaxel with or without carboplatin first line in HER2 positive metastatic breast cancer (MBC). J Clin Oncol. 2006;24(8):516. https://doi.org/10.1200/jco.2006.24.18_suppl.lba516.

186. Wardley AM, Pivot X, Morales-Vasquez F, Zetina LM, Gaui MFD, Jassem DOR, Barton C, Button P, Hersberger V, Torres AA. Randomized phase II trial of first-line trastuzumab plus docetaxel and capecitabine compared with trastuzumab plus docetaxel in HER2-Positive metastatic breast cancer. J Clin Oncol. 2010;28(6):976–83. https://doi.org/10.1200/JCO.2008.21.6531.

187. Mendonça AB, Pereira ER, Magnago C, Barreto BMF, Goes TRP, Silva RM. Sequencing of antineoplastic drug administration: contributions to evidence-based oncology nursing practice. Rev Eletron Enferm. 2018;20:20–51. https://doi.org/10.5216/ree.v20.52232.

188. Kilany LAA, Gaber AAS, Aboulwafa MM, Zedan HH. Trastuzumab immunogenicity development in patients' sera and in laboratory animals. BMC Immunol. 2021;22:15. https://doi.org/10.1186/s12865-021-00405-z.

189. Waller CF, Mobius J, Fuentes-Alburo A. Intravenous and subcutaneous formulations of trastuzumab, and trastuzumab biosimilars: implications for clinical practice. Br J Cancer. 2021;124:1346–52. https://doi.org/10.1038/s41416-020-01255-z.

190. Nabholtz JM, Smylie M, Mackey JR, Noel D, Paterson AH, Al Tweigeri T, Au D, Sansregret E, Delorme F, Riva A. Docetaxel/doxorubicin/cyclophosphamide in the treatment of metastatic breast cancer. Oncology. 1997;11(8):37–41.

191. Martin M. Docetaxel, doxorubicin and cyclophosphamide (the TAC regimen): an effective adjuvant treatment for operable breast cancer. Womens Health. 2006;2(4):527–37. https://doi.org/10.2217/17455057.2.4.527.

192. NCT00074139. Docetaxel, doxorubicin, and cyclophosphamide in treating women with advanced breast cancer. Clinical Trials. 2014. Available https://clinicaltrials.gov/ct2/show/NCT00074139. Accessed Aug 4, 2021.

193. NCT00121992. Docetaxel, doxorubicin (A), cyclophosphamide (C) (TAC) vs 5-fluorouracil, A, C (5FAC) breast cancer adjuvant treatment. Clinical Trials, 2020. Available https://clinicaltrials.gov/ct2/show/NCT00121992. Accessed Aug 4, 2021.

194. Bear HD, Anderson S, Smith RE, Geyer CE Jr, Mamounas EP, Fisher B, Brown AM, Robidoux A, Margolese R, Kahlenberg MS, Paik S, Soran A, Wickerham DL, Wolmark N. Sequential preoperative or postoperative docetaxel added to preoperative doxorubicin plus cyclophosphamide for operable breast cancer: national surgical adjuvant breast and bowel project protocol B-27. J Clin Oncol. 2006;24(13):2019–27. https://doi.org/10.1200/JCO.2005.04.1665.

195. Baltali E, Ozisik Y, Guler N, Firat D, Altundag K. Combination of docetaxel and doxorubicin as first-line chemotherapy in metastatic breast cancer. Tumori J. 2001;87(1):18–9.

196. Zeng S, Chen YZ, Fu L, Johnson KR, Fan W. *In vitro* evaluation of schedule-dependent interactions between docetaxel and doxorubicin against human breast and ovarian cancer cells. Clin Cancer Res. 2000;6(9):3766–73.

197. Itoh K, Sasaki Y, Fujii H, Minami H, Ohtsu T, Wakita H, Igarashi T, Watanabe Y, Onozawa Y, Kashimura M, Ohashi Y. Study of dose escalation and sequence switching of administration of the combination of docetaxel and doxorubicin in advanced breast cancer. Clin Cancer Res. 2000;6(10):4082–90.

198. NHS. Chemotherapy protocol. Breast cancer. Cyclophosphamide-docetaxel-doxorubicin. NHS, University Hospital Southampton, NHS Foundation Trust, England, 2014. Available https://www.uhs.nhs.uk/Media/SUHTExtranet/Services/Chemotherapy-SOPs/Breastcancer/BreastCyclophosphamideDocetaxelDoxorubicin(TAC)Ver11.pdf. Accessed Aug 4, 2021.

199. Chang TK, Weber GF, Crespi CL, Waxman DJ. Differential activation of cyclophosphamide and ifosfamide by cytochromes P-450 2B and 3A in human liver microsomes. Cancer Res. 1993;53(23):5629–37.

200. Miyoshi Y, Ando A, Takamura Y, Taguchi T, Tamaki Y, Noguchi S. Prediction of response to docetaxel by CYP3A4 mRNA expression in breast cancer tissues. Int J Cancer. 2002;97(1):129–32. https://doi.org/10.1002/ijc.1568.

201. Ando Y. Possible metabolic interaction between docetaxel and ifosfamide. Br J Cancer. 2000;82(2):497. https://doi.org/10.1054/bjoc.1999.0949.

202. NHS. Chemotherapy protocol. Breast cancer. Cyclophosphamide-docetaxel. NHS, University Hospital Southampton, NHS Foundation Trust, England, 2014. Available https://www.uhs.nhs.uk/Media/SUHTExtranet/Services/Chemotherapy-SOPs/Breastcancer/BreastCyclophosphamideDocetaxelVer11.pdf. Accessed Aug 4, 2021.

203. Eppler S, Gordon MS, Redfern CH, Trudeau C, Xu N, Han K, Lum BL. Lack of a pharmacokinetic interaction between trastuzumab and carboplatin in the presence of docetaxel: results from a phase Ib study in patients with HER2-positive metastatic or locally advanced inoperable solid tumors. Anti-Cancer Drugs. 2015;26(4):448–55. https://doi.org/10.1097/CAD.0000000000000214.

204. NCT00047255. Docetaxel and trastuzumab with or without carboplatin in treating women with HER2-positive breast cancer. Clinical Trials. 2020. Available https://clinicaltrials.gov/ct2/show/NCT00047255. Accessed Aug 4, 2021.

205. Wu D, Xiong L. Efficacy analysis of trastuzumab, carboplatin and docetaxel in HER-2-positive breast cancer patients. Oncol Lett. 2020;19:2539–46. https://doi.org/10.3892/ol.2020.11277.

206. Sousa GF, Wlodarczyk SR, Monteiro G. Carboplatin: molecular mechanisms of action associated with chemoresistance. Braz J Pharm Sci. 2014;50(4):693–701. https://doi.org/10.1590/S1984-82502014000400004.

207. Almeida VL, Leitão A, Reina LCB, Montanari CA, Donnici CL, Lopes MTP. Câncer e agentes antineoplásicos não específicos do ciclo celular que interagem com o DNA: uma introdução. Química Nova. 2005;28(1):118–29. https://doi.org/10.1590/S0100-40422005000100021.

208. Xu N, Redfern CH, Gordon M, Eppler S, Lum BL, Trudeau C. Trastuzumab, in combination with carboplatin and docetaxel, does not prolong the QT interval of patients with HER2-positive metastatic or locally advanced inoperable solid tumors: results from a phase Ib study. Cancer Chemother Pharmacol. 2014;74(6):1251–60. https://doi.org/10.1007/s00280-014-2603-9.

209. NHS. Chemotherapy protocol. Breast cancer. Carboplatin(AUC6)-docetaxel-trastuzumab(TCH). NHS, University Hospital Southampton, NHS Foundation Trust, England, 2014. Available https://www.uhs.nhs.uk/Media/SUHTExtranet/Services/Chemotherapy-SOPs/Breastcancer/BreastCarboplatinDocetaxelTrastuzumabVer11.pdf. Accessed Aug 4, 2021.

210. Aguiar PHW, Pinheiro LGP, Mota RMS, Margotti NHG, Rocha JIX. Sentinel lymph node biopsy in patients with locally advanced breast cancer after neoadjuvant chemotherapy. Acta Cir Bras. 2012;27(12):912–6. https://doi.org/10.1590/S0102-86502012001200014.

211. Koca E, Kuzan TY, Dizdar O, Babacan T, Sahin I, Ararat E, Altundag K. Outcomes of locally advanced breast cancer patients with ≥ 10 positive axillary lymph nodes. Med Oncol. 2013;30(3):615. https://doi.org/10.1007/s12032-013-0615-7.

212. Lane DL, Adeyefa MM, Yang WT. Role of sonography for the locoregional staging of breast cancer. AJR Am Roent Ray Soc. 2014;203(5):1132–41. https://doi.org/10.2214/AJR.13.12311.

213. Pan H, Wang H, Qian M, Mao X, Shi G, Ma G, Yu M, Xie H, Ling L, Ding Q, Zhang K, Wang S, Zhou W. Comparison of survival outcomes among patients with breast cancer with distant

vs ipsilateral supraclavicular lymph node metastases. JAMA Netw Open. 2021;4(3):e211809. https://doi.org/10.1001/jamanetworkopen.2021.1809.

214. Barni S, Mandalà M. Locally advanced breast cancer. Curr Opin Obstet Gynecol. 2006;18(1):47–52. https://doi.org/10.1097/01.gco.0000192998.04793.ba.

215. Cláudia S, Mafalda C, Ana N, Kayla P, Marta P, Joana B, Mónica H, Domingos R, Rui M, Cristina M, Gilberto M, Gabriela S, Paulo F, Paula A. Neoadjuvant radiotherapy in the approach of locally advanced breast cancer. ESMO Open. 2020;5(2):E000640. https://doi.org/10.1136/esmoopen-2019-000640.

216. Scholl SM, Asselain B, Palangie T, Dorval T, Jouve M, Garcia Giralt E, Vilcoq J, Durand JC, Pouillart P. Neoadjuvant chemotherapy in operable breast cancer. Eur J Cancer. 1991;27(12):1668–71. https://doi.org/10.1016/0277-5379(91)90442-g.

217. Gaui MFD, Amorim G, Arcuri RA, Pereira G, Moreira D, Djahjah C, Biasoli I, Spector N. A phase II study of second-line neoadjuvant chemotherapy with capecitabine and radiation therapy for anthracycline-resistant locally advanced breast cancer. Am J Clin Oncol. 2007;30(1):78–81. https://doi.org/10.1097/01.coc.0000245475.41324.6d.

218. Carrara GFA, Scapulatempo-Neto C, Abrahão-Machado LF, Brentani MM, Nunes JS, Folgueira MAAK, Vieira RAC. Breast-conserving surgery in locally advanced breast cancer submitted to neoadjuvant chemotherapy. Safety and effectiveness based on ipsilateral breast tumor recurrence and long-term follow-up. Clinics. 2017;72(3):134–42. https://doi.org/10.6061/clinics/2017(03)02.

219. Callahan R, Hurvitz S. HER2-positive breast cancer: current management of early, advanced, and recurrent disease. Curr Opin Obstet Gynecol. 2011;23(1):37–43.

220. Rugo HS, Rumble RB, Macrae E, Barton DL, Connolly HK, Dickler MN, Fallowfield L, Fowble B, Ingle JN, Jahanzeb M, Johnston SRD, Korde LA, Khatcheressian JL, Mehta RS, Muss HB, Burstein HJ. Endocrine therapy for hormone receptor–positive metastatic breast cancer: American Society of Clinical Oncology Guideline. J Clin Oncol. 2016;34(25):3069–103. https://doi.org/10.1200/JCO.2016.67.1487.

221. Montagna E, Colleoni M. Hormonal treatment combined with targeted therapies in endocrine-responsive and HER2-positive metastatic breast cancer. Therap Adv Med Oncol. 2019;11:1758835919894105. https://doi.org/10.1177/1758835919894105.

222. Remick J, Amin NP. Postmastectomy breast cancer radiation therapy. Treasure Island: StatPearls Publishing; 2021.

223. Schlam I, Swain SM. HER2-positive breast cancer and tyrosine kinase inhibitors: the time is now. NPJ Breast Cancer. 2021;7:56. https://doi.org/10.1038/s41523-021-00265-1.

224. Smith RE, Anderson SJ, Brown A, Scholnik AP, Desai AM, Kardinal CG, Lembersky BC, Mamounas EP. Phase II trial of doxorubicin/docetaxel/cyclophosphamide for locally advanced and metastatic breast cancer: results from NSABP trial BP-58. Clin Breast Cancer. 2002;3(5):333–40. https://doi.org/10.3816/CBC.2002.n.036.

225. Diéras V, Fumoleau P, Romieu G, Tubiana-Hulin M, Namer M, Mauriac L, Guastalla JP, Pujade-Lauraine E, Kerbrat P, Maillart P, Pénault-Llorca F, Buyse M, Pouillart P. Randomized parallel study of doxorubicin plus paclitaxel and doxorubicin plus cyclophosphamide as neoadjuvant treatment of patients with breast cancer. J Clin Oncol. 2004;22(24):4958–65. https://doi.org/10.1200/JCO.2004.02.122.

226. Wonders KY, Reigle BS. Trastuzumab and doxorubicin-related cardiotoxicity and the cardioprotective role of exercise. Integr Cancer Ther. 2009;8(1):17–21. https://doi.org/10.1177/1534735408330717.

227. Ewer MS, Ewer SM. The anthracycline-trastuzumab interaction: a lesson in not jumping to confusion. Trends Pharmacol Sci. 2015;36(6):321–2. https://doi.org/10.1016/j.tips.2015.04.007.

228. Mohan N, Jiang J, Dokmanovic M, Wu WJ. Trastuzumab-mediated cardiotoxicity: current understanding challenges, and frontiers. Antibody Ther. 2018;1(1):13–7. https://doi.org/10.1093/abt/tby003.

229. Gelmon K. BC cancer protocol summary for treatment of locally advanced breast cancer using DOXOrubicin and cyclophosphamide followed by DOCEtaxel and trastuzumab.

BC Cancer, British Columbia, 2021. Available http://www.bccancer.bc.ca/chemotherapy-protocols-site/Documents/Breast/BRLAACDT_Protocol.pdf. Accessed Aug 5, 2021.

230. Baldo BA. Monoclonal antibodies approved for cancer therapy. Saf Biol Ther. 2016;13:57–140. https://doi.org/10.1007/978-3-319-30472-4_3.

231. Chia S. BC cancer protocol summary for NEOAdjuvant therapy for triple negative breast cancer using carboplatin and weekly PACLitaxel followed by DOXOrubicin and cyclophosphamide. BC Cancer, British Columbia, 2021. Available http://www.bccancer.bc.ca/chemotherapy-protocols-site/Documents/Breast/BRLACTWAC_Protocol.pdf.   Accessed Aug 5, 2021.

232. Calvert AH. A review of the pharmacokinetics and pharmacodynamics of combination carboplatin/paclitaxel. Semin Oncol. 1997;24(1):85–90.

233. Guminski AD, Harnett PR, DeFazio A. Carboplatin and paclitaxel interact antagonistically in a megakaryoblast cell line–a potential mechanism for paclitaxel-mediated sparing of carboplatin-induced thrombocytopenia. Cancer Chemother Pharmacol. 2001;48(3):229–34. https://doi.org/10.1007/s002800100279.

234. Scripture CD, Figg WD, Sparreboom A. Peripheral neuropathy induced by paclitaxel: recent insights and future perspectives. Curr Neuropharmacol. 2006;4(2):165–72. https://doi.org/10.2174/157015906776359568.

235. Bhutani M, Colucci PM, Laird-Fick H, Conley BA. Management of paclitaxel-induced neurotoxicity. Oncol Rev. 2010;4:107–15. https://doi.org/10.1007/s12156-010-0048-x.

236. Amptoulach S, Tsavaris N. Neurotoxicity caused by the treatment with platinum analogues. Chemother Res Pract. 2011;2011:843019. https://doi.org/10.1155/2011/843019.

237. Avan A, Postma TJ, Ceresa C, Avan A, Cavaletti G, Giovannetti E, Peters GJ. Platinum-induced neurotoxicity and preventive strategies: past, present, and future. Oncologist. 2015;20(4):411–32. https://doi.org/10.1634/theoncologist.2014-0044.

238. Pentheroudakis G, Razis E, Athanassiadis A, Pavlidis N, Fountzilas G. Paclitaxel-carboplatin combination chemotherapy in advanced breast cancer: accumulating evidence for synergy, efficacy, and safety. Med Oncol. 2006;23(2):147–60. https://doi.org/10.1385/MO:23:2:147.

239. Yu KD, Ye FG, He M, Fan L, Ma D, Mo M, Wu J, Liu GY, Di GH, Zeng XH, He PQ, Wu KJ, Hou YF, Wang J, Wang C, Zhuang ZG, Song CG, Lin XY, Toss A, Ricci F, Shen ZZ, Shao ZM. Effect of adjuvant paclitaxel and carboplatin on survival in women with triple-negative breast cancer: a phase 3 randomized clinical trial. JAMA Oncol. 2020;6(9):1390–6. https://doi.org/10.1001/jamaoncol.2020.2965.

240. NHS. Chemotherapy protocol. Breast cancer. Carboplatin (AUC 5)-Paclitaxel (7 day). NHS, University Hospital Southampton, NHS Foundation Trust, England, 2020. Available https://www.uhs.nhs.uk/Media/SUHTExtranet/Services/Chemotherapy-SOPs/Breastcancer/CarboplatinAUC5-Paclitaxel-7day.pdf. Accessed Aug 5, 2021.

241. Chen W, Hoffmann AD, Liu H, Liu X. Organotropism: new insights into molecular mechanisms of breast cancer metastasis. NPJ Precis Oncol. 2018;2:4. https://doi.org/10.1038/s41698-018-0047-0.

242. Liedtke C, Kolberg HC. Systemic therapy of advanced/metastatic breast cancer - current evidence and future concepts. Breast Care. 2016;11:275–81. https://doi.org/10.1159/000447549.

243. Loibl S, Poortmans P, Morrow M, Denkert C, Curigliano G. Breast cancer. Lancet. 2021;397(10286):1750–69. https://doi.org/10.1016/S0140-6736(20)32381-3.

244. Harrington SE, Smith TJ. The role of chemotherapy at the end of life. JAMA. 2008;299(22):2667–78. https://doi.org/10.1001/jama.299.22.2667.

245. Shrestha A, Martin C, Burton M, Walters S, Collins K, Wyld L. Quality of life versus length of life considerations in cancer patients: a systematic literature review. Psycho-Oncology. 2019;28(7):1367–80. https://doi.org/10.1002/pon.5054.

246. NCT03691493. Radiation therapy, palbociclib, and hormone therapy in treating breast cancer patients with bone metastasis (ASPIRE). Clinical Trials. 2020. Available https://clinicaltrials.gov/ct2/show/NCT03691493. Accessed Aug 5, 2021.

247. Cardoso F, Bedard PL, Winer EP, Pagani O, Senkus-Konefka E, Fallowfield LJ, Kyriakides S, Costa A, Cufer T, Albain KS. International guidelines for management of metastatic breast cancer: combination vs sequential single-agent chemotherapy. J Natl Cancer Inst. 2009;101(17):1174–81.

248. Im AS, Lu YS, Bardia A, Harbeck N, Colleoni M, Franke F, Chow L, Sohn J, Lee KS, Campos-Gomez S, Villanueva-Vazquez R, Jung KH, Chakravartty A, Hughes G, Gounaris I, Rodriguez-Lorenc K, Taran T, Hurvitz S, Tripathy D. Overall survival with ribociclib plus endocrine therapy in breast cancer. N Engl J Med. 2019;381:307–16. https://doi.org/10.1056/NEJMoa1903765.

249. Si W, Zhu YY, Li Y, Gao P, Han C, You JH, Linghu RX, Jiao SC, Yang JL. Capecitabine maintenance therapy in patients with recurrent or metastatic breast cancer. Braz J Med Biol Res. 2013;46(12):1074–81. https://doi.org/10.1590/1414-431X20133168.

250. Mehta RS, Barlow WE, Albain KS, Vandenberg TA, Dakhil SR, Tirumali NR, Lew DL, Hayes DF, Gralow JR, Linden HH, Livingston RB, Hortobagyi GN. Overall survival with fulvestrant plus anastrozole in metastatic breast cancer. N Engl J Med. 2019;380(13):1226–34. https://doi.org/10.1056/NEJMoa1811714.

251. Fisusi FA, Akala EO. Drug combinations in breast cancer therapy. Pharm Nanotechnol. 2019;7(3):3–23. https://doi.org/10.2174/2211738507666190122111224.

252. Heinemann V. Gemcitabine plus cisplatin for the treatment of metastatic breast cancer. Clin Breast Cancer. 2002;3:24–9. https://doi.org/10.3816/cbc.2002.s.006.

253. Koshy N, Quispe D, Shi R, Mansour R, Burton GV. Cisplatin–gemcitabine therapy in metastatic breast cancer: Improved outcome in triple negative breast cancer patients compared to non-triple negative patients. Breast. 2010;19(3):246–8. https://doi.org/10.1016/j.breast.2010.02.003.

254. Kohail H, Shehata S, Mansour O, Gouda Y, Gaafar R, Hamid TA, El Nowieam S, Al Khodary A, El Zawahry H, Wareth AA, Halim IA, Taleb FA, Hamada E, Barsoum M, Abdullah M, Meshref M. A phase 2 study of the combination of gemcitabine and cisplatin in patients with locally advanced or metastatic breast cancer previously treated with anthracyclines with/without taxanes. Hematology. 2012;5(1):42–8. https://doi.org/10.5144/1658-3876.2012.42.

255. Ozkan M, Berk V, Kaplan MA, Benekli M, Coskun U, Bilici A, Gumus M, Alkis N, Dane F, Ozdemir NY, Colak D, Dikilitas M. Gemcitabine and cisplatin combination chemotherapy in triple negative metastatic breast cancer previously treated with a taxane/anthracycline chemotherapy; multicenter experience. Neoplasma. 2012;59(1):38–42. https://doi.org/10.4149/neo_2012_005.

256. NCT01585805. Gemcitabine hydrochloride and cisplatin with or without veliparib or veliparib alone in treating patients with locally advanced or metastatic pancreatic cancer. Clinical Trials. 2021. Available https://clinicaltrials.gov/ct2/show/NCT01585805. Accessed Aug 5, 2021.

257. Alexopoulos A, Tryfonopoulos D, Karamouzis MV, Gerasimidis G, Karydas I, Kandilis K, Stavrakakis J, Stavrinides H, Georganta C, Ardavanis A, Rigatos G. Evidence for in vivo synergism between docetaxel and gemcitabine in patients with metastatic breast cancer. Ann Oncol. 2004;15:95–9. https://doi.org/10.1093/annonc/mdh028.

258. Seidman AD. Gemcitabine and docetaxel in metastatic breast cancer. Oncology. 2004;18(14):13–6.

259. Galmarini CM, Mackey JR, Dumontet C. Nucleoside analogues: mechanisms of drug resistance and reversal strategies. Leukemia. 2001;15:875–90. https://doi.org/10.1038/sj.leu.2402114.

260. Pourquier P, Gioffre C, Kohlhagen G, Urasaki Y, Goldwasser F, Hertel LW, Yu S, Pon RT, Gmeiner WH, Pommier Y. Gemcitabine (2',2'-Difluoro-2'-Deoxycytidine), an antimetabolite that poisons topoisomerase I. Clin Cancer Res. 2002;8(8):2499–504.

261. Sampath D, Rao VA, Plunkett W. Mechanisms of apoptosis induction by nucleoside analogs. Oncogene. 2003;22:9063–74. https://doi.org/10.1038/sj.onc.1207229.

262. Ciccolini J, Serdjebi C, Peters GJ, Giovannetti E. Pharmacokinetics and pharmacogenetics of gemcitabine as a mainstay in adult and pediatric oncology: an EORTC-PAMM perspective. Cancer Chemother Pharmacol. 2016;78:1–12. https://doi.org/10.1007/s00280-016-3003-0.
263. Harada H, Shibuya K, Hiraoka M. Combinations of antimetabolites and ionizing radiation. In: Multimodal concepts for integration of cytotoxic drugs. Berlin: Springer; 2006.
264. Corrigan A, Gorski L, Hankins J, Perucca R. Infusion nursing: an evidence-based approach. Berlin: Elsevier; 2009.
265. Ferrazzi E, Stievano L. Gemcitabine: monochemotherapy of breast cancer. Ann Oncol. 2006;17(5):169–72. https://doi.org/10.1093/annonc/mdj975.
266. Chan S, Romieu G, Huober J, Delozier T, Tubiana-Hulin M, Schneeweiss A, Lluch A, Llombart A, du Bois A, Kreienberg R, Mayordomo JI, Antón A, Harrison M, Jones A, Carrasco E, Vaury AT, Frimodt-Moller B, Fumoleau P. Phase III study of gemcitabine plus docetaxel compared with capecitabine plus docetaxel for anthracycline-pretreated patients with metastatic breast cancer. J Clin Oncol. 2009;27(11):1753–60. https://doi.org/10.1200/JCO.2007.15.8485.
267. Rizvi NA, Spiridonidis CH, Davis TH, Bhargava P, Marshall JL, Dahut W, Figuera M, Hawkins MJ. Docetaxel and gemcitabine combinations in non-small cell lung cancer. Semin Oncol. 1999;26(5):27–31.
268. Leu KM, Ostruszka LJ, Shewach D, Zalupski M, Sondak V, Biermann JS, Lee JSJ, Couwlier C, Palazzolo K, Baker LH. Laboratory and clinical evidence of synergistic cytotoxicity of sequential treatment with gemcitabine followed by docetaxel in the treatment of sarcoma. J Clin Oncol. 2004;22(9):1706–12. https://doi.org/10.1200/JCO.2004.08.043.
269. Harita S, Watanabe Y, Kiura K, Tabata M, Takigawa N, Kuyama S, Kozuki T, Kamei H, Tada A, Okimoto N, Genba K, Tada S, Ueoka H, Hiraki S, Tanimoto M. Influence of altering administration sequence of docetaxel, gemcitabine and cisplatin in patients with advanced non-small cell lung cancer. Anticancer Res. 2006;26(2B):1637–41.
270. Chia S. BC cancer protocol summary for palliative therapy for metastatic breast cancer using gemcitabine and DOCEtaxel. BC Cancer, British Columbia, 2021. Available http://www.bccancer.bc.ca/chemotherapy-protocols-site/Documents/Breast/BRAVGEMD_Protocol.pdf. Accessed Aug 6, 2021.
271. NCT00002998. Gemcitabine and cisplatin in treating patients with metastatic breast cancer. Clinical Trials. 2016. Available https://clinicaltrials.gov/ct2/show/NCT00002998. Accessed Aug 6, 2021.
272. Dasari S, Tchounwou PB. Cisplatin in cancer therapy: molecular mechanisms of action. Eur J Pharmacol. 2014;740:364–78. https://doi.org/10.1016/j.ejphar.2014.07.025.
273. Li LY, Guan YD, Chen XS, Yang JM, Cheng Y. DNA repair pathways in cancer therapy and resistance. Front Pharmacol. 2021;11:629266. https://doi.org/10.3389/fphar.2020.629266.
274. Li X, Liu Y, Tian H. Current developments in Pt(IV) prodrugs conjugated with bioactive ligands. Bioinorg Chem Appl. 2018;2018:8276139. https://doi.org/10.1155/2018/8276139.
275. O'Donnell D, Leahy M, Marples M, Protheroe A, Selby P. Problem solving in oncology. Witney: Evidence-based Networks Ltd.; 2007.
276. Basu A, Krishnamurthy S. Cellular responses to cisplatin-induced DNA damage. J Nucl Acids. 2010;2010:201367. https://doi.org/10.4061/2010/201367.
277. Kreidieh FY, Moukadem HA, El Saghir NS. Overview, prevention and management of chemotherapy extravasation. World J Clin Oncol. 2016;7(1):87–97. https://doi.org/10.5306/wjco.v7.i1.87.
278. Zhang J, Wang Z, Hu X, Wang B, Wang L, Yang W, Liu Y, Liu G, Di G, Hu Z, Wu J, Shao Z. Cisplatin and gemcitabine as the first line therapy in metastatic triple negative breast cancer. Int J Cancer. 2015;136(1):204–11. https://doi.org/10.1002/ijc.28966.
279. Hu XC, Zhang J, Xu BH, Cai L, Ragaz J, Wang ZH, Wang BY, Teng YE, Tong ZS, Pan YY, Yin YM, Wu CP, Jiang ZF, Wang XJ, Lou GY, Liu DG, Feng JF, Luo JF, Sun K, Gu YJ, Wu J, Shao ZM. Cisplatin plus gemcitabine versus paclitaxel plus gemcitabine as first-line therapy for metastatic triple-negative breast cancer (CBCSG006): a randomised, open-

label, multicentre, phase 3 trial. Lancet Oncol. 2015;16(4):436–46. https://doi.org/10.1016/S1470-2045(15)70064-1.

280. Chitapanarux I, Lorvidhaya V, Kamnerdsupaphon P, Tharavichitkul E, Trakultivakorn H, Somwangprasert A, Sumitsawan S. Gemcitabine plus cisplatin (GC): a salvage regimen for breast cancer patients who failed anthracycline and/or taxanes. J Clin Oncol. 2005;23(16):757. https://doi.org/10.1200/jco.2005.23.16_suppl.757.

281. Peters GJ, Bergman AM, Ruiz van Haperen VW, Veerman G, Kuiper CM, Braakhuis BJ. Interaction between cisplatin and gemcitabine in vitro and in vivo. Semin Oncol. 1995;22(4):72–9.

282. Bergman AM, Ruiz van Haperen VW, Veerman G, Kuiper CM, Peters GJ. Synergistic interaction between cisplatin and gemcitabine in vitro. Clin Cancer Res. 1996;2(3):521–30.

283. Kroep JR, Peters GJ, van Moorsel CJ, Catik A, Vermorken JB, Pinedo HM, van Groeningen CJ. Gemcitabine-cisplatin: a schedule finding study. Ann Oncol. 1999;10(12):1503–10. https://doi.org/10.1023/a:1008339425708.

284. Colomer R. Gemcitabine in combination with paclitaxel for the treatment of metastatic breast cancer. Womens Health. 2005;1(3):323–9. https://doi.org/10.2217/17455057.1.3.323.

285. NCT00334802. Combination chemotherapy of gemcitabine and paclitaxel for metastatic breast cancer. Clinical Trials. 2010. Available https://clinicaltrials.gov/ct2/show/NCT00334802. Accessed Aug 6, 2021.

286. Rau KM, Li SH, Chen SMS, Tang Y, Huang CH, Wu SC, Chen YY. Weekly paclitaxel combining with gemcitabine is an effective and safe treatment for advanced breast cancer patients. Jpn J Clin Oncol. 2011;41(4):455–61. https://doi.org/10.1093/jjco/hyq232.

287. NCT00006459. Paclitaxel with or without gemcitabine in treating women with advanced breast cancer. 2012. Available https://clinicaltrials.gov/ct2/show/NCT00006459. Accessed Aug 6, 2021.

288. Allouache D, Gawande SR, Tubiana-Hulin M, Tubuana-Mathieu N, Piperno-Neumann S, Mefti F, Bozec L, Genot JT. First-line therapy with gemcitabine and paclitaxel in locally, recurrent or metastatic breast cancer: a phase II study. BMC Cancer. 2005;5:151. https://doi.org/10.1186/1471-2407-5-151.

289. Albain KS, Nag SM, Calderillo-Ruiz G, Jordaan JP, Llombart AC, Pluzanska A, Rolski J, Melemed AS, Reyes-Vidal JM, Sekhon JS, Simms L, O'Shaughnessy J. Gemcitabine plus Paclitaxel versus Paclitaxel monotherapy in patients with metastatic breast cancer and prior anthracycline treatment. J Clin Oncol. 2008;26(24):3950–7. https://doi.org/10.1200/JCO.2007.11.9362.

290. Demiray M, Kurt E, Evrensel T, Kanat O, Arslan M, Saraydaroglu O, Ercan I, Gonullu G, Gokgoz S, Topal U, Tolunay S, Tasdelen I, Manavoglu O. Phase II study of gemcitabine plus paclitaxel in metastatic breast cancer patients with prior anthracycline exposure. Cancer Investig. 2005;23:386–91. https://doi.org/10.1081/CNV-200067133.

291. Swain SM, Baselga J, Kim SB, Ro J, Semiglazov V, Campone M, Ciruelos E, Ferrero JM, Schneeweiss A, Heeson S, Clark E, Ross G, Benyunes MC, Cortés J. Pertuzumab, trastuzumab, and docetaxel in HER2-positive metastatic breast cancer. N Engl J Med. 2015;372:724–34. https://doi.org/10.1056/NEJMoa1413513.

292. Shao Z, Pang D, Yang H, Li W, Wang S, Cui S, Liao N, Wang Y, Wang C, Chang YC, Wang H, Kang SY, Seo JH, Shen K, Laohawiriyakamol S, Jiang Z, Li J, Zhou J, Althaus B, Mao Y, Eng-Wong J. Efficacy, safety, and tolerability of pertuzumab, trastuzumab, and docetaxel for patients with early or locally advanced ERBB2-positive breast cancer in Asia: the PEONY phase 3 randomized clinical trial. JAMA Oncol. 2020;6(3):e193692. https://doi.org/10.1001/jamaoncol.2019.3692.

293. Swain SM, Miles D, Kim SB, Im YH, Im SA, Semiglazov V, Ciruelos E, Schneeweiss A, Loi S, Monturus E, Clark E, Knott A, Restuccia E, Benyunes MC, Cortés J. Pertuzumab, trastuzumab, and docetaxel for HER2-positive metastatic breast cancer (CLEOPATRA): end-of-study results from a double-blind, randomised, placebo-controlled, phase 3 study. Lancet Oncol. 2020;21(4):519–30. https://doi.org/10.1016/S1470-2045(19)30863-0.

294. Ramagopalan SV, Pisoni R, Rathore LS, Ray J, Sammon C. Association of pertuzumab, trastuzumab, and docetaxel combination therapy with overall survival in patients with metastatic breast cancer. JAMA Netw Open. 2021;4(1):e2027764. https://doi.org/10.1001/jamanetworkopen.2020.27764.

295. Hubalek M, Brantner C, Marth C. Role of pertuzumab in the treatment of HER2-positive breast cancer. Breast Cancer Targets Ther. 2012;4:65–73. https://doi.org/10.2147/BCTT.S23560.

296. Boix-Perales H, Borregaard J, Jensen KB, Ersboll J, Galluzzo S, Giuliani R, Ciceroni C, Melchiorri D, Salmonson T, Bergh J, Schellens JH, Pignatti F. The European medicines agency review of pertuzumab for the treatment of adult patients with HER2-positive metastatic or locally recurrent unresectable breast cancer: summary of the scientific assessment of the committee for medicinal products for human use. Oncologist. 2014;19(7):766–73. https://doi.org/10.1634/theoncologist.2013-0348.

297. Gama CS, Nobre SMPC, Neusquen LPDG. Extravasamento de medicamentos antineoplásicos. São Paulo: Eurofarma; 2016.

298. Swain SM, Ewer MS, Viale G, Delaloge S, Ferrero JM, Verrill M, Colomer R, Vieira C, Werner TL, Douthwaite H, Bradley D, Waldron-Lynch M, Kiermaier A, Eng-Wong J, Dang C. Pertuzumab, trastuzumab, and standard anthracycline- and taxane-based chemotherapy for the neoadjuvant treatment of patients with HER2-positive localized breast cancer (BERENICE): a phase II, open-label, multicenter, multinational cardiac safety study. Ann Oncol. 2018;29(3):646–53. https://doi.org/10.1093/annonc/mdx773.

299. NHS. Chemotherapy protocol. Breast cancer. Docetaxel-pertuzumab-trastuzumab. NHS, University Hospital Southampton, NHS Foundation Trust, England, 2015. Available https://www.uhs.nhs.uk/Media/SUHTExtranet/Services/Chemotherapy-SOPs/Breastcancer/Docetaxel-Pertuzumab-Trastuzumab.pdf. Accessed Aug 7, 2021.

300. Bachelot T, Ciruelos E, Schneeweiss A, Puglisi F, Peretz-Yablonski T, Bondarenko I, Paluch-Shimon S, Wardley A, Merot JL, du Toit Y, Easton V, Lindegger N, Miles D. Preliminary safety and efficacy of first-line pertuzumab combined with trastuzumab and taxane therapy for HER2-positive locally recurrent or metastatic breast cancer (PERUSE). Ann Oncol. 2019;30(5):766–73. https://doi.org/10.1093/annonc/mdz061.

301. Wang R, Smyth LM, Iyengar N, Chandarlapaty S, Modi S, Jochelson M, Patil S, Norton L, Hudis CA, Dang CT. Phase II study of weekly paclitaxel with trastuzumab and pertuzumab in patients with human epidermal growth receptor 2 overexpressing metastatic breast cancer: 5-year follow-up. Oncologist. 2019;24(8):e646–52. https://doi.org/10.1634/theoncologist.2018-0512.

302. NCT01276041. Paclitaxel, trastuzumab, and pertuzumab in the treatment of metastatic HER2-positive breast cancer. Clinical Trials. 2020. Available https://www.clinicaltrials.gov/ct2/show/NCT01276041. Accessed Aug 7, 2021.

303. Smyth LM, Iyengar NM, Chen MF, Popper SM, Patil S, Wasserheit-Lieblich C, Argolo DF, Singh JC, Chandarlapaty S, Sugarman SM, Comen EA, Drullinsky PR, Traina TA, Troso-Sandoval T, Baselga J, Norton L, Hudis CA, Dang CT. Weekly paclitaxel with trastuzumab and pertuzumab in patients with HER2-overexpressing metastatic breast cancer: overall survival and updated progression-free survival results from a phase II study. Breast Cancer Res Treat. 2016;158(1):91–7. https://doi.org/10.1007/s10549-016-3851-7.

304. Gupta NK, Giblin E, Leagre CA, Govert K, Givens S, Chichester T, Locker M, Bhayani P, Burnett R, Spivey T, Cohen S, Paul R. Effect of a combination of pertuzumab, trastuzumab, and weekly paclitaxel on pCR rates and side-effect profile as a neoadjuvant treatment regimen for HER2-positive breast cancer. J Clin Oncol. 2018;36(15):e12652. https://doi.org/10.1200/JCO.2018.36.15_suppl.e12652.

305. Sun S. BC Cancer protocol summary for palliative therapy for metastatic breast cancer using PERTuzumab, trastuzumab (HERCEPTIN), and PACLitaxel as first-line treatment for advanced breast cancer. BC Cancer, British Columbia, 2021. Available http://www.bccancer.bc.ca/chemotherapy-protocols-site/Documents/Breast/BRAVPTRAT_Protocol.pdf. Accessed Aug 7, 2021.

306. Suzuki Y, Tokuda Y, Saito Y, Ohta M, Tajima T. Combination of trastuzumab and vinorelbine in metastatic breast cancer. Jpn J Clin Oncol. 2003;33(10):514–7. https://doi.org/10.1093/jjco/hyg101.
307. NCT01185509. Trastuzumab and vinorelbine in advanced breast cancer. Clinical Trials. 2019. Available https://clinicaltrials.gov/ct2/show/NCT01185509. Accessed Aug 7, 2021.
308. Burstein HJ, Harris LN, Marcom PK, Lambert-Falls R, Havlin K, Overmoyer B, Friedlander RJ Jr, Gargiulo J, Strenger R, Vogel CL, Ryan PD, Ellis MJ, Nunes RA, Bunnell CA, Campos SM, Hallor M, Gelman R, Winer EP. Trastuzumab and vinorelbine as first-line therapy for HER2-overexpressing metastatic breast cancer: multicenter phase II trial with clinical outcomes, analysis of serum tumor markers as predictive factors, and cardiac surveillance algorithm. J Clin Oncol. 2003;21(15):2889–95. https://doi.org/10.1200/JCO.2003.02.018.
309. Stravodimou A, Zaman K, Voutsadakis IA. Vinorelbine with or without trastuzumab in metastatic breast cancer: a retrospective single institution series. Int Sch Res Notices. 2014;2014:289836. https://doi.org/10.1155/2014/289836.
310. Chan A, Martin M, Untch M, Gil MG, Guillem-Porta V, Wojtukiewicz M, Kellokumpu-Lehtinen P, Sommer HL, Georgoulias V, Battelli N, Pawlocki M, Aubert D, Bourlard T, Gasmi J, Villanova G, Petruzelka L. Vinorelbine plus trastuzumab combination as first-line therapy for HER 2-positive metastatic breast cancer patients: an international phase II trial. Br J Cancer. 2006;95:788–93. https://doi.org/10.1038/sj.bjc.6603351.
311. Burstein HJ, Kuter I, Campos SM, Gelman RS, Tribou L, Parker LM, Manola J, Younger J, Matulonis U, Bunnell CA, Partridge AH, Richardson PG, Clarke K, Shulman LN, Winer EP. Clinical activity of trastuzumab and vinorelbine in women with HER2-overexpressing metastatic breast cancer. J Clin Oncol. 2001;19(10):2722–30. https://doi.org/10.1200/JCO.2001.19.10.2722.

Chapter 5
Chemotherapeutic Protocols for the Treatment of Gastrointestinal Tract Cancer

5.1 Epidemiological Profile of Cancers of the Gastrointestinal Tract

The gastrointestinal tract extends from the mouth to the anus, being responsible for food digestion and nutrient extraction, where waste is removed from the body through the colon and rectum [1–3]. Tumor formation may be from a mutation in the DNA causing abnormal cells to grow, where this mutation may be induced by conditions underlying lifestyle choices and genetics factors [4, 5]. Gastrointestinal tract cancer develops in the digestive system and can affect the esophagus, stomach, small and large intestines, and rectum, with more than 70% of cases occurring in the stomach or intestine [6–11]. Figure 5.1 presents the estimated data for 2040 of incidence of cases and mortality of cancers of the gastrointestinal tract.

Gastrointestinal tract cancers account for 26% of the global cancer incidence and 35% of cancer-related deaths [13–15]. As for signs and symptoms, they may not exist at the beginning of the tumor, but in the long term, it can cause anemia, inducing fatigue and weakness, and it can also cause bleeding in the digestive system, which can be identified in feces or vomiting [16–18]. In addition, gastrointestinal cancers can induce stomach or abdominal pain, bloating in the abdomen, loss of appetite, weight loss, difficulty in swallowing, among others [19, 20].

Diagnosis is based on imaging tests such as ultrasound, computed tomography, and magnetic resonance imaging, in addition to endoscopy and colonoscopy used to locate possible tumors in the stomach and intestine [21–23]. Biopsy is indicated to confirm the tumor. As for the therapeutic modality, they may include chemotherapy, target therapy, surgery, tumor ablation, embolization, and radiotherapy [24–26].

© The Author(s), under exclusive license to Springer Nature
Switzerland AG 2022
I. D. Lima Cavalcanti, *Chemotherapy Protocols and Infusion Sequence*,
https://doi.org/10.1007/978-3-031-10839-6_5

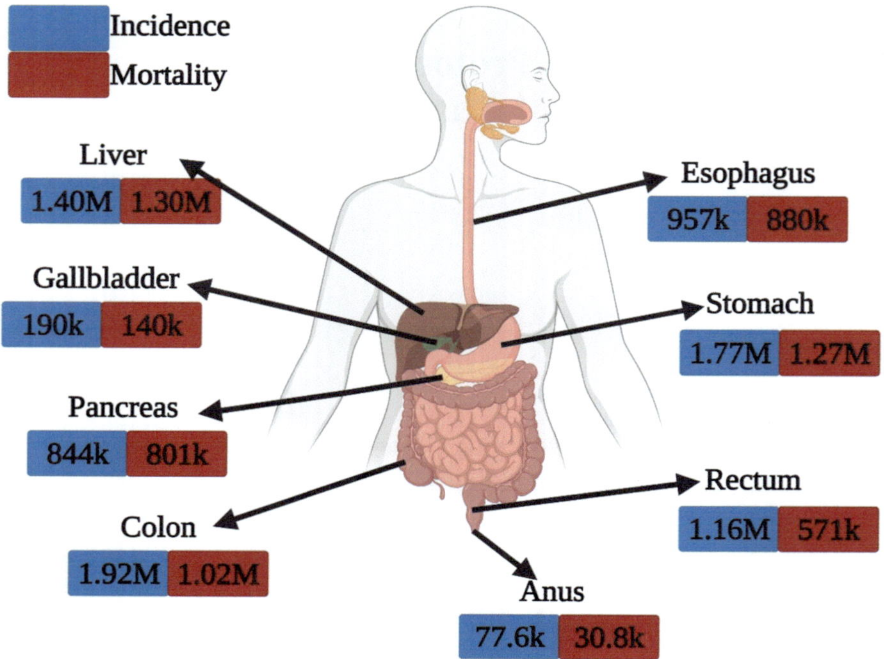

Fig. 5.1 Estimate data for the year 2040 of incidence of cases and mortality of cancers of the gastrointestinal tract. (Source: Created with BioRender.com and data were extracted from [12])

5.2   Pathophysiology of Colorectal Cancer

Colorectal cancer starts in the colon or rectum and may also be called colon cancer or rectal cancer depending on where the tumor starts. These cancers are often grouped together because of the characteristics they have in common. Physiologically, the colon and rectum make up the large intestine, for which the colon accounts for most, measuring about 1.5 meters in length. The colon is divided into four parts into the ascending, transverse, descending, and sigmoid colon, which the latter joins the rectum that connects to the anus [27–31].

The colon is responsible for absorbing water and salt from the remaining food material after it passes through the small intestine, while the remaining waste forms the feces, passing through the rectum and anus for disposal [2, 32].

The growth of colorectal cancer most often starts with the growth of polyps (Fig. 5.2). Not all polyps can induce the development of cancer; examples are the hyperplastic and inflammatory polyps, which, although more common, do not usually induce the development of cancer. On the other hand, sessile serrated polyps and traditional serrated adenomas have an increased risk of developing colorectal cancer [33–39].

Colorectal cancer initially develops in the polyp, which can grow into the wall of the colon or rectum, which is composed of several layers, and can grow out of some

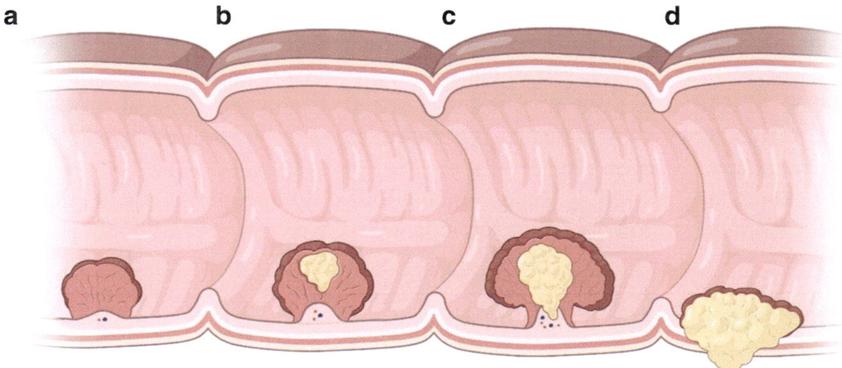

Fig. 5.2 Development of colorectal cancer. (**a**) Polyp, (**b**) precancerous lesion, (**c**) colorectal cancer, and (**d**) advanced colorectal cancer. (Source: Created with BioRender.com)

or all of the layers (Fig. 5.2d) and can transform in blood vessels or lymphatic vessels, thus spreading to other organs [27, 40–42].

There are several types of colorectal cancer, which the most common is adenocarcinoma; they also include carcinoid tumors, gastrointestinal stromal tumors, and colorectal lymphoma [41, 43, 44]. Adenocarcinomas start in the lining of the internal organs in cells with glandular properties or cells that secrete; they can start from small adenomatous polyps that continue to grow and can then develop into malignant cancers [29, 41, 45].

Colorectal cancer can also be classified into resectable and unresectable cancers [46, 47]. Resectable cancers can be treated with tumor removal surgery with a margin of safety for adjacent healthy tissue, where the cancer is localized. In cases where the tumor has invaded the bowel wall or has spread to nearby lymph nodes, there is the possibility of indicating treatment with chemotherapy or radiotherapy, seeking to destroy the cancer cells remaining from the surgery [48–52].

Tumors are classified as unresectable when they spread to nearby tissues or other organs, where the indication for surgery is no longer curative, with the objective of unblocking the intestine, thereby improving symptoms such as nausea, vomiting, or even pain abdominal [53, 54]. Patients with unresectable colorectal cancer undergo chemotherapy treatment, whereas radiotherapy is indicated for the treatment of organs where there has been dissemination, such as the brain or bones [55–57].

5.2.1 Adjuvant Chemotherapy for the Treatment of Resectable Colorectal Cancer

Depending on the stage of colorectal cancer, the 5-year survival rate increases, with stage I being 90%, stage II 70–80%, and stage III 40–65%. An important fact is that about 80% of patients with colorectal cancer have localized and resectable disease, allowing for a surgical approach with the objective of cure [58–60].

Surgical resection is the treatment of choice for the treatment of liver or lung metastases. Performing the surgery is important because it benefits the overall 5-year survival rate, which can range from 28 to 38% in patients who have had complete resection of liver metastases. Associated with the surgical procedure, some pharmacological therapies have been indicated for the adjuvant treatment of colorectal cancer, such as the use of monotherapy with capecitabine or associated with radiotherapy, as well as some combinations of antineoplastic agents that we will discuss in the following topics [60–68].

5.2.1.1   CAPOX Protocol (Oxaliplatin and Capecitabine)

One of the protocols used for the treatment of resectable colorectal cancer is CAPOX, which is a combination of oxaliplatin and capecitabine [69–70]. Oxaliplatin is one of the most used antineoplastics for the treatment of colorectal cancer, being part of the class of drugs composed of platinum, which acts as an alkylating agent on DNA, forming inter- and intra-filament bridges, thereby inhibiting DNA synthesis. Like other alkylating agents, it is also classified as a nonspecific agent, and its dermatological toxicity is characterized as an irritant [71–75].

Capecitabine, on the other hand, is a drug of the antimetabolite class, derived from the fluoropyrimidine carbamate, where it is metabolized in the body into its cytotoxic fraction 5-fluorouracil. Unlike other drugs, capecitabine comes in tablet form and is administered orally [76, 77].

Li et al. [70] evaluated the efficacy of the combination of capecitabine and oxaliplatin in colorectal cancer with liver metastases. The authors observed a response rate of 40%, proving to be a safe protocol with survival benefits and can convert colorectal cancer with potentially resectable liver metastases into resectable ones.

Hattori et al. [78] evaluated the effectiveness of the CAPOX protocol in locally advanced rectal cancer as postoperative adjuvant therapy. The results showed a relapse-free survival rate and a 3-year overall survival rate of 75% and 96%, respectively. Gil-Delgado et al. [79] carried out a pharmacokinetic study of the CAPOX protocol in colorectal cancer, showing a combination that is well tolerated, without significant neurological toxicity after administration of oxaliplatin for more than 6 h.

According to the study by Satake et al. [80], the combination of capecitabine with oxaliplatin after hepatectomy in patients with colorectal cancer with liver metastases has been shown to be tolerable and may be a promising strategy for post-curative resection. The results showed a 5-year recurrence-free survival of 65.2% and an overall survival of 87.2%.

Administration of the CAPOX protocol is based on the infusion of oxaliplatin on the first day intravenously followed by the administration of capecitabine orally twice daily for 14 days (Fig. 5.3) [78, 81].

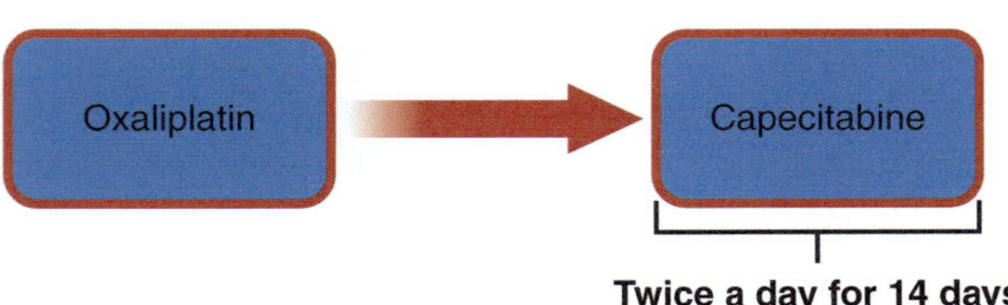

Fig. 5.3 CAPOX protocol administration schedule with oral administration of capecitabine

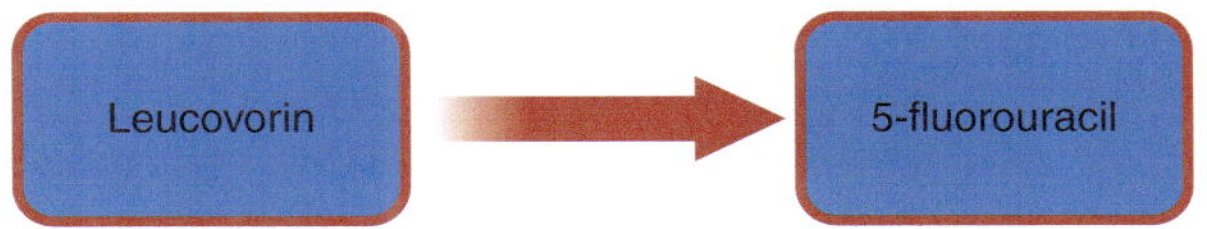

Fig. 5.4 FL protocol infusion sequence

5.2.1.2   FL Protocol (5-Fluorouracil and Leucovorin)

The combination of 5-fluorouracil and leucovorin is very common in the treatment of colorectal cancer [82–84]. As discussed in Chap. 1, leucovorin enhances the cytotoxic action of 5-fluorouracil. Leucovorin is the 5-formyl derivative of tetrahydrofolic acid, an active form of folic acid that is essential for nucleic acid synthesis, being a basic factor for cell reproduction, especially in fast-growing cells. Unlike 5-fluorouracil, leucovorin is not an antineoplastic drug, but it plays a fundamental role in enhancing the anticancer effects of 5-fluoro-uracil [84–87].

Borner et al. [88] noted that the addition of low-dose leucovorin to 5-fluorouracil had great benefits in the treatment of colorectal cancer, increasing the response rate from 9% (5-fluorouracil alone) to 22% with the combination, also with increased of progression-free survival from 3.9 to 6.2 months. When toxicity, fatal events were not observed, presenting only cases of stomatitis, diarrhea, and nausea. Porschen et al. [89] and Arkenau et al. [90] also observed the benefits of the association of 5-fluorouracil with leucovorin, improving disease-free survival, decreasing overall mortality, and being well tolerated.

Portier et al. [91] observed that the combination of 5-fluorouracil with leucovorin promoted a disease-free 5-year survival rate of 33.5% and an overall 5-year survival rate of 51.1%, proving to be an effective therapy for the treatment of colorectal cancer with resected liver metastases. Due to the benefits of 5-fluorouracil action, it is important that leucovorin is administered prior to 5-fluorouracil administration (Fig. 5.4) [84, 92, 93].

5.2.1.3   FOLFOX Protocol (Oxaliplatin, Leucovorin, 5-Fluorouracil, and 5-Fluorouracil in Continuous Infusion)

The inclusion of oxaliplatin combined with 5-fluorouracil and leucovorin is also a widely used combination for the treatment of colorectal cancer [94–97]. As we saw in Sect. 5.2.1.1, oxaliplatin is an alkylating agent, acting in a nonspecific manner in the cell cycle, whose action is based on the inhibition of DNA synthesis [74, 98]. The inclusion of oxaliplatin promoted an improvement in the efficiency of the combination of the FL protocol, where according to André et al. [99] promoted a 3-year free survival rate of 78.2%. Regarding adverse events, the authors observed cases of febrile neutropenia, gastrointestinal effects, and sensory neuropathy, proving to be a safe protocol for the adjuvant treatment of colon cancer.

Alberts et al. [100] found that the combination of oxaliplatin, 5-fluorouracil, and leucovorin promoted a high response rate in patients with liver metastases from colorectal cancer, allowing for successful resection. However, the authors observed a high recurrence rate. Goldberg et al. [101] report in their study that the FOLFOX protocol is active and safe in the treatment of advanced colorectal cancer, with a response rate of 45% and a mean survival time of 19.5 months, with low cases of severe nausea, vomiting, diarrhea, febrile neutropenia, and dehydration. André et al. [97] also shows the benefits of the FOLFOX protocol in stage III colon cancer, promoting an increase in overall survival of 67.1%.

In a phase I/II study, Yamada et al. [102] observed the efficacy of the FOLFOX protocol with administration of oxaliplatin with weekly bolus of 5-fluorouracil and high-dose leucovorin as a first-line treatment for colorectal cancer. The study showed a response rate of 61% with a median time to progression of 171 days and an overall survival time of 603 days. As for toxicity, some patients had limiting toxicity, with cases of thrombocytopenia and neutropenia, thus postponing chemotherapy and all patients had sensory neuropathy.

As for the infusion schedule of the FOLFOX protocol, it is preferable that oxaliplatin is administered initially, and it can be administered concomitantly with leucovorin, since both are compatible when administered concomitantly in a Y-infusion device. The concomitant administration of oxaliplatin with leucovorin (Fig. 5.5a) can reduce the patient's length of stay in the chemotherapy sector, but sequential administration, starting with oxaliplatin followed by leucovorin (Fig. 5.5b), is also possible and finally the infusion of 5-fluorouracil in bolus followed by the infusion of 5-fluorouracil in continuous infusion (Fig. 5.5). Because oxaliplatin is incompatible with 0.9% sodium chloride, as we saw in Chap. 3, and can precipitate, ideally, all drugs that make up the FOLFOX protocol are diluted in glucose serum [99, 102–106].

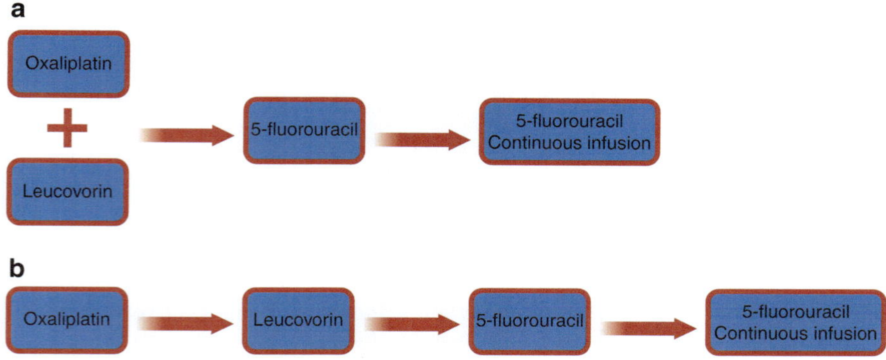

Fig. 5.5 FOLFOX protocol infusion sequence. (**a**) Concomitant infusion of oxaliplatin with leucovorin followed by 5-fluorouracil bolus and 5-fluorouracil continuous infusion. (**b**) Infusion of oxaliplatin followed by administration of leucovorin and finally 5-fluorouracil in bolus and 5-fluorouracil in continuous infusion

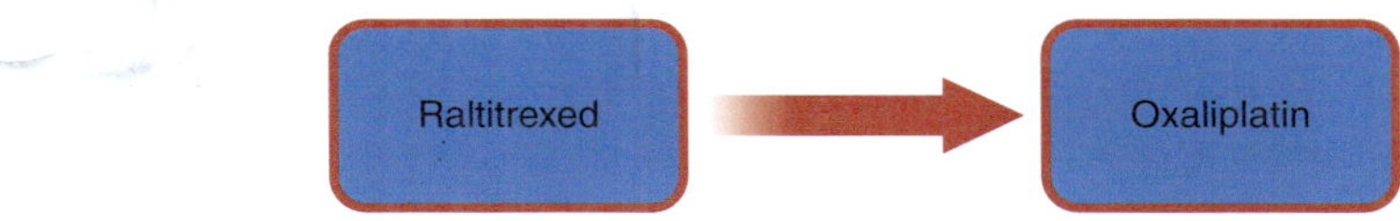

Fig. 5.6 RALOX protocol infusion sequence

5.2.1.4 RALOX Protocol (Oxaliplatin and Raltitrexed)

Some studies have demonstrated the effectiveness of the RALOX protocol in the treatment of colorectal cancer [107–109]. Raltitrexed is an antimetabolite drug, and, like 5-fluorouracil, it acts by inhibiting the enzyme thymidylate synthase, thereby inhibiting the formation of DNA and RNA, inducing cells to apoptosis. Despite similar mechanisms of action, raltitrexed is more specific and has a different toxicity profile than 5-fluorouracil. Therefore, some protocols have replaced 5-fluorouracil with raltitrexed, as well as being used as monotherapy [110–114].

In a phase II study, Cascinu et al. [107] evaluated the efficacy of the combination of raltitrexed plus oxaliplatin as a first-line treatment for metastatic colorectal cancer, proving to be an effective and well-tolerated protocol. The combination promoted an overall response rate of 50%, median overall survival of >9 months, and median time to progression of 6.5 months. As for the toxicity profile, the patients presented neutropenia as the main hematological toxicity and as the non-hematological toxicity cases of transient transaminitis, asthenia, neurotoxicity, and diarrhea.

Cortinovis et al. [108] also demonstrated the effectiveness of the RALOX protocol in the treatment of metastatic colorectal cancer, with a toxicity profile similar to that presented in the study by Cascinu et al. [107], with cases of transaminitis, diarrhea, asthenia, nausea, and vomiting.

As for the infusion sequence, most studies have evaluated the effectiveness of the combination by administering raltitrexed for 15 min followed by oxaliplatin (Fig. 5.6). This sequence seems adequate for promoting the protocol's efficacy in the treatment of colorectal cancer without inducing an increase in the toxicity profile [108, 114, 115].

5.2.2 Chemotherapy for the Treatment of Advanced Unresectable Colorectal Cancer

In advanced unresectable colorectal cancer, surgery is not the first therapeutic option, chemotherapy being the first indication. Several antineoplastics are indicated for the treatment of unresectable advanced colorectal cancer, whether they are indicated as monotherapy, such as capecitabine, irinotecan, raltitrexed, and panitu-mumab, as well as some drugs that can be associated with radiotherapy [116–119].

Combination antineoplastics are also indicated, and some protocols such as FL, CAPOX, and FOLFOX that are indicated for the treatment of resectable colorectal cancer may also be indicated for the treatment of advanced unresectable colorectal cancer. Some of these protocols have helped to reduce tumor mass and allow unresectable colorectal tumors to become resectable [120–123]. In the following topics, we will discuss protocols that are also indicated for the treatment of advanced unresectable colorectal cancer.

5.2.2.1   CAPB Protocol (Capecitabine and Bevacizumab)

The CAPB protocol is based on the combination of the drugs capecitabine and bevacizumab in the treatment of metastatic or unresectable colorectal cancer in patients not suitable for receiving combination therapy with irinotecan or oxaliplatin [124–127]. Bevacizumab is a monoclonal antibody that specifically binds to vascular endothelial growth factor (VEGF), thereby preventing its binding to its receptors on the surface of endothelial cells and inhibiting the formation of new blood vessels [128–131].

The combination of bevacizumab with capecitabine has been beneficial in the treatment of advanced unresectable colorectal cancer. According to the study by Bang et al. [127], the CAPB protocol promoted a median overall survival of 9.7 months, progression-free survival of 4.6 months, and an overall response rate of 14% in patients with metastatic colorectal cancer refractory to irinotecan, oxaliplatin, and fluoropyrimidines.

Larsen et al. [132] evaluated the combination of capecitabine with bevacizumab in patients pretreated for advanced colorectal cancer, proving to be a well-tolerated combination, with progression-free survival of 5.4 months and median overall survival of 12.2 months, with an acceptable toxicity profile. Goey et al. [133] demonstrated the benefits of the CAPB protocol in the treatment of metastatic colorectal cancer, especially in patients with wild-type RAS/BRAF mutation tumors.

One of the problems for the application of the protocol in the clinic is due to its high cost, where according to the study by Sherman et al. [134] it would be necessary to reduce the price of the protocol by 93% to make it economical, thereby limiting its use in clinical practice. As per the CAPB protocol schedule, bevacizumab is administered on the first day by infusion combined with capecitabine, which is administered orally for 14 consecutive days (Fig. 5.7) [125, 135].

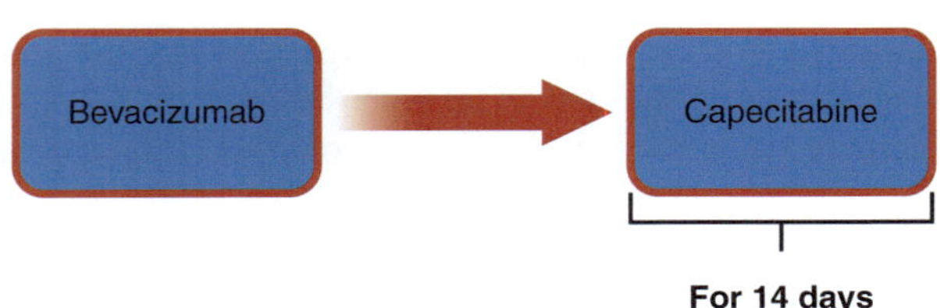

Fig. 5.7 CAPB protocol administration schedule with oral administration of capecitabine

5.2.2.2 CETIR Protocol (Cetuximab and Irinotecan)

Another monoclonal antibody also used in the treatment of unresectable advanced colorectal cancer is cetuximab, which acts on the epidermal growth factor receptor (EGFR), inducing its internalization, thereby leading to a reduction in EGFR regulation. In addition, cetuximab also sends cytotoxic immuneffector cells against tumor cells that express the EGFR [136–138].

The use of cetuximab in the CETIR protocol is combined with irinotecan in the treatment of colorectal cancer. Irinotecan is an antineoplastic agent that inhibits the action of topoisomerase I, thereby preventing DNA strand religation by inducing the binding of topoisomerase I to the DNA complex. The formation of the complex will prevent DNA replication and induce the breakage of the DNA double chain, thereby leading the cell to apoptosis. The differences in the mechanisms of action of these drugs when combined favor the treatment of advanced colorectal cancer [139–143].

Wilke et al. [139] highlighted the benefits of combining cetuximab with irinotecan in metastatic colorectal cancer. The protocol proved to be well-tolerated, with acceptable adverse events such as diarrhea, neutropenia, rash, and asthenia. The 12-week progression-free survival results from 61% and median survival of 9.2 months, proving to be an effective and safe protocol in metastatic colorectal cancer.

According to Cunningham et al. [136], the response rate of the combination seems to be higher than cetuximab monotherapy. The authors noted that the response rate increased 12% with the combination, with an increase in median time to progression and median survival time as well. As for the toxicity profile, the combination therapy between irinotecan and cetuximab showed more toxic effects, but the severity and incidence of the effects were similar to those expected from the isolated use of irinotecan.

In phase II clinical trial, Martín-Martorell et al. [144] report the benefits of the combination of irinotecan and cetuximab, obtaining an overall response rate of 22.5%, disease control rate of 60%, time to progression of 3.4 months, and overall survival of 8 months. The toxicity profile was acceptable, similar to that obtained in other protocols with reports of diarrhea, rash, anemia, and neutropenia.

Vincenzi et al. [145] used the CETIR protocol in the third-line treatment of advanced colorectal cancer. The authors report that the combination led to a 25.4% response rate, with an overall tumor control rate of 63.6%, with a median time to progression of 4.7 months, and a median survival time of 9.8 months. The toxicity profile was similar to other studies with cases of diarrhea, fatigue, stomatitis, and skin toxicity.

Pfeiffer et al. [146] also tested the combination of the CETIR protocol as third-line therapy in patients with advanced colorectal cancer who failed with irinotecan, oxaliplatin, and 5-fluorouracil. The protocol had a response rate similar to the other studies of 20%, with a time to progression of 5.5 months and overall survival of 10.4 months. This therapy has been shown to be effective as rescue therapy in patients pretreated with irinotecan and oxaliplatin.

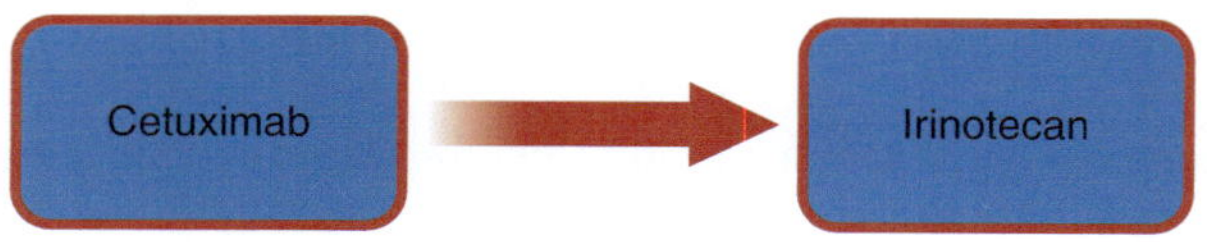

Fig. 5.8 Infusion sequence of the CETIR protocol

Seeking to identify some pharmacokinetic interaction, Czejka et al. [147] evaluated the pharmacokinetic profile of the CETIR protocol. According to the authors, the combination appears to have no pharmacokinetic interactions. Given the results presented, the infusion sequence of the CETIR protocol starting with cetuximab seems to be more appropriate as it is a target-directed drug followed by the infusion of irinotecan (Fig. 5.8) [144, 148].

5.2.2.3　FOLFIRI Protocol (Irinotecan, Leucovorin, 5-Fluorouracil, and 5-Fluorouracil in Continuous Infusion)

Similar to the FOLFOX protocol (Sect. 5.2.1.3), the FOLFIRI protocol is based on the combination of irinotecan with 5-fluorouracil and leucovorin for the treatment of advanced colorectal cancer [149–151]. As we saw in the previous topic, irinotecan is a natural product that is part of the class of drugs that act on topoisomerase I, being a cycle-specific antineoplastic agent [152–154].

Glynne-Jones et al. [155] in a phase I/II study evaluated the use of irinotecan combined with 5-fluorouracil and leucovorin and pelvic radiation in locally advanced rectal cancer. The results showed that the combination induced an acceptable toxicity profile with cases of diarrhea, neutropenia, febrile neutropenia, and anemia. As for the response to the tumor, the protocol promoted a clear circumferential resection margin in 80% of the patients who were resected.

Barone et al. [156] evaluated the benefits of the FOLFIRI protocol in patients with colorectal cancer with unresectable liver metastases, showing that surgical resection of liver metastases after neoadjuvant treatment with the FOLFIRI protocol brought important results in terms of survival, with median survival results of 31 0.5 months for unresected patients and disease-free survival of 52.2 months for resected patients.

As for the data regarding the infusion schedule, the administration of irinotecan with 5-fluorouracil concomitantly is not adequate because they are incompatible when administered in a Y device. Despite this, irinotecan when administered first seems to provide a synergistic effect to 5-fluorouracil, increasing DNA damage, and protocol toxicity seems to be more acceptable when irinotecan is administered first. As we saw in Sect. 5.2.1.2, leucovorin also potentiates the effects of 5-fluorouracil, and it should be administered before and as in the FOLFOX protocol (Sect. 5.2.1.3); because leucovorin is compatible with irinotecan, they can be infused concomitant, with this, reducing the length of stay of the patient in the chemotherapy sector [151, 154, 157]. In Fig. 5.9, I present two infusion sequence options that can be used in the FOLFIRI protocol.

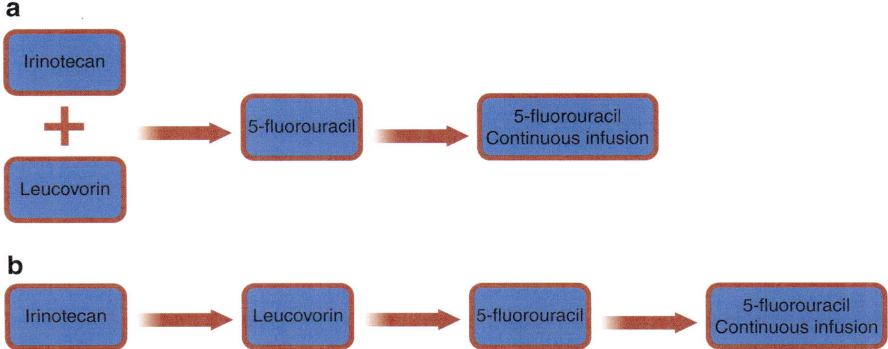

Fig. 5.9 FOLFIRI protocol infusion sequence. (**a**) Concomitant infusion of irinotecan with leucovorin followed by 5-fluorouracil bolus and 5-fluorouracil continuous infusion. (**b**) Infusion of irinotecan followed by administration of leucovorin and finally 5-fluorouracil in bolus and 5-fluorouracil in continuous infusion

5.2.2.4 CAPIRI Protocol (Capecitabine and Irinotecan)

The CAPIRI protocol is based on the combination of capecitabine and irinotecan as palliative therapy in patients unsuitable for FOLFIRI therapy in metastatic colorectal cancer [158]. The combination between capecitabine and irinotecan demonstrated a synergistic effect in vitro, showing that the association was much more active than the drugs alone against tumor models of colon cancer, salivary gland, and hypopharyngeal squamous cell carcinoma. The synergistic effects appear to be tumor dependent and independent of p53 expression [159, 160]. Despite the synergistic effects, the drugs have a pharmacokinetic interaction and need to be activated by the enzyme carboxylesterases, where capecitabine can induce the delayed conversion of irinotecan into SN-38 (active metabolite) [160, 161]. However, according to Goel et al. [160], the combination appears to be safe and well tolerated.

Czejka et al. [161] in a pharmacokinetic study in patients with advanced colorectal cancer found that capecitabine did not change the plasma disposition of irinotecan during treatment with the CAPIRI protocol, but there was a decrease in SN-38 plasma concentrations in the first 3 h after initiation of irinotecan infusion, with time-dependent differences in concentration. Despite this, there was no significant impact on the pharmacokinetics of irinotecan.

According to the study by Tewes et al. [162], the CAPIRI protocol as the first line in metastatic colorectal cancer promoted a response rate of 38% with a median response duration of 8.7 months, proving to be a protocol with significant therapeutic efficacy, in addition to controllable toxicity. The CAPIRI protocol is based on the infusion of irinotecan on the first day followed by oral administration of capecitabine twice daily for 14 days (Fig. 5.10) [163].

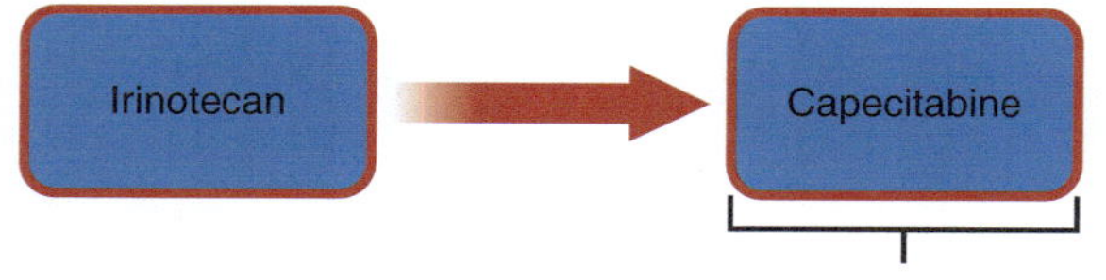

Fig. 5.10 CAPIRI protocol administration schedule with oral administration of capecitabine

5.2.2.5 CAPIRIB Protocol (Capecitabine, Irinotecan, and Bevacizumab)

With the efficacy results important of the CAPIRI protocol, some studies have invested in analyzing the efficacy of the combination with bevacizumab. Therefore, the CAPIRIB protocol has been indicated for the treatment of advanced colorectal cancer [164–168]. As we saw in Sect. 5.2.2.1, bevacizumab is a monoclonal antibody that acts specifically on VEGF binding, where the combination with capecitabine and irinotecan has brought benefits for the treatment of colorectal cancer, being a well-tolerated regimen with effective control tumor growth, with rare severe toxic effects [130, 164, 165, 169].

Behourah, Bousahba, and Djellali [170] evaluated the use of the CAPIRIB protocol in patients with previously untreated metastatic colorectal cancer. The authors noted that the protocol led to a median overall survival of 20.8 months and a 12-month progression-free survival rate of 44.2%. As for the toxicity profile, the patients had diarrhea, neutropenia, asthenia, vomiting, and refeeding syndrome.

In a phase II study, Garcia-Alfonso et al. [171] used the combination of capecitabine and biweekly irinotecan with bevacizumab as therapy for metastatic colorectal cancer. The results showed that the protocol was effective and tolerable, with a progression-free survival time of 11.9 months, overall survival of 24.8 months, overall response rate of 51%, and disease control rate of 84%. The main adverse events were similar to the study by Behourah, Bousahba, and Djellali [170], with cases of asthenia, diarrhea, and neutropenia.

The benefits of the CAPIRIB protocol were also demonstrated in the study by García-Alfonso et al. [172] with an overall response rate of 67.4%, disease control rate of 93.5%, progression-free survival of 12.3 months, and overall survival of 23.7 months, with toxic effects similar to previous studies with asthenia, diarrhea, nausea, and vomiting.

As for possible drug interactions, according to Denlinger et al. [173], bevacizumab does not affect the pharmacokinetics of irinotecan, with normal plasma concentrations of irinotecan and its active metabolite SN-38 when compared when given alone or in combination with bevacizumab. Because bevacizumab is a target-targeted drug, it is ideally given first, followed by irinotecan, and finally capecitabine orally for 14 days (Fig. 5.11) [174, 175].

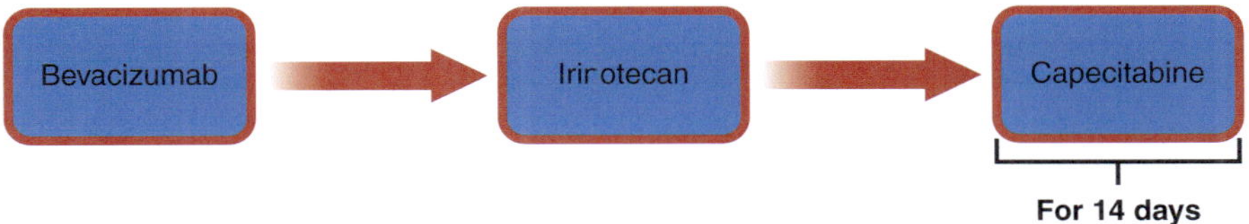

Fig. 5.11 Schedule of administration of the CAPIRIB protocol with oral administration of capecitabine

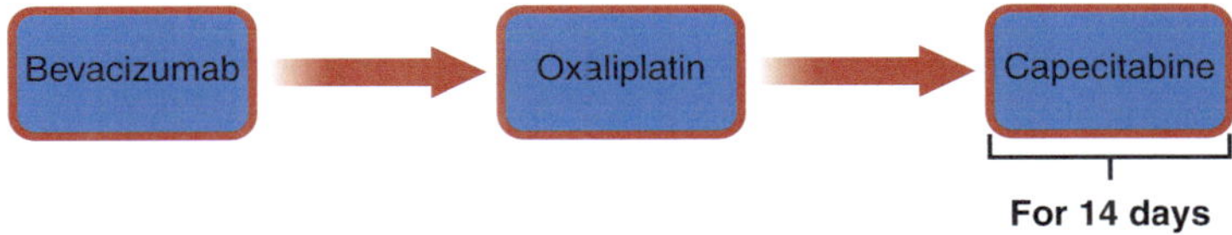

Fig. 5.12 Schedule of administration of the CAPOXB protocol with oral administration of capecitabine

5.2.2.6   CAPOXB Protocol (Oxaliplatin, Bevacizumab, and Capecitabine)

The CAPOXB protocol is based on a combination of oxaliplatin, bevacizumab, and capecitabine for the treatment of advanced colorectal cancer [176, 177]. Gruenberger et al. [178] evaluated the use of the CAPOXB protocol as neoadjuvant therapy in patients with metastatic colorectal cancer, showing that the use of bevacizumab 5 weeks before liver resection is safe in patients with metastatic colorectal cancer without increasing the rate of surgical complications or healing of wounds or severity of bleeding.

Feliu et al. [179] also report the benefits of the CAPOXB protocol in elderly patients with metastatic colorectal cancer, being effective and well tolerated with a time to progression of 11.1 months, overall survival of 20.4 months, and an overall response rate of 46%. The most frequent adverse events were the same presented by other protocols such as diarrhea and asthenia.

Munemoto et al. [180] presented the feasibility of using the CAPOXB protocol in elderly patients aged at least 75 years with metastatic colorectal cancer. The authors reported a progression-free survival time of 11.7 months and median overall survival of 22.9 months. The response rate was 55.6%, and disease control was 91.7%. The main toxicities were cases of neutropenia and neuropathy.

So far, there are no reports of drug interactions between bevacizumab and schedule-dependent oxaliplatin, so the CAPOXB protocol infusion order is more appropriate starting with bevacizumab, which is a target-targeted drug, followed by oxaliplatin and capecitabine via oral for 14 days (Fig. 5.12) [181, 182].

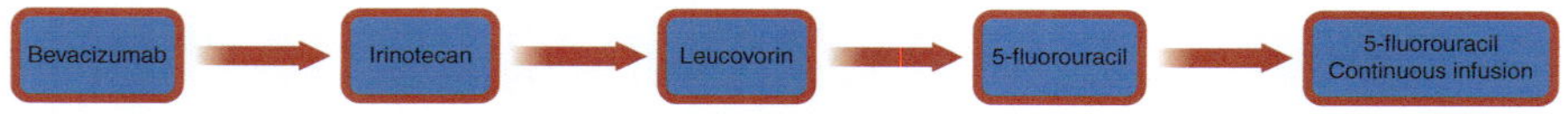

Fig. 5.13 Infusion sequence of the FOLFIRIB protocol

5.2.2.7   FOLFIRIB Protocol (5-Fluorouracil, 5-Fluorouracil in Continuous Infusion, Leucovorin, Irinotecan, and Bevacizumab)

Another protocol for the treatment of advanced colorectal cancer is the FOLFIRIB protocol, which is based on a combination of the FOLFIRI protocol (Sect. 5.2.2.3) plus bevacizumab [183, 184]. According to Deng et al. [185], the inclusion of bevacizumab in the FOLFIRI protocol for the second-line treatment of metastatic colorectal cancer led to a response rate of 31% and a controlled disease rate of 76.4%. Median progression-free survival was 6 months and overall survival was 17 months. The protocol also showed tolerable toxicity, with cases of neutropenia.

The FOLFIRIB protocol has also been shown to be effective in treating patients with metastatic colorectal cancer who have been treated with regimens containing oxaliplatin [186]. Moriwaki et al. [186] demonstrated that in this group of patients the protocol promoted a progression-free survival of 7.8–8.3 months, overall survival of 16.5–21.6 months, and an overall response rate of 25–29%.

Hurwitz et al. [183], as well as other studies, also proved the benefits of the FOLFIRIB protocol in patients with metastatic colorectal cancer, with results of median survival duration of 20.3 months, progression-free survival of 10.6 months, and mean duration of response of 10.4 months. The results of Hurwitz et al. [183] highlighted the improvement in the treatment of metastatic colorectal cancer with the addition of bevacizumab with the FOLFIRI protocol. Fyfe et al. [187] highlight that the FOLFIRIB protocol brought benefits in the survival of patients with metastatic colorectal cancer.

In a phase IV study, Sobrero et al. [188], as well as other studies, highlight the efficacy and safety of the FOLFIRIB protocol, showing a progression-free survival of 11.1 months, overall survival of 22.2 months, an overall response rate of 53.1%, and control rate 85.6% of the disease. As for toxicity, the vast majority of adverse events were manageable with cases of neutropenia, venous thromboembolic events, diarrhea, and fatigue. Regarding the infusion sequence of the FOLFIRIB protocol, it is similar to the infusion sequence of the FOLFIRI protocol but starts the infusion with bevacizumab (Fig. 5.13) [189].

5.2.2.8   FOLFIRIPAN Protocol (5-Fluorouracil, Leucovorin, Irinotecan, and Panitumumab)

The FOLFIRI protocol can also be combined with the drug panitumumab for the treatment of advanced colorectal cancer. Panitumumab is also a monoclonal antibody that acts by binding to the EGFR ligand-binding domain, which is the same

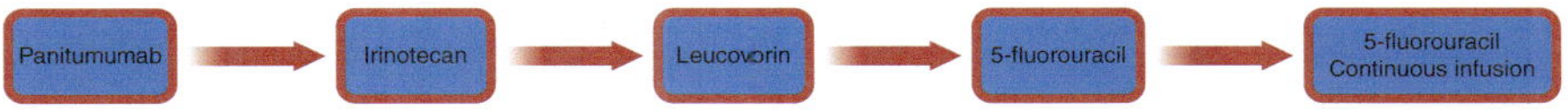

Fig. 5.14 FOLFIRIPAN protocol infusion sequence

target as cetuximab. The toxicity profile of panitumumab is similar to that of cetuximab with the main side effects being acneiform rash and diarrhea, which can also cause allergic or anaphylactic reactions [190–194].

Berlin et al. [195] and Berlin et al. [196] evaluated the use of the FOLFIRIPAN protocol as a first-line treatment for metastatic colorectal cancer, showing it to be well tolerated and with promising activity. Results showed a response rate of 42%, disease control rate of 79%, median progression-free survival of 10.9 months, and median overall survival of 22.5 months. The main toxicity was diarrhea in 25% of patients.

Efficacy results of the FOLFIRIPAN protocol were also observed by Kohne et al. [197], being more favorable to patients with wild-type KRAS metastatic colorectal cancer, with an objective response rate of 56%, response duration of 13 months, and progression-free survival of 8.9 months. As for the toxicity profile, it was similar to other protocols with tegumentary toxic effects, diarrhea, and oral stomatitis/mucositis. More recently, Pietrantonio et al. [198] compared the use of panitumumab in monotherapy and the combination with 5-fluorouracil and leucovorin in patients with RAS wild-type metastatic colorectal cancer. The use of panitumumab as monotherapy was inferior to panitumumab combined with 5-fluorouracil and leucovorin with 10-month progression-free survival outcomes of 49% and 59.9%, respectively.

In a phase 3 study, Peeters et al. [199] evaluated the benefits of the FOLFIRIPAN protocol as a second-line treatment for metastatic colorectal cancer. In patients with wild-type KRAS gene, the protocol induced a significant increase in progression-free survival, as demonstrated by Pietrantonio et al. [198], at 6.7 months and overall survival of 14.5 months, with a response rate of 36%. As for the infusion sequence, it is similar to the FOLFIRIB protocol, starting the infusion with the monoclonal antibody due to its specific action, highlighting the importance of evaluating the risk of developing allergic reactions due to the use of the monoclonal antibody (Fig. 5.14) [200].

5.2.2.9   FOLFOXB Protocol (Oxaliplatin, Leucovorin, 5-Fluorouracil, 5-Fluorouracil in Continuous Infusion, and Bevacizumab)

As with the FOLFIRI protocol, there is also a combination of the FOLFOX protocol with bevacizumab for the treatment of metastatic colorectal cancer [201, 202]. The effectiveness of the FOLFOXB protocol is similar to the effectiveness of the CAPOXB protocol, being highlighted in the study by Buchler et al. [203], who, when comparing these two protocols, observed a median overall survival of 27 months for FOLFOXB and 30.6 months for CAPOXB and progression-free survival of 11.4 months for FOLFOXB and 11.5 months for CAPOXB.

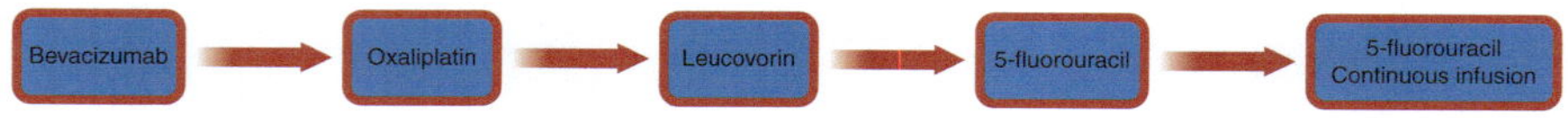

Fig. 5.15 Infusion sequence of the FOLFOXB protocol

Giantonio et al. [204] report that the FOLFOXB protocol improved the duration of survival in patients with previously treated metastatic colorectal cancer, resulting in progression-free survival of 7.3 months and an overall response rate of 22.7%. In a phase II multicenter study, Emmanouilides et al. [205] evaluated the effectiveness of the FOLFOXB protocol as a first line in metastatic colorectal cancer. The authors observed that the protocol promoted a complete response of 15.1% and a partial response of 52.8%. As for toxic effects, cases of neutropenia, febrile neutropenia, diarrhea, and neurotoxicity have been reported.

The FOLFOXB protocol also seems to benefit patients when combined with hyperthermia, where Ranieri et al. [206] report that the combination promoted a progression-free survival prolongation of 2.7 months compared with standard treatment without profound electrohypertemia, with progression-free survival of 12.1 months, and overall survival of 21.4 months.

Regarding the infusion schedule of the FOLFOXB protocol, it is similar to the infusion of the FOLFIRIB protocol (Sect. 5.2.2.7) starting with bevacizumab followed by oxaliplatin and other drugs as shown in Fig. 5.15 [207].

5.2.2.10   FOLFOXPAN Protocol (Oxaliplatin, 5-Fluorouracil, 5-Fluorouracil in Continuous Infusion, Leucovorin, and Panitumumab)

The combination of FOLFOX with panitumumab has also shown good results for the treatment of advanced colorectal cancer. Douillard et al. [208] evaluated the efficacy of the FOLFOXPAN protocol in colorectal cancer with RAS mutations. The authors noted that the protocol promoted a progression-free survival of 10.1 months and overall survival of 26 months. The authors highlight that patients with colorectal cancer without RAS mutations had better overall survival outcomes with the FOLFOXPAN protocol.

The FOLFOXPAN protocol may be an option in patients with wild-type RAS due to the addition of panitumumab. The study by Lonardi et al. [209] found that the combination promoted a progression-free survival of 9.6 months and a response rate of 65%. Regarding the toxicity profile, the most prevalent adverse events were neutropenia, diarrhea, stomatitis, neurotoxicity, fatigue, skin rash, and hypomagnesemia.

As for the infusion sequence of the FOLFOXPAN protocol, as well as the FOLFIRIPAN protocol (Sect. 5.2.2.8), it starts the infusion with panitumumab, as it is the monoclonal antibody, acting in a target-directed manner (Fig. 5.16) [210].

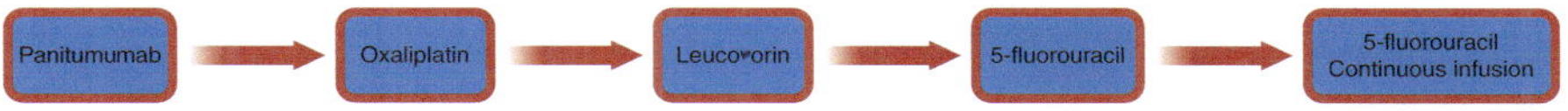

Fig. 5.16 FOLFOXPAN protocol infusion sequence

5.3   Pathophysiology of Esophageal and Stomach Cancers

Esophageal and stomach cancers are one of the most prevalent gastrointestinal cancers (Fig. 5.1) and are also the most lethal malignancies worldwide. The increased incidence of esophageal cancer seems to be related to an increased incidence of adenocarcinoma, being more prevalent in men. Gastric cancer is one of the most common cancers of the gastrointestinal tract worldwide, where its prevalence varies according to geographic location, being more common in Japan, Korea, and in regions of South and Central America. Like esophageal cancer, gastric cancer is also more prevalent in men [12, 211, 212].

Esophageal cancer is classified according to histological subtype into squamous cell carcinoma or adenocarcinoma (Fig. 5.17) [212–214]. The esophagus is lined with nonkeratinized stratified squamous epithelium; differentiation into these cells can lead to the development of squamous cell carcinoma, which develops in the upper and middle part of the esophagus [213, 215–217].

Adenocarcinoma results from intestinal epithelial metaplasia and is secondary to chronic gastroesophageal reflux. This type of tumor develops in the dysplastic columnar epithelium, starting in glandular cells, responsible for the production of mucus in the lower part of the esophagus, mainly at the esophagogastric and cardia junction [218–222]. The esophageal tumor can be located in the epithelium, as well as in an advanced stage, it can grow in the pleura or diaphragm and spread to lymph nodes, trachea, aorta, spine, and among other organs and/or tissues [223–225].

Gastric cancer refers to a neoplasm that develops in the region that extends between the gastroesophageal junction and the pylorus. Gastric cancer has two histological types described by the World Health Organization with distinct clinical entities, namely intestinal and diffuse. Well-differentiated intestinal cancer presents cohesive neoplastic cells, with tubular structures similar to glands that usually ulcerate, while the poorly differentiated, diffuse type is characterized by infiltration and thickening of the stomach wall without the formation of a discrete mass. Some patients can have mixed gastric carcinoma with both intestinal and diffuse components [226–229].

Invasive gastric carcinoma develops from a gradual evolution, with a cumulative series of genetic alterations, with sequential histopathological changes in the gastric mucosa including atrophic gastritis leading to a loss of parietal cell mass, intestinal metaplasia, and dysplasia, and finally in the development of the carcinoma. In addition to genetic alterations, the development of gastric polyps due to the use of non-steroidal anti-inflammatory drugs or drugs that inhibit the proton pump can also induce the development of gastric cancer [228, 230–234]. Figure 5.18 shows the growth patterns of advanced gastric cancer.

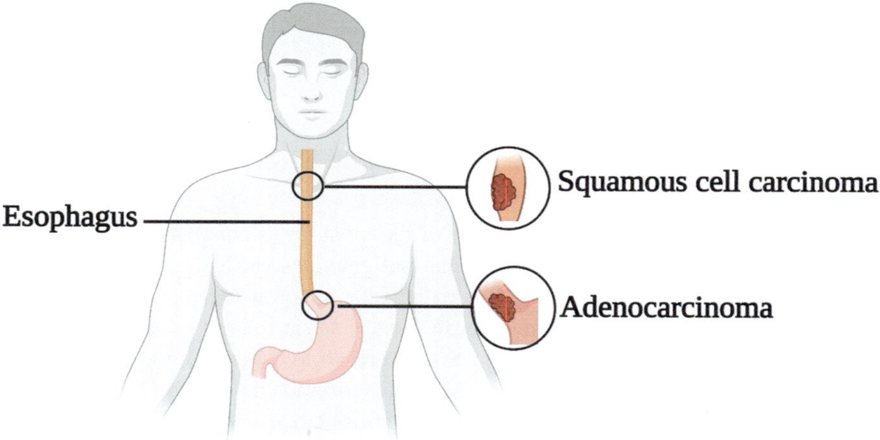

Fig. 5.17 Histological subtypes of esophageal cancer. Source: Created with BioRender.com

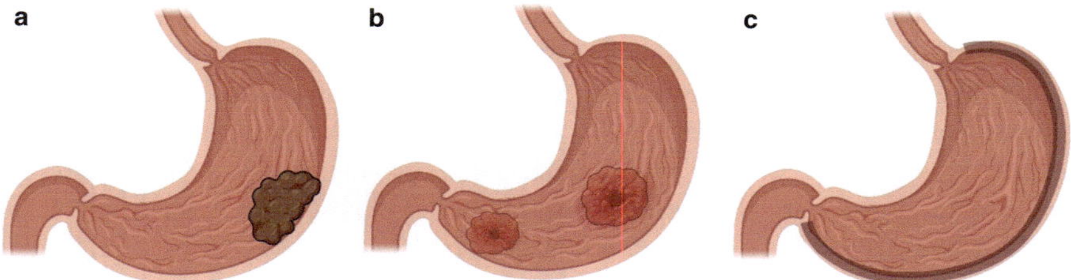

Fig. 5.18 Growth pattern of advanced gastric cancer. (**a**) Polypoid, (**b**) ulcerated, and (**c**) infiltrative. (Source: Created with BioRender.com)

5.3.1 *Chemotherapy for the Treatment of Esophageal and Stomach Cancer*

The treatment of esophageal and stomach cancer was based on the use of chemotherapy, surgery, radiotherapy, and targeted therapy. As for chemotherapy, it can be neoadjuvant (before the surgical approach), adjuvant (after the surgical procedure), and palliative chemotherapy, in cases of more advanced cancers with the presence of metastases in other organs [235–239]. Chemotherapy can be based on drug administration as monotherapy with docetaxel, palliative treatment of metastatic esophagogastric adenocarcinoma, trastuzumab in the palliative treatment of metastatic or inoperable adenocarcinoma, locally advanced gastric or gastroesophageal adenocarcinoma, and among other antineoplastic agents [240–244].

As for combinations, some protocols that are used in the treatment of colorectal cancer can also be indicated for gastric and esophageal cancers, such as the CAPOX protocol that combines oxaliplatin and capecitabine (Sect. 5.2.1.1), the FOLFIRI protocol (Sect. 5.2.2.3), which is indicated in second-line palliative therapy for metastatic gastric or esophageal adenocarcinoma, and the FOLFOX protocol (Sect. 5.2.1.3), which is indicated in the treatment of gastric and esophageal cancers and may be associated with radiotherapy in the treatment of esophageal cancer locally advanced [245–248]. In the following topics, we will approach some protocols [65, 67, 68] indicated for the therapy of esophageal and stomach cancers.

5.3.1.1   FOLFOXT Protocol (Oxaliplatin, 5-Fluorouracil, 5-Fluorouracil in Continuous Infusion, Leucovorin, and Trastuzumab)

In addition to combining the FOLFOX protocol with radiotherapy, this protocol can also be combined with trastuzumab in the palliative treatment of HER-2 positive metastatic or locally advanced gastric or esophageal adenocarcinoma. We discussed in Chap. 4 that some breast cancers have overexpression of HER2 receptors and that is why these patients were indicated for treatment with targeted therapy. Gastric, esophageal, or gastroesophageal adenocarcinoma may also have HER2-positive receptors, and for these patients, the use of targeted therapy has been indicated, as in the case of trastuzumab [249–252]. The inclusion of trastuzumab in the treatment of gastric or esophageal cancer has been associated with significant improvement in progression-free survival and overall survival [253, 254].

Soularue et al. [255] highlighted the efficacy and safety of combining oxaliplatin with 5-fluorouracil and trastuzumab in the treatment of HER2-positive metastatic gastric adenocarcinoma and adenocarcinoma of the gastroesophageal junction. The authors observed an overall response rate of 41%, with a median duration of treatment of 7.5 months, median progression-free survival of 9 months, and overall survival of 17.3 months. The protocol was well tolerated, presenting neutropenia and neuropathy as the main toxicity.

Regarding the order of infusion, the ideal is to start with trastuzumab as it is target directed, followed by the standard sequence of the FOLFOX protocol presented in Sect. 5.2.1.3, followed by the infusion of oxaliplatin, leucovorin, and 5-fluorouracil (Fig. 5.19) [256].

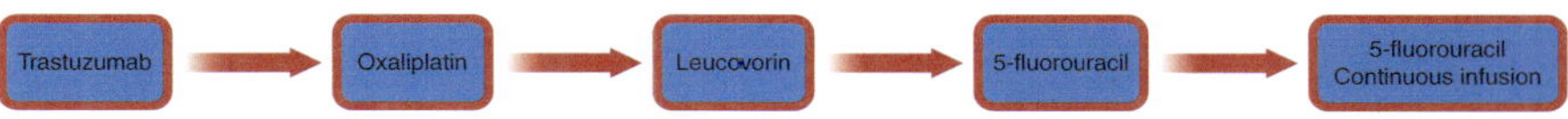

Fig. 5.19 FOLFOXT protocol infusion sequence

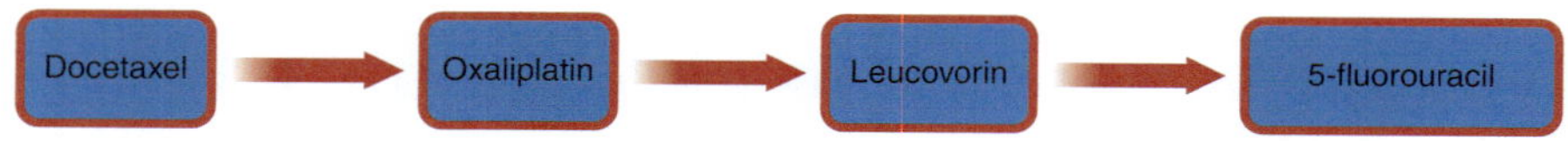

Fig. 5.20 FLOT protocol infusion sequence

5.3.1.2   FLOT Protocol (Oxaliplatin, 5-Fluorouracil, Leucovorin, and Docetaxel)

The combination of the FLOX protocol (oxaliplatin, 5-fluorouracil, and leucovorin) with docetaxel has also been indicated for the perioperative treatment of resectable adenocarcinoma of the stomach, gastroesophageal junction, or 1/3 lower esophagus [257–260]. Pernot et al. [261] evaluated the combination in the first-line treatment of advanced gastric cancer and adenocarcinoma of the gastroesophageal junction. The authors noted that the protocol was safe and effective, with a response rate of 66%, progression-free survival of 6.3 months, and overall survival of 12.1 months, with tolerable toxicity in cases of neutropenia and neuropathy.

In a phase II study, Al-Batran et al. [262] evaluated the combination of FLOX with docetaxel in metastatic adenocarcinoma of the stomach or gastroesophageal junction. The toxicities induced by the combination were cases of leukopenia, neutropenia, anemia, febrile neutropenia, peripheral neuropathy, nausea, vomiting, diarrhea, and fatigue. According to Rosenberg et al. [258], the combination of modified FLOX with docetaxel showed high activity in advanced gastric cancer. The results showed an overall response rate of 73.2%, overall survival of 10.3 months, and the toxicity profile was similar to other studies with cases of neutropenia, diarrhea, and neurological toxicity.

Wang et al. [259] observed the effectiveness of the FLOT protocol in patients with locally advanced gastric cancer, noting that the protocol promoted a 3-year survival rate of 30.9–58.7%, showing that the use of the protocol in the preoperative period is safe and viable. The infusion sequence of the FLOT protocol starts with the infusion of docetaxel, which is a specific cycle drug and presents an irritant and/or vesicant characteristic, and then continues with the infusion of oxaliplatin, leucovorin, and 5-fluorouracil (Fig. 5.20) [263].

5.3.1.3   CTRT Protocol (Carboplatin, Paclitaxel, and Radiotherapy)

Another protocol indicated for the neoadjuvant treatment of esophageal and gastroesophageal carcinomas is the CTRT, which is based on a combination of carboplatin, paclitaxel, and radiotherapy. The combination of chemotherapy and radiotherapy has been a standard of care for locally advanced cancer of the esophagus or gastroesophageal junction, and the combination of paclitaxel with carboplatin and radiotherapy has stood out in the neoadjuvant treatment of squamous esophageal cancer and adenocarcinoma [264–267]. According to Platz et al. [265], the CTRT protocol

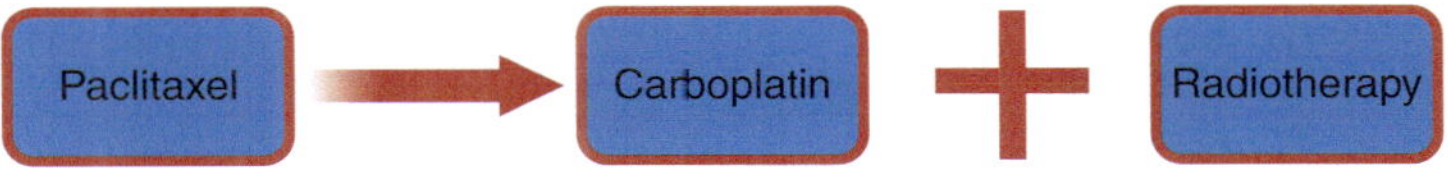

Fig. 5.21   CTRT protocol infusion sequence

in the treatment of esophageal/gastroesophageal carcinoma promoted a complete pathological response in 38% of patients, being well tolerated.

van Hagen et al. [268] evaluated the effectiveness of the CTRT protocol in the preoperative treatment of esophageal or junctional cancer. The authors noted that the main toxic effects were similar to other chemotherapy protocols in inducing leukopenia, neutropenia, fatigue, and anorexia. The protocol showed a complete pathological response in 29% of patients and overall survival of 49.4 months.

One of the advantages of the combination of paclitaxel and carboplatin is in the reduction of antiplatelet toxicity induced by carboplatin; in addition, when combined, they have additive antitumor activity [269]. As for the infusion sequence, it starts with the infusion of paclitaxel followed by carboplatin combined with radiotherapy for 5 days a week (Fig. 5.21) [270, 271].

5.3.1.4   FUC Protocol (5-Fluorouracil and Cisplatin)

The FUC protocol is a combination of cisplatin and 5-fluorouracil and is indicated as palliative therapy for upper gastrointestinal cancer (gastric, esophageal, gallbladder carcinoma, and cholangiocarcinoma) and metastatic anal cancer [272]. Cisplatin is part of the class of platinum compounds, being one of the most used drugs in the treatment of cancer, acting as an alkylating agent, binding to DNA with the formation of adducts, forming intra- and interchain bonds, thereby inducing structural changes. Therefore, cisplatin induces the inhibition of DNA transcription and replication, leading the cell to apoptosis. As for dermatological toxicity, cisplatin may present irritating or vesicant characteristics depending on the amount of extravasated drug [273–278].

The combination of cisplatin with 5-fluorouracil induce drug interactions that will depend on the infusion time of 5-fluorouracil, where when infused for 2 h it appears to have antagonistic effects and when infused within 24 h the combination appears to be more active, with cytotoxicity synergistic that may be related to a greater degree of fragmentation of nascent and parental DNA [279–281]. According to Nishiyama et al. [282], low doses of cisplatin combined with continuous infusion of 5-fluorouracil reduces the increase in gene expression related to the resistance of these drugs and induces synergistic cytotoxic effects in gastrointestinal cancer cells.

Levard et al. [283] evaluated the efficacy of the combination 5-fluorouracil and cisplatin in the palliative treatment of advanced esophageal squamous cell carcinoma, but the combination was not effective for this type of tumor, which induced an increase in neurological complications. According to Steber et al. [284], the combination of cisplatin and 5-fluorouracil had similar results with the combination of

Fig. 5.22 FUC protocol infusion sequence

carboplatin and paclitaxel in the preoperative treatment of esophageal cancer in terms of overall survival and progression-free survival.

The indication of the combination of 5-fluorouracil and cisplatin seems to bring good results when administered preoperatively with response rates of 14–64% with complete resection performed in 47–80% of cases, with mean survival numbers of 8–23 months [285]. The FUC protocol is based on the infusion of cisplatin followed by a continuous infusion of 5-fluorouracil (Fig. 5.22) [272, 286].

5.3.1.5   CCAPRT Protocol (Cisplatin, Capecitabine, and Radiotherapy)

The CCAPRT protocol combines cisplatin with capecitabine and radiotherapy in the adjuvant treatment of completely resected gastric cancer. The combination of capecitabine and cisplatin appears to have a synergistic effect in vitro [287, 288]. Kim et al. [289], in a phase II study, evaluated the efficacy of the combination of cisplatin and capecitabine in advanced gastric cancer. As a result, the authors observed an overall response rate of 54.8%, the median time to progression of 6.3 months, and overall survival of 10.1 months. As toxic effects, neutropenia, hand-foot syndrome, thrombocytopenia, stomatitis, and diarrhea were observed.

In a phase III study, Lee et al. [287] compared the efficacy of the combination of cisplatin and capecitabine with or without associated radiotherapy, where they observed that the inclusion of radiotherapy does not seem to promote a significant reduction in recurrence after curative resection and lymph node dissection in completely resected gastric cancer. According to Zhi et al. [290], chemoradiotherapy in the treatment of gastric cancer in patients with lymph node metastasis provides a better prognosis compared to the isolated surgical approach. The combination of capecitabine and cisplatin is indicated for postoperative treatment after D2 lymph node dissection [291].

Ustaalioglu et al. [292] observed that the CCAPRT protocol was well tolerated and less toxic when compared to the combination of 5-fluorouracil and leucovorin with radiotherapy in the adjuvant treatment of locally advanced lymph node-positive gastric cancer.

Regarding the administration schedule of the CCAPRT protocol, cisplatin is infused on the first day with oral administration of capecitabine for 21 days associated with radiotherapy (Fig. 5.23) [293]

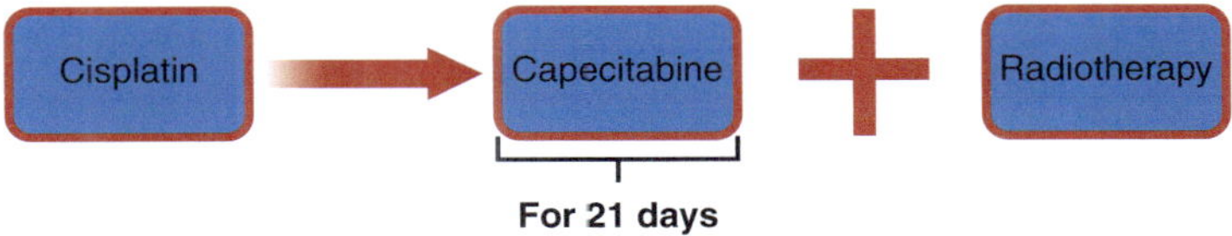

Fig. 5.23 Schedule of administration of the CCAPRT protocol with oral administration of capecitabine

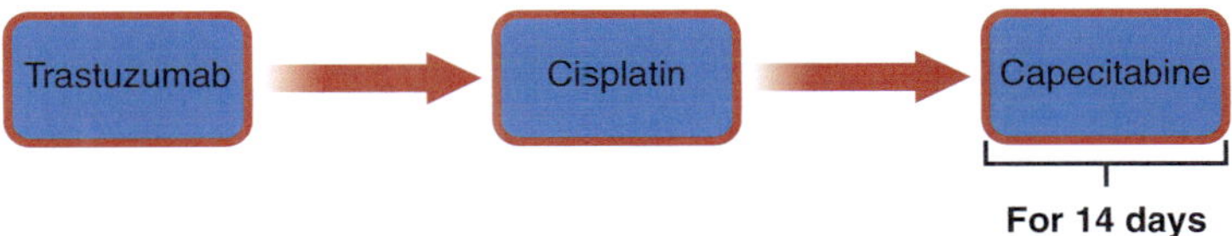

Fig. 5.24 Schedule of administration of the CCAPT protocol with oral administration of capecitabine

5.3.1.6   CCAPT Protocol (Cisplatin, Capecitabine, and Trastuzumab)

The combination of cisplatin, capecitabine, and trastuzumab is also an alternative in the palliative treatment of esophageal or metastatic or locally advanced gastric adenocarcinoma, gastroesophageal, or esophageal junction with HER2 overexpression [239, 294–297]. The combination between capecitabine, cisplatin, and trastuzumab does not seem to suffer pharmacokinetic interactions. According to the study by Satoh et al. [293], the pharmacokinetic profile of capecitabine combined was consistent with the profile of the drug alone.

The inclusion of trastuzumab combined with cisplatin and capecitabine has been shown to be effective in the treatment of advanced gastric cancer or HER2-positive gastroesophageal junction [298, 299]. The study by Bang et al. [298] found that the combination led to an increase in median overall survival from 11.1 months to 13.8 months. Regarding the CCAPT protocol administration schedule, the administration of the monoclonal antibody trastuzumab initiates the protocol due to its target-directed action, followed by cisplatin and oral administration of capecitabine for 14 days (Fig. 5.24) [300].

5.3.1.7   CFUT Protocol (Cisplatin, 5-Fluorouracil, and Trastuzumab)

Trastuzumab combined with cisplatin and 5-fluorouracil has been indicated for the palliative treatment of locally advanced metastatic or inoperable adenocarcinoma of the gastric or gastroesophageal junction. As with other protocols that include targeted therapy with trastuzumab, patients need to have HER2 receptor overexpression to be eligible [301–303].

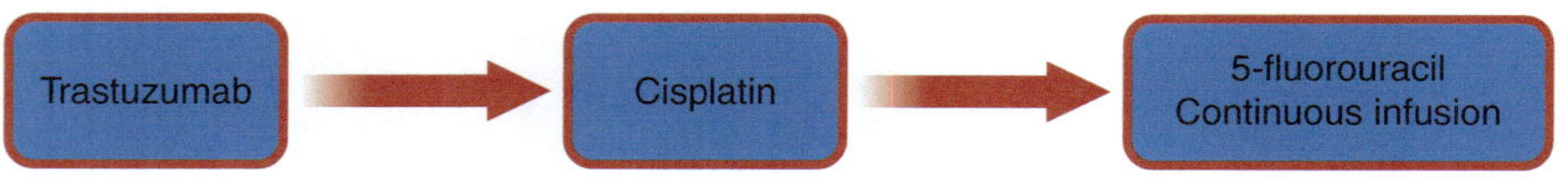

Fig. 5.25 CFUT protocol infusion sequence

As we saw in Sect. 5.3.1.4, the infusion of 5-fluorouracil for a long time favors the synergistic cytotoxic effects with cisplatin; thus, in this protocol, 5-fluorouracil is administered by continuous infusion over 24 h [279, 280, 281]. As for the infusion sequence, the protocol starts with trastuzumab followed by cisplatin and finally the infusion of 5-fluorouracil in continuous infusion (Fig. 5.25) [303, 304].

5.3.1.8   CAPOXT Protocol (Capecitabine, Oxaliplatin, and Trastuzumab)

The combination of the CAPOX protocol with trastuzumab has been used for the palliative treatment of esophageal or metastatic or locally advanced gastric adenocarcinoma, a gastroesophageal or esophageal junction that present HER2 receptor overexpression [305–307]. Ryu et al. [308] evaluated the use of the combination of trastuzumab, capecitabine, and oxaliplatin in the treatment of advanced gastric cancer. The use of the protocol in this group of patients promoted a response rate of 67%, with a progression-free survival of 9.8 months and overall survival of 21 months. Regarding the toxicity profile, the main ones were neutropenia, anemia, and peripheral neuropathy.

In a HER2-positive receptor gastric cancer xenograft model, Harada et al. [309] verified the antitumor activity of the CAPOXT protocol. As a result, the authors noted that the combination demonstrated significantly stronger activity compared to trastuzumab treatment or the CAPOX protocol alone. The interaction of trastuzumab with capecitabine increases the expression of thymidine phosphorylase, which is responsible for generating 5-fluorouracil from the metabolism of capecitabine, which may increase its cytotoxic activity.

Gong et al. [310] evaluated the effectiveness of the CAPOXT protocol as a first-line treatment in HER2-positive advanced gastric cancer. The protocol promoted a response rate of 66.7%, with a progression-free survival of 9.2 months and overall survival of 19.5 months, with toxic effects that included thrombocytopenia, neutropenia, anemia, and leukopenia.

In a more recent study, Rivera et al. [311] evaluated the effect of the CAPOXT protocol in the perioperative period in patients with resectable gastric or HER2-positive gastroesophageal junction adenocarcinoma. As a result, 38% of patients achieved a partial response and 50% had stable disease, with overall survival of 60 months of 58%. As for the toxicity profile, the main toxic effects were diarrhea, nausea, and vomiting.

Regarding the infusion schedule, it starts with trastuzumab, which acts specifically on HER2 receptors, followed by oxaliplatin and oral administration of capecitabine for 14 days (Fig. 5.26) [306, 312].

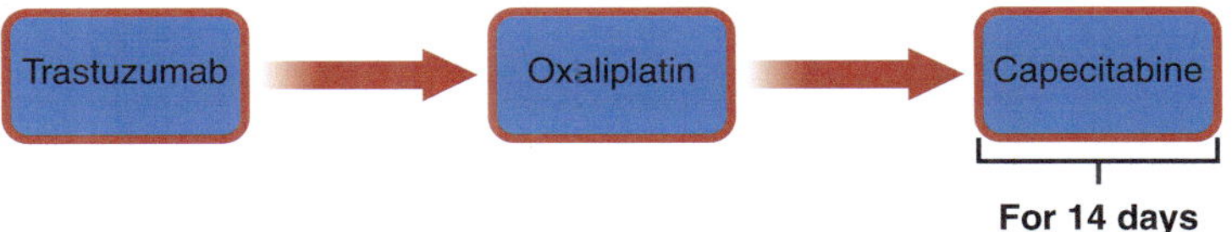

Fig. 5.26 Schedule of administration of the CAPOXT protocol with oral administration of capecitabine

5.3.1.9   RAMP Protocol (Paclitaxel and Ramucirumab)

The RAMP protocol is based on the combination of paclitaxel and ramucirumab and is indicated as second-line therapy for metastatic or locally advanced gastric cancer or gastroesophageal junction cancer [313–315]. Ramucirumab is a monoclonal antibody that acts on the vascular endothelial growth factor 2 (VEGFR2) receptor, blocking its activation and thereby inhibiting neovascularization and tumor growth, and is indicated for the treatment of advanced gastric or gastric cancers after the use of fluoropyrimidines or platinum [316–318].

Ramucirumab can be used alone or combined with paclitaxel. The concomitant administration of ramucirumab with paclitaxel does not seem to present pharmacokinetic interactions. According to Chow et al. [319], it is unlikely that the concomitant administration of these drugs affects the pharmacokinetics of both drugs, as well as the incidence and severity of adverse events, which were consistent with the safety profile of the drugs when administered alone.

According to Refolo et al. [320], the combination of ramucirumab and paclitaxel have synergistic action on gastric cancer cell lines, where ramucirumab was able to increase the inhibitory action of paclitaxel on cell cycle progression, as well as on the expression of proteins responsible for cell motility, organization of microtubules, and epithelial-mesenchymal transition. In addition, the combination also promoted synergistic inhibition in VEGFR2 expression, demonstrating the benefits of the combination in the treatment of gastric cancer.

Zang et al. [315] evaluated the use of the RAMP protocol in the second-line treatment of patients with advanced gastric or gastroesophageal junction adenocarcinoma. This study showed that the combination promoted a response rate of 15.1%, disease control rate of 57.7%, progression-free survival of 4.03 months, and overall survival of 10.3 months. As for the toxic effects, the patients had neutropenia, anemia, neuropathy, fatigue, and anorexia. The results evidence the protocol's effectiveness in treating patients with locally advanced metastatic or unresectable gastric adenocarcinoma.

Vita et al. [321] evaluated the use of the combination of ramucirumab and paclitaxel in patients with gastric cancer who had previously received trastuzumab. The results of the study showed that the combination was superior to the use of ramucirumab alone, with overall survival results of 11.4 months, longer progression-free survival, and a manageable safety profile. As for the infusion sequence, the infusion of ramucirumab should be before the infusion of paclitaxel (Fig. 5.27) [322].

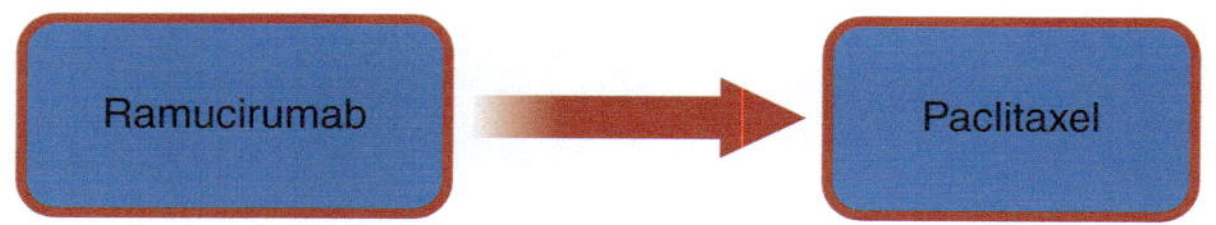

Fig. 5.27 RAMP protocol infusion sequence

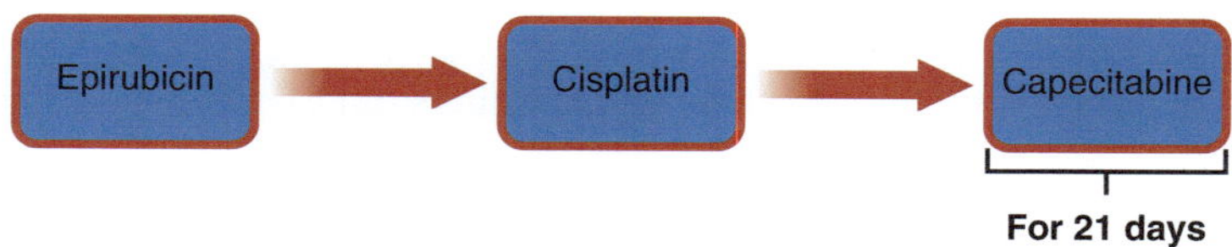

Fig. 5.28 Schedule of administration of the ECCAP protocol with oral administration of capecitabine

5.3.1.10   ECCAP Protocol (Epirubicin, Cisplatin, and Capecitabine)

Another combination used in the perioperative treatment of resectable adenocarcinoma of the stomach, gastroesophageal junction, or lower 1/3 of the esophagus is an association between epirubicin, cisplatin, and capecitabine [323, 324]. The superiority of the ECCAP protocol in the treatment of advanced gastric cancer was observed by Ocvirk et al. [325] compared to the combination of epirubicin, cisplatin, and 5-fluorouracil. The ECCAP protocol showed an objective response rate of 30% and a disease control rate of 73%. The overall survival was 8.3 months, and the time to progression was 6 months. The toxicity profile was similar to other protocols, with cases of neutropenia, fatigue, vomiting, nausea, and anemia.

ECCAP protocol efficacy results were also presented in the study by Evans et al. [326] in the treatment of patients with inoperable esophagogastric adenocarcinoma. The protocol was tolerable, with esophagitis, diarrhea, neutropenia, stomatitis, and thrombocytopenia as toxic effects. The response rate was 24%, progression-free survival 22 weeks, and overall survival 34 weeks. Also according to the study by Evans et al. [326], the combination did not influence the pharmacokinetic profile of capecitabine, being rapidly absorbed after administration and with plasma concentrations of its metabolites similar to the results presented in monotherapy with capecitabine.

In a phase II study, Cho et al. [327] evaluated the efficacy of the ECCAP protocol in metastatic gastric cancer. The use of this protocol in advanced gastric cancer promoted an overall response rate of 59%, with a mean duration of response of 5.8 months and time to progression of 6 months. As for the toxicity profile, cases of neutropenia, febrile neutropenia, nausea, vomiting, and stomatitis were observed. Regarding the infusion schedule, epirubicin is initially infused as it is a vesicant drug, followed by cisplatin, and finally capecitabine is administered orally for 21 days (Fig. 5.28) [328, 329].

5.4   Pathophysiology of Pancreatic, Biliary Tract, and Gallbladder Cancers

Pancreaticobiliary cancers account for about 4–5% of all cancers, but they tend to be more aggressive with a high mortality rate, accounting for nearly 6% of cancer-related deaths. Pancreatic cancer is more common in Western countries and predominant in men and blacks, with twice the risk for smokers and diabetic patients. On the other hand, cancer of the biliary tract is highest in Latin Americans and American Indians, being more common in women worldwide except Chinese and Japanese [330, 331].

Biliary tract cancer starts in the biliary epithelium of the small intrahepatic ducts and the main hilar (extrahepatic) ducts (Fig. 5.29). Bile tract cancer can develop in any region of the bile duct, where its classification is based on where primary cancer started, for example, when cancer starts in the bile duct in the liver is called intrahepatic cancers and when that start in the ducts outside the liver are called extrahepatic cancers [332–335].

Cancers of the gallbladder, ampoules, and pancreatic bile ducts are part of extrahepatic biliary tract cancers. Gallbladder cancer starts in the inner layer of the gallbladder mucosa and spreads to the outer layers. Gallbladder cancer is classified according to the type of cells it affects, and adenocarcinomas are the most common to which they affect the cells of the gland that lines the gallbladder. Adenocarcinomas can be subclassified into non-papillary adenocarcinomas, which are the most common, and papillary and mucinous adenocarcinomas [334, 336–340].

Regarding pancreatic cancer, it develops in the pancreas, being mainly exocrine tumors including adenosquamous, colloid, acinar cell, signet ring cell, pancreatoblastoma, cystadenocarcinoma, and hepatoid carcinomas, in which the most frequent cancer of the pancreas is adenocarcinoma ductal. Pancreatic cancer tends to arise in the head of the pancreas (Fig. 5.30) and is commonly seen in patients with pancreatitis and jaundice due to blockage in the common bile duct that results in jaundice, thereby leading to symptoms such as nausea, vomiting, dark urine, and clear stools. Cancers in the body and tail of the pancreas are less frequent and have a worse prognosis [341–345].

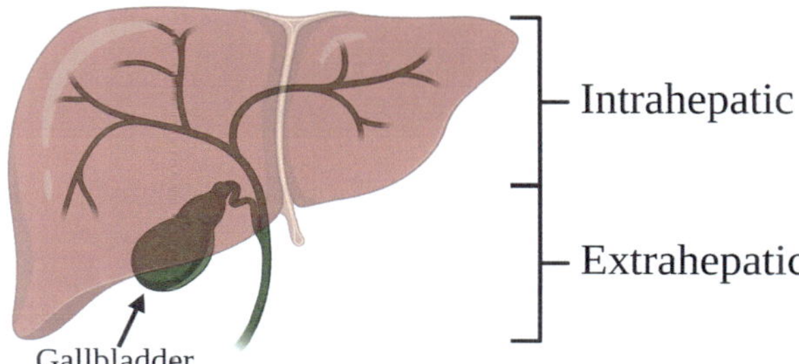

Fig. 5.29 Distribution of the biliary tract and location of the gallbladder. Source: Created with BioRender.com

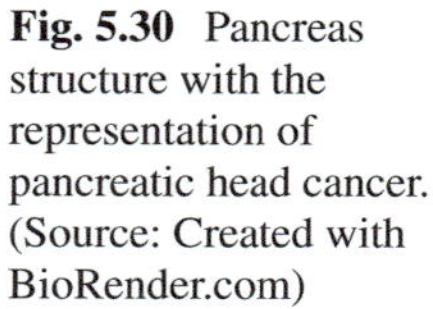

Fig. 5.30 Pancreas structure with the representation of pancreatic head cancer. (Source: Created with BioRender.com)

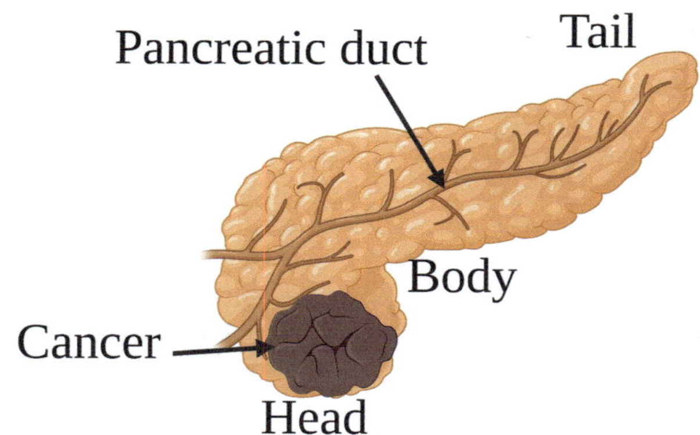

5.4.1 Chemotherapy for the Treatment of Pancreatic, Biliary Tract, and Gallbladder Cancers

Pancreatic, biliary tract, and gallbladder cancers are aggressive and highly fatal, where treatment may be indicated for surgery, radiotherapy, and/or chemotherapy. Surgery is the only potentially curative therapy, but disease recurrence is frequent. The use of chemotherapy as monotherapy or even as a combination therapy has brought benefits in overall survival and relapse-free survival [346–349].

As monotherapy, capecitabine has been indicated in the adjuvant therapy of biliary cancer and in the second-line treatment of metastatic or unresectable pancreatic adenocarcinoma. Another drug also used as monotherapy is gemcitabine, which is indicated in adjuvant therapy in pancreatic adenocarcinoma and as palliative therapy in pancreatic adenocarcinoma, gallbladder cancer, and cholangiocarcinoma [350–352].

Some protocols that are indicated for other types of cancers of the gastrointestinal tract may also be indicated in the treatment of pancreatic, biliary tract, and gallbladder cancers. The FOLFIRI protocol (Sect. 5.2.2.3) is indicated in the second-line treatment of metastatic pancreatic cancer, the FOLFOX protocol (Sect. 5.2.1.3) is indicated in palliative therapy for metastatic pancreatic cancer as well as the FUC protocol (Sect. 5.3.1.4). In the following topics, we will talk about other protocols also used in the treatment of pancreatic, biliary tract, and gallbladder cancers [65, 67, 68, 353–357].

5.4.1.1   GEMCIS Protocol (Gemcitabine and Cisplatin)

The GEMCIS protocol combines cisplatin and gemcitabine in first-line palliative therapy for advanced gallbladder cancer and cholangiocarcinoma [358–360]. According to Valle et al. [358], the GEMCIS protocol promotes a significant improvement in progression-free survival and overall survival in the treatment of

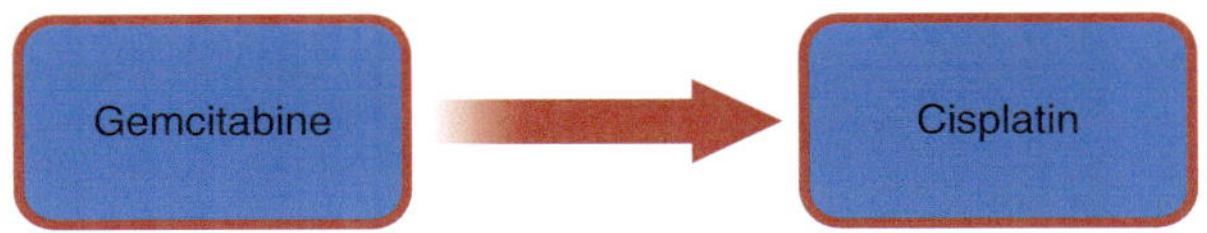

Fig. 5.31 GEMCIS protocol infusion sequence

advanced biliary tract cancer and in the treatment of intra- and extrahepatic cholangiocarcinomas and gallbladder cancer.

You et al. [361] evaluated the effectiveness of the GEMCIS protocol in treating unresectable gallbladder cancer, noting that the protocol promoted a disease control rate of 59.9%, overall survival of 8.1 months, and progression-free survival of 5.6 months. The results obtained by You et al. [361] demonstrated a high rate of cancer control with the GEMCIS protocol.

The combination of gemcitabine and cisplatin was associated with a significant survival advantage in the study by Valle et al. [362], with no added toxicity when compared to gemcitabine monotherapy in the treatment of biliary tract cancer. The GEMCIS protocol conferred an overall survival of 11.7 months, a progression-free survival of 8 months, and a tumor control rate of 81.4%, with adverse events similar to gemcitabine monotherapy.

In a study of four cases, Lee et al. [363] observed that the GEMCIS protocol can also be effective in the second-line treatment of intrahepatic cholangiocarcinoma, in which two patients had a partial response to the treatment and two had stable disease, with a mean time to progression of 5 months, median survival of 9 months, and tolerable toxicity. According to Malik et al. [364], the combination of gemcitabine and cisplatin has been shown to be highly effective in the treatment of advanced gallbladder cancer. The protocol in these patients achieved an overall response rate of 64%, with manageable toxicity.

In patients with unresectable biliary tract cancer, Dierks et al. [365] evaluated the use of the combination of gemcitabine and cisplatin as palliative therapy. As a result, the authors observed that the protocol proved to be effective and safe in patients with unresectable biliary tract cancer. As we saw in Chap. 4, gemcitabine is a deoxycytidine nucleoside analog, and when combined with cisplatin depending on the infusion sequence, it can increase the toxicity profile. Thus, the most appropriate infusion sequence would be starting with gemcitabine followed by cisplatin (Fig. 5.31), as we saw in Sect. 4.6.2 of Chap. 4 [366–368].

5.4.1.2   FOLFIRINOX Protocol (Irinotecan, Oxaliplatin, 5-Fluorouracil, 5-Fluorouracil in Continuous Infusion, and Leucovorin)

The FOLFOX protocol combined with irinotecan has been used as palliative therapy for advanced pancreatic adenocarcinoma [369, 370]. The FOLFIRINOX protocol showed efficacy in the treatment of advanced pancreatic adenocarcinoma, in the

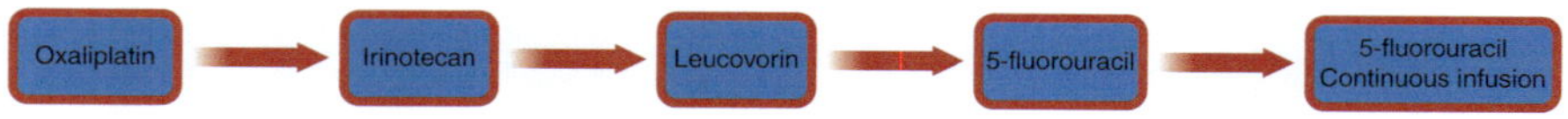

Fig. 5.32 Infusion sequence of the FOLFIRINOX protocol

study by Mota et al. [370], with a response rate of 39.3%, despite having a high prevalence of toxic effects that included neuropathy, fatigue, and diarrhea.

Berger et al. [369] also evaluated the efficacy of the combination as palliative therapy for pancreatic adenocarcinoma, proving to be effective with overall survival of 10.2 months, even with a dose reduction in 57% of patients. According to Zhang et al. [371], the combination may improve the overall survival rate in patients with metastatic pancreatic cancer, but it did not show progression-free survival benefits. Despite this, the FOLFIRINOX protocol brings benefits in the prognosis of patients with metastatic pancreatic cancer.

In the study by Chllamma et al. [372], the FOLFIRINOX protocol in advanced pancreatic cancer induced an overall survival of 13.1 months and progression-free survival of 6.2 months. Regarding toxicity, 43% had hematological adverse events and 28% had non-hematological adverse events. As for drug interactions, Zoetemelk et al. [373] highlight the need for an interaction study by proposing a chemotherapy protocol for a better use of the efficacy of each drug, where administration in clinical doses resulted in antagonistic interactions compared to low doses. The authors also highlight the synergistic effects between leucovorin and 5-fluorouracil, as well as the benefits of oxaliplatin or the active metabolite of irinotecan that appear to sensitize cells to the combination of leucovorin and 5-fluorouracil. As for the infusion sequence, the protocol starts with oxaliplatin followed by irinotecan, leucovorin, and 5-fluorouracil in bolus and continuous infusion (Fig. 5.32) [374].

5.4.1.3   GEMCAP Protocol (Capecitabine and Gemcitabine)

The combination of gemcitabine and capecitabine may be an alternative for adjuvant treatment for resected pancreatic adenocarcinoma [375, 376]. In a phase I/II study, Hess et al. [377] evaluated the effectiveness of the GEMCAP protocol in advanced pancreatic cancer, showing a combination with apparent efficacy and well tolerated, with toxic effects consisting of myelotoxicity and mucositis.

Kaur et al. [378] found that the combination of gemcitabine and capecitabine was effective and tolerable in the treatment of resected pancreatic cancer. As a result, the authors observed an overall survival of 20.2 months and progression-free survival of 19.3 months. As toxic effects, the protocol induced more hematological than non-hematological effects.

Neoptolemos et al. [379] compared the GEMCAP protocol with gemcitabine monotherapy in resected pancreatic cancer. The authors observed that the combination was superior to gemcitabine monotherapy, with overall survival of 28 months, with a similar toxicity profile with cases of anemia, diarrhea, fatigue, neutropenia, hand-foot syndrome, and among others.

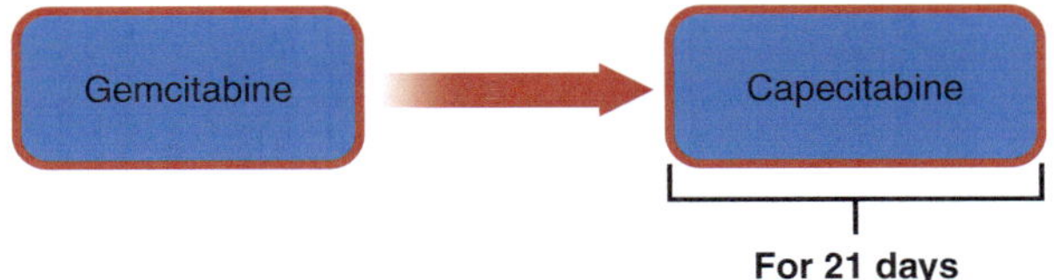

Fig. 5.33 Schedule of administration of the GEMCAP protocol with oral administration of capecitabine

Regarding the infusion schedule of the GEMCAP protocol, gemcitabine is infused on the first day, on the eighth day, and the 15th day, and capecitabine are administered orally twice a day for 21 days, starting on the first day after the infusion of gemcitabine (Fig. 5.33) [380].

5.4.1.4 GEMABR Protocol (Gemcitabine and Nab-Paclitaxel)

The GEMABR protocol combines gemcitabine and nab-paclitaxel (Abraxane) in the first-line treatment of locally advanced and metastatic pancreatic cancer [381–384]. Nab-paclitaxel is a drug that is based on paclitaxel in albumin nanoparticles. The encapsulation of paclitaxel in albumin nanoparticles increases its distribution among the endothelial cells, thereby promoting the increase in the accumulation of paclitaxel in the area of the tumor mediated by albumin receptors SPARC (secreted protein acidic and rich in cysteine) [385–388].

The combination of nab-paclitaxel with gemcitabine increased pancreatic cancer survival [389]. Von Hoff et al. [389] found that the GEMABR protocol combination improved overall survival (8.5 months), progression-free survival (5.5 months), and response rate (35%) in patients with metastatic pancreatic adenocarcinoma. According to Zhang et al. [383], the combination of nab-paclitaxel and gemcitabine led to a tumor reduction and an acceptable toxicity profile in metastatic pancreatic cancer, thereby demonstrating its efficacy and safety.

Petrioli et al. [384] evaluated the effectiveness of the GEMABR protocol followed by maintenance treatment with gemcitabine monotherapy in the treatment of locally advanced or metastatic pancreatic cancer. The authors noted that the protocol induced a partial response in 50% of patients, with a 6-month disease control rate of 61%, progression-free survival of 6.4 months, and overall survival of 13.4 months. As for toxicity, patients had neutropenia, anemia, and thrombocytopenia.

Zhang et al. [390] evaluated the use of the combination of gemcitabine and nab-paclitaxel in advanced pancreatic cancer after applying the FOLFIRINOX protocol as the first line. The authors noted that the use of the GEMABR protocol as a second line showed modest activity and clinical benefit in the treatment of advanced pancreatic cancer, with overall survival of 23 weeks and a partial response rate of 17.9%.

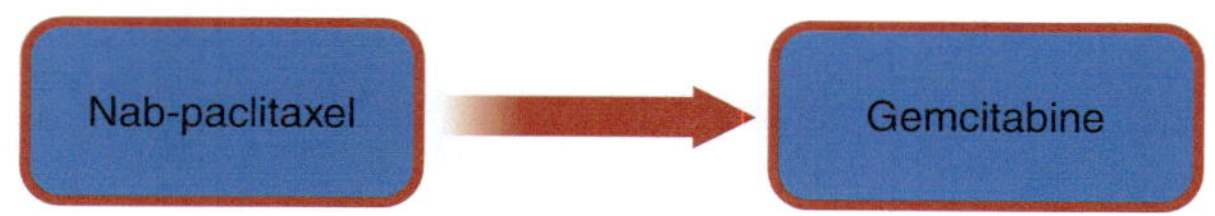

Fig. 5.34 Infusion sequence of the GEMABR protocol

In another study, Dean et al. [391] verified the effectiveness of retreatment with the GEMABR protocol as second line for the treatment of advanced pancreatic adenocarcinoma after using FOLFIRINOX as a second line. As a result, the authors observed a median overall survival of 18 months, showing that retreatment was tolerable and effective, with good performance status in patients with advanced pancreatic cancer.

Regarding the GEMABR protocol infusion sequence, nab-paclitaxel has been administered initially followed by gemcitabine infusion (Fig. 5.34). The beginning of the protocol with nab-paclitaxel may be interesting due to its target-directed action to albumin receptors on tumor cells promoted by albumin nanoparticles, in addition to its high binding rate with plasma proteins that favor its distribution fast [392–394].

5.5   Pathophysiology of Liver Cancer

Liver cancer is the seventh most common cancer in the world, with the highest rates in Asia and Africa. As for mortality, it is the fourth leading cause of cancer-related death worldwide, second only to lung, colorectal, and stomach cancers. Liver cancer is considered a highly fatal cancer, with the vast majority of cases being detected in the late stages [395, 396].

Several types of cancers can form in the liver, which includes hepatocellular carcinoma, intrahepatic cholangiocarcinoma, and hepatoblastoma. The most common is hepatocellular carcinoma that starts in hepatocytes, from chronic liver disease, having a strong association with chronic hepatitis B and C virus infections with other risk factors such as coinfection with hepatitis D, consumption of alcohol, and smoking. Some genetic mutations can also contribute to the development of liver cancer, such as mutations in genes for hemochromatosis (*HFE*), alpha 1-antitrypsin deficiency (*SERPINA1*), porphyria (*HMBS*, *UROD*), tyrosinemia (*FAH*), among others [396–398].

Repeated inflammation in the liver favors carcinogenesis, where hepatocellular carcinoma arises in a cirrhotic liver where repeated inflammation associated with fibrogenesis predisposes the liver to dysplasia, with the perpetuation of the healing response activated by the death of parenchymal cells and the inflammatory cascade, consequently leading to the development of cancer [397, 399, 400]. Fig. 5.35 provides a schematic of the evolution of liver tissue characteristics in the development of cancer.

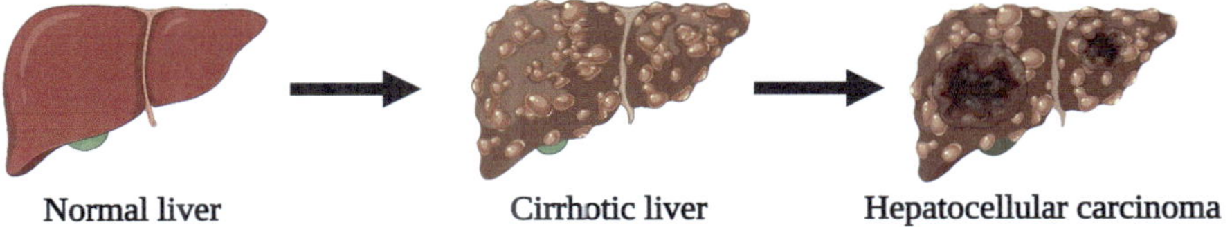

Fig. 5.35 Tissue evolution in the development of liver cancer. (Source: Created with BioRender.com)

5.5.1 Chemotherapy for the Treatment of Liver Cancer

The choice of the therapeutic modality for liver cancer will depend on the stage of cancer, as well as the patient's clinical condition and age. Treatment modalities include surgery, embolization therapy, ablation, radiation therapy, target-directed therapy, immunotherapy, and chemotherapy [26, 401–403]. In potentially resectable or transplantable liver cancer, the surgical approach can be an alternative curative treatment, aiming to remove the tumor or in liver transplantation [404, 405].

Some localized treatments are also possible in liver cancer that is potentially transplantable, intending to keep cancer under control until the time of transplantation. Ablation is a technique that can be used, which is based on the destruction of the liver tumor without removing it, which may be by radiofrequency, microwave, cryotherapy, or ethanol ablation [406, 407]. Another localized treatment technique is embolization, which is based on injecting substances directly into an artery in the liver to block or reduce blood flow to the liver tumor. In unresectable liver tumors, ablation and embolization can also be a therapeutic alternative, as well as targeted therapy, immunotherapy, chemotherapy, and radiotherapy [405, 408, 409].

In advanced liver cancer, when there is spread to lymph nodes or other organs, the drugs of choice are usually based on immunotherapy in the case of atezolizumab and/or targeted drugs such as bevacizumab, sorafenib, cabozantinib, ramucirumab, or lenvatinib, as well as anticancer chemotherapy [410–412]. Doxorubicin monotherapy has been indicated as palliative therapy in hepatoma, as well as transarterial chemoembolization in hepatocellular carcinoma. Lenvatinib, regorafenib, and sorafenib have been indicated in the treatment of advanced hepatocellular carcinoma [413–415].

There are few combination protocols used in liver cancer, generally based on the combination of immunotherapeutic and target-directed drugs. Below, we cover some of the protocols [65, 67–68].

5.5.1.1 Nivolumab and Ipilimumab Protocol

The combination of nivolumab and ipilimumab has been approved by the FDA for the treatment of advanced liver cancer. The use of the combination has been used as a second-line treatment in patients who were previously treated with sorafenib.

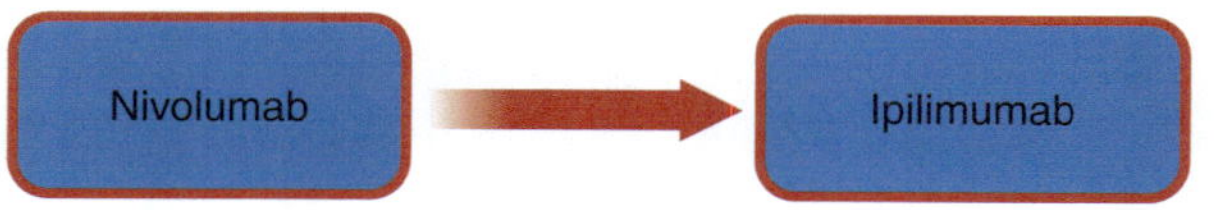

Fig. 5.36 Infusion sequence of the combination between nivolumab and ipilimumab

Nivolumab is a monoclonal antibody that acts by binding to programmed death receptors-1 (PD-1), thereby blocking the interaction with PD-L1 and PD-L2. The PD-1 receptor is responsible for negatively regulating T-cell activities, controlling their immune response, in which the binding of PD-L1 and PD-L2 inhibits T-cell proliferation. With the blockade of PD-1 receptors by nivolumab, there is a potentiation of T cells, with an increase in antitumor responses [416–420].

Ipilimumab also potentiates the T cell–mediated immune response through an indirect mechanism. Ipilimumab is also a monoclonal antibody, but it works by binding to cytotoxic T lymphocyte antigen-4 (CTLA4), thereby blocking the inhibitory signals of CTLA4-induced T cells, increasing the number of reactive effector T cells that will counteract cancer cells through a direct attack of T cells. The combination of these two monoclonal antibodies has brought benefits for the treatment of hepatocellular carcinoma, especially in patients who have previously used sorafenib [419–425].

Yau et al. [419] evaluated the efficacy and safety of a combination between ipilimumab and nivolumab in second-line advanced hepatocellular carcinoma after treatment with sorafenib. The combination led to a 32% response rate, with a high overall survival rate (22.8 months) and a manageable safety profile. The infusion sequence used by Yau et al. [419] in hepatocellular carcinoma was nivolumab followed by ipilimumab. According to Weber et al. [426], sequential infusion of nivolumab followed by ipilimumab showed greater benefits compared to the reverse order, inducing an increase in overall survival of patients with advanced melanoma, despite having a higher frequency of adverse events. Figure 5.36 presents an infusion suggestion according to the study by Weber et al. [426] and Yau et al. [419].

5.5.1.2 Atezolizumab and Bevacizumab Protocol

The combination atezolizumab and bevacizumab has been approved by the FDA for the treatment of hepatocellular carcinoma [410, 427, 428]. Atezolizumab is a monoclonal antibody that binds to PD-L1, inducing a double blockade of PD-1 and B7.1 receptors, thus triggering an immune response with consequent reactivation of the immune response in cancer cells. On the other hand, as we have seen in previous topics, bevacizumab works by binding to VEGF, thereby preventing the growth of blood vessels [417, 429, 430].

Yang et al. [431] evaluated the effectiveness of the combination in the treatment of unresectable liver cancer. The results obtained showed a response rate of 36%, progression-free survival of 5–6 months, with longer overall survival than treatment

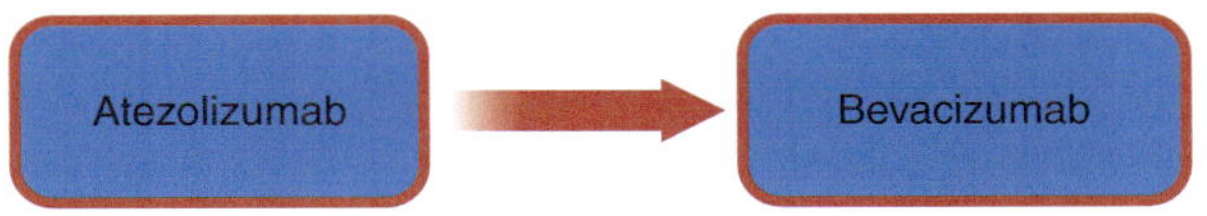

Fig. 5.37 Sequence of infusion of the combination of atezolizumab and bevacizumab

with sorafenib monotherapy, being indicated as first-line therapy. Finn et al. [432] found that atezolizumab combined with bevacizumab improved overall survival (from 54.6% to 67.2%) and progression-free survival (from 4.3 months to 6.8 months) compared with sorafenib monotherapy.

According to Vogel et al. [433], the combination of atezolizumab and bevacizumab has a superior overall survival compared to other protocols used in the first-line treatment of unresectable hepatocellular carcinoma. Zhang et al. [434] also noted the benefits of the combination in metastatic or unresectable hepatocellular carcinoma, but it was not cost-effective compared with sorafenib monotherapy. According to Liu, Lu, and Qin [435], the double blockade of VEGF and PD-L1 offers survival benefits, an example being the combination between atezolizumab and bevacizumab, in addition to presenting a manageable toxicity profile.

As for the infusion sequence, studies such as the one by Lee et al. [427] and Finn et al. [432] administered atezolizumab followed by bevacizumab showing its benefits in overall survival and progression-free survival, and this protocol was approved by the FDA in this infusion sequence [436]. In Fig. 5.37, the infusion sequence of the combination is shown.

5.6   Pathophysiology of Carcinoid and Neuroendocrine Tumors

Neuroendocrine tumors are rare, but according to Dasari et al. [437] from 1973 to 2012, there was an increase in the incidence rate of 6.4 times, mainly in early-stage tumors. The 5-year survival rate is 97% in patients who do not have metastatic disease, whereas in patients where the disease has spread to nearby tissue or regional lymph nodes, the 5-year survival rate is 95%, and in patients with that the tumor has spread to distant areas the survival rate is 67%.

Regarding carcinoid tumors of the gastrointestinal tract, the incidence has also been constantly increasing, as well as the 5-year mortality rate, although according to Mocellin and Nitti [438], the survival rate of patients dying of carcinoid is better than that reported for other cancers of the gastrointestinal tract. Ellis, Shale, and Coleman [439] believe that the increased incidence of these tumors is related to changes in anatomical distribution, with changes in the classification and detection of these cancers. Carcinoid and neuroendocrine tumors can manifest throughout the body, but approximately 2/3 of tumors arise in the gastrointestinal tract [440].

Neuroendocrine tumors have three main subtypes, which include carcinoid, pancreatic endocrine, and lung carcinoid tumors, and arise from cells of the neuroendocrine system. Despite the better prognosis of gastrointestinal carcinoid cancer, diagnosis is usually made late, so there is a relatively high proportion of patients with advanced or metastatic cancer [24, 438, 441, 442].

Neuroendocrine cancers are derived from enterochromaffin cells present mainly in the gastrointestinal tract. These tumors can be classified into well-differentiated and poorly differentiated neuroendocrine tumors. About 30–40% of cases of well-differentiated neuroendocrine tumors present the carcinoid syndrome, which is responsible for the secretion of several humoral factors, such as amines and biologically active peptides, which escape the first-pass metabolism in the liver [443, 444].

There is no exact cause of what can lead to the development of neuroendocrine tumors, but the development starts with mutations in the DNA of neuroendocrine cells, where the risk factor is linked to people who inherit genetic syndromes. Small bowel neuroendocrine tumors are the most common, two-thirds of which occur in the terminal ileum. Patients with small bowel neuroendocrine tumors are more likely to develop distant metastases than other neuroendocrine tumors in other organs. Other neuroendocrine tumors include gastric, duodenal, jejunal-ileal, appendix, colon, rectal, and others (Fig. 5.38) [445–447].

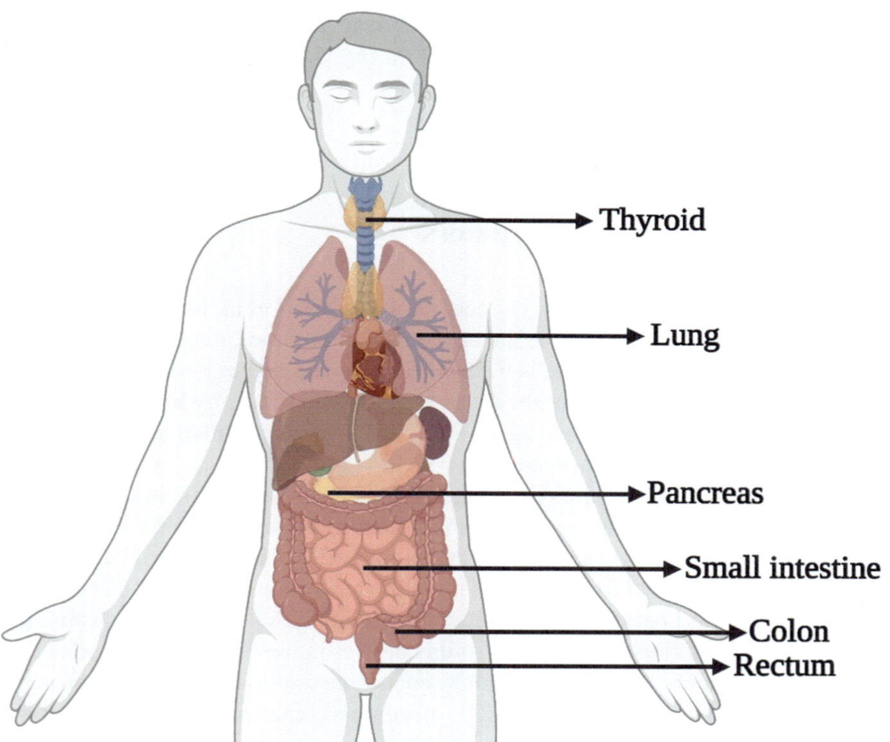

Fig. 5.38 Some organs that are affected by neuroendocrine tumors. (Source: Created with BioRender.com)

5.6.1 Chemotherapy for the Treatment of Carcinoid and Neuroendocrine Tumors

There are several treatment modalities for carcinoid and neuroendocrine tumors. In an early stage, the removal of the tumor by the surgical procedure is indicated. Other treatment modalities include radiation therapy, chemotherapy, and targeted therapy. In liver neuroendocrine tumors, ablation and embolization techniques can also be used, as seen in Sect. 5.5 [448–452].

Drug treatment can be through monotherapy with lanreotide in the symptomatic management of carcinoid and functional neuroendocrine tumors of the gastrointestinal tract, everolimus in the treatment of advanced neuroendocrine tumors of gastrointestinal origin (non-functional), and the palliative treatment of advanced pancreatic neuroendocrine tumors. Octreotide is indicated in the treatment of non-functional neuroendocrine tumors and the symptomatic management of carcinoid and functional neuroendocrine tumors of the gastrointestinal tract and sunitinib used in the palliative treatment of advanced pancreatic neuroendocrine tumors [452–459].

Treatment can also be with drugs given orally such as a combination of temozolomide and capecitabine in the palliative therapy of metastatic neuroendocrine cancer [460, 461]. Other protocols [65, 67, 68] used for the treatment of carcinoid and neuroendocrine tumors will be cited in the next topics.

5.6.1.1 ETCIS Protocol (Etoposide and Cisplatin)

One of the combinations used as palliative therapy for neuroendocrine tumors is the combination of etoposide and cisplatin [462–464]. Cisplatin, as we have seen, is a drug that acts as an alkylating agent, forming adducts with DNA. On the other hand, etoposide is a natural semisynthetic product derived from podophyllotoxin, whose pharmacological action is from the inhibition of topoisomerase II, thereby inhibiting and/or altering DNA synthesis [465–468]. According to Soranzo, Pratesi, and Zunino [469], the interaction of cisplatin with etoposide enhances the antitumor effects of both drugs with synergistic effects both in in vitro studies and in in vivo studies. Despite the synergistic effects, the drugs can have additive toxicity since both are nephrotoxic and can induce renal toxicity, requiring the monitoring of renal function during treatment.

Mitry et al. [470] highlighted that poorly differentiated neuroendocrine tumors are chemosensitive to the ETCIS protocol. The protocol promoted an objective response rate of 41.5%, with a response duration of 9.2 months, overall survival of 15 months, and progression-free survival of 8.9 months. As for toxicity, the patients did not present renal toxicity, but the authors observed auditory and neurological toxicity.

Fjallskog et al. [471] evaluated the benefits of the combination in neuroendocrine tumors, noting that etoposide with cisplatin can produce a significant response in pretreated and poorly differentiated patients. However, one must be aware of the

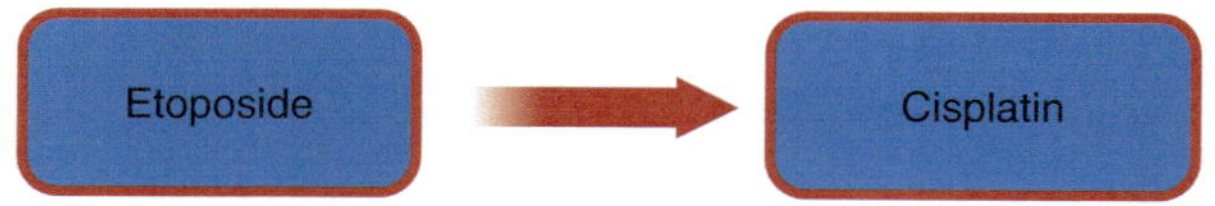

Fig. 5.39 ETCIS protocol infusion sequence

toxicity of the protocol, especially concerning nephrotoxicity, which is a dose-limiting factor.

Iwasa et al. [462] evaluated the efficacy of the combination of cisplatin and etoposide in poorly differentiated neuroendocrine carcinoma of the hepatobiliary tract and pancreas. The combination was not very effective in this type of tumor with marginal antitumor activity, with a response rate of 14%, progression-free survival of 1.8 months and overall survival of 5.8 months, and a relatively severe toxicity profile with neutropenia of grade 3 or 4 in 90% of patients.

According to Patta and Fakih [463], the combination of cisplatin and etoposide showed a high response rate in patients with high-grade metastatic neuroendocrine tumors of the colon and rectum. The authors observed a progression-free survival of 4.5 months and overall survival of 9.5 months. In grade 3 gastroenteropancreatic neuroendocrine carcinoma, Yoon et al. [472] found that the combination promoted a response rate of 27.9% and progression-free survival of 3.5 months.

As for the infusion sequence of the ETCIS protocol (Fig. 5.39), the studies used cisplatin on day 1 followed by etoposide on day 1 and administered alone on days 2 and 3 [462, 471, 472].

5.6.1.2 DS Protocol (Doxorubicin and Streptozotocin)

The DS protocol combines doxorubicin with streptozotocin in the palliative therapy of pancreatic endocrine tumors. As we have seen in other topics, doxorubicin is part of the drugs belonging to the class of cytotoxic antibiotics, being an anthracycline, which is indicated for the treatment of various cancers such as breast cancer and some cancers of the gastrointestinal tract. Streptozotocin, on the other hand, is a glucosamine-nitrosourea whose function is to inhibit the synthesis and secretion of insulin, being toxic to insulin-producing beta cells in the pancreas, acting as an alkylating agent [473–478].

The combination of doxorubicin and streptozotocin has been an alternative treatment for neuroendocrine tumors, where Pavel et al. [479] report that although the combination has low response rates in patients with progressive neuroendocrine tumors, it can prolong the life of patients who have a tumor response. The authors noted with their results that the combination promoted survival of 50 months in patients who responded to treatment and 8 months in patients who did not respond.

Delaunoit et al. [473] suggest that the DS protocol may be a first-line treatment option in advanced pancreatic endocrine carcinoma. The authors noted that the combination induced an objective response rate of 36%, with a median duration of

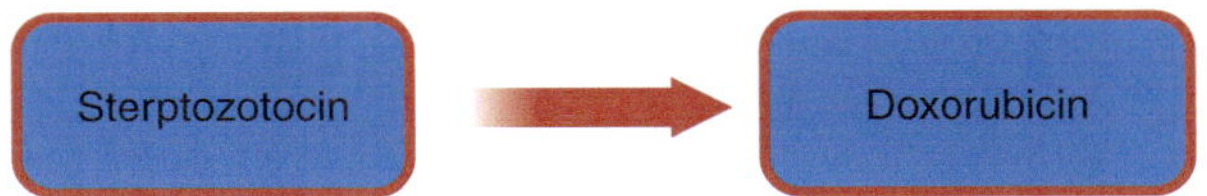

Fig. 5.40 DS protocol infusion sequence

partial response of 19.7 months and overall 2-year survival of 50.2%, and 3-year survival of 24.4%. As the main toxicities, patients had neutropenia and vomiting.

Fjallskog et al. [480] combined the streptozotocin with liposome-encapsulated doxorubicin in the metastatic pancreatic endocrine tumors. The efficacy profile, according to the study, appears to be similar to the combination with unencapsulated doxorubicin, but the use of liposomal doxorubicin reduced cardiac toxicity. The 2-year progression-free survival was 18%, while the 2-year overall survival was 72% with the combination of streptozotocin and liposomal doxorubicin.

The toxicity of doxorubicin may be increased with concomitant use with streptozotocin. According to Eriksson et al. [481], streptozotocin is administered for 5 days every 6 weeks combined with doxorubicin on days 1 and 22. It is not clear whether there is any interaction or toxic effect of the protocol depending on the infusion schedule, as to dermatological toxicity, both drugs are vesicants. The infusion of both drugs only occurs on the first day of the protocol cycle, so perhaps the infusion sequence most used in the cited articles is the most appropriate, starting with streptozotocin followed by doxorubicin (Fig. 5.40) [479, 481, 482].

5.7 Pathophysiology of Anal Cancer

Anal cancer is quite rare, far less common than colorectal cancer. The number of cases is increasing every year, being rarer in people under 35 years old and more incidents in elderly people with an average age of 60 years, being more common in white women and black men [483, 484].

Among anal canal cancers, around 85% are of squamous cell origin, while the other cases are of adenocarcinoma (10%) and 5% of rare tumors such as melanoma, small cell carcinoma, and metastatic tumors. Anal cancer accounts for 2.7% of all digestive cancers and less than 0.5% of all diagnosed malignancies [485].

Anal cancer appears to be directly linked to a complex inflammatory process secondary to infections, as in the case of human papillomavirus (HPV) infections, where the progression of the inflammatory process induces the development of anal intraepithelial neoplasms or squamous cell carcinoma in situ, which is a condition premalignant. Anal intraepithelial neoplasms can progress to the development of invasive squamous cell carcinoma, occurring in about 10–11% of cases. Tumors of the anus tend to spread by local extension, but they can also cause distant metastases [486–489]. Figure 5.41 shows the location of anal cancer.

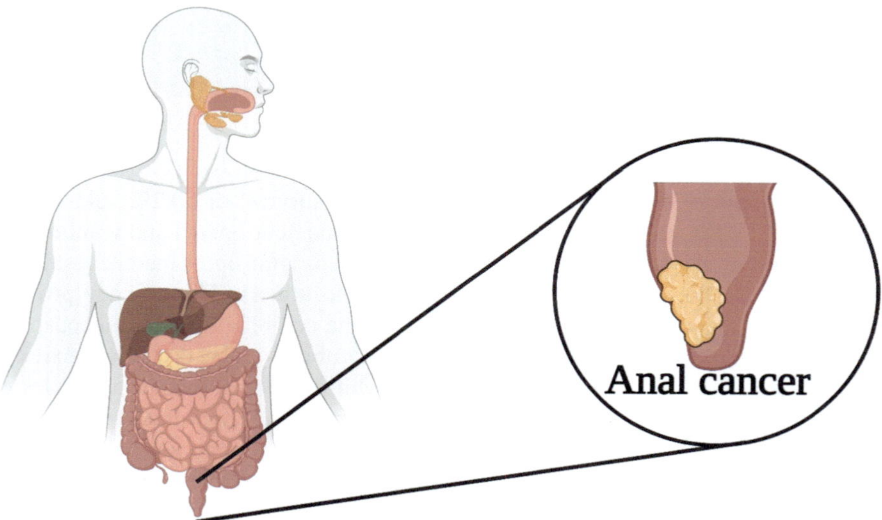

Fig. 5.41 Tumor in the anal canal. (Source: Created with BioRender.com)

5.7.1   *Chemotherapy in the Treatment of Anal Cancer*

As with other types of cancer, treatment for anal cancer will depend on the stage of the disease. In stage 0, surgery is indicated to remove all the lesions that can induce the development of cancer, since at this stage the precancerous cells are located in the inner lining of the anus. In stages I and II, however, the cancer is located in the anal wall, without dissemination to other organs or lymph nodes; thus, the surgical procedure for removal of small tumors is also indicated, and in some cases, it can be followed by treatment with radiotherapy and/or chemotherapy [487, 490, 491].

In a more advanced stage, in the case of stage III, anal cancer has already spread to nearby organs and/or nearby lymph nodes, and radiotherapy associated with chemotherapy is indicated in most cases. In stage IV, the patient presents metastasis, with tumor dissemination in distant organs, which may be in the liver, lungs, bones, and distant lymph nodes. In this case, the probability of cure is very low, where the treatment is based on the control and relief of symptoms, where the standard treatment is often based on a combination of chemotherapy and radiotherapy [490–492].

Some protocols that are indicated for other tumors of the gastrointestinal tract are also used in the treatment of anal cancer. The combination of carboplatin and paclitaxel (Sect. 5.3.1.3) has been indicated as first-line palliative therapy for metastatic anal squamous cell carcinoma, whereas the combination of cisplatin and capecitabine (Sect. 5.3.1.5) has been used in the treatment of carcinoma of the anal canal, and as palliative therapy in anal cancer for metastatic or locally advanced anal squamous cell carcinoma, and the FUC protocol (5-fluorouracil and cisplatin) plus radiotherapy (Sect. 5.3.1.4) has been indicated in curative therapy for carcinoma of the anal canal [65, 67, 68, 493–497].

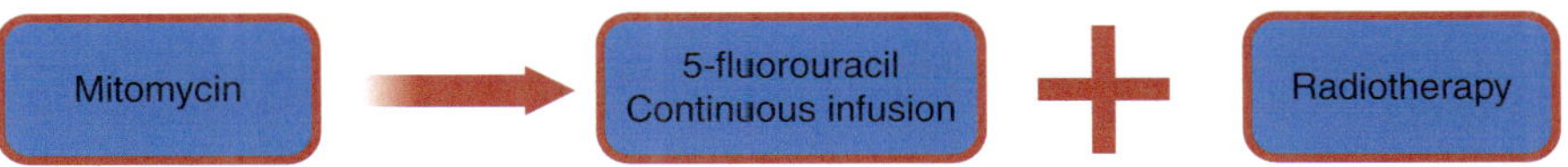

Fig. 5.42 Infusion sequence of the FUMRT protocol

5.7.1.1 FUMRT Protocol (5-Fluorouracil, Mitomycin C, and Radiotherapy)

The combination of 5-fluorouracil with mitomycin C has been indicated as curative therapy for anal canal carcinoma [498, 499]. Mitomycin C is an antineoplastic antibiotic that works by inhibiting DNA synthesis and at higher concentrations is also capable of inhibiting RNA and protein synthesis [500, 501]. The association of 5-fluorouracil with mitomycin C appears to have synergistic effects in vitro [502].

Ajani et al. [498] compared the effectiveness of the combination of 5-fluorouracil and mitomycin C with the combination of 5-fluorouracil and cisplatin, where both protocols were associated with radiotherapy. As a result, the authors observed that the combination of 5-fluorouracil, mitomycin C, and radiotherapy had better results in 5-year disease-free survival (60%) and in the cumulative colostomy rate (10%), with overall survival of 5 years of 75%.

Saint et al. [503] proposed the use of the FUMRT protocol as second line of metastatic squamous cell carcinoma of the anal canal. As a result, the authors observed complete response in 31.6% of patients with 3-month progression-free survival and 7-month overall survival, showing that the protocol provides tumor control with acceptable tolerance.

As for the infusion sequence of the FUMRT protocol, it starts with the infusion of mitomycin C, which is a vesicant drug, followed by 5-fluorouracil by continuous infusion with subsequent administration of radiotherapy, which should be at least two hours after the infusion of 5-fluorouracil (Fig. 5.42) [504].

5.7.1.2 CAPMRT Protocol (Capecitabine, Mitomycin C, and Radiotherapy)

Replacing 5-fluorouracil with capecitabine is another alternative treatment with the combination of capecitabine and mitomycin C associated with radiotherapy for anal canal carcinoma [505, 506]. The combination of mitomycin C with capecitabine proved to be effective in the treatment of anal cancer, where according to Thind et al. [503], the combination was well tolerated with a reasonable activity profile in patients with stage I–III anal squamous cell carcinoma.

Meulendijks et al. [507] and Peixoto et al. [508] highlight that the combination of capecitabine and mitomycin C associated with radiotherapy has similar efficacy to chemoradiotherapy with 5-fluorouracil, mitomycin C, and radiotherapy. In the study by Meulendijks et al. [507], the combination promoted an overall 3-year survival of 86% and a colostomy-free survival of 79%. In the study by Peixoto et al.

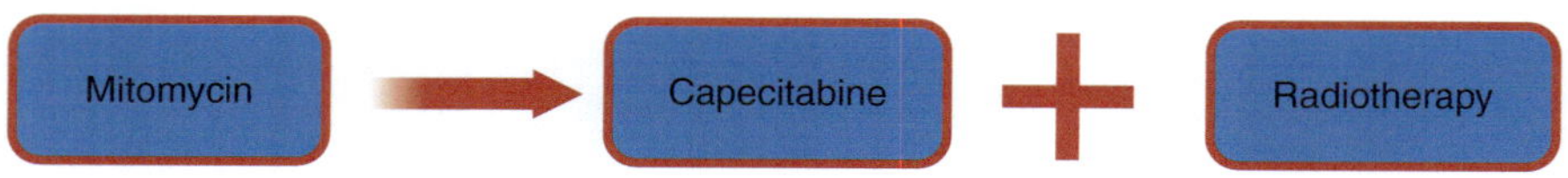

Fig. 5.43 Schedule of administration of the CAPMRT protocol with oral administration of capecitabine

[508], the combination promoted a disease-free survival of 79.7% and an anal cancer-specific survival of 88.7%. According to the study by Goodman et al. [506], the combination appears to reduce acute hematologic toxicity and treatment delays in patients who have undergone definitive chemoradiotherapy in anal cancer using intensity-modulated radiotherapy.

Regarding the infusion schedule of the CAPMRT protocol, care must be taken with the infusion of mitomycin C as it presents a vesicant characteristic, being infused in bolus; the administration of capecitabine is done orally, indicated twice a day, on the days when the patient is undergoing radiotherapy (Fig. 5.43) [509].

References

1. Muto T. Digestion and absorption. Tokyo: Daiichishuppan Co. Ltd; 1988.
2. Molnar C, Gair J (2013) 15.1 Digestive systems. Concepts of biology-1st Canadian edition. Canada.
3. Capuano E. The behavior of dietary fiber in the gastrointestinal tract determines its physiological effect. Crit Rev Food Sci Nutr. 2017;57(16):3543–64. https://doi.org/10.1080/10408398.2016.1180501.
4. Anand P, Kunnumakara AB, Sundaram C, Harikumar KB, Tharakan ST, Lai OS, Sung B, Aggarwal BB. Cancer is a preventable disease that requires major lifestyle changes. Pharm Res. 2008;25(9):2097–116. https://doi.org/10.1007/s11095-008-9661-9.
5. Cofre J, Abdelhay E. Cancer is to embryology as mutation is to genetics: hypothesis of the cancer as embryological phenomenon. Sci World J. 2017;2017:3578090. https://doi.org/10.1155/2017/3578090.
6. Ghai S, Pattison J, Ghai S, O'Malley ME, Khalili K, Stephens M. Primary gastrointestinal lymphoma: spectrum of imaging findings with pathologic correlation. Radiographics. 2007;27(5):1371–88. https://doi.org/10.1148/rg.275065151.
7. Zilberstein B, Quintanilha AG, Santos MAA, Pajecki D, Moura EG, Alves PRA, Maluf Filho F, Souza JAU, Gama-Rodrigues J. Digestive tract microbiota in healthy volunteers. Clinics. 2007;62(1):47–54. https://doi.org/10.1590/S1807-59322007000100008.
8. Matsuda NM, Miller SM, Evora PRB. The chronic gastrointestinal manifestations of Chagas disease. Clinics. 2009;64(12):1219–24. https://doi.org/10.1590/S1807-59322009001200013.
9. Linhares E, Gonçalves R, Valadão M, Vilhena B, Herchenhorn D, Romano S, Ferreira MA, Ferreira CG, Ramos CA, Jesus JP. Gastrointestinal stromal tumor: analysis of 146 cases of the center of reference of the National Cancer Institute—INCA. Rev Col Bras Cir. 2011;38(6):398–406. https://doi.org/10.1590/S0100-69912011000600006.
10. Kang HC, Menias CO, Gaballah AH, Shroff S, Taggart MW, Garg N, Elsayes KM. Beyond the GIST: mesenchymal tumors of the stomach. Radiographics. 2013;33(6):1673–90. https://doi.org/10.1148/rg.336135507.
11. Passos MCF, Moraes-Filho JP. Intestinal microbiota in digestive diseases. Arq Gastroenterol. 2017;54(3):255–62. https://doi.org/10.1590/S0004-2803.201700000-31.

12. WHO – World Health Organization (2020) Estimated number of incident cases from 2018 to 2040. International Agency for Research on Cancer. Available in: https://gco.iarc.fr/tomorrow/graphic-isotype?type=0&type_sex=0&mode=population&sex=0&populations=900&cancers=36&age_group=value&apc_male=0&apc_female=0&single_unit=100000&print=0. Accessed Aug 12 2021.

13. Bray F, Ferlay J, Soerjomataram I, Siegel RL, Torre LA, Jemal A. Global cancer statistics 2018: GLOBOCAN estimates of incidence and mortality worldwide for 36 cancers in 185 countries. CA Cancer J Clin. 2018;68:394–424. https://doi.org/10.3322/caac.21492.

14. Arnold M, Abnet CC, Neale RE, Vignat J, Giovannucci EL, McGlynn KA, Bray F. Global burden of 5 major types of gastrointestinal cancer. Gastroenterology. 2020;159(1):335–49. https://doi.org/10.1053/j.gastro.2020.02.068.

15. Sung H, Ferlay J, Siegel RL, Laversanne M, Soerjomataram I, Jemal A, Bray F. Global cancer statistics 2020: GLOBOCAN estimates of incidence and mortality worldwide for 36 cancers in 185 countries. CA Cancer J Clin. 2021.71(3):209–49. https://doi.org/10.3322/caac.21660.

16. Jones SL, Blikslager AT. Disorders of the gastrointestinal system. Equine Inter Med. 2004:769–949. https://doi.org/10.1016/B0-72-169777-1/50015-9.

17. Bower JE. Cancer-related fatigue: mechanisms, risk factors, and treatments. Nat Rev Clin Oncol. 2014;11(10):597–609. https://doi.org/10.1038/nrclinonc.2014.127.

18. Ber Y, García-Lopez S, Gargallo-Puyuelo CJ, Gomollón F. Small and large intestine (II): inflammatory bowel disease, short bowel syndrome, and malignant tumors of the digestive tract. Nutrients. 2021;13(7):2325. https://doi.org/10.3390/nu13072325.

19. Talley NJ, Phung N, Kalantar JS. Indigestion: when is it functional? BMJ. 2001;323(7324):1294–7. https://doi.org/10.1136/bmj.323.7324.1294.

20. Zali H, Rezaei-Tavirani M, Azodi M. Gastric cancer: prevention, risk factors and treatment. Gastroenterol Hepatol Bed Bench. 2011;4(4):175–85.

21. Kekelidze M, D'Errico L, Pansini M, Tyndall A, Hohmann J. Colorectal cancer: current imaging methods and future perspectives for the diagnosis, staging and therapeutic response evaluation. World J Gastroenterol. 2013;19(46):8502–14. https://doi.org/10.3748/wjg.v19.i46.8502.

22. Ratin RF, Melão S, Lima DMR, Sagae EU, Kurachi G. Gastrointestinal stromal tumor of rectum diagnosed by three-dimensional anorectal ultrasound. J Coloproctol. 2015;36(1):45–9. https://doi.org/10.1016/j.jcol.2015.03.003.

23. Yu XZ, Yang YN, Li JG. Application of ultrasound in the diagnosis of gastrointestinal tumors. European J Inflam. 2020;18:1–8. https://doi.org/10.1177/2058739220961194.

24. van der Lely AJ, Herder WW. Carcinoid syndrome: diagnosis and medical management. Arq Bras Endocrinol Metabol. 2005;49(5):850–60. https://doi.org/10.1590/S0004-27302005000500028.

25. Zhou J, Sun H, Wang Z, Cong W, Wang J, Zeng M, Zhou W, Bie P, Liu L, Wen T, Han G, Wang M, Liu R, Lu L, Ren Z, Chen M, Zeng Z, Liang P, Liang C, Chen M, Yan F, Wang W, Ji Y, Yun J, Cai D, Chen Y, Cheng W, Cheng S, Dai C, Guo W, Hua B, Huang X, Jia W, Li Y, Li Y, Liang J, Liu T, Lv G, Mao Y, Peng T, Ren W, Shi H, Shi G, Tao K, Wang W, Wang X, Wang Z, Xiang B, Xing B, Xu J, Yang J, Yang J, Yang Y, Yang Y, Ye S, Yin Z, Zhang B, Zhang L, Zhang S, Zhang T, Zhao Y, Zheng H, Zhu J, Zhu K, Liu R, Shi Y, Xiao Y, Dai Z, Teng G, Cai J, Wang W, Cai X, Li Q, Shen F, Qin S, Dong J, Fan J. Guidelines for the diagnosis and treatment of hepatocellular carcinoma (2019 edition). Liver Cancer. 2020;9:682–720. https://doi.org/10.1159/000509424.

26. Llovet JM, Kelley RK, Villanueva A, Singal AG, Pikarsky E, Roayaie S, Lencioni R, Koike K, Zucman-Rossi J, Finn RS. Hepatocellular carcinoma. Nat Rev Dis Primers. 2021;7:6. https://doi.org/10.1038/s41572-020-00240-3.

27. Araujo SEA, Alves PRA, Habr-Gama A. Role of colonoscopy in colorectal cancer. Revista do Hospital das Clínicas. 2001;56(1):25–35. https://doi.org/10.1590/S0041-87812001000100005.

28. Conteduca V, Sansonno D, Russi S, Dammacco F. Precancerous colorectal lesions (review). Int J Oncol. 2013;43(4):973–84. https://doi.org/10.3892/ijo.2013.2041.

29. Kuipers EJ, Grady WM, Lieberman D, Seufferlein T, Sung JJ, Boelens PG, van de Velde CJH, Watanabe T. Colorectal Cancer. Nat Rev Dis Primers. 2015;1:15065. https://doi.org/10.1038/nrdp.2015.65.

30. Kiela PR, Ghishan FK. Physiology of intestinal absorption and secretion. Best Pract Res Clin Gastroenterol. 2016;30(2):145–59. https://doi.org/10.1016/j.bpg.2016.02.007.

31. Yavuz A, Hacifazlioğlu Ç, Akkurt G, Aydin A, Ataş H. Diagnosis and management of rectosigmoid perforations. London United Kingdom: Intechopen; 2016.

32. Azzouz LL, Sharma S. Physiology, Large Intestine. Treasure Island USA: StatPearls Publishing; 2020.

33. Shussman N, Wexner SD. Colorectal polyps and polyposis syndromes. Gastroenterol Rep. 2014;2(1):1–15. https://doi.org/10.1093/gastro/got041.

34. Baldin RKS, Anselmi Júnior RA, Azevedo M, Sebastião APM, Montemor M, Tullio LF, Soares LFP, Noronha L. Interobserver variability in histological diagnosis of serrated colorectal polyps. J Coloproctol. 2015;35(4):193–7. https://doi.org/10.1016/j.jcol.2015.06.008.

35. Obuch JC, Pigott CM, Ahnen DJ. Sessile serrated polyps: detection, eradication, and prevention of the evil twin. Curr Treat Options Gastroenterol. 2015;13(1):156–70. https://doi.org/10.1007/s11938-015-0046-y.

36. Erichsen R, Baron JA, Hamilton-Dutoit SJ, Snover DC, Torlakovic EE, Pedersen L, Froslev T, Vyberg M, Hamilton SR, Sorensen HT. Increased risk of colorectal cancer development among patients with serrated polyps. Gastroenterology. 2016;150(4):895–902. https://doi.org/10.1053/j.gastro.2015.11.046.

37. Campos FGCM, Figueiredo MN, Monteiro M, Nahas SC, Cecconello I. Incidence of colorectal cancer in young patients. Rev Col Bras Cir. 2017;44(2):208–15. https://doi.org/10.1590/0100-69912017002004.

38. Wright M, Beaty JS, Ternent CA. Molecular markers for colorectal cancer. Surg Clin N Am. 2017;97:683–701. https://doi.org/10.1016/j.suc.2017.01.014.

39. Witold K, Anna K, Maciej T, Jakub J. Adenomas – genetic factors in colorectal cancer prevention. Rep Pract Oncol Radiother. 2018;23(2):75–83. https://doi.org/10.1016/j.rpor.2017.12.003.

40. Bujanda L, Cosme A, Gil I, Arenas-Mirave JI. Malignant colorectal polyps. World J Gastroenterol. 2010;16(25):3103–11. https://doi.org/10.3748/wjg.v16.i25.3103.

41. Fleming M, Ravula S, Tatishchev SF, Wang HL. Colorectal carcinoma: pathologic aspects. J Gastrointest Oncol. 2012;3(3):153–73. https://doi.org/10.3978/j.issn.2078-6891.2012.030.

42. Bach C (2021) Understanding your pathology report: colon cancer. OncoLink. Available in: https://www.oncolink.org/print/pdf/2007?print_2007.pdf. Accessed Aug 14 2021.

43. Fry LC, Gutierres JP, Jovanovic I, Monkemuller K. Small bowel Neoplasias: current options for diagnosis, staging and therapeutic management. Gastroinstestinal Tumors. 2014;1:9–17. https://doi.org/10.1159/000355210.

44. Surabhi VR, Menias CO, Amer AM, Elshikh M, Katabathina VS, Hara AK, Baughman WC, Kielar A, Elsayes KM, Siegel CL. Tumors and Tumorlike conditions of the Anal Canal and perianal region: MR imaging findings. Radiographics. 2016;36(5):1339–53. https://doi.org/10.1148/rg.2016150209.

45. Valarini SBM, Bortoli VT, Wassano NS, Pukanski MF, Maggi DC, Bertollo LA. Correlation between location, size and histologic type of colorectal polyps at the presence of dysplasia and adenocarcinoma. J Coloproctol. 2011;31(3):241–7. https://doi.org/10.1590/S2237-93632011000300003.

46. Oki E, Ando K, Nakanishi R, Sugiyama M, Nakashima Y, Kubo N, Kudou K, Saeki H, Nozoe T, Emi Y, Maehara Y. Recent advances in treatment for colorectal liver metastasis. Ann Gastroenterol Surg. 2018;2:167–75. https://doi.org/10.1002/ags3.12071.

47. Li J, Barbosa LER. Rectal carcinoma with synchronous liver metastases. J Coloproctol. 2019;39(4):365–72. https://doi.org/10.1016/j.jcol.2019.06.001.

48. Nelson H, Petrelli N, Carlin A, Couture J, Fleshman J, Guillem J, Miedema B, Ota D, Sargent D. Guidelines 2000 for colon and rectal cancer surgery. J Natl Cancer Inst. 2001;93(8):583–96. https://doi.org/10.1093/jnci/93.8.583.

49. Barbaro B, Vitale R, Leccisotti L, Vecchio FM, Santoro L, Valentini V, Coco C, Pacelli F, Crucitti A, Persiani R, Bonomo L. Restaging locally advanced rectal cancer with MR imaging after Chemoradiation therapy. Radiographics. 2010;30(3):699–721. https://doi.org/10.1148/rg.303095085.

50. Bonjer HJ, Deijen CL, Abis GA, Cuesta MA, van der Pas MHGM, Klerk ESML, Lacy AM, Bernelman WA, Andersson J, Angenete E, Rosenberg J, Fuerst A, Haglind E. A randomized trial of laparoscopic versus open surgery for rectal cancer. N Engl J Med. 2015;372:1324–32. https://doi.org/10.1056/NEJMoa1414882.

51. Ong MLH, Schofield JB. Assessment of lymph node involvement in colorectal cancer. World J Gastrointest Surg. 2016;8(3):179–92. https://doi.org/10.4240/wjgs.v8.i3.179.

52. Horvat N, Rocha CCT, Oliveira BC, Petkovska I, Gollub MJ. MRI of rectal cancer: tumor staging, imaging techniques, and management. Radiographics. 2019;39(2):367–87. https://doi.org/10.1148/rg.2019180114.

53. Yang XF, Pan K. Diagnosis and management of acute complications in patients with colon cancer: bleeding, obstruction, and perforation. Chin J Cancer Res. 2014;26(3):331–40. https://doi.org/10.3978/j.issn.1000-9604.2014.06.11.

54. Baer C, Menon R, Bastawrous S, Bastawrous A. Emergency presentations of colorectal cancer. Surg Clin N Am. 2017;97:529–45. https://doi.org/10.1016/j.suc.2017.01.004.

55. Tirumani SH, Kim KW, Nishino M, Howard SA, Krajewski KM, Jagannathan JP, Cleary JM, Ramaiya NH, Shinagare AB. Update on the role of imaging in management of metastatic colorectal cancer. Radiographics. 2014;34(7):1908–28. https://doi.org/10.1148/rg.347130090.

56. Stewart CL, Warner S, Ito K, Raoof M, Wu GX, Lu WP, Kessler J, Kim JY, Fong Y. Cytoreduction for colorectal metastases: liver, lung, peritoneum, lymph nodes, bone, brain. When does it palliate, prolong survival, and potentially cure? Curr Probl Surg. 2018;55(9):330–79. https://doi.org/10.1057/j.cpsurg.2018.08.004.

57. Sgouros G, Bodei L, McDevitt MR, Nedrow JR. Radiopharmaceutical therapy in cancer: clinical advances and challenges. Nat Rev Drug Discov. 2020;19:589–608. https://doi.org/10.1038/s41573-020-0073-9.

58. Petrelli NJ. Perioperative or adjuvant therapy for resectable colorectal hepatic metastases. J Clin Oncol. 2008;26(30):4862–3. https://doi.org/10.1200/JCO.2008.18.5868.

59. Moghimi-Dehkordi B, Safaee A. An overview of colorectal cancer survival rates and prognosis in Asia. World J Gastrointest Oncol. 2012;4(4):71–5. https://doi.org/10.4251/wjgo.v4.i4.71.

60. Brandi G, Lorenzo SD, Nannini M, Curti S, Ottone M, Dall'Olio FG, Barbera MA, Pantaleo MA, Biasco G. Adjuvant chemotherapy for resected colorectal cancer metastases: literature review and meta-analysis. World J Gastroenterol. 2016;22(2):519–33. https://doi.org/10.3748/wjg.v22.i2.519.

61. McGavin JK, Goa KL. Capecitabine: a review of its use in the treatment of advanced or metastatic colorectal cancer. Drugs. 2001;61(150):2309–26. https://doi.org/10.2165/00003495-200161150-00015.

62. Mitry E, Fields ALA, Bleiberg H, Labianca R, Portier G, Tu D, Nitti D, Torri V, Elias D, O'Callaghan C, Langer B, Martignoni G, Bouché O, Lazorthes F, Cutsem EV, Bedenne L, Moore MJ, Rougier P. Adjuvant chemotherapy after potentially curative resection of metastases from colorectal cancer: a pooled analysis of two randomized trials. J Clin Oncol. 2008;26(30):4906–11. https://doi.org/10.1200/JCO.2008.17.3781.

63. Petersen SH, Harling H, Kirkeby LT, Jorgensen PW, Mocellin S. Postoperative adjuvant chemotherapy in rectal cancer operated for cure. Cochrane Library. 2012;2012(3):CD004078. https://doi.org/10.1002/14651858.CD004078.pub2.

64. Figueiredo Junior AG, Forones NM. Study on adherence to capecitabine among patients with colorectal cancer and metastatic breast cancer. Arq Gastroenterol. 2014;51(3):186–91. https://doi.org/10.1590/S0004-28032014000300004.

65. Kuehr T, Thaler J, Woell E (2017) Chemotherapy protocols 2017: current protocols and "targeted therapies". Klinikum Wels-Grieskirchen and Caritas Christi URGET NOS. Austria. www.chemoprotocols.eu.

66. Xie YH, Chen YX, Fang JY. Comprehensive review of targeted therapy for colorectal cancer. Signal Transduct Target Ther. 2020;5:22. https://doi.org/10.1038/s41392-020-0116-z.

67. BC Cancer (2021) Supportive care protocols. BC Cancer. British Columbia. Available in: http://www.bccancer.bc.ca/health-professionals/clinical-resources/chemotherapy-protocols/supportive-care. Accessed July 2 2021.

68. NHS (2021) Chemotherapy Protocols. NHS. University Hospital Southampton. NHS Foundation Trust. England. Available in: https://www.uhs.nhs.uk/HealthProfessionals/Chemotherapy-protocols/Chemotherapy-protocols.aspx. Access July 2 2021.

69. NCT00070265 (2013) Neoadjuvant and Adjuvant Capecitabine and Oxaliplatin in Treating Patients With Resectable Liver Metastases Secondary to Colorectal Cancer. Clinical Trials. Available in: https://www.clinicaltrials.gov/ct2/show/NCT00070265. Access Aug 15 2021.

70. Li Y, Li GX, Chu ZH, Hao CY, Jiang ZW, Chen HQ, Lin JJ, Li DC, Hu B, Wang XS, Lin F. Conversion chemotherapy with capecitabine and oxaliplatin for colorectal cancer with potentially resectable liver metastases: a phase II, open-label, single-arm study. J Cancer Res Ther. 2018;14(4):772–9. https://doi.org/10.4103/jcrt.JCRT_738_17.

71. Wiseman LR, Adkins JC, Plosker GL, Goa KL. Oxaliplatin: a review of its use in the management of metastatic colorectal cancer. Drugs Aging. 1999;14(6):459–75. https://doi.org/10.2165/00002512-199914060-00006.

72. Almeida VL, Leitão A, Reina LCB, Montanari CA, Donnici CL, Lopes MTP. Cancer and cell cycle-specific and cell cycle nonspecific anticancer DNA-interactive agents: an introduction. Química Nova. 2005;28(1):118–29. https://doi.org/10.1590/S0100-40422005000100021.

73. Pericay C, López A, Soler JR, Bonfill T, Dotor E, Saigí E. Extracasation of oxaliplatin: na infrequente and irritant toxicity. Clin Transl Oncol. 2009;11(2):114–6. https://doi.org/10.1007/s12094-009-0324-z.

74. Alcindor T, Beauger N. Oxaliplatin: a review in the era of molecularly targeted therapy. Curr Oncol. 2011;18(1):18–25. https://doi.org/10.3747/co.v18i1.708.

75. Moskovitz M, Wollner M, Haim N. Oxaliplatin-induced pulmonary toxicity in gastrointestinal malignancies: two case reports and review of the literature. Case Rep Oncol Med. 2015;2015:341064. https://doi.org/10.1155/2015/341064.

76. van Cutsem E, Twelves C, Cassidy J, Allman D, Bajetta E, Boyer M, Bugat R, Findlay M, Frings S, Jahn M, McKendrick J, Osterwalder B, Perez-Manga G, Rosso R, Rougier P, Schmiegel WH, Seitz JF, Thompson P, Vieitez C, Harper P. Oral capecitabine compared with intravenous fluorouracil plus leucovorin in patients with metastatic colorectal cancer: results of a large phase III study. J Clin Oncol. 2001;19(21):4097–106. https://doi.org/10.1200/JCO.2001.19.21.4097.

77. Walko CM, Lindley C. Capecitabine: a review. Clin Ther. 2005;27(1):23–44. https://doi.org/10.1016/j.clinthera.2005.01.005.

78. Hattori N, Nakayama G, Uehara K, Aiba T, Ishigure K, Sakamoto E, Tojima Y, Kanda M, Kobayashi D, Tanaka C, Yamada S, Koike M, Fujiwara M, Nagino M, Kodera Y. Phase II study of capecitabine plus oxaliplatin (CapOX) as adjuvant chemotherapy for locally advanced rectal cancer (CORONA II). Int J Clin Oncol. 2020;25:118–25. https://doi.org/10.1007/s10147-019-01546-3.

79. Gil-Delgado M, Bastian G, Paule B, Urien S, Spano JP, Deguetz G, Chouania K, Saintini P, Breau JL, Khayat D. Pharmacokinetic study of oxaliplatin (lohp) and capecitabine combination in advanced colorectal cancer. J Clin Oncol. 2004;22(14):2108. https://doi.org/10.1200/jco.2004.22.90140.2108.

80. Satake H, Hashida H, Tanioka H, Miyake Y, Yoshioka S, Watanabe T, Matsuura M, Kyogoku T, Inukai M, Kotake T, Okita Y, Matsumoto T, Yasui H, Kotaka M, Kato T, Kaihara S, Tsuji A. Hepatectomy followed by adjuvant chemotherapy with 3-month Capecitabine plus Oxaliplatin for colorectal cancer liver metastases. Oncologist. 2021;26(7):e1125–32. https://doi.org/10.1002/onco.13816.

81. NHS (2020) Chemotherapy Protocol. Colorectal cancer. Capecitabine and oxaliplatin. NHS. University Hospital Southampton. NHS Foundation Trust. England. Available in:

https://www.uhs.nhs.uk/Media/SUHTExtranet/Services/Chemotherapy-SOPs/Colorectal/Capecitabine-Oxaliplatin.pdf. Accessed Aug 15 2021.

82. Machover D. A comprehensive review of 5-fluorouracil and leucovorin in patients with metastatic colorectal carcinoma. Cancer 1997;80(7):1179–87. https://doi.org/10.1002/(sici)1097-0142(19971001)80:7<1179::aid-cncr1>3.0.co;2-g.

83. Tsalic M, Bar-Sela G, Beny A, Visel B, Haim N. Severe toxicity related to the 5-fluorouracil/leucovorin combination (the Mayo Clinic regimen): a prospective study in colorectal cancer patients. Am J Clin Oncol. 2003;26(1):103–6. https://doi.org/10.1097/01.COC.0000017526.55135.6D.

84. Hegde VS, Nagalli S. Leucovorin. Treasure Island USA: StatPearls Publishing; 2021.

85. Madhyastha S, Prabhu LV, Saralaya V, Rai R. A comparison of vitamin a and leucovorin for the prevention of methotrexate-induced micronuclei production in rat bone marrow. Clinics. 2008;63(6):821–6. https://doi.org/10.1590/S1807-59322008000600019.

86. Saif MW, Makrilia N, Syrigos K. CoFactor: folate requirement for optimization of 5-Fluouracil activity in anticancer chemotherapy. J Oncol. 2010;2010:934359. https://doi.org/10.1155/2010/934359.

87. Lemire M, Zaidi SHE, Zanke BW, Gallinger S, Hudson TJ, Cleary SP. The effect of 5-fluorouracil/leucovorin chemotherapy on CpG methylation, or the confounding role of leukocyte heterogeneity: An illustration. Genomics. 2015;106(6):340–7. https://doi.org/10.1016/j.ygeno.2015.09.003.

88. Borner MM, Castiglione M, Bacchi M, Weber W, Herrmann R, Fey MF, Pagani O, Leyvraz S, Morant R, Pestalozzi B, Hanselmann S, Goldhirsch A. The impact of adding low-dose leucovorin to monthly 5-fluorouracil in advanced colorectal carcinoma: results of a phase III trial. Ann Oncol. 1998;9(5):535–41. https://doi.org/10.1023/A:1008270916325.

89. Porschen R, Bermann A, Loffler T, Haack G, Rettig K, Anger Y, Strohmeyer G. Fluorouracil plus Leucovorin as effective adjuvant chemotherapy in curatively resected stage III colon cancer: results of the trial adjCCA-01. J Clin Oncol. 2001;19(6):1787–94. https://doi.org/10.1200/JCO.2001.19.6.1787.

90. Arkenau HT, Bermann A, Rettig K, Strohmeyer G, Porschen R. 5-fluorouracil plus leucovorin is an effective adjuvant chemotherapy in curatively resected stage III colon cancer:long-term follow-up results of the adjCCA-01 trial. Ann Oncol. 2003;14(3):395–9. https://doi.org/10.1093/annonc/mdg100.

91. Portier G, Elias D, Bouche O, Rougier P, Bosset JF, Saric J, Belghiti J, Piedbois P, Guimbaud R, Nordlinger B, Bugat R, Lazorthes F, Bedenne L. Multicenter randomized trial of adjuvant fluorouracil and folinic acid compared with surgery alone after resection of colorectal liver metastases: FFCD ACHBTH AURC 9002 trial. J Clin Oncol. 2006;24(31):4976–82. https://doi.org/10.1200/JCO.2006.06.8353.

92. Jolivet J. Role of leucovorin dosing and administration schedule. Eur J Cancer. 1995;31(7–8):1311–5. https://doi.org/10.1016/0959-8049(95)00140-E.

93. NHS (2020) Chemotherapy Protocol. Colorectal cancer. Fluorouracil and folinic acid (Modified de Gramont). NHS. University Hospital Southampton. NHS Foundation Trust. England. Available in: https://www.uhs.nhs.uk/Media/SUHTExtranet/Services/Chemotherapy-SOPs/Colorectal/Fluorouracil-Folinic-Acid.pdf. Accessed Aug 15 2021.

94. Rothenberg ML, Oza AM, Bigelow RH, Berlin JD, Marshall JL, Ramanathan RK, Hart LL, Gupta S, Garay CA, Burger BG, Bail NL, Haller DG. Superiority of Oxaliplatin and fluorouracil-Leucovorin compared with either therapy alone in patients with progressive colorectal cancer after irinotecan and fluorouracil-Leucovorin: interim results of a phase III trial. J Clin Oncol. 2003;21(11):2059–69. https://doi.org/10.1200/JCO.2003.11.126.

95. Jonker D, Rumble RB, Maroun J. Role of oxaliplatin combined with 5-fluorouracil and folinic acid in the first- and second-line treatment of advanced colorectal cancer. Curr Oncol. 2006;13(5):173–84.

96. Healey E, Stillfried GE, Eckermann S, Dawber JP, Clingan PR, Ranson M. Comparative effectiveness of 5-fluorouracil with and without Oxaliplatin in the treatment of colorectal cancer in clinical practice. Anticancer Res. 2013;33(3):1053–60.

97. André T, Gramont A, Vernerey D, Chibaudel B, Bonnetain F, Tiheras-Raballand A, Scriva A, Hickish T, Tabernero J, Van Laethem JL, Banzi M, Maartense E, Shmueli E, Carisson GU, Scheithauer W, Papamichael D, Moehler M, Landolfi S, Demetter P, Colote S, Tournigand C, Louvet C, Duval A, Fléjou JF, Gramont A. Adjuvant fluorouracil, Leucovorin, and Oxaliplatin in stage II to III colon cancer: updated 10-year survival and outcomes according to BRAF mutation and mismatch repair status of the MOSAIC study. J Clin Oncol. 2015;33(35):4176–87. https://doi.org/10.1200/JCO.2015.63.4238.

98. Weber GF. DNA damaging drugs. Mol Therapies Cancer. 2014;8:9–112. https://doi.org/10.1007/978-3-319-13278-5_2.

99. André T, Boni C, Mounedji-Boudiaf L, Navarro M, Tabernero J, Hickish T, Topham C, Zaninelli M, Clingan P, Bridgewater J, Tabah-Fisch I, Gramont A. Oxaliplatin, fluorouracil, and leucovorin as adjuvant treatment for colon cancer. N Engl J Med. 2004;350(23):2343–51. https://doi.org/10.1056/NEJMoa032709.

100. Alberts SR, Horvath WL, Sternfeld WC, Goldberg RM, Mahoney MR, Dakhil SR, Levitt R, Rowland K, Nair S, Sargent DJ, Donohue JH. Oxaliplatin, fluorouracil, and Leucovorin for patients with Unresectable liver-only metastases from colorectal cancer: a north central cancer treatment group phase II study. J Clin Oncol. 2005;23(36):9243–9. https://doi.org/10.1200/JCO.2005.07.740.

101. Goldberg RM, Sargent DJ, Morton RF, Fuchs CS, Ramanathan RK, Williamson SK, Findlay BP, Pitot HC, Alberts SR. A randomized controlled trial of fluorouracil plus Leucovorin, irinotecan, and Oxaliplatin combinations in patients with previously untreated metastatic colorectal cancer. J Clin Oncol. 2004;22(1):23–30. https://doi.org/10.1200/JCO.2004.09.046.

102. Yamada Y, Ohtsu A, Boku N, Miyata Y, Shimada Y, Doi T, Muro K, Muto M, Hamaguchi T, Mera K, Yano T, Tanigawara Y, Shirao K. Phase I/II study of Oxaliplatin with weekly bolus fluorouracil and high-dose Leucovorin (ROX) as first-line therapy for patients with colorectal cancer. Jpn J Clin Oncol. 2006;36(4):218–23. https://doi.org/10.1093/jjco/hyl020.

103. Jerremalm E, Hedeland M, Wallin I, Bondesson U, Ehrsson H. Oxaliplatin degradation in the presence of chloride: identification and cytotoxicity of the Monochloro Monooxalato complex. Pharm Res. 2004;21(5):891–4. https://doi.org/10.1023/b:pham.0000026444.67883.83.

104. Eto S, Yamamoto K, Shimazu K, Sugiura T, Baba K, Sato A, Goromaru T, Hagiwara Y, Hara K, Shinohara Y, Takahashi K. Formation of oxalate in oxaliplatin injection diluted with infusion solutions. Gan To Kagaku Ryoho. 2014;41(1):71–5.

105. Mehta AM, Van den Hoven JM, Rosing H, Hillebrand MJX, Nuijen B, Huitema ADR, Beijnen JH, Verwaal VJ. Stability of oxaliplatin in chloride-containing carrier solutions used in hyperthermic intraperitoneal chemotherapy. Int J Pharm. 2015;479(1):23–7. https://doi.org/10.1016/j.ijpharm.2014.12.025.

106. NHS (2020) Chemotherapy Protocol. Colorectal cancer. Fluorouracil, folinic acid (modified de gramont) and oxaliplatin (FOLFOX). NHS. University Hospital Southampton. NHS Foundation Trust. England. Available in: https://www.uhs.nhs.uk/Media/SUHTExtranet/Services/Chemotherapy-SOPs/Colorectal/Fluorouracil-FolinicAcid-Oxaliplatin.pdf. Access Aug 16 2021.

107. Cascinu S, Graziano F, Ferraù F, Catalano V, Massacesi C, Santini D, Silva RR, Barni S, Zaniboni A, Battelli N, Siena S, Giordani P, Mari D, Baldelli AM, Antognoli S, Maisano R, Priolo D, Pessi MA, Tonini G, Rota S, Labianca R. Raltitrexed plus oxaliplatin (TOMOX) as first-line chemotherapy for metastatic colorectal cancer. A phase II study of the Italian Group for the Study of gastrointestinal tract carcinomas (GISCAD). Ann Oncol. 2002;13(5):716–20. https://doi.org/10.1093/annonc/mdf091.

108. Cortinovis D, Bajetta E, Bartolomeo MD, Dognini G, Beretta E, Ferrario E, Ricotta R, Buzzoni R. Raltitrexed plus Oxaliplatin in the treatment of metastatic colorectal cancer. Tumori J. 2004;90(2):186–91. https://doi.org/10.1177/030089160409000205.

109. NCT02557490 (2015) Oxaliplatin and Raltitrexed Treatment of Colorectal Cancer With Liver Metastases. Clinical Trials. Available in: https://clinicaltrials.gov/ct2/show/NCT02557490. Accessed Aug 17 2021.

110. Gunasekara NS, Faulds D. Raltitrexed. A review of its pharmacological properties and clinical efficacy in the management of advanced colorectal cancer. Drugs. 1998;55(3):423–35. https://doi.org/10.2165/00003495-199855030-00012.

111. Comella P, Casaretti R, Crucitta E, De Vita F, Palmeri S, Avallone A, Orditura M, De Lucia L, Del Prete S, Catalano G, Lorusso V, Comella G. Oxaliplatin plus raltitrexed and leucovorin-modulated 5-fluorouracil i.v. bolus: a salvage regimen for colorectal cancer patients. Br J Cancer. 2002;86:1871–5. https://doi.org/10.1038/sj.bjc.6600414.

112. van Cutsem E, Cunningham D, Maroun J, Cervantes A, Glimelius B. Raltitrexed: current clinical status and future directions. Ann Oncol. 2002;13(4):513–22. https://doi.org/10.1093/annonc/mdf054.

113. Rivory LP. New drugs for colorectal cancer – mechanisms of action. Aust Prescr. 2002;25:108–10. https://doi.org/10.18773/austprescr.2002.110.

114. Feliu J, Castañón C, Salud A, Mel JR, Escudero P, Pelegrín A, López-Gómes L, Ruiz M, González E, Juárez F, Lizón J, Castro J. González-Barón M. Phase II randomised trial of raltitrexed–oxaliplatin vs raltitrexed–irinotecan as first-line treatment in advanced colorectal cancer. Br J Cancer. 2005;93(11):1230–5. https://doi.org/10.1038/sj.bjc.6602860.

115. BC Cancer (2016) BC Cancer Protocol Summary for Adjuvant Combination Chemotherapy for Node Positive Colon Cancer Using Oxaliplatin and Raltitrexed in Patients Intolerant to Fluorouracil or Capecitabine. BC Cancer. British Columbia. Available in: http://www.bccancer.bc.ca/chemotherapy-protocols-site/Documents/Gastrointestinal/GIAJRALOX_Protocol.pdf. Accessed Aug 17 2021.

116. Keating GM. Panitumumab: a review of its use in metastatic colorectal cancer. Drugs. 2010;70(8):1059–78. https://doi.org/10.2165/11205090-000000000-00000.

117. Chibaudel B. Therapeutic strategy in unresectable metastatic colorectal cancer. Ther Adv Med Oncol. 2012;4(2):75–89. https://doi.org/10.1177/1758834011431592.

118. Chibaudel B, Tournigand C, Bonnetain F, Richa H, Benetkiewicz M, André T, Gramont A. Therapeutic strategy in unresectable metastatic colorectal cancer: an updated review. Ther Adv Med Oncol. 2015;7(3):153–69. https://doi.org/10.1177/1758834015572343.

119. Feo L, Polcino M, Nash GM. Resection of the primary tumor in stage IV colorectal cancer: when is it necessary? Surg Clin N Am. 2017;97:657–69. https://doi.org/10.1016/j.suc.2017.01.012.

120. Giacchetti S, Itzhaki M, Gruia G, Adam R, Zidani R, Kunstlinger F, Brienza S, Alafaci E, Bertheault-Cvitkovic F, Jasmin C, Reyres M, Bismuth H, Misset JL, Lévi F. Long-term survival of patients with unresectable colorectal cancer liver metastases following infusional chemotherapy with 5-fluorouracil, leucovorin, oxaliplatin and surgery. Ann Oncol. 1999;10:663–9. https://doi.org/10.1023/a:1008347829017.

121. Ishibashi K, Yoshimatsu K, Yokomizo H. Umehara A, Yoshida K, Fujimoto T, Watanabe K, Katsube T, Naritaka Y, Ogawa K. Low-dose Leucovorin and 5-fluorouracil for Unresectable multiple liver metastasis from colorectal cancer. Anticancer Res. 2005;25:4747–52.

122. Cassidy J, Clarke S, Díaz-Rubio E, Scheithauer W, Figer A, Wong R, Koski S, Lichinitser M, Yang TS, Rivera F, Couture F, Sirzén F, Saltz L. Randomized phase III study of Capecitabine plus Oxaliplatin compared with fluorouracil/Folinic acid plus Oxaliplatin as first-line therapy for metastatic colorectal cancer. J Clin Oncol. 2008;26(12):2006–12. https://doi.org/10.1200/JCO.2007.14.9898.

123. Koukourakis GV, Zacharias G, Tsalafoutas J, Theodoridis D, Kouloulias V. Capecitabine for locally advanced and metastatic colorectal cancer: a review. World J Gastrointest Oncol. 2010;2(8):311–21. https://doi.org/10.4251/wjgo.v2.i8.311.

124. NCT00623805 (2014) A Study of Avastin (Bevacizumab) and Xeloda (Capecitabine) as Maintenance Treatment in Patients With Metastatic Colorectal Cancer. Clinical Trials. Available in: https://clinicaltrials.gov/ct2/show/NCT00623805. Accessed Aug 17 2021.

125. BC Cancer (2018) BC Cancer Protocol Summary for Palliative Therapy of Metastatic Colorectal Cancer using Capecitabine and Bevacizumab. BC Cancer. British Columbia. Available in: http://www.bccancer.bc.ca/chemotherapy-protocols-site/Documents/Gastrointestinal/GIAVCAPB_Protocol.pdf. Accessed Aug 17 2021.

126. Sonbol MB, Mountjoy LJ, Firwana B, Liu AJ, Almader-Dougls D, Mody K, Hubbard J, Borad M, Ahn DH, Murad MH, Bekaii-Saab T. The role of maintenance strategies in metastatic colorectal cancer- a systematic review and network meta-analysis of randomized clinical trials. JAMA Oncol. 2020;6(3):e194489. https://doi.org/10.1001/jamaoncol.2019.4489.

127. Bang YH, Kim JE, Lee JS, Kim SY, Kim KP, Kim TW, Hong YS. Bevacizumab plus capecitabine as later-line treatment for patients with metastatic colorectal cancer refractory to irinotecan, oxaliplatin, and fluoropyrimidines. Sci Rep. 2021;11:7118. https://doi.org/10.1038/s41598-021-86482-x.

128. Hicklin DJ, Ellis LM. Role of the vascular endothelial growth factor pathway in tumor growth and angiogenesis. J Clin Oncol. 2005;23(5):1011–27. https://doi.org/10.1200/JCO.2005.06.081.

129. Ranieri G, Patruno R, Ruggieri E, Montemurro S, Valerio P, Ribatti D. Vascular endothelial growth factor (VEGF) as a target of bevacizumab in cancer: from the biology to the clinic. Curr Med Chem. 2006;13(16):1845–57. https://doi.org/10.2174/092986706777585059.

130. Bock F, Onderka J, Dietrich T, Bachmann B, Kruse FE, Paschke M, Zahn G, Cursiefen C. Bevacizumab as a potent inhibitor of inflammatory corneal angiogenesis and Lymphangiogenesis. Invest Ophthalmol Vis Sci. 2007;48(6):2545–52. https://doi.org/10.1167/iovs.06-0570.

131. Teleanu RI, Chircov C, Grumezescu AM, Teleanu DM. Tumor angiogenesis and anti-angiogenic strategies for cancer treatment. J Clin Med. 2020;9:84. https://doi.org/10.3390/jcm9010084.

132. Larsen FO, Boisen MK, Fromm AL, Jensen BV. Capecitabine and bevacizumab in heavily pre-treated patients with advanced colorectal cancer. Acta Oncol. 2011;51(2):231–3. https://doi.org/10.3109/0284186X.2011.614637.

133. Goey KKH, Elias SG, van Tinteren H, Laclé MM, Willems SM, Offerhaus GJA, Leng WWJ, Strengman E, ten Tije AJ, Creemers GJM, van der Velden A, Jongh FE, Erdkamp FLG, Tanis BC, Punt CJA, Koopman M. Maintenance treatment with capecitabine and bevacizumab versus observation in metastatic colorectal cancer: updated results and molecular subgroup analyses of the phase 3 CAIRO3 study. Ann Oncol. 2017;28(9):2128–34. https://doi.org/10.1093/annonc/mdx322.

134. Sherman SK, Lange JJ, Dahdaleh FS, Rajeev R, Gamblin TC, Polite BN, Turaga KK. Cost-effectiveness of maintenance capecitabine and bevacizumab for metastatic colorectal cancer. JAMA Oncol. 2019;5(2):236–42. https://doi.org/10.1001/jamaoncol.2018.5070.

135. NHS (2020) Chemotherapy Protocol. Colorectal cancer. Bevacizumab-Capecitabine. NHS. University Hospital Southampton. NHS Foundation Trust. England. Available in: https://www.uhs.nhs.uk/Media/SUHTExtranet/Services/Chemotherapy-SOPs/Colorectal/Bevacizumab-Capecitabine.pdf. Accessed Aug 17 2021.

136. Cunningham D, Humblet Y, Siena S, Khayat D, Bleiberg H, Santoro A, Bets D, Mueser M, Harstrick A, Verslype C, Chau I, Cutsem EV. Cetuximab monotherapy and Cetuximab plus irinotecan in irinotecan-refractory metastatic colorectal cancer. N Engl J Med. 2004;351:337–45. https://doi.org/10.1056/NEJMoa033025.

137. Harding J, Burtness B. Cetuximab: an epidermal growth factor receptor chemeric human-murine monoclonal antibody. Drugs Today (Barc). 2005;41(2):107–27. https://doi.org/10.1358/dot.2005.41.2.882662.

138. Lenz HJ. Cetuximab in the management of colorectal cancer. Biologics. 2007;1(2):77–91.

139. Wilke H, Glynne-Jones R, Thaler J, Adenis A, Preusser P, Ahuilar EA, Aapro MS, Esser R, Loos AH, Siena S. Cetuximab plus irinotecan in heavily pretreated metastatic colorectal cancer progressing on irinotecan: MABEL study. J Clin Oncol. 2008;26(33):5335–43. https://doi.org/10.1200/JCO.2008.16.3758.

140. BC Cancer (2009) BC Cancer Protocol Summary Third Line Treatment of Metastatic Colorectal Cancer Using Cetuximab in Combination with Irinotecan. BC Cancer. British Columbia. Available in: http://www.bccancer.bc.ca/chemotherapy-protocols-site/Documents/Gastrointestinal/GIAVCETIR_Protocol.pdf. Accessed Aug 17 2021.

141. NCT00005076 (2013) Cetuximab and Irinotecan in Treating Patients With Advanced Colorectal Cancer. Clinical Trials. Available in: https://clinicaltrials.gov/ct2/show/NCT00005076. Accessed Aug 17 2021.

142. Xu Y, Her C. Inhibition of topoisomerase (DNA) I (TOP1): DNA damage repair and anticancer therapy. Biomol Ther. 2015;5(3):1652–70. https://doi.org/10.3390/biom5031652.

143. Kciuk M, Marciniak B, Kontek R. Irinotecan—still an important player in cancer chemotherapy: a comprehensive overview. Int J Mol Sci. 2020;21(14):4919. https://doi.org/10.3390/ijms21144919.

144. Martín-Martorell P, Roselló S, Rodríguez-Braun E, Chirivella I, Bosch A, Cervantes A. Biweekly cetuximab and irinotecan in advanced colorectal cancer patients progressing after at least one previous line of chemotherapy: results of a phase II single institution trial. Br J Cancer. 2008;99(3):455–8. https://doi.org/10.1038/sj.bjc.6604530.

145. Vincenzi B, Santini D, Rabitti C, Coppola R, Zobel BB, Trodella L, Tonini G. Cetuximab and irinotecan as third-line therapy in advanced colorectal cancer patients: a single Centre phase II trial. Br J Cancer. 2006;94:792–7. https://doi.org/10.1038/sj.bjc.6603018.

146. Pfeiffer P, Nielsen D, Yilmaz M, Iversen A, Vejlo C, Jensen BV. Cetuximab and irinotecan as third line therapy in patients with advanced colorectal cancer after failure of irinotecan, oxaliplatin and 5-fluorouracil. Acta Oncol. 2009;46(5):697–701. https://doi.org/10.1080/02841860601009455.

147. Czejka M, Gruenberger B, Kiss A, Farkouh A, Schueller J. Pharmacokinetics of irinotecan in combination with biweekly Cetuximab in patients with advanced colorectal cancer. Anticancer Res. 2010;30(6):2355–60.

148. NHS (2020) Chemotherapy Protocol. Colorectal cancer. Cetuximab-Irinotecan. NHS. University Hospital Southampton. NHS Foundation Trust. England. Available in: https://www.uhs.nhs.uk/Media/SUHTExtranet/Services/Chemotherapy-SOPs/Colorectal/Cetuximab-Irinotecan14day.pdf. Accessed Aug 17 2021.

149. NCT00654160 (2017) Irinotecan, Fluorouracil, and Leucovorin in Treating Patients With Advanced Gastrointestinal Cancer. Clinical Trials. Available in: https://clinicaltrials.gov/ct2/show/NCT00654160. Accessed Aug 18 2021.

150. BC Cancer (2020) BC Cancer Protocol Summary for Palliative Combination Chemotherapy for Metastatic Colorectal Cancer Using Irinotecan, Fluorouracil and Leucovorin. BC Cancer. British Columbia. Available in: http://www.bccancer.bc.ca/chemotherapy-protocols-site/Documents/Gastrointestinal/GIFOLFIRI_Protocol.pdf. Accessed Aug 18 2021.

151. NHS (2020) Chemotherapy Protocol. Colorectal cancer. Fluorouracil, folinic acid (modified de gramont) and irinotecan (FOLFIRI). NHS. University Hospital Southampton. NHS Foundation Trust. England. Available in: https://www.uhs.nhs.uk/Media/SUHTExtranet/Services/Chemotherapy-SOPs/Colorectal/Fluorouracil-FolinicAcid-Irinotecan.pdf. Accessed Aug 18 2021.

152. Jain CK, Majumder HK, Roychoudhury S. Natural compounds as anticancer agents targeting DNA topoisomerases. Curr Genomics. 2017;18(1):75–92. https://doi.org/10.2174/1389202917666160808125213.

153. Delgado JL, Hsieh CM, Chan NL, Hiasa H. Topoisomerases as anticancer targets. Biochem J. 2018;475(2):373–98. https://doi.org/10.1042/BCJ20160583.

154. Silva AA, Carlotto J, Rotta I. Padronização da ordem de infusão de medicamentos antineoplásicos utilizados no tratamento dos cânceres de mama e colorretal. Einstein. 2018;16(2):1–9. https://doi.org/10.1590/S1679-45082018RW4074.

155. Glynne-Jones R, Falk S, Maughan TS, Meadows HM, Sebag-Montefiore D. A phase I/II study of irinotecan when added to 5-fluorouracil and leucovorin and pelvic radiation in locally advanced rectal cancer: a colorectal clinical oncology group study. Br J Cancer. 2007;96(4):551–8. https://doi.org/10.1038/sj.bjc.6603570.

156. Barone C, Nuzzo G, Cassano A, Basso M, Schinzari G, Giuliante F, D'Argento E, Trigila N, Astone A, Pozzo C. Final analysis of colorectal cancer patients treated with irinotecan and 5-fluorouracil plus folinic acid neoadjuvant chemotherapy for unresectable liver metastases. Br J Cancer. 2007;97:1035–9. https://doi.org/10.1038/sj.bjc.6603988.

157. Rodrigues R (2015) Ordem de infusão de medicamentos antineoplásicos – sistematização de informações para auxiliar a discussão e criação de protocolos assistenciais. Atheneu. São Paulo. Brazil.
158. BC Cancer (2021) BC Cancer Protocol Summary for Palliative Combination Chemotherapy for Metastatic Colorectal Cancer using Irinotecan and Capecitabine in Patients Unsuitable for GIFOLFIRI. BC Cancer. British Columbia. Available in: http://www.bccancer.bc.ca/chemotherapy-protocols-site/Documents/Gastrointestinal/GICAPIRI_Protocol.pdf. Accessed Aug 18 2021.
159. Cao S, Durrani FA, Rustum YM. Synergistic antitumor activity of capecitabine in combination with irinotecan. Clin Colorectal Cancer. 2005;4(5):336–43. https://doi.org/10.3816/ccc.2005.n.007.
160. Goel S, Desai K, Karri S, Gollamudi R, Chaudhary I, Bulgaru A, Kaubisch A, Goldberg G, Einstein M, Camacho F, Baker S, Mani S. Pharmacokinetic and safety study of weekly irinotecan and oral capecitabine in patients with advanced solid cancers. Investig New Drugs. 2007;25(3):237–45. https://doi.org/10.1007/s10637-006-9028-1.
161. Czejka M, Schueller J, Hauer K, Ostermann E. Pharmacokinetics and metabolism of irinotecan combined with capecitabine in patients with advanced colorectal cancer. Anticancer Res. 2005;25(4):2985–90.
162. Tewes M, Schleucher N, Achterrath W, Wilke HJ, Frings S, Seeber S, Harstrick A, Rustum YM, Vanhoefer U. Capecitabine and irinotecan as first-line chemotherapy in patients with metastatic colorectal cancer: results of an extended phase I study†. Ann Oncol. 2003;14(9):1442–8. https://doi.org/10.1093/annonc/mdg376.
163. NHS (2020) Chemotherapy Protocol. Colorectal cancer. Capecitabine and irinotecan (XELIRI). NHS. University Hospital Southampton. NHS Foundation Trust. England. Available in: https://www.uhs.nhs.uk/Media/SUHTExtranet/Services/Chemotherapy-SOPs/Colorectal/Capecitabine-Irinotecan.pdf. Accessed Aug 18 2021.
164. Moehler M, Sprinzl MF, Abdelfattah M, Schimanski CC, Adami B, Godderz W, Majer K, Flieger D, Teufel A, Siebler J, Hoehler T, Galle PR, Kanzler S. Capecitabine and irinotecan with and without bevacizumab for advanced colorectal cancer patients. World J Gastroenterol. 2009;15(4):449–56. https://doi.org/10.3748/wjg.15.449.
165. Schmiegel W, Reinacher-Schick A, Arnold D, Kubicka S, Freier W, Dietrich G, Geißler M, Hegewisch-Becker S, Tannapfel A, Pohl M, Hinke A, Schmoll HJ, Graeven U. Capecitabine/irinotecan or capecitabine/oxaliplatin in combination with bevacizumab is effective and safe as first-line therapy for metastatic colorectal cancer: a randomized phase II study of the AIO colorectal study group. Ann Oncol. 2013;24(6):1580–7. https://doi.org/10.1093/annonc/mdt028.
166. NCT00717990 (2015) Irinotecan, Capecitabine and Avastin for Metastatic Colorectal Cancer as Salvage Treatment. Clinical Trials. Available in: https://clinicaltrials.gov/ct2/show/NCT00717990. Accessed Aug 19 2021.
167. NCT00875771 (2017) Irinotecan, Capecitabine and Bevacizumab in Metastatic Colorectal Cancer Patients (AVAXIRI). Clinical Trials. Available in: https://clinicaltrials.gov/ct2/show/NCT00875771. Accessed Aug 19 2021.
168. NCT00483834 (2019) A Phase II Study of Bevacizumab, Irinotecan and Capecitabine in Patients With Previously Untreated Metastatic Colorectal Cancer. Clinical Trials. Available in: https://clinicaltrials.gov/ct2/show/NCT00483834. Accessed Aug 19 2021.
169. Tsiros D, Sheehy CE, Nugent MA. Heparin-avastin complexes show enhanced VEGF binding and inhibition of VEGF-mediated cell migration. Int J Transl Med. 2021;10:101–15. https://doi.org/10.3390/ijtm1020008.
170. Behourah Z, Bousahba A, Djellali L. Capecitabine, irinotecan, and bevacizumab in patients with previously untreated metastatic colorectal cancer: experience of the oncology department of the university hospital of Oran, Algeria. Ann Oncol. 2018;29(Supplement 5):V70. https://doi.org/10.1093/annonc/mdy151.249.

171. García-Alfonso P, Muñoz-Martin AJ, Alvarez-Suarez S, Jerez-Gilarranz Y, Riesco-Martinez M, Khosravi P, Martin M. Bevacizumab in combination with biweekly capecitabine and irinotecan, as first-line treatment for patients with metastatic colorectal cancer. Br J Cancer. 2010;103:1524–8. https://doi.org/10.1038/sj.bjc.6605907.

172. Garcia-Alfonso P, Chaves M, Muñoz A, Salud A, García-Gonzalez M, Grávalos C, Massuti B, González-Flores E, Queralt B, López-Ladrón A, Losa F, Gómez MJ, Oltra A, Aranda E. Capecitabine and irinotecan with bevacizumab 2-weekly for metastatic colorectal cancer: the phase II AVAXIRI study. BMC Cancer. 2015;15:327. https://doi.org/10.1186/s12885-015-1293-y.

173. Denlinger CS, Blanchard R, Xu L, Bernaards C, Litwin S, Spittle C, Berg DJ, McLaughlin S, Redlinger M, Dorr A, Hambleton J, Holden S, Kearns A, Kenkare-Mitra S, Lum B, Meropol NJ, O'Dwyer PJ. Pharmacokinetic analysis of irinotecan plus bevacizumab in patients with advanced solid tumors. Cancer Chemother Pharmacol. 2009;65(1):97–105. https://doi.org/10.1007/s00280-009-1008-7.

174. NHS (2014a) Chemotherapy Protocol. Colorectal cancer. Bevacizumab-irinotecan. NHS. University Hospital Southampton. NHS Foundation Trust. England. Available in: https://www.uhs.nhs.uk/Media/SUHTExtranet/Services/Chemotherapy-SOPs/Colorectal/Bevacizumab-IrinotecanVer11.pdf. Accessed Aug 19 2021.

175. BC Cancer (2021b) BC Cancer Protocol Summary for Palliative Combination Chemotherapy for Metastatic Colorectal Cancer using Irinotecan, Bevacizumab and Capecitabine. BC Cancer. British Columbia. Available in: http://www.bccancer.bc.ca/chemotherapy-protocols-site/Documents/Gastrointestinal/GICIRB_Protocol.pdf. Accessed Aug 19 2021.

176. NCT00159432 (2014) Study of Oxaliplatin, Capecitabine and Bevacizumab as First Line Treatment for Patients With Advanced Colorectal Cancer. Clinical Trials. Available in: https://clinicaltrials.gov/ct2/show/NCT00159432. Accessed Aug 19 2021.

177. Garrett MJ, Waddell JA, Solimando DA Jr. Capecitabine, oxaliplatin, and bevacizumab (BCaoOx) regimen for metastatic colorectal cancer. Hosp Pharm. 2017;52(5):341–7. https://doi.org/10.1177/0018578717715353.

178. Gruenberger B, Tamandl D, Schueller J, Scheithauer W, Zielinski C, Herbst F, Gruenberger T. Bevacizumab, Capecitabine, and Oxaliplatin as neoadjuvant therapy for patients with potentially curable metastatic colorectal cancer. J Clin Oncol. 2008;26(11):1830–5. https://doi.org/10.1200/JCO.2007.13.7679.

179. Feliu J, Salud A, Safont MJ, García-Girón C, Aparicio J, Vera R, Serra O, Casado E, Jorge M, Escudero P, Bosch C, Bohn U, Pérez-Carrión R, Carmona A, Martínez-Marín V, Maurel J. First-line bevacizumab and capecitabine–oxaliplatin in elderly patients with mCRC: GEMCAD phase II BECOX study. Br J Cancer. 2014;111:241–8. https://doi.org/10.1038/bjc.2014.346.

180. Munemoto Y, Kanda M, Ishibashi K, Hata T, Kobayashi M, Hasegawa J, Fukunaga M, Takagane A, Otsuji T, Miyake Y, Nagase M, Sakamoto J, Matsuoka M, Oba K, Mishima H. Capecitabine and oxaliplatin combined with bevacizumab are feasible for treating selected Japanese patients at least 75 years of age with metastatic colorectal cancer. BMC Cancer. 2015;15:786. https://doi.org/10.1186/s12885-015-1712-0.

181. NHS (2020) Chemotherapy Protocol. Colorectal cancer. Bevacizumab-capecitabine-oxaliplatin. NHS. University Hospital Southampton. NHS Foundation Trust. England. Available in: https://www.uhs.nhs.uk/Media/SUHTExtranet/Services/Chemotherapy-SOPs/Colorectal/Bevacizumab-Capecitabine-Oxaliplatin.pdf. Accessed Aug 19 2021.

182. BC Cancer (2021) BC Cancer Protocol Summary for Palliative Combination Chemotherapy for Metastatic Colorectal Cancer using Oxaliplatin, Bevacizumab and Capecitabine. BC Cancer. British Columbia. Available in: http://www.bccancer.bc.ca/chemotherapy-protocols-site/Documents/Gastrointestinal/GICOXB_Protocol.pdf. Accessed Aug 19 2021.

183. Hurwitz H, Fehrenbacher L, Novotny W, Cartweight T, Hainsworth J, Heim W, Berlin J, Baron A, Griffing S, Holmgren E, Ferrara N, Fyfe G, Rogers B, Ross R, Kabbinavar

F. Bevacizumab plus irinotecan, fluorouracil, and leucovorin for metastatic colorectal cancer. N Engl J Med. 2004;350:2335–42. https://doi.org/10.1056/NEJMoa032691.

184. NCT01183494 (2019) A Genotype-guided Study of Irinotecan Administered in Combination With 5-fluorouracil/Leucovorin (FOLFIRI) and Bevacizumab in Advanced Colorectal Cancer Patients. Clinical Trials. Available in: https://clinicaltrials.gov/ct2/show/NCT01183494. Accessed Aug 19 2021.

185. Deng T, Zhang L, Liu XJ, Xu JM, Bai YX, Wang Y, Han Y, Li YH, Ba Y. Bevacizumab plus irinotecan, 5-fluorouracil, and leucovorin (FOLFIRI) as the second-line therapy for patients with metastatic colorectal cancer, a multicenter study. Med Oncol. 2013;30(4):752. https://doi.org/10.1007/s12032-013-0752-z.

186. Moriwaki T, Bando H, Takashima A, Yamazaki K, Esaki T, Yamashita K, Fukunaga M, Miyake Y, Katsumata K, Kato S, Satoh T, Ozeki M, Baba E, Yoshida S, Boku N, Hyodo I. Bevacizumab in combination with irinotecan, 5-fluorouracil, and leucovorin (FOLFIRI) in patients with metastatic colorectal cancer who were previously treated with oxaliplatin-containing regimens: a multicenter observational cohort study (TCTG 2nd-BV study). Med Oncol. 2012;29(4):2842–8. https://doi.org/10.1007/s12032-011-0151-2.

187. Fyfe GA, Hurwitz H, Fehrenbacher L, Cartwright T, Hainsworth J, Heim W, Berlin J, Kabbinavar F, Holmgren E, Novotny W. Bevacizumab plus irinotecan/5-FU/leucovorin for treatment of metastatic colorectal cancer results in survival benefit in all pre-specified patient subgroups. J Clin Oncol. 2004;22(14):3617. https://doi.org/10.1200/jco.2004.22.90140.3617.

188. Sobrero A, Ackland S, Clarke S, Perez-Carrión R, Chiara S, Gapski J, Mainwaring P, Langer B, Young S. Phase IV study of bevacizumab in combination with Infusional fluorouracil, Leucovorin and irinotecan (FOLFIRI) in first-line metastatic colorectal cancer. Oncology. 2009;77:113–9. https://doi.org/10.1159/000229787.

189. NHS (2020) Chemotherapy Protocol. Colorectal cancer. Bevacizumab-fluorouracil-folinic acid (modified de gramont)-irinotecan. NHS. University Hospital Southampton. NHS Foundation Trust. England. Available in: https://www.uhs.nhs.uk/Media/SUHTExtranet/Services/Chemotherapy-SOPs/Colorectal/Bevacizumab-Fluorouracil-FolinicAcid-Irinotecan.pdf. Accessed Aug 19 2021.

190. Cartenì G, Fiorentino R, Vecchione L, Chiurazzi B, Battista C. Panitumumab a nove drug in cancer treatment. Ann Oncol. 2007;18(Supplement 6):vi16–21. https://doi.org/10.1093/annonc/mdm218.

191. Vieira FMAC, Sena VOD. Câncer colorretal metastático: papel atual dos anticorpos monoclonais e a individualização de seu uso. ABCD Arquivos Brasileiros de Cirurgia Digestiva (São Paulo). 2009;22(1):45–9. https://doi.org/10.1590/S0102-67202009000100010.

192. Françoso A, Simioni PU. Immunotherapy for the treatment of colorectal tumors: focus on approved and in-clinical-trial monoclonal antibodies. Drug Des Devel Ther. 2017;11:177–84. https://doi.org/10.2147/DDDT.S119036.

193. Silvinato A, Pedreira IS, Reis JCB, Marcondes JGZ, Bernardo WM. Metastatic colorectal cancer: treatment with panitumumab. Rev Assoc Med Bras. 2018;64(7):568–74. https://doi.org/10.1590/1806-9282.64.07.568.

194. NCT00508404 (2019) Panitumumab Plus FOLFIRI in First-line Treatment of Metastatic Colorectal Cancer. Clinical Trials. Available in: https://clinicaltrials.gov/ct2/show/NCT00508404. Accessed Aug 20 2021.

195. Berlin J, Posey J, Tchekmedyian S, Hu E, Chan D, Malik I, Yang L, Amado RG, Hecht JR. Panitumumab with irinotecan/leucovorin/5-fluorouracil for first-line treatment of metastatic colorectal cancer. Clin Colorectal Cancer. 2007;6(6):427–32. https://doi.org/10.3816/CCC.2007.n.011.

196. Berlin J, Posey J, Tchekmedyian S, Hu E, Chan D, Malik I, Yang L, Amado RG, Hecht JR. Panitumumab with irinotecan/leucovorin/5-fluorouracil for first-line treatment of metastatic colorectal cancer. Clin Colorectal Cancer. 2009;8:9–14. https://doi.org/10.1016/S1533-0028(11)70550-3.

197. Kohne CH, Hofheinz R, Mineur L, Letocha H, Greil R, Thaler J, Fernebro E, Gamelin E, Decosta L, Karthaus M. First-line panitumumab plus irinotecan/5-fluorouracil/leucovorin treatment in patients with metastatic colorectal cancer. J Cancer Res Clin Oncol. 2012;138(1):65–72. https://doi.org/10.1007/s00432-011-1061-6.

198. Pietrantonio F, Morano F, Corallo S, Miceli R, Lonardi S, Raimondi A, Cremolini C, Rimassa L, Bergamo F, Sartore-Bianchi A, Tampellini M, Racca P, Clavarezza M, Berenato R, Caporale M, Antista M, Niger M, Smiroldo V, Murialdo R, Zaniboni A, Adamo V, Tomasello G, Giordano M, Petrelli F, Longarini R, Cinieri S, Falcone A, Zagonel V, Bartolomeo MD, Braud F. Maintenance therapy with Panitumumab alone vs Panitumumab plus fluorouracil-Leucovorin in patients with RAS wild-type metastatic colorectal cancer - a phase 2 randomized clinical trial. JAMA Oncol. 2019;5(9):1268–75. https://doi.org/10.1001/jamaoncol.2019.1467.

199. Peeters M, Price TJ, Cervantes A, Sobrero AF, Ducreux M, Hotko Y, André T, Chan E, Lordick F, Punt CJA, Strickland AH, Wilson G, Ciuleanu TE, Roman L, van Cutsem E, Tian Y, Sidhu R. Final results from a randomized phase 3 study of FOLFIRI ± panitumumab for second-line treatment of metastatic colorectal cancer. Ann Oncol. 2014;25(1):107–16. https://doi.org/10.1093/annonc/mdt523.

200. NHS (2020j) Chemotherapy Protocol. Colorectal cancer. Fluorouracil, folinic acid (modified de gramont), irinotecan and panitumumab (FOLFIRI-Panitumumab). NHS. University Hospital Southampton. NHS Foundation Trust. England. Available in: uhs.nhs.uk/Media/SUHTExtranet/Services/Chemotherapy-SOPs/Colorectal/Fluorouracil-Folinic-acidMdG-Irinotecan-Panitumumab.pdf. Accessed Aug 20 2021.

201. Lièvre A, Samalin E, Mitry E, Assenat E, Boyer-Gestin C, Lepère C, Bachet JB, Portales F, Vaillant JN, Ychou M, Rougier P. Bevacizumab plus FOLFIRI or FOLFOX in chemotherapy-refractory patients with metastatic colorectal cancer: a retrospective study. BMC Cancer. 2009;9:347. https://doi.org/10.1186/1471-2407-9-347.

202. NCT00062426 (2013) Oxaliplatin and Bevacizumab (Avastin™) With Either Fluorouracil and Leucovorin or Capecitabine in Treating Patients With Advanced Colorectal Cancer. Clinical Trials. Available in: https://clinicaltrials.gov/ct2/show/NCT00062426. Accessed Aug 20 2021.

203. Buchler T, Pavlik T, Melichar B, Bortlicek Z, Usiakova Z, Dusek L, Kiss I, Kohoutek M, Benesova V, Vyzula R, Abrahamova J, Obermannova R. Bevacizumab with 5-fluorouracil, leucovorin, and oxaliplatin versus bevacizumab with capecitabine and oxaliplatin for metastatic colorectal carcinoma: results of a large registry-based cohort analysis. BMC Cancer. 2014;14:323. https://doi.org/10.1186/1471-2407-14-323.

204. Giantonio BJ, Catalano PJ, Meropol NJ, O'Dwyer PJ, Mitchell EP, Alberts SR, Schwartz MA, Benson AB. Bevacizumab in combination with Oxaliplatin, fluorouracil, and Leucovorin (FOLFOX4) for previously treated metastatic colorectal cancer: results from the eastern cooperative oncology group study E3200. J Clin Oncol. 2007;25(12):1539–44. https://doi.org/10.1200/JCO.2006.09.6305.

205. Emmanouilides C, Sfakiotaki G, Androulakis N, Kalbakis K, Christophylakis C, Kalykaki A, Vamvakas L, Kotsakis A, Agelaki S, Diamandidou E, Touroutoglou N, Chatzidakis A, Georgoulias V, Mavroudis D, Souglakos J. Front-line bevacizumab in combination with oxaliplatin, leucovorin and 5-fluorouracil (FOLFOX) in patients with metastatic colorectal cancer: a multicenter phase II study. BMC Cancer. 2007;7:91. https://doi.org/10.1186/1471-2407-7-91.

206. Ranieri G, Laface C, Laforgia M, Summa SD, Porcelli M, Macina F, Ammendola M, Molinari P, Lautetta G, Palo AD, Rubini G, Ferrari C, Gadaleta CD. Bevacizumab plus FOLFOX-4 combined with deep electro-hyperthermia as first-line therapy in metastatic colon cancer: a pilot study. Front Oncol. 2020;10:590707. https://doi.org/10.3389/fonc.2020.590707.

207. NHS (2020) Chemotherapy Protocol. Colorectal cancer. Bevacizumab-fluorouracil-folinic acid (modified de gramont)-oxaliplatin. NHS. University Hospital Southampton. NHS

Foundation Trust. England. Available in: https://www.uhs.nhs.uk/Media/SUHTExtranet/Services/Chemotherapy-SOPs/Colorectal/Bevacizumab-Fluorouracil-FolinicAcid-Oxaliplatin.pdf. Accessed Aug 20 2021.

208. Douillard JY, Oliner KS, Siena S, Tabernero J, Burkes R, Barugel M, Humblet Y, Bodoky G, Cunningham D, Jassem J, Rivera F, Kocákova I, Ruff P, Błasińska-Morawiec M, Šmakal M, Canon JL, Rother M, Williams R, Rong A, Wiezorek J, Sidhu R, Patterson SD. Panitumumab-FOLFOX4 treatment and RAS mutations in colorectal cancer. N Engl J Med. 2013;369:1023–34. https://doi.org/10.1056/NEJMoa1305275.

209. Lonardi S, Schirripa M, Buggin F, Antonuzzo L, Merelli B, Boscolo G, Cinieri S, Donato SD, Lobefaro R, Moretto R, Formica V, Passardi A, Ricci V, Pella N, Scartozzi M, Zustovich F, Zagonel V, Fassan M, Boni L, Loupakis F, Grouo G. First-line FOLFOX plus panitumumab versus 5FU plus panitumumab in RAS-BRAF wild-type metastatic colorectal cancer elderly patients: the PANDA study. J Clin Oncol. 2020;38(15_suppl):4002. https://doi.org/10.1200/JCO.2020.38.15_suppl.4002.

210. NHS (2020l) Chemotherapy Protocol. Colorectal cancer. Fluorouracil, folinic acid (modified de gramont), oxaliplatin and panitumumab (FOLFOX-Panitumumab). NHS. University Hospital Southampton. NHS Foundation Trust. England. Available in: https://www.uhs.nhs.uk/Media/SUHTExtranet/Services/Chemotherapy-SOPs/Colorectal/Fluorouracil-FolinicAcidMdG-Oxaliplatin-Panitumumab.pdf. Accessed Aug 20 2021.

211. Gallo A, Cha C. Updates on esophageal and gastric cancers. World J Gastroenterol. 2006;12(20):3237–42. https://doi.org/10.3748/wjg.v12.i20.3237.

212. Hajmanoochehri F, Mohammadi N, Nasirian N, Hosseinkhani M. Patho-epidemiological features of esophageal and gastric cancers in an endemic region: a 20-year retrospective study. Asian Pac J Cancer Prev. 2013;14(6):3491–7. https://doi.org/10.7314/apjcp.2013.14.6.3491.

213. Henry MACA, Lerco MM, Ribeiro PW, Rodrigues MAM. Epidemiological features of esophageal cancer. Squamous cell carcinoma versus adenocarcinoma. Acta Cir Bras. 2014;29(1):877–81. https://doi.org/10.1590/S0102-86502014000600007.

214. Abbas G, Krasna M. Overview of esophageal cancer. Ann Cardiothorac Surg. 2017;6(2):131–6. https://doi.org/10.21037/acs.2017.03.03.

215. Hao J, Liu B, Yang CS, Chen X. Gastroesophageal reflux leads to esophageal cancer in a surgical model with mice. BMC Gastroenterol. 2009;9:59. https://doi.org/10.1186/1471-230X-59.

216. Sánchez-Danés A, Blanpain C. Deciphering the cells of origin of squamous cell carcinomas. Nat Rev Cancer. 2018;18(9):549–61. https://doi.org/10.1038/s41568-018-0024-5.

217. Soliman SA, Madkour FA. Developmental events and cellular changes occurred during esophageal development of quail embryos. Sci Rep. 2021;11:7257. https://doi.org/10.1038/s41598-021-86503-9.

218. DeMeester SR, DeMeester TR. Columnar mucosa and intestinal metaplasia of the esophagus. Ann Surg. 2000;231(3):303–21. https://doi.org/10.1097/00000658-200003000-00003.

219. Szachnowicz S, Cecconello I, Iriya K, Marson AG, Takeda FR, Gama-Rodrigues JJ. Origin of adenocarcinoma in Barrett's esophagus: P53 and Ki67 expression and histopathologic background. Clinics. 2005;60(2):103–12. https://doi.org/10.1590/S1807-59322005000200005.

220. Dietz J, Silva SC, Meurer L, Sekine S, Souza AR, Meine GC. Short segment Berrett's esophagus and distal gastric intestinal metaplasia. Arq Gastroenterol. 2006;43(2):117–20. https://doi.org/10.1590/S0004-28032006000200011.

221. Naini BV, Souza RF, Odze RD. Barrett's esophagus: a comprehensive and contemporary review for pathologists. Am J Surg Pathol. 2016;40(5):e45–66. https://doi.org/10.1097/PAS.0000000000000598.

222. Tercioti-Junior V, Lopes LR, Coelho-Neto JS. Adenocarcinoma versus carcinoma epidermóide: análise de 306 pacientes em hospital universitário. ABCD Arquivos Brasileiros de Cirugia Digestiva. 2011;24(4):272–6.

223. Kuwano H, Sadanaga N, Watanabe M, Yasuda M, Nozoe T, Sugimachi K. Esophageal squamous cell carcinoma occurring in the surface epithelium over a benign tumor. J Surg Oncol. 1995;59(4):268–72. https://doi.org/10.1002/jso.2930590414.

224. Shaheen O, Ghibour A, Alsaid B. Esophageal cancer metastases to unexpected sites: a systematic review. Gastroenterol Res Pract. 2017;2017:1657310. https://doi. org/10.1155/2017/1657310.

225. Tamura H, Saiki H, Amano T, Yamamoto M, Hayashi S, Ando H, Doi R, Nishida T, Yamamoto K, Adachi S. Esophageal carcinoma originating in the surface epithelium with immunohistochemically proven esophageal gland duct differentiation: a case report. World J Gastroenterol. 2017;23(21):3928–33. https://doi.org/10.3748/wjg.v23.i21.3928.

226. Layke JC, Lopez PP. Gastric cancer: diagnosis and treatment options. Am Fam Physician. 2004;69(5):1133–41.

227. Hu B, Haji NE, Sittler S, Lammert N, Barnes R, Meloni-Ehrig A. Gastric cancer: classification, histology and application of molecular pathology. J Gastrointest Oncol. 2012;3(3):251–61. https://doi.org/10.3978/j.issn.2078-6891.2012.021.

228. Nagini S. Carcinoma of the stomach: a review of epidemiology, pathogenesis, molecular genetics and chemoprevention. World J Gastrointest Oncol. 2012;4(7):156–69. https://doi. org/10.4251/wjgo.v4.i7.156.

229. Virmani V, Khandelwal A, Sethi V, Fraser-Hill M, Fasih N, Kielar A. Neoplastic stomach lesions and their mimickers: spectrum of imaging manifestations. Cancer Imaging. 2012;12(1):269–78. https://doi.org/10.1102/1470-7330.2012.0031.

230. Riva S, Muñoz-Navas M, Sola JJ. Gastric carcinogenesis. Rev Esp Enferm Dig. 2003;96(4):265–76.

231. Kuipers EJ. Proton pump inhibitors and gastric neoplasia. Gut. 2006;55(9):1217–21. https:// doi.org/10.1136/gut.2005.090514.

232. Banks M, Graham D, Jansen M, Gotoda T, Coda S, Pietro M, Uedo N, Bhandari P, Pritchard DM, Kuipers EJ, Rodriguez-Justo M, Novelli MR, Ragunath K, Shepherd N, Dinis-Ribeiro M. British Society of Gastroenterology guidelines on the diagnosis and management of patients at risk of gastric adenocarcinoma. Gut. 2019;68:1545–75. https://doi.org/10.1136/ gutjnl-2018-318126.

233. Cheung KS, Leung WK. Long-term use of proton-pump inhibitors and risk of gastric cancer: a review of the current evidence. Ther Adv Gastroenterol. 2019;12:1756284819834511. https://doi.org/10.1177/1756284819834511.

234. Jeong CY, Kim N, Lee HS, Yoon H, Shin CM, Park YS, Kim JW, Lee DH. Risk factors of multiple gastric polyps according to the histologic classification: prospective observational cohort study. Korean J Gastroenterol. 2019;74(1):17–29. https://doi.org/10.4166/ kjg.2019.74.1.17.

235. Ilson DH. Esophageal cancer chemotherapy: recent advances. Gastrointest Cancer Res. 2008;2(2):85–92.

236. Tai P, Yu E. Esophageal cancer management controversies: radiation oncology point of view. World J Gastrointest Oncol. 2014;6(8):263–74. https://doi.org/10.4251/wjgo.v6.i8.263.

237. Deng HY, Wang WP, Wang YC, Hu WP, Ni PZ, Lin YD, Chen LQ. Neoadjuvant chemoradiotherapy or chemotherapy? A comprehensive systematic review and meta-analysis of the options for neoadjuvant therapy for treating oesophageal cancer. Eur J Cardiothorac Surg. 2017;51(3):421–31. https://doi.org/10.1093/ejcts/ezw315.

238. Ramos MFKP, Pereira MA, Charruf AZ, Dias AR, Castria TB, Barchi LC, Ribeiro-Júnior U, Zilberstein B, Cecconello I. Conversion therapy for gastric cancer: expanding the treatment possibilities. ABCD Arquivos Brasileiros de Cirurgia Digestiva. 2019;32(2):e1435.

239. Yang YM, Hong P, Xu WW, He QY, Li B. Advances in targeted therapy for esophageal cancer. Signal Transduct Target Ther. 2020;5:229. https://doi.org/10.1038/s41392-020-00323-3.

240. Okines AFC, Cunningham D. Trastuzumab: a novel standard option for patients with HER-2-positive advanced gastric or gastro-oesophageal junction cancer. Ther Adv Gastroenterol. 2012;5(5):301–18. https://doi.org/10.1177/1756283X12450246.

241. Park SC, Chun HJ. Chemotherapy for advanced gastric cancer: review and update of current practices. Gut Liver. 2013;7(4):385–93. https://doi.org/10.5009/gnl.2013.7.4.385.

242. Ford H, Gounaris I. Docetaxel and its potential in the treatment of refractory esophagogastric adenocarcinoma. Ther Adv Gastroenterol. 2015;8(4):189–205. https://doi.org/10.117 7/1756283X15585468.

243. Ilhan-Mutlu A, Taghizadeh H, Beer A, Dolak W, Ba-Ssalamah A, Schoppmann SF, Hejna M, Birner P, Preusser M. Correlation of trastuzumab-based treatment with clinical characteristics and prognosis in HER2-positive gastric and gastroesophageal junction cancer: a retrospective single center analysis. Cancer Biol Ther. 2018;19(3):169–74. https://doi.org/10.108 0/15384047.2017.1414759.

244. Woll E, Eisterer W, Gerger A, Kuhr T, Prager GW, Rumpold H, Ulrich-Pur H, Vogl U, Winder T, Weiss L, Greil R. Treatment algorithm for patients with gastric adenocarcinoma: an Austrian consensus on systemic therapy. Anticancer Res. 2019;39(9):4589–96. https://doi.org/10.21873/anticanres.13638.

245. Al-Batran SE, Hartmann JT, Probst S, Schmalenberg H, Hollerbach S, Hofheinz R, Rethwisch V, Seipelt G, Homann N, Wilhelm G, Schuch G, Stoehlmacher J, Derigs HG, Hegewisch-Becker S, Grossmann J, Pauligk C, Atmaca A, Bokemeyer C, Knuth A, Jager E. Phase III trial in metastatic gastroesophageal adenocarcinoma with fluorouracil, Leucovorin plus either Oxaliplatin or cisplatin: a study of the Arbeitsgemeinschaft Internistische Onkologie. J Clin Oncol. 2008;26(9):1435–42. https://doi.org/10.1200/JCO.2007.13.9378.

246. Qin TJ, An GL, Zhao XH, Tian F, Li XH, Lian JW, Pan BR, Gu SZ. Combined treatment of oxaliplatin and capecitabine in patients with metastatic esophageal squamous cell cancer. World J Gastroenterol. 2009;15(7):871–6. https://doi.org/10.3748/wjg.15.871.

247. Guimbaud R, Louvet C, Ries P, Ychou M, Maillard E, André T, Gornet JM, Aparicio T, Nguyen S, Azzedine A, Etienne PL, Boucher E, Rebischung C, Hammel P, Rougier P, Bedenne L, Bouché O. Prospective, randomized, multicenter, phase III study of fluorouracil, Leucovorin, and irinotecan versus Epirubicin, cisplatin, and Capecitabine in advanced gastric adenocarcinoma: a French intergroup (Fédération francophone de Cancérologie digestive, Fédération Nationale des Centres de Lutte Contre le cancer, and Groupe Coopérateur Multidisciplinaire en Oncologie) study. J Clin Oncol. 2014;32(31):3520–6. https://doi.org/10.1200/JCO.2013.54.1011.

248. Yoshii T, Hara H, Asayama M, Kumekawa Y, Miyazawa S, Takahashi N, Matsushima T, Shimizu S, Saito Y. Chemoradiotherapy with FOLFOX for esophageal squamous cell cancer with synchronous rectal cancer: four case reports and a literature review. Mol Clin Oncol. 2020;12(1):23–30. https://doi.org/10.3892/mco.2019.1945.

249. Janjigian YY, Werner D, Pauligk C, Steinmetz K, Kelsen DP, Jager E, Altmannsberger HM, Robinson E, Tafe LJ, Tang LH, Shah MA, Al-Batran SE. Prognosis of metastatic gastric and gastroesophageal junction cancer by HER2 status: a European and USA international collaborative analysis. Ann Oncol. 2012;23(10):2656–62. https://doi.org/10.1093/annonc/mds104.

250. Kim JW, Im SA, Kim M, Cha Y, Lee KH, Keam B, Kim MA, Han SW, Oh DY, Kim TY, Kim WH, Bang YJ. The prognostic significance of HER2 positivity for advanced gastric cancer patients undergoing first-line modified FOLFOX-6 regimen. Anticancer Res. 2012;32(4):1547–53.

251. Aguiar Junior PN, Artigiani Neto R, Forones NM. HER2 expression as a prognostic fator in metastatic gastric cancer. Arq Gastroenterol. 2016;53(2):62–7. https://doi.org/10.1590/S0004-28032016000200003.

252. Zhao D, Klempner SJ, Chao J. Progress and challenges in HER2-positive gastroesophageal adenocarcinoma. J Hematol Oncol. 2019;12:50. https://doi.org/10.1186/s13045-019-0737-2.

253. Press MF, Ellis CE, Gagnon RC, Grob TJ, Buyse M, Villalobos I, Liang Z, Wu S, Bang YJ, Qin SK, Chung HC, Xu J, Park JO, Jeziorski K, Afenjar K, Ma Y, Estrada MC, Robinson DM, Scherer SJ, Sauter G, Hecht JR, Slamon DJ. HER2 status in advanced or metastatic gastric, esophageal, or gastroesophageal adenocarcinoma for entry to the TRIO-013/LOGiC trial of Lapatinib. Mol Cancer Ther. 2017;16(1):228–38. https://doi.org/10.1158/1535-7163.MCT-15-0887.

254. Hackshaw MD, Bui CL, Ladner A, Tu N, Islam Z, Ritchey ME, Salas M. Review of survival, safety, and clinical outcomes in HER2+ metastatic gastric cancer following the administration of trastuzumab post-Trastuzumab gastric cancer. Cancer Treat Res Commun. 2020;24:100189. https://doi.org/10.1016/j.ctarc.2020.100189.

255. Soularue E, Cohen R, Tournigand C, Zaanan A, Louvet C, Bachet JB, Hentic O, Samalin E, Chibaudell B, Gramont A, André T. Efficacy and safety of trastuzumab in combination with oxaliplatin and fluorouracil-based chemotherapy for patients with HER2-positive metastatic gastric and gastro-oesophageal junction adenocarcinoma patients: a retrospective study. Bull Cancer. 2015;102(4):324–31. https://doi.org/10.1016/j.bulcan.2014.08.001.

256. BC Cancer (2021) BC Cancer Protocol Summary for Palliative Treatment of Metastatic or Locally Advanced Gastric, Gastroesophageal Junction, or Esophageal Adenocarcinoma using Oxaliplatin, Fluorouracil, Leucovorin, and Trastuzumab. BC Cancer. British Columbia. Available in: http://www.bccancer.bc.ca/chemotherapy-protocols-site/Documents/Gastrointestinal/GIGAVFFOXT_Protocol.pdf. Accessed Aug 25 2021.

257. NCT00526110 (2016) Docetaxel, 5-Fluorouracil and Oxaliplatin in Adenocarcinoma of the Stomach or Gastroesophageal Junction Patients. Clinical Trials. Available in: https://www.clinicaltrials.gov/ct2/show/NCT00526110. Accessed Aug 25 2021.

258. Rosenberg AJ, Rademaker A, Hochster HS, Ryan T, Hensing T, Shankaran V, Baddi L, Mahalingam D, Mulcahy MF, Benson AB. Docetaxel, Oxaliplatin, and 5-fluorouracil (DOF) in metastatic and Unresectable gastric/gastroesophageal junction adenocarcinoma: a phase II study with long-term follow-up. Oncologist. 2019;24(8):1039–e642. https://doi.org/10.1634/theoncologist.2019-0330.

259. Wang KS, Ren YX, Ma ZJ, Li F, Cheng XC, Xiao JY, Zhang SZ, Yu ZY, Yang HT, Zhou HN, Li YM, Liu HB, Jiao ZY. Docetaxel, oxaliplatin, leucovorin, and 5-fluorouracil (FLOT) as preoperative and postoperative chemotherapy compared with surgery followed by chemotherapy for patients with locally advanced gastric cancer: a propensity score-based analysis. Cancer Manag Res. 2019;11:3009–20. https://doi.org/10.2147/CMAR.S200883.

260. BC Cancer (2021) BC Cancer Protocol Summary For Perioperative Treatment of Resectable Adenocarcinoma of the Stomach, Gastroesophageal Junction or Lower 1/3 Esophagus using DOCEtaxel, Oxaliplatin, Infusional Fluorouracil, and Leucovorin. BC Cancer. British Columbia. Available in: http://www.bccancer.bc.ca/chemotherapy-protocols-site/Documents/Gastrointestinal/GIGFLODOC_Protocol.pdf. Accessed Aug 25 2021.

261. Pernot S, Mitry E, Samalin E, Dahan L, Dalban C, Ychou M, Seitz JF, Turki H, Mazard T, Zaanan A, Lepère C, Vaillant JN, Landi B, Rougier P, Taieb J. Biweekly docetaxel, fluorouracil, leucovorin, oxaliplatin (TEF) as first-line treatment for advanced gastric cancer and adenocarcinoma of the gastroesophageal junction: safety and efficacy in a multicenter cohort. Gastric Cancer. 2014;17(2):341–7. https://doi.org/10.1007/s10120-013-0266-6.

262. Al-Batran S, Hartmann JT, Hofheinz R, Mahlberg R, Homann N, Probst S, Stoehlmacher J, Fritz M, Rethwisch V, Seipelt G, Jager E. Modified FOLFOX in combination with docetaxel for patients with metastatic adenocarcinoma of the stomach or gastroesophageal junction: a multicenter phase II study of the Arbeitsgemeinschaft Internistische Onkologie (AIO). J Clin Oncol. 2007;25(18_suppl):4545. https://doi.org/10.1200/jco.2007.25.18_suppl.4545.

263. NHS (2020) Chemotherapy Protocol. UPPER Gastrointestinal Cancer. Docetaxel-fluorouracil-folinic acid-oxaliplatin (FLOT). NHS. University Hospital Southampton. NHS Foundation Trust. England. Available in: https://www.uhs.nhs.uk/Media/SUHTExtranet/Services/Chemotherapy-SOPs/Upper-gastro-intestinal/Docetaxel-Fluorouracil-Folinic-Acid-Oxaliplatin-FLOT.pdf. Accessed Aug 25 2021.

264. Berger AC, Farma J, Scott WJ, Freedman G, Weiner L, Cheng JD, Wang H, Goldberg M. Complete response to neoadjuvant Chemoradiotherapy in esophageal carcinoma is associated with significantly improved survival. J Clin Oncol. 2005;23(19):4330–7. https://doi.org/10.1200/JCO.2005.05.017.

265. Platz TA, Nurkin SJ, Fong MK, Groman A, Flaherty L, Malhotra U, LeVea CM, Yendamuri S, Warren GW, Nava HR, May KS. Neoadjuvant chemoradiotherapy for esophageal/gastroesophageal carcinoma. J Gastrointest Oncol. 2013;4(2):137–43. https://doi.org/10.3978/j.issn.2078-6891.2013.007.

266. Tomasello G, Ghidini M, Barni S, Passalacqua R, Petrelli F. Overview of different available chemotherapy regimens combined with radiotherapy for the neoadjuvant and definitive treat-

ment of esophageal cancer. Expert Rev Clin Pharmacol. 2017;10(6):649–60. https://doi.org/1 0.1080/17512433.2017.1313112.

267. Munch S, Pigorsch SU, Devecka M, Dapper H, Feith M, Friess H, Weichert W, Jesinghaus M, Braren R, Combs SE, Habermehl D. Neoadjuvant versus definitive chemoradiation in patients with squamous cell carcinoma of the esophagus. Radiat Oncol. 2019;14:66. https://doi.org/10.1186/s13014-019-1270-8.

268. van Hagen P, Hulshof MCCM, van Lanschot JJB, Steyerberg EW, van Berge Henegouwen MI, Wijnhoven BPL, Richel DJ, Nieuwenhuijzen GAP, Hospers GAP, Bonenkamp JJ, Cuesta MA, Blaisse RJB, Busch ORC, ten Kate FJ, Creemers GJ, Punt CJ, Plukker JT, Verheul HM, Spillenaar Bilgen EJ, van Dekken H, van der Sangen MJ, Rozema T, Biermann K, Beukema JC, Piet AH, van Rij CM, Reinders JG, Tilanus HW, van der Gaast A. Preoperative chemo-radiotherapy for esophageal or junctional cancer. N Engl J Med. 2012;366:2074–84. https://doi.org/10.1056/NEJMoa1112088.

269. Guminski AD, Harnett PR, deFazio A. Carboplatin and paclitaxel interact antagonistically in a megakaryoblast cell line--a potential mechanism for paclitaxel-mediated sparing of carboplatin-induced thrombocytopenia. Cancer Chemother Pharmacol. 2001;48(3):229–34. https://doi.org/10.1007/s002800100279.

270. NHS (2020) Chemotherapy Protocol. Gastrointestinal (UPPER) Cancer. Carboplatin (AUC2)-paclitaxel-radiotherapy. NHS. University Hospital Southampton. NHS Foundation Trust. England. Available in: https://www.uhs.nhs.uk/Media/SUHTExtranet/Services/Chemotherapy-SOPs/Upper-gastro-intestinal/CarboplatinAUC2-Paclitaxel-RT.pdf. Accessed Aug 25 2021.

271. BC Cancer (2021) BC Cancer Protocol Summary for Neoadjuvant Treatment of Esophageal and Gastroesophageal Carcinomas Using CARBOplatin, PACLitaxel and Radiation Therapy. BC Cancer. British Columbia. Available in: http://www.bccancer.bc.ca/chemotherapy--protocols-site/Documents/Gastrointestinal/GIENACTRT_Protocol.pdf. Accessed Aug 25 2021.

272. BC Cancer (2021) BC Cancer Protocol Summary for Palliative Chemotherapy for Upper Gastrointestinal Tract Cancer (Gastric, Esophageal, Gall Bladder, Pancreas Carcinoma and Cholangiocarcinoma) and Metastatic Anal using Infusional Fluorouracil and CISplatin. BC Cancer. British Columbia. Available in: http://www.bccancer.bc.ca/chemotherapy-protocols-site/Documents/Gastrointestinal/GIFUC_Protocol.pdf. Accessed Aug 26 2021.

273. Boulikas T, Vougiouka M. Cisplatin and platinum drugs at the molecular level (review). Oncol Rep. 2003;10(6):1663–82. https://doi.org/10.3892/or.10.6.1663.

274. Sedletska Y, Giraud-Panis MJ, Malinge JM. Cisplatin is a DNA-damaging antitumour compound triggering multifactorial biochemical responses in cancer cells: importance of apoptotic pathways. Curr Med Chem Anticancer Agents. 2005;5(3):251–65. https://doi.org/10.2174/1568011053765967.

275. O'Donnell D, Leahy M, Marples M, Protheroe A, Selby P. Problem solving in oncology. Witney. UK: Evidence-based Networks Ltd.; 2007.

276. Florea AM, Busselberg D. Cisplatin as an anti-tumor drug: cellular mechanisms of activity, drug resistance and induced side effects. Cancers (Basel). 2011;3(1):1351–71. https://doi.org/10.3390/cancers3011351.

277. Farrell NP. Multi-platinum anti-cancer agents. Substitution-inert compounds for tumor selectivity and new targets. Chem Soc Rev. 2012;00:1–3. https://doi.org/10.1039/x0xx00000x.

278. Kreidieh FY, Moukadem HA, El Saghir NS. Overview, prevention and management of chemotherapy extravasation. World J Clin Oncol. 2016;7(1):87–97. https://doi.org/10.5306/wjco.v7.i1.87.

279. Johnston PG, Geoffrey F, Drake J, Voeller D, Grem JL, Allegra CJ. The cellular interaction of 5-fluorouracil and cisplatin in a human colon carcinoma cell line. Eur J Cancer. 1996;32(12):2148–54. https://doi.org/10.1016/S0959-8049(96)00266-3.

280. Harstrick A, Vanhoefer U, Heidemann A, Druyen H, Wilke H, Seeber S. Drug interactions of 5-fluorouracil with either cisplatin or lobaplatin--a new, clinically active platinum ana-

log in established human cancer cell lines. Anti-Cancer Drugs. 1997;8(4):391–5. https://doi.org/10.1097/00001813-199704000-00013.

281. Tang WX, Cheng PY, Luo YP, Wang RX. Interaction between cisplatin, 5-fluorouracil and vincristine on human hepatoma cell line (7721). World J Gastroenterol. 1998;4(5):418–20. https://doi.org/10.3748/wjg.v4.i5.418.

282. Nishiyama M, Yamamoto W, Park JS, Okamoto R, Hanaoka H, Takano H, Saito N, Matsukawa M, Shirasaka T, Kurihara M. Low-dose cisplatin and 5-fluorouracil in combination can repress increased gene expression of cellular resistance determinants to themselves. Clin Cancer Res. 1999;5(9):2620–8.

283. Levard H, Pouliquen X, Hay JM, Fingerhut A, Langlois-Zantain O, Huguier M, Lozach P, Testart J. 5-fluorouracil and cisplatin as palliative treatment of advanced oesophageal squamous cell carcinoma. A multicentre randomised controlled trial. The French associations for surgical research. Eur J Surg. 1998;164(11):849–57. https://doi.org/10.1080/110241598750005273.

284. Steber C, Hughes RT, McTyre ER, Scike M, Farris M, Levine BJ, Pasche B, Levine E, Blackstock AW. Cisplatin/5-fluorouracil (5-FU) versus carboplatin/paclitaxel Chemoradiotherapy as definitive or pre-operative treatment of esophageal cancer. Cureus. 2021;13(1):e12574. https://doi.org/10.7759/cureus.12574.

285. Thomas AL, O'Byrne K, Steward WP. Chemotherapy for upper gastrointestinal tumours. Postgrad Med J. 1999;76:321–7. https://doi.org/10.1136/pmj.76.896.321.

286. NHS (2020) Chemotherapy Protocol. Gastrointestinal (UPPER) Cancer. Cisplatin and fluorouracil. NHS. University Hospital Southampton. NHS Foundation Trust. England. Available in: https://www.uhs.nhs.uk/Media/SUHTExtranet/Services/Chemotherapy-SOPs/Upper-gastro-intestinal/Cisplatin-Fluorouracil.pdf. Accessed Aug 26 2021.

287. Lee J, Lim DH, Kim S, Park SH, Park JO, Park YS, Lim HY, Choi MG, Sohn TS, Noh JH, Bae JM, Ahn YC, Sohn I, Jung SH, Park CK, Kim KM, Kang WK. Phase III trial comparing capecitabine plus cisplatin versus capecitabine plus cisplatin with concurrent capecitabine radiotherapy in completely resected gastric cancer with D2 lymph node dissection: the ARTIST trial. J Clin Oncol. 2012;30(3):268–73. https://doi.org/10.1200/JCO.2011.39.1953.

288. Xiao X, Wang T, Li L, Zhu Z, Zhang W, Cui G, Li W. Co-delivery of cisplatin (IV) and capecitabine as an effective and non-toxic cancer treatment. Front Pharmacol. 2019;10:110. https://doi.org/10.3389/fphar.2019.00110.

289. Kim TW, Kang YK, Ahn JH, Chang HM, Yook JH, Oh ST, Kim BS, Lee JS. Phase II study of capecitabine plus cisplatin as first-line chemotherapy in advanced gastric cancer. Ann Oncol. 2002;13:1893–8. https://doi.org/10.1093/annonc/mdf323.

290. Zhi Y, Lin Z, Ma J, Mou W, Chen X. Distinguish the role of radiotherapy from Chemoradiotherapy for gastric cancer with behavior of metastasis-indolent in lymph node. Technol Cancer Res Treat. 2020;19:1–13. https://doi.org/10.1177/1533033820959400.

291. Kim IH. Current status of adjuvant chemotherapy for gastric cancer. World J Gastrointest Oncol. 2019;11(9):679–85. https://doi.org/10.4251/wjgo.v11.i9.679.

292. Ustaalioglu BBO, Bilici A, Tilki M, Surmelioglu A, Erkol B, Figen M, Uyar S. Capecitabine-cisplatin versus 5-fluorouracil/leucovorin in combination with radiotherapy for adjuvant therapy of lymph node positive locally advanced gastric cancer. J Cancer Res Ther. 2018;14(Supplement):S736–41. https://doi.org/10.4103/0973-1482.183548.

293. NHS (2020p) Chemotherapy Protocol. Gastrointestinal (UPPER) Cancer. Capecitabine-cisplatin (Radiotherapy). NHS. University Hospital Southampton. NHS Foundation Trust. England. Available in: https://www.uhs.nhs.uk/Media/SUHTExtranet/Services/Chemotherapy-SOPs/Upper-gastro-intestinal/Capecitabine-Cisplatin-Radiotherapy.pdf. Accessed Aug 26 2021.

294. Norman G, Rice S, Spackman E, Stirk L, Danso-Appiah A, Suh D, Palmer S, Eastwood A. Trastuzumab for the treatment of HER2-positive metastatic adenocarcinoma of the stomach or gastro-oesophageal junction. Health Technol Assess. 2011;15(Suppl 1):33–42. https://doi.org/10.3310/hta15suppl1/04.

295. Satoh T, Omuro Y, Sasaki Y, Hamamoto Y, Boku N, Tamura T, Ohtsu A. Pharmacokinetic analysis of capecitabine and cisplatin in combination with trastuzumab in Japanese patients with advanced HER2-positive gastric cancer. Cancer Chemother Pharmacol. 2012;69(4):949–55. https://doi.org/10.1007/s00280-011-1783-9.

296. Zhu B, Wu JR, Zhou XP. A retrospective comparison of Trastuzumab plus cisplatin and Trastuzumab plus Capecitabine in elderly HER2-positive advanced gastric cancer patients. Medicine (Baltimore). 2015;94(34):e1428. https://doi.org/10.1097/MD.0000000000001428.

297. NCT01450696 (2016) A Study of Herceptin (Trastuzumab) in Combination With Cisplatin/Capecitabine Chemotherapy in Participants With Human Epidermal Growth Factor Receptor 2 (HER2)-Positive Metastatic Gastric or Gastro-Esophageal Junction Cancer (HELOISE). Clinical Trials. Available in: https://clinicaltrials.gov/ct2/show/NCT01450696. Accessed Aug 26 2021.

298. Bang YJ, van Cutsem E, Feyereislova A, Chung HC, Shen L, Sawaki A, Lordick F, Ohtsu A, Omuro Y, Satoh T, Aprile G, Kulikov E, Hill J, Lehle M, Ruschoff J, Kang YK. Trastuzumab in combination with chemotherapy versus chemotherapy alone for treatment of HER2-positive advanced gastric or gastro-oesophageal junction cancer (ToGA): a phase 3, open-label, randomised controlled trial. Lancet. 2010;376(9742):687–97. https://doi.org/10.1016/S0140-6736(10)61121-X.

299. Davidson M, Starling N. Trastuzumab in the management of gastroesophageal cancer: patient selection and perspectives. Onco Targets Ther. 2016;9:7235–45. https://doi.org/10.2147/OTT.S100643.

300. NHS (2020) Chemotherapy Protocol. Gastrointestinal (UPPER) Cancer. Capecitabine-cisplatin-trastuzumab. NHS. University Hospital Southampton. NHS Foundation Trust. England. Available in: https://www.uhs.nhs.uk/Media/SUHTExtranet/Services/Chemotherapy-SOPs/Upper-gastro-intestinal/Capecitabine-Cisplatin-Trastuzumab.pdf. Accessed Aug 26 2021.

301. Pasini F, Fraccon AP, Manzoni G. The role of chemotherapy in metastatic gastric cancer. Anticancer Res. 2011;31:3543–54.

302. Salati M, Emidio KD, Tarantino V, Cascinu S. Second-line treatments: moving towards an opportunity to improve survival in advanced gastric cancer? ESMO Open. 2017;2(3):e000206. https://doi.org/10.1136/esmoopen-2017-000206.

303. BC Cancer (2021) BC Cancer Summary for Palliative Treatment of Metastatic or Inoperable, Locally Advanced Gastric or Gastroesophageal Junction Adenocarcinoma using CISplatin, Infusional Fluorouracil and Trastuzumab. BC Cancer. British Columbia. Available in: http://www.bccancer.bc.ca/chemotherapy-protocols-site/Documents/Gastrointestinal/GIGAVCFT_Protocol.pdf. Accessed Aug 26 2021.

304. NHS (2020) Chemotherapy Protocol. Gastrointestinal (UPPER) Cancer. Cisplatin-fluorouracil-trastuzumab. NHS. University Hospital Southampton. NHS Foundation Trust. England. Available in: https://www.uhs.nhs.uk/Media/SUHTExtranet/Services/Chemotherapy-SOPs/Upper-gastro-intestinal/Cisplatin-Fluorouracil-Trastuzumab.pdf. Accessed Aug 26 2021.

305. NCT01396707 (2020) Trastuzumab in Combination With Capecitabine and Oxaliplatin(XELOX) in Patients With Advanced Gastric Cancer(AGC): Her+XELOX. Clinical Trials. Available in: https://clinicaltrials.gov/ct2/show/NCT01396707. Accessed Aug 27 2021.

306. BC Cancer (2021) BC Cancer Protocol Summary for Palliative Treatment of Metastatic or Locally Advanced Gastric, Gastroesophageal Junction, or Esophageal Adenocarcinoma using Capecitabine, Oxaliplatin, and Trastuzumab. BC Cancer. British Columbia. Available in: http://www.bccancer.bc.ca/chemotherapy-protocols-site/Documents/Gastrointestinal/GIGAVCOXT_Protocol.pdf. Accessed Aug 27 2021.

307. Hassan MS, Makuru V, von Holzen U. Targeted therapy in esophageal cancer. Dig Med Res. 2021;4:29. https://doi.org/10.21037/dmr-21-16.

308. Ryu MH, Yoo C, Kim JG, Ryoo BY, Park YS, Park SR, Han HS, Chung IJ, Song EK, Lee KH, Kang SY, Kang YK. Multicenter phase II study of trastuzumab in combination with capecitabine and oxaliplatin for advanced gastric cancer. Eur J Cancer. 2015;51(4):482–8. https://doi.org/10.1016/j.ejca.2014.12.015.

309. Harada S, Yanagisawa M, Kaneko S, Yorozu K, Yamamoto K, Moriya Y, Harada N. Superior antitumor activity of trastuzumab combined with capecitabine plus oxaliplatin in a human epidermal growth factor receptor 2-positive human gastric cancer xenograft model. Mol Clin Oncol. 2015;3(5):987–94. https://doi.org/10.3892/mco.2015.609.

310. Gong J, Liu T, Fan Q, Bai L, Bi F, Qin S, Wang J, Xu N, Cheng Y, Bai Y, Liu W, Wang L, Shen L. Optimal regimen of trastuzumab in combination with oxaliplatin/ capecitabine in first-line treatment of HER2-positive advanced gastric cancer (CGOG1001): a multicenter, phase II trial. BMC Cancer. 2016;16:68. https://doi.org/10.1186/s12885-016-2092-9.

311. Rivera F, Izquierdo-Manuel M, García-Alfonso P, Castro EM, Gallego J, Limón ML, Alsina M, López L, Galán M, Falcó E, Manzano JL, González E, Muñoz-Unceta N, López C, Aranda E, Fernández E, Jorge M, Jiménez-Fonseca P. Perioperative trastuzumab, capecitabine and oxaliplatin in patients with HER2-positive resectable gastric or gastro-oesophageal junction adenocarcinoma: NEOHX phase II trial. Eur J Cancer. 2021;145:158–67. https://doi.org/10.1016/j.ejca.2020.12.005.

312. Cancer Institute NSW (2021) Gastric and gastroesophageal metastatic CAPOX (XELOX) (capecitabine and oxaliplatin) and trastuzumab. NSW government. Australia. Available in: https://www.Eviq.Org.Au/medical-oncology/upper-gastrointestinal/gastric-and-oesophageal/3896-gastric-and-gastroesophageal-metastatic-capox#interactions. Accessed Aug 27 2021.

313. Yen CJ, Bai LY, Cheng R, Hsiao F, Orlando M. Ramucirumab in patients with advanced gastric and gastroesophageal junction cancer: learnings from east Asian data. J Cancer Res Pract. 2018;5(2):43–6. https://doi.org/10.1016/j.jcrpr.2018.03.001.

314. NCT04192734 (2021) Retrospective Study of Ramucirumab and Paclitaxel in Gastric or Gastroesophageal Junction Adenocarcinoma. Clinical Trials. Available in: https://clinicaltrials.gov/ct2/show/NCT04192734. Accessed Aug 27 2021.

315. Zang DY, Han HS, Kim BJ, Jee HJ, Suh YJ, An H, Byun JH, Kim DS, Park SH, Rha SY, Oh DY, Kim JG, Bae WK, Kim IH, Sym SJ, Oh SY, Kim HS, Lee KW, Ryu MH. Real-world outcomes of second-line ramucirumab plus paclitaxel in patients with advanced gastric or gastroesophageal junction adenocarcinoma: a nationwide retrospective study in Korea (KCSG-ST19-16). J Clin Oncol. 2021;39(15_suppl):4056. https://doi.org/10.1200/JCO.2021.39.15_suppl.4056.

316. Chiorean EG, Hurwitz HI, Cohen RB, Schwartz JD, Dalal RP, Fox FE, Gao L, Sweeney CJ. Phase I study of every 2- or 3-week dosing of ramucirumab, a human immunoglobulin G1 monoclonal antibody targeting the vascular endothelial growth factor receptor-2 in patients with advanced solid tumors. Ann Oncol. 2015;26(6):1230–7. https://doi.org/10.1093/annonc/mdv144.

317. Young K, Smyth E, Chau I. Ramucirumab for advanced gastric cancer or gastro-oesophageal junction adenocarcinoma. Ther Adv Gastroenterol. 2015;8(6):373–83. https://doi.org/10.1177/1756283X15592586.

318. Falcon BL, Chintharlapalli S, Uhlik MT, Pytowski B. Antagonist antibodies to vascular endothelial growth factor receptor 2 (VEGFR-2) as anti-angiogenic agents. Pharmacol Ther. 2016;164:204–25. https://doi.org/10.1016/j.pharmthera.2016.06.001.

319. Chow LQM, Smith DC, Tan AR, Denlinger CS, Wang D, Shepard DR, Chaudhary A, Lin Y, Gao L. Lack of pharmacokinetic drug-drug interaction between ramucirumab and paclitaxel in a phase II study of patients with advanced malignant solid tumors. Cancer Chemother Pharmacol. 2016;78(2):433–41. https://doi.org/10.1007/s00280-016-3098-3.

320. Refolo MG, Lotesoriere C, Lolli IR, Messa C, D'Alessandro R. Molecular mechanisms of synergistic action of Ramucirumab and paclitaxel in gastric cancers cell lines. Sci Rep. 2020;10:7162. https://doi.org/10.1038/s41598-020-64195-x.

321. Vita F, Borg C, Farina G, Geva R, Carton I, Cuku H, Wei R, Muro K. Ramucirumab and pacli-taxel in patients with gastric cancer and prior trastuzumab: subgroup analysis from RAINBOW study. Future Oncol. 2019;15(23):2723–31. https://doi.org/10.2217/fon-2019-0243.
322. Stenger M (2014) Ramucirumab in combination with paclitaxel in advanced gastric or gastro-esophageal junction adenocarcinoma. The ASCO post. New York. USA. Available in: https://ascopost.Com/issues/november-15-2014/ramucirumab-in-combination-with-paclitaxel-in-advanced-gastric-or-gastroesophageal-junction-adenocarcinoma/. Accessed Aug 27 2021.
323. Corporaal S, Smit WM, Russel MGVM, van der Palen J, Boot H, Legdeur MCJC. Capecitabine, epirubicin and cisplatin in the treatment of oesophagogastric adenocarcinoma. Neth J Med. 2006;64(5):141–6.
324. BC Cancer (2021j) BC Cancer Protocol Summary for Perioperative Treatment of Resectable Adenocarcinoma of the Stomach, Gastroesophageal Junction or Lower 1/3 Esophagus using Epirubicin, CISplatin and Capecitabine. BC Cancer. British Columbia. Available in: http://www.bccancer.bc.ca/chemotherapy-protocols-site/Documents/Gastrointestinal/GIGECC_Protocol.pdf. Accessed Aug 27 2021.
325. Ocvirk J, Rebersek M, Skof E, Hlebanja Z, Boc M. Randomized prospective phase II study to compare the combination chemotherapy regimen epirubicin, cisplatin, and 5-fluorouracil with epirubicin, cisplatin, and capecitabine in patients with advanced or metastatic gastric cancer. Am J Clin Oncol. 2012;35(3):237–41. https://doi.org/10.1097/COC.0b013e31820dc0b0.
326. Evans TRJ, Pentheroudakis G, Paul J, McInnes A, Blackie R, Raby N, Morrison R, Fullarton GM, Soukop M, McDonald AC. A phase I and pharmacokinetic study of capecitabine in combination with epirubicin and cisplatin in patients with inoperable oesophago-gastric adenocarcinoma. Ann Oncol. 2002;13(9):1469–78. https://doi.org/10.1093/annonc/mdf243.
327. Cho EK, Lee WK, Im SA, Lee SN, Park SH, Bang SM, Park DK, Park YH, Shin DB, Lee JH. A phase II study of epirubicin, cisplatin and capecitabine combination chemotherapy in patients with metastatic or advanced gastric cancer. Oncology. 2005;68(4–6):333–40. https://doi.org/10.1159/000086972.
328. Cancer Research UK (2018) Epirubicin, cisplatin and capecitabine (ECX). Cancer research. London. UK. Available in: https://www.Cancerresearchuk.Org/about-cancer/cancer-in-general/treatment/cancer-drugs/drugs/ecx. Accessed Aug 27 2021.
329. NHS (2020) Chemotherapy Protocol. Gastrointestinal (UPPER) Cancer. Capecitabine, cis-platin and epirubicin (ECX). NHS. University Hospital Southampton. NHS Foundation Trust. England. Available in: https://www.uhs.nhs.uk/Media/SUHTExtranet/Services/Chemotherapy-SOPs/Upper-gastro-intestinal/Capecitabine-Cisplatin-Epirubicin.pdf. Accessed Aug 27 2021.
330. Fraumeni JF Jr. Cancers of the pancreas and biliary tract: epidemiological considerations. Cancer Res. 1975;35(11):3437–46.
331. Alberts SR, Kelly JJ, Ashokkumar R, Lanier AP. Occurrence of pancreatic, biliary tract, and gallbladder cancers in Alaska native people, 1973-2007. Int J Circumpolar Health. 2012;71:17521. https://doi.org/10.3402/IJCH.v71i0.17521.
332. Curley SA. Bile duct cancer. In: Kufe DW, Pollock RE, Weichselbaum RR, et al., editors. Holland-Frei cancer medicine. 6th ed. Hamilton. Canada: BC Decker; 2003.
333. Patel T. Cholangiocarcinoma-controversies and challenges. Nat Rev Gastroenterol Hepatol. 2011;8(4):189–200. https://doi.org/10.1038/nrgastro.2011.20.
334. Bridgewater JA, Goodman KA, Kalyan A, Mulcahy MF. Biliary tract cancer: epidemiology, radiotherapy, and molecular profiling. Am Soc Clin Oncol Educ Book. 2016;36:e194–203. https://doi.org/10.1200/EDBK_160831.
335. Banales JM, Marin JJG, Lamarca A, Rodrigues PM, Khan AS, Roberts LR, Cardinale V, Carpino G, Andersen JB, Braconi C, Calvisi DF, Perugorria MJ, Fabris L, Boulter L, Macias RIR, Gaudio E, Alvaro D, Gradilone AS, Strazzabosco M, Marzioni M, Coulouarn C, Fouassier L, Raggi C, Invernizzi P, Mertens JC, Moncsek A, Rizvi S, Heimbach J, Koerkamp BG, Bruix J, Forner A, Bridgewater J, Valle JW, Gores GJ. Cholangiocarcinoma 2020: the next horizon in mechanisms and management. Nat Rev Gastroenterol Hepatol. 2020;17:557–88. https://doi.org/10.1038/s41575-020-0310-z.

336. Kobari M, Egawa SI, Shibuya K, Shimamura H, Sunamura M, Takeda K, Matsuno S, Furukawa T. Intraductal papillary mucinous tumors of the pancreas comprise 2 clinical subtypes: differences in clinical characteristics and surgical management. JAMA Surg. 1999;134(10):1131–6. https://doi.org/10.1001/archsurg.134.10.1131.

337. Zen Y, Fujii T, Itatsu K, Nakamura K, Minato H, Kasashima S, Kurumaya H, Katayanagi K, Kawashima A, Masuda S, Niwa H, Mitsui T, Asada Y, Miura S, Ohta T, Nakanuma Y. Biliary papillary tumors share pathological features with intraductal papillary mucinous neoplasm of the pancreas. Hepatology. 2006;44(5):1333–43. https://doi.org/10.1002/hep.21387.

338. Henson DE, Schwartz AM, Nsouli H, Albores-Saavedra J. Carcinomas of the pancreas, gallbladder, extrahepatic bile ducts, and ampulla of vater share a field for carcinogenesis: a population-based study. Arch Pathol Lab Med. 2009;133(1):67–71. https://doi.org/10.5858/133.1.67.

339. Dwivedi AND, Jain S, Dixit R. Gall bladder carcinoma: aggressive malignancy with protean loco-regional and distant spread. World J Clin Cases. 2015;3(3):231–44. https://doi.org/10.12998/wjcc.v3.i3.231.

340. Kanthan R, Senger JL, Ahmed S, Janthan SC. Gallbladder cancer in the 21st century. J Oncol. 2015;2015:967472. https://doi.org/10.1155/2015/967472.

341. Bowles MJ, Benjamin IS. Cancer of the stomach and pancreas. BMJ. 2001;323(7326):1413–6. https://doi.org/10.1136/bmj.323.7326.1413.

342. Kusumayanti RR, Simadibrata M, Abdullah M, Gani RA, Luthariana L. Problems in diagnosis approach for carcinoma of pancreatic head. Indonesian J Gastroenterol Hepatol Dig Endos. 2008;9(2):64–9.

343. Dariya B, Alam A, Nagaraju GP. Biology, pathophysiology, and epidemiology of pancreatic cancer. Theranost Approach Pancreat Cancer. 2019:1–50. https://doi.org/10.1016/B978-0-12-819457-7.00001-3.

344. Bazzichetto C, Luchini C, Conciatori F, Vaccaro V, Cello ID, Mattiolo P, Falcone I, Ferretti G, Scarpa A, Cognetti F, Milella M. Morphologic and molecular landscape of pancreatic cancer variants as the basis of new therapeutic strategies for precision oncology. Int J Mol Sci. 2020;21:8841. https://doi.org/10.3390/ijms21228841.

345. Schawkat K, Manning MA, Glickman JN, Mortele KJ. Pancreatic ductal adenocarcinoma and its variants: pearls and perils. Radiographics. 2020;40(5):e190184. https://doi.org/10.1148/rg.2020190184.

346. Bridgewater J, Imber C. New advances in the management of biliary tract cancer. HPB (Oxford). 2007;9(2):104–11. https://doi.org/10.1080/13651820701216216.

347. Riechelmann R, Coutinho AK, Weschenfelder RF, Paulo GA, Fernandes GS, Gifoni M, Oliveira ML, Gansl R, Gil R, Luersen G, Lucas L, Reisner M, Vieira FM, Machado MA, Murad A, Osvaldt A, Brandão M, Carvalho E, Souza T, Pfiffer T, Prolla G. Guideline for the management of bile duct cancers by the Brazilian gastrointestinal tumor group. Arq Gastroenterol. 2016;53(1):5–9. https://doi.org/10.1590/S0004-28032016000100003.

348. Gkika E, Hawkins MA, Grosu AL, Brunner TB. The evolving role of radiation therapy in the treatment of biliary tract cancer. Front Oncol. 2020;10:604387. https://doi.org/10.3389/fonc.2020.604387.

349. Gómez-España A, Montes AF, Garcia-Carbonero R, Mercadé TM, Maurel J, Martín AM, Pazo-Cid R, Vera R, Carrato A, Feliu J. SEOM clinical guidelines for pancreatic and biliary tract cancer (2020). Clin Transl Oncol. 2021;23(5):988–1000. https://doi.org/10.1007/s12094-021-02573-1.

350. Herrmann R, Bodoky G, Ruhstaller T, Glimelius B, Bajetta E, Schuller J, Saletti P, Bauer J, Figer A, Pestalozzi B, Kohne CH, Mingrone W, Stemmer SM, Tàmas K, Kornek GV, Koeberle D, Cina S, Bernhard J, Dietrich D, Scheithauer W. Gemcitabine plus Capecitabine compared with gemcitabine alone in advanced pancreatic cancer: a randomized, multicenter, phase III trial of the Swiss Group for Clinical Cancer Research and the central European cooperative oncology group. J Clin Oncol. 2007;25(16):2212–7. https://doi.org/10.1200/JCO.2006.09.0886.

351. Ramírez-Merino N, Aix SP, Cortés-Funes H. Chemotherapy for cholangiocarcinoma: na update. World J Gastroint Oncol. 2013;5(7):171–6. https://doi.org/10.4251/wjgo.v5.i7.171.
352. Doherty MK, Knox JJ. Adjuvant therapy for resected biliary tract cancer: a review. Chin Clin Oncol. 2016;5(5):64. https://doi.org/10.21037/cco.2016.08.05.
353. Novarino A, Satolli MA, Chiappino I, Giacobino A, Bellone G, Rahimi F, Milanesi E, Bertetto O, Ciuffreda L. Oxaliplatin, 5-fluorouracil, and leucovorin as second-line treatment for advanced pancreatic cancer. Am J Clin Oncol. 2009;32(1):44–8. https://doi.org/10.1097/COC.0b013e31817be5a9.
354. Dahan L, Bonnetain F, Ychou M, Mitry E, Gasmi M, Raoul JL, Cattan S, Phelip JM, Hammel P, Chauffert B, Michel P, Legoux JL, Rougier P, Bedenne L, Seitz JF. Combination 5-fluorouracil, folinic acid and cisplatin (LV5FU2-CDDP) followed by gemcitabine or the reverse sequence in metastatic pancreatic cancer: final results of a randomised strategic phase III trial (FFCD 0301). Gut. 2010;59(11):1527–34. https://doi.org/10.1136/gut.2010.216135.
355. Neuzillet C, Hentic O, Rousseau B, Rebours V, Bengrine-Lefèvre L, Bonnetain F, Lévy P, Raymond E, Ruszniewski P, Louvet C, Hammel P. FOLFIRI regimen in metastatic pancreatic adenocarcinoma resistant to gemcitabine and platinum-salts. World J Gastroenterol. 2012;18(33):4533–41. https://doi.org/10.3748/wjg.v18.i33.4533.
356. Zaniboni A, Aitini E, Barni S, Ferrari D, Cascinu S, Catalano V, Valmadre G, Ferrara D, Veltri E, Codignola C, Labianca R. FOLFIRI as second-line chemotherapy for advanced pancreatic cancer: a GISCAD multicenter phase II study. Cancer Chemother Pharmacol. 2012;69(6):1641–5. https://doi.org/10.1007/s00280-012-1875-1.
357. Abbassi R, Algul H. Palliative chemotherapy in pancreatic cancer-treatment sequences. Transl Gastroenterol Hepatol. 2019;4:56. https://doi.org/10.21037/tgh.2019.06.09.
358. Valle JW, Furuse J, Jitlal M, Beare S, Mizuno N, Wasan H, Bridgewater J, Okusaka T. Cisplatin and gemcitabine for advances biliary tract cancer: a meta-analysis of two randomized trials. Ann Oncol. 2014;25(2):391–8. https://doi.org/10.1093/annonc/mdt540.
359. Doherty MK, McNamara MG, Aneja P, McInerney E, Moignard S, Horgan AM, Jiang H, Panzarella T, Jang R, Dhani N, Hedley D, Knox JJ. Long term responders to palliative chemotherapy for advanced biliary tract cancer. J Gastrointest Oncol. 2017;8(2):352–60. https://doi.org/10.21037/jgo.2017.03.06.
360. Azizi AA, Lamarca A, Valle JW. Systemic therapy of gallbladder cancer: review of first line, maintenance, neoadjuvant and second line therapy specific to gallbladder cancer. Chin Clin Oncol. 2019;8(4):43. https://doi.org/10.21037/cco.2019.07.05.
361. You MS, Ryu JK, Choi YH, Choi JH, Huh G, Paik WH, Lee SH, Kim YT. Therapeutic outcomes and prognostic factors in unresectable gallbladder cancer treated with gemcitabine plus cisplatin. BMC Cancer. 2019;19:10. https://doi.org/10.1186/s12885-018-5211-y.
362. Valle J, Wasan H, Palmer DH, Cunningham D, Anthoney A, Maraveyas A, Madhusudan S, Iveson T, Hughes S, Pereira SP, Roughton M, Bridgewater J. Cisplatin plus gemcitabine versus gemcitabine for biliary tract cancer. N Engl J Med. 2010;362:1273–81. https://doi.org/10.1056/NEJMoa0908721.
363. Lee MA, Woo IS, Kang JH, Hong YS, Lee KS. Gemcitabine and cisplatin combination chemotherapy in intrahepatic cholangiocarcinoma as second-line treatment: report of four cases. Jpn J Clin Oncol. 2004;34(9):547–50. https://doi.org/10.1093/jjco/hyh099.
364. Malik IA, Aziz Z, Zaidi SHM, Sethuraman G. Gemcitabine and cisplatin is a highly effective combination chemotherapy in patients with advanced cancer of the gallbladder. Am J Clin Oncol. 2003;26(2):174–7. https://doi.org/10.1097/00000421-200304000-00015.
365. Dierks J, Gaspersz MP, Belkouz A, van Vugt JLA, Coelen RJS, Groot JWB, Ten Tije AJ, Meijer WG, Pruijt JFM, van Voorthuizen T, van Spronsen DJ, Rentinck M, Ten Oever D, Smit JM, Otten HM, van Gulik TM, Wilmink JW, Groot Koerkamp B, Klumpen H. Translating the ABC-02 trial into daily practice: outcome of palliative treatment in patients with unresectable biliary tract cancer treated with gemcitabine and cisplatin. Acta Oncol. 2018;57(6):807–12. https://doi.org/10.1080/0284186X.2017.1418532.

366. Peters GJ, Bergman AM, Ruiz van Haperen VW, Veerman G, Kuiper CM, Braakhuis BJ. Interaction between cisplatin and gemcitabine in vitro and in vivo. Semin Oncol. 1995;22(4 Suppl 11):72–9.

367. Kroep JR, Peters GJ, van Moorsel CJ, Catik A, Vermorken JB, Pinedo HM, van Groeningen CJ. Gemcitabine-cisplatin: a schedule finding study. Ann Oncol. 1999;10(12):1503–10. https://doi.org/10.1023/a:1008339425708.

368. NHS (2014) Chemotherapy Protocol. Pancreatic Cancer. Cisplatin-gemcitabine (Radiotherapy). NHS. University Hospital Southampton. NHS Foundation Trust. England. Available in: https://www.uhs.nhs.uk/Media/SUHTExtranet/Services/Chemotherapy-SOPs/Pancreas/Cisplatin-GemcitabineVer21.pdf. Accessed Aug 28 2021.

369. Berger AK, Haag GM, Ehmann M, Byl A, Jager D, Springfeld C. Palliative chemotherapy for pancreatic adenocarcinoma: a retrospective cohort analysis of efficacy and toxicity of the FOLFIRINOX regimen focusing on the older patient. BMC Gastroenterol. 2017;17:143. https://doi.org/10.1186/s12876-017-0709-3.

370. Mota JM, Silva AHC, Franco AS, Talans A, Riveiro-Ferreira F, Castria TB, Sabbaga J, Hoff PM. FOLFIRINOX for advanced pancreatic adenocarcinoma in Brazil: a single-institution experience. Braz J Oncol. 2018;14(47):1–10. https://doi.org/10.26790/BJO20181447A197.

371. Zhang B, Zhou F, Hong J, Ng DM, Yang T, Zhou X, Jin J, Zhou F, Chen P, Xu Y. The role of FOLFIRINOX in metastatic pancreatic cancer: a meta-analysis. World J Surg Oncol. 2021;19:182. https://doi.org/10.1186/s12957-021-02291-6.

372. Chllamma MK, Cook N, Dhani NC, Giby K, Dodd A, Wang L, Hedley DW, Moore MJ, Knox JJ. FOLFIRINOX for advanced pancreatic cancer: the Princess Margaret cancer Centre experience. Br J Cancer. 2016;115:649–54. https://doi.org/10.1038/bjc.2016.222.

373. Zoetemelk M, Ramzy GM, Rausch M, Nowak-Sliwinska P. Drug-drug interactions of irinotecan, 5-fluorouracil, Folinic acid and Oxaliplatin and its activity in colorectal carcinoma treatment. Molecules. 2020;25(11):2614. https://doi.org/10.3390/molecules25112614.

374. NHS (2020) Chemotherapy Protocol Pancreatic Cancer. Fluorouracil-folinic acid-irinotecan-oxaliplatin (FOLFIRINOX). NHS. University Hospital Southampton. NHS Foundation Trust. England. Available in: https://www.uhs.nhs.uk/Media/SUHTExtranet/Services/Chemotherapy-SOPs/Pancreas/Fluorouracil-Folinic-Acid-Irinotecan-Oxaliplatin.pdf. Accessed Aug 29 2021.

375. NHS England (2017) Evidence review: Gemcitabine plus capecitabine for adjuvant treatment in resected pancreatic cancer. NHS. University Hospital Southampton. NHS Foundation Trust. England. Available in: https://www.nice.org.uk/Media/Default/About/NICE-Communities/Medicines-prescribing/ER-NHSE-gemcitabine-capecitabine.pdf. Accessed Aug 29 2021.

376. Chen H, He R, Shi X, Zhou M, Zhao C, Zhang H, Qin R. Meta-analysis on resected pancreatic cancer: a comparison between adjuvant treatments and gemcitabine alone. BMC Cancer. 2018;18:1034. https://doi.org/10.1186/s12885-018-4948-7.

377. Hess V, Salzberg M, Borner M, Morant R, Roth AD, Ludwig C, Herrmann R. Combining capecitabine and gemcitabine in patients with advanced pancreatic carcinoma: a phase I/II trial. J Clin Oncol. 2003;21(1):66–8. https://doi.org/10.1200/JCO.2003.04.029.

378. Kaur G, Jahangiri V, Park SJ, Wegner RE, Monga DK. Efficacy and tolerability of adjuvant gemcitabine and capecitabine in patients with resected pancreatic cancer in US population: a single network experience. J Clin Oncol. 2019;37(15_suppl) https://doi.org/10.1200/JCO.2019.37.15_suppl.e15789.

379. Neoptolemos JP, Palmer DH, Ghaneh P, Psarelli EE, Valle JW, Halloran CM, Faluyi O, O'Reilly DA, Cunningham D, Wadsley J, Darby S, Meyer T, Gillmore R, Anthoney A, Lind P, Glimelius B, Falk S, Izbicki JR, Middleton GW, Cummins S, Ross PJ, Wasan H, McDonald A, Crosby T, Ma YT, Patel K, Sherriff D, Soomal R, Borg D, Sothi S, Hammel P, Hackert T, Jackson R Buchler MW (2017) Comparison of adjuvant gemcitabine and capecitabine with gemcitabine monotherapy in patients with resected pancreatic cancer (ESPAC-4): a multicentre, open-label, randomised, phase 3 trial. Lancet 389(10073):1011–1024. doi: https://doi.org/10.1016/S0140-6736(16)32409-6.

380. NHS (2020) Chemotherapy Protocol. Pancreatic Cancer. Capecitabine and gemcitabine. NHS. University Hospital Southampton. NHS Foundation Trust. England. Available in: https://www.uhs.nhs.uk/Media/SUHTExtranet/Services/Chemotherapy-SOPs/Pancreas/Capecitabine-Gemcitabine.pdf. Accessed Aug 29 2021.
381. NCT00691054 (2017) Abraxane Therapy in Patients With Pancreatic Cancer Who Failed First-Line Gemcitabine Therapy. Clinical Trials. Available in: https://clinicaltrials.gov/ct2/show/NCT00691054. Accessed Aug 29 2021.
382. NCT02043730 (2019) Abraxane and Gemcitabine Versus Gemcitabine Alone in Locally Advanced Unresectable Pancreatic Cancer. (GAP). Clinical Trials. Available in: https://clinicaltrials.gov/ct2/show/NCT02043730. Accessed Aug 29 2021.
383. Zhang Y, Xu J, Hua J, Liu J, Liang C, Meng Q, Ni Q, Shi S, Yu X. Nab-paclitaxel plus gemcitabine as first-line treatment for advanced pancreatic cancer: a systematic review and meta-analysis. J Cancer. 2019;10(18):4420–9. https://doi.org/10.7150/jca.29898.
384. Petrioli R, Torre P, Pesola G, Paganini G, Paolelli L, Miano ST, Martellucci I, Francini G, Francini E. Gemcitabine plus nab-paclitaxel followed by maintenance treatment with gemcitabine alone as first-line treatment for older adults with locally advanced or metastatic pancreatic cancer. J Geriatr Oncol. 2020;11(4):647–51. https://doi.org/10.1016/j.jgo.2019.08.008.
385. Iglesias J. *Nab*-paclitaxel (Abraxane®): an albumin-bound cytotoxic exploiting natural delivery mechanisms into tumors. Breast Cancer Res. 2009;11:S21. https://doi.org/10.1186/bcr2282.
386. Cucinotto I, Fiorillo L, Gualtieri S, Arbitrio M, Ciliberto D, Staropoli N, Grimaldi A, Luce A, Tassone P, Caraglia M, Tagliaferri P. Nanoparticle albumin bound paclitaxel in the treatment of human cancer: Nanodelivery reaches prime-time? J Drug Deliv. 2013;2013:905091. https://doi.org/10.1155/2013/905091.
387. Zhao M, Lei C, Yang Y, Bu X, Ma H, Gong H, Liu J, Fang X, Hu Z, Fang Q. Abraxane, the nanoparticle formulation of paclitaxel can induce drug resistance by up-regulation of P-gp. PLoS One. 2015;10(7):e0131429. https://doi.org/10.1371/journal.pone.0131429.
388. Hama M, Ishima Y, Chuang VTG, Ando H, Shimizu T, Ishida T. Evidence for delivery of abraxane via a denatured-albumin transport system. ACS Appl Mater Interfaces. 2021;13(17):19736–44. https://doi.org/10.1021/acsami.1c03065.
389. Von Hoff DD, Ervin T, Arena FP, Chiorean EG, Infante J, Moore M, Seay T, Tijulandin SA, Ma WW, Saleh MN, Harris M, Reni M, Dowden S, Laheru D, Bahary N, Ramanathan RK, Tabernero J, Hidalgo M, Goldstein D, Cutsem EV, Wei X, Iglesias J, Renschler MF. Increased survival in pancreatic cancer with nab-paclitaxel plus gemcitabine. N Engl J Med. 2013;369:1691–703. https://doi.org/10.1056/NEJMoa1304369.
390. Zhang Y, Hochster H, Stein S, Lacy J. Gemcitabine plus nab-paclitaxel for advanced pancreatic cancer after first-line FOLFIRINOX: single institution retrospective review of efficacy and toxicity. Exp Hematol Oncol. 2015;4:29. https://doi.org/10.1186/s40164-015-0025-y.
391. Dean AP, Das A, McNulty M, Higgs D. Gemcitabine and nab-paclitaxel retreatment as a third-line therapy following second-line FOLFIRINOX for advanced pancreatic adenocarcinoma. J Clin Oncol. 2019;37(15_suppl):e15794. https://doi.org/10.1200/JCO.2019.37.15_suppl.e15794.
392. NHS (2014) Chemotherapy Protocol. Pancreatic Cancer. Gemcitabine-paclitaxel albumin bound. NHS. University Hospital Southampton. NHS Foundation Trust. England. Available in: https://www.uhs.nhs.uk/Media/SUHTExtranet/Services/Chemotherapy-SOPs/Pancreas/Gemcitabine-Paclitaxel-Albumin-Bound-(Abraxane)-Ver1.pdf. Accessed Aug 29 2021.
393. Narayanan V, Weekes C. Nanoparticle albumin-bound (nab)-paclitaxel for the treatment of pancreas ductal adenocarcinoma. Gastrointestinal Cancer. 2015;5:11–9. https://doi.org/10.2147/GICTT.S55158.
394. Spada A, Emami J, Tuszynski JÁ, Lavasanifar A. The uniqueness of albumin as a carrier in nanodrug delivery. Mol Pharm. 2021;18(5):1862–94. https://doi.org/10.1021/acs.molpharmaceut.1c00046.

395. Singal AG, Lampertico P, Nahon P. Epidemiology and surveillance for hepatocellular carcinoma: new trends. J Hepatol. 2020;72(2):250–61. https://doi.org/10.1016/j.jhep.2019.08.025.

396. McGlynn KA, Petrick JL, El-Serag HB. Epidemiology of hepatocellular carcinoma. Hepatology. 2021;73(Suppl 1):4–13. https://doi.org/10.1002/hep.31288.

397. Waller LP, Deshpande V, Pyrsopoulos N. Hepatocellular carcinoma: a comprehensive review. World J Hepatol. 2015;7(26):2648–63. https://doi.org/10.4254/wjh.v7.i26.2648.

398. Recio-Boiles A, Babiker HM. Liver cancer. Treasure Island USA: StatPearls Publishing; 2021.

399. Ramakrishna G, Rastogi A, Trehanpati N, Sen B, Khosla R, Sarin SK. From cirrhosis to hepatocellular carcinoma: new molecular insights on inflammation and cellular senescence. Liver Cancer. 2013;2(3–4):367–83. https://doi.org/10.1159/000343852.

400. Bishayee A. The inflammation and liver cancer. In: Aggarwal B, Sung B, Gupta S, editors. Inflammation and cancer. Advances in experimental medicine and biology 816. Basel: Springer; 2014. https://doi.org/10.1007/978-3-0348-0837-8_16.

401. França AVC, Elias Junior J, Lima BLG, Martinelli ALC, Carrilho FJ. Diagnosis, staging and treatment of hepatocellular carcinoma. Braz J Med Biol Res. 2004;37(11):1689–705. https://doi.org/10.1590/S0100-879X2004001100015.

402. Gosalia AJ, Martin P, Jones PD. Advances and future directions in the treatment of hepatocellular carcinoma. Gastroenterol Hepatol. 2017;13(7):398–410.

403. Weeda VB, Murawski M. The future of pediatric hepatocellular carcinoma: a combination of surgical, locoregional, and targeted therapy. Hepatoma Res. 2021;7:43. https://doi.org/10.20517/2394-5079.2021.10.

404. Kow AWC. Transplantation versus liver resection in patients with hepatocellular carcinoma. Transl Gastroenterol Hepatol. 2019;4:33. https://doi.org/10.21037/tgh.2019.05.06.

405. Lurje I, Czigany Z, Bednarsch J, Roderburg C, Isfort P, Neumann UP, Lurje G. Treatment strategies for hepatocellular carcinoma—a multidisciplinary approach. Int J Mol Sci. 2019;20(6):1465. https://doi.org/10.3390/ijms20061465.

406. Ansari D, Andersson R. Radiofrequency ablation or percutaneous ethanol injection for the treatment of liver tumors. World J Gastroenterol. 2012;18(10):1003–8. https://doi.org/10.3748/wjg.v18.i10.1003.

407. Tombesi P, Vece FD, Sartori S. Radiofrequency, microwave, and laser ablation of liver tumors: time to move toward a tailored ablation technique? Hepatoma Res. 2015;1:52–7. https://doi.org/10.4103/2394-5079.155697.

408. Shin SW. The current practice of Transarterial chemoembolization for the treatment of hepatocellular carcinoma. Korean J Radiol. 2009;10(5):425–34. https://doi.org/10.3348/kjr.2009.10.5.425.

409. Tsurusaki M, Murakami T. Surgical and locoregional therapy of HCC: TACE. Liver Cancer. 2015;4(3):165–75. https://doi.org/10.1159/000367739.

410. NIH – National Cancer Institute (2020) Atezolizumab plus bevacizumab approved to treat liver cancer. National Cancer Institute. USA. Available in: https://www.cancer.gov/contact. Accessed Aug 30 2021.

411. Armstrong S, Prins P, He AR. Immunotherapy and immunotherapy biomarkers for hepatocellular carcinoma. Hepatoma Res. 2021;7:18. https://doi.org/10.20517/2394-5079.2020.118.

412. Koulouris A, Tsagkaris C, Spyrou V, Pappa E, Troullinou A, Nikolaou M. Hepatocellular carcinoma: An overview of the changing landscape of treatment options. J Hepatocell Carcinoma. 2021;8:387–401. https://doi.org/10.2147/JHC.S300182.

413. Grazie ML, Biagini MR, Tarocchi M, Polvani S, Galli A. Chemotherapy for hepatocellular carcinoma: the present and the future. World J Hepatol. 2017;9(21):907–20. https://doi.org/10.4254/wjh.v9.i21.907.

414. Kudo M. A new era of systemic therapy for hepatocellular carcinoma with Regorafenib and Lenvatinib. Liver Cancer. 2017;6:177–84. https://doi.org/10.1159/000462153.

415. Koroki K, Kanogawa N, Maruta S, Ogasawara S, Lino Y, Obu M, Okubo T, Itokawa N, Maeda T, Inoue M, Haga Y, Seki A, Okabe S, Koma Y, Azemoto R, Atsukawa M, Itobayashi T, Ito K,

Sugiura N, Mizumoto H, Unozawa H, Iwanaga T, Sakuma T, Fujita N, Kanzaki H, Kobayashi K, Kiyono S, Nakamura M, Saito T, Kondo T, Suzuki E, Ooka Y, Nakamoto S, Tawada A, Chiba T, Arai M, Kanda T, Maruyama H, Kato J, Kato N. Posttreatment after lenvatinib in patients with advanced hepatocellular carcinoma. Liver Cancer. 2021;10(5):473–84. https://doi.org/10.1159/000515552.

416. Guo L, Zhang H, Chen B. Nivolumab as programmed death-1 (PD-1) inhibitor for targeted immunotherapy in tumor. J Cancer. 2017;8(3):410–6. https://doi.org/10.7150/jca.17144.

417. Han Y, Liu D, Li L. PD-1/PD-L1 pathway: current researches in cancer. Am J Cancer Res. 2020;10(3):727–42.

418. Stenger M (2020) Nivolumab/Ipilimumab in patients with Sorafenib-pretreated hepatocellular carcinoma. The ASCO post. New York. USA. Available in: https://ascopost.Com/issues/april-25-2020/nivolumabipilimumab-in-patients-with-sorafenib-pretreated-hepatocellular-carcinoma/. Accessed Aug 31 2021.

419. Yau T, Kang YK, Kim TY, El-Khoueiry AB, Santoro A, Sangro B, Melero I, Kudo M, Hou MM, Matilla A, Tovoli F, Knox JJ, He AR, El-Rayes BF, Acosta-Rivera M, Lim HY, Neely J, Shen Y, Wisniewski T, Anderson J, Hsu C. Efficacy and safety of Nivolumab plus Ipilimumab in patients with advanced hepatocellular carcinoma previously treated with Sorafenib: the CheckMate 040 randomized clinical trial. JAMA Oncol. 2020;6(11):e204564. https://doi.org/10.1001/jamaoncol.2020.4564.

420. Tsang J, Wong JSL, Kwok GGW, Li BCW, Leung R, Chiu J, Cheung TT, Yau T. Nivolumab + Ipilimumab for patients with hepatocellular carcinoma previously treated with Sorafenib. Expert Rev Gastroenterol Hepatol. 2021;15(6):589–98. https://doi.org/10.1080/17474124.2021.1899808.

421. Giacomo AMD, Danielli R, Guidobini M, Calabrò L, Carlucci D, Miracco C, Volterrani L, Mazzei MA, Biagioli M, Altomonte M, Maio M. Therapeutic efficacy of ipilimumab, an anti-CTLA-4 monoclonal antibody, in patients with metastatic melanoma unresponsive to prior systemic treatments: clinical and immunological evidence from three patient cases. Cancer Immunol Immunother. 2009;58(8):1297–306. https://doi.org/10.1007/s00262-008-0642-y.

422. Leung AM, Lee AF, Ozao-Choy J, Ramos RI, Hamid O, O'Day SJ, Shin-Sim M, Morton DL, Faries MB, Sieling PA, Lee DJ. Clinical benefit from ipilimumab therapy in melanoma patients may be associated with serum CTLA4 levels. Front Oncol. 2014;4:110. https://doi.org/10.3389/fonc.2014.00110.

423. Kooshkaki O, Derakhshani A, Hosseinkhani N, Torabi M, Safaei S, Brunetti O, Racanelli V, Silvestris N, Baradaran B. Combination of ipilimumab and nivolumab in cancers: from clinical practice to ongoing clinical trials. Int J Mol Sci. 2020;21(12):4427. https://doi.org/10.3390/ijms21124427.

424. Waldman AD, Fritz JM, Lenardo MJ. A guide to cancer immunotherapy: from T cell basic science to clinical practice. Nat Rev Immunol. 2020;20:651–68. https://doi.org/10.1038/s41577-020-0306-5.

425. Donisi C, Puzzoni M, Ziranu P, Lai E, Mariani S, Saba G, Impera V, Dubois M, Persano M, Migliari M, Pretta A, Liscia N, Astara G, Scartozzi M. Immune checkpoint inhibitors in the treatment of HCC. Front Oncol. 2021;10:601240. https://doi.org/10.3389/fonc.2020.601240.

426. Weber JS, Gibney G, Sullivan RJ, Sosman JA, Slingluff CL, Lawrence DP, Logan TF, Schuchter LM, Nair S, Fecher L, Buchbinder EI, Berghorn E, Ruisi M, Kong G, Jiang J, Horak C, Hodi FS. Sequential administration of nivolumab and ipilimumab with a planned switch in patients with advanced melanoma (CheckMate 064): an open-label, randomised, phase 2 trial. Lancet Oncol. 2016;17(7):943–55. https://doi.org/10.1016/S1470-2045(16)30126-7.

427. Lee MS, Ryoo BY, Hsu CH, Numata K, Stein S, Verret W, Hack SP, Spahn J, Liu B, Abdullah H, Wang Y, Ruth A, Lee KH. Atezolizumab with or without bevacizumab in unresectable hepatocellular carcinoma (GO30140): an open-label, multicentre, phase 1b study. Lancet Oncol. 2020;21(6):808–20. https://doi.org/10.1016/S1470-2045(20)30156-X.

428. Casak SJ, Donoghue M, Fashoyin-Aje L, Jiang X, Rodriguez L, Shen YL, Xu Y, Jiang X, Liu J, Zhao H, Pierce WF, Mehta S, Goldberg KB, Theoret MR, Kluetz PG, Pazdur R, Lemery SJ. FDA approval summary: Atezolizumab plus bevacizumab for the treatment of patients with advanced Unresectable or metastatic hepatocellular carcinoma. Clin Cancer Res. 2021;27(7):1836–41. https://doi.org/10.1158/1078-0432.CCR-20-3407.

429. Kazazi-Hyseni F, Beijnen JH, Schellens JHM. Bevacizumab. Oncologist. 2010;15(8):819–25. https://doi.org/10.1634/theoncologist.2009-0317.

430. Qin W, Hu L, Zhang X, Jiang S, Li J, Zhang Z, Wang X. The diverse function of PD-1/PD-L pathway beyond cancer. Front Immunol. 2019;10:2298. https://doi.org/10.3389/fimmu.2019.02298.

431. Yang X, Wang D, Lin J, Yang X, Zhao H. Atezolizumab plus bevacizumab for unresectable hepatocellular carcinoma. Lancet Oncol. 2020;21(9):E412. https://doi.org/10.1016/S1470-2045(20)30430-7.

432. Finn RS, Qin S, Ikeda M, Galle PR, Ducreux M, Kim TY, Kudo M, Breder V, Merle P, Kaseb AO, Li D, Verret W, Xu DZ, Hernandez S, Liu J, Huang C, Mulla S, Wang Y, Lim HY, Zhu AX, Cheng AL. Atezolizumab plus bevacizumab in unresectable hepatocellular carcinoma. N Engl J Med. 2020;382:1894–905. https://doi.org/10.1056/NEJMoa1915745.

433. Vogel A, Rimassa L, Sun HC, Abou-Alfa GK, El-Khoueiry A, Pinato DJ, Sanchez Alvarez J, Daigl M, Orfanos P, Leibfried M, Blanchet Zumofen MH, Gaillard VE, Merle P. Comparative efficacy of Atezolizumab plus bevacizumab and other treatment options for patients with Unresectable hepatocellular carcinoma: a network meta-analysis. Liver Cancer. 2021;10:240–8. https://doi.org/10.1159/000515302.

434. Zhang X, Wang J, Shi J, Jia X, Dang S, Wang W. Cost-effectiveness of Atezolizumab plus bevacizumab vs Sorafenib for patients with Unresectable or metastatic hepatocellular carcinoma. JAMA Netw Open. 2021;4(4):e214846. https://doi.org/10.1001/jamanetworkopen.2021.4846.

435. Liu X, Lu Y, Qin S. Atezolizumab and bevacizumab for hepatocellular carcinoma: mechanism, pharmacokinetics and future treatment strategies. Future Oncol. 2021;17(17):2243–56. https://doi.org/10.2217/fon-2020-1290.

436. FDA – Food & Drug Administration (2020) FDA approves atezolizumab plus bevacizumab for unresectable hepatocellular carcinoma. Available in: https://www.fda.gov/drugs/resources-information-approved-drugs/fda-approves-atezolizumab-plus-bevacizumab-unresectable-hepatocellular-carcinoma. Accessed Aug 31 2021.

437. Dasari A, Shen C, Halperin D, Zhao B, Zhou S, Xu Y, Shih T, Yao JC. Trends in the incidence, prevalence, and survival outcomes in patients with neuroendocrine tumors in the United States. JAMA Oncol. 2017;3(10):1335–42. https://doi.org/10.1001/jamaoncol.2017.0589.

438. Mocellin S, Nitti D. Gastrointestinal carcinoid: epidemiological and survival evidence from a large population-based study (n = 25 531). Ann Oncol. 2013;24(12):3040–4. https://doi.org/10.1093/annonc/mdt377.

439. Ellis L, Shale MJ, Coleman MP. Carcinoid tumors of the gastrointestinal tract: trends in incidence in England since 1971. Am J Gastroenterol. 2010;105(12):2563–9. https://doi.org/10.1038/ajg.2010.341.

440. Uhlig J, Nie J, Stein S, Cecchini M, Lacy J, Kim HS. Neuroendocrine and carcinoid tumors of the gastrointestinal tract: epidemiology and outcomes from the National Cancer Database. J Clin Oncol. 2020;38(4_suppl):609. https://doi.org/10.1200/JCO.2020.38.4_suppl.609.

441. Pinchot SN, Holen K, Sippel RS, Chen H. Carcinoid tumors. Oncologist. 2008;13(12):1255–69. https://doi.org/10.1634/theoncologist.2008-0207.

442. Baxi AJ, Chintapalli K, Katkar A, Restrepo CS, Betancourt SL, Sunnapwar A. Multimodality imaging findings in carcinoid tumors: a head-to-toe spectrum. Radiographics. 2017;37(2):516–36. https://doi.org/10.1148/rg.2017160113.

443. Ferrari ACRC, Glasberg J, Riechelmann RP. Carcinoid syndrome: update on the pathophysiology and treatment. Clinics. 2018;73(Suppl 1):e490s. https://doi.org/10.6061/clinics/2018/e490s.

444. Clement D, Ramage J, Srirajaskanthan R. Update on pathophysiology, treatment, and complications of carcinoid syndrome. J Oncol. 2020;2020:8341426. https://doi.org/10.1155/2020/8341426.

445. Pea A, Hruban RH, Wood LD. Genetics of pancreatic neuroendocrine tumors: implications for the clinic. Expert Rev Gastroenterol Hepatol. 2015;9(11):1407–19. https://doi.org/10.1586/17474124.2015.1092383.

446. O'Shea T, Druce M. When should genetic testing be performed in patients with neuroendocrine tumors? Rev Endocr Metab Disord. 2017;18(4):499–515. https://doi.org/10.1007/s11154-017-9430-3.

447. Ahmed M. Gastrointestinal neuroendocrine tumors in 2020. World J Gastrointest Oncol. 2020;12(8):791–807. https://doi.org/10.4251/wjgo.v12.i8.791.

448. Steward MJ, Warbey VS, Malhotra A, Caplin ME, Buscombe JR, Yu D. Neuroendocrine tumors: role of interventional radiology in therapy. Radiographics. 2008;28(4):1131–45. https://doi.org/10.1148/rg.284075170.

449. Sahani DV, Bonaffini PA, Castillo CFD, Blake MA. Gastroenteropancreatic neuroendocrine tumors: role of imaging in diagnosis and management. Radiology. 2013;266(1):38–61. https://doi.org/10.1148/radiol.12112512.

450. Alagusundaramoorthy SS, Gedaly R. Role of surgery and transplantation in the treatment of hepatic metastases from neuroendocrine tumor. World J Gastroenterol. 2014;20(39):14348–58. https://doi.org/10.3748/wjg.v20.i39.14348.

451. Limani P, Tschuor C, Gort L, Balmer B, Gu A, Ceresa C, Raptis DA, Lesurtel M, Puhan M, Breitenstein S. Nonsurgical strategies in patients with NET liver metastases: a protocol of four systematic reviews. JMIR Res Protoc. 2014;3(1):e9. https://doi.org/10.2196/resprot.2893.

452. Wang R, Zheng-Pywell R, Chen HA, Bibb JA, Chen H, Rose JB. Management of gastrointestinal neuroendocrine tumors. Clin Med Insights Endocrinol Diabetes. 2019;12:1179551419884058. https://doi.org/10.1177/1179551419884058.

453. Chadha MK, Lombardo J, Mashtare T, Wilding GE, Litwin A, Raczyk C, Gibbs JF, Kuvshinoff B, Javle MM, Iyer RV. High-dose octreotide acetate for Management of Gastroenteropancreatic Neuroendocrine Tumors. Anticancer Res. 2009;29(10):4127–30.

454. Raymond E, Dahan L, Raoul JL, Bang YJ, Borbath I, Lombard-Bohas C, Valle J, Metrakos P, Smith D, Vinik A, Chen JS, Horsch D, Hammel P, Wiedenmann B, van Cutsem E, Patyna S, Lu DR, Blanckmeister C, Chao R, Ruszniewski P. Sunitinib malate for the treatment of pancreatic neuroendocrine tumors. N Engl J Med. 2011;364:501–13. https://doi.org/10.1056/NEJMoa1003825.

455. Delbaldo C, Faivre S, Dreyer C, Raymond E. Sunitinib in advanced pancreatic neuroendocrine tumors: latest evidence and clinical potential. Ther Adv Med Oncol. 2012;4(1):9–18. https://doi.org/10.1177/1758834011428147.

456. Yao JC, Fazio N, Singh S, Buzzoni R, Carnaghi C, Wolin E, Tomasek J, Raderer M, Lahner H, Voi M, Pacaud LB, Rouyrre N, Sachs C, Valle JW, Fave GD, van Cutsem E, Tesselaar M, Shimada Y, Oh DY, Strosberg J, Kulke MH, Pavel ME. Everolimus for the treatment of advanced, non-functional neuroendocrine tumours of the lung or gastrointestinal tract (RADIANT-4): a randomised, placebo-controlled, phase 3 study. Lancet. 2016;387(10022):968–77. https://doi.org/10.1016/S0140-6736(15)00817-X.

457. Yao JC, Oh DY, Qian J, Park YS, Herbst F, Ridolfi A, Izquierdo M, Ito T, Jia L, Komoto I, Sriuranpong V, Shimada Y. Everolimus for the treatment of advanced gastrointestinal or lung nonfunctional neuroendocrine tumors in east Asian patients: a subgroup analysis of the RADIANT-4 study. Onco Targets Ther. 2019;12:1717–28. https://doi.org/10.2147/OTT.S182259.

458. McAuliffe JC, Wolin EM. Randomized controlled trials in neuroendocrine tumors. Surg Oncol Clin N Am. 2017;26:751–65. https://doi.org/10.1016/j.soc.2017.05.012.

459. Hofland J, Herrera-Martínez AD, Zandee WT, Herder WW. Management of carcinoid syndrome: a systematic review and meta-analysis. Endocr Relat Cancer. 2019;26(3):R145–56. https://doi.org/10.1530/ERC-18-0495.

460. Lu Y, Zhao Z, Wang J, Lv W, Lu L, Fu W, Li W. Safety and efficacy of combining capecitabine and temozolomide (CAPTEM) to treat advanced neuroendocrine neoplasms: a meta-analysis. Medicine. 2018;97(41):e12784. https://doi.org/10.1097/MD.0000000000012784.

461. Jeong H, Shin J, Jeong JH, Kim KP, Hong SM, Kim YI, Ryu JS, Ryoo BY, Yoo C. Capecitabine plus temozolomide in patients with grade 3 unresectable or metastatic gastroenteropancreatic neuroendocrine neoplasms with Ki-67 index <55%: single-arm phase II study. ESMO Open. 2021;6(3):100119. https://doi.org/10.1016/j.esmoop.2021.100119.

462. Iwasa S, Morizane C, Okusaka T, Ueno H, Ikeda M, Kondo S, Tanaka T, Nakachi K, Mitsunaga S, Kojima Y, Hagihara A, Hiraoka N. Cisplatin and etoposide as first-line chemotherapy for poorly differentiated neuroendocrine carcinoma of the hepatobiliary tract and pancreas. Jpn J Clin Oncol. 2010;40(4):313–8. https://doi.org/10.1093/jjco/hyp173.

463. Patta A, Fakih M. First-line cisplatin plus etoposide in high-grade metastatic neuroendocrine tumors of colon and Rectum (MCRC NET): review of 8 cases. Anticancer Res. 2011;31(3):975–8.

464. NCT03963193 (2019) Etoposide/Cisplatin Compared With Irinotecan/Cisplatin for Advanced Gastrointestinal Neuroendocrine Tumor G3 Type. Clinical Trials. Available in: https://clinicaltrials.gov/ct2/show/NCT03963193. Accessed Sep 2 2021.

465. Damayanthi Y, Lown JW. Podophyllotoxins: current status and recent developments. Curr Med Chem. 1998;5(3):205–52.

466. Baldwin EL, Osheroff N. Etoposide, topoisomerase II and cancer. Curr Med Chem Anticancer Agents. 2005;5(4):363–72. https://doi.org/10.2174/1568011054222364.

467. Dasari S, Tchounwou PB. Cisplatin in cancer therapy: molecular mechanisms of action. Eur J Pharmacol. 2014;740:364–78. https://doi.org/10.1016/j.ejphar.2014.07.025.

468. Montecucco A, Zanetta F, Biamonti G. Molecular mechanisms of etoposide. EXCLI J. 2015;14:95–108. https://doi.org/10.17179/excli2015-561.

469. Soranzo C, Pratesi G, Zunino F. Different interaction of cisplatin and etoposide on in vivo and in vitro tumor systems. Anti-Cancer Drugs. 1990;1(1):23–8. https://doi.org/10.1097/00001813-199010000-00004.

470. Mitry E, Baudin E, Ducreux M, Sabourin JC, Rufié P, Aparicio T, Lasser P, Elias D, Duvillard P, Schlumberger M, Rougier P. Treatment of poorly differentiated neuroendocrine tumours with etoposide and cisplatin. Br J Cancer. 1999;81:1351–5. https://doi.org/10.1038/sj.bjc.6690325.

471. Fjallskog ML, Granberg DP, Welin SL, Eriksson C, Oberg KE, Janson ET, Eriksson BK. Treatment with cisplatin and etoposide in patients with neuroendocrine tumors. Cancer. 2001;92(5):1101–7. https://doi.org/10.1002/1097-0142(20010901)92:5<1101::aid-cncr1426>3.0.co;2-v.

472. Yoon SE, Kim JH, Lee SJ, Lee J, Park SH, Park JO, Lim HY, Kang WK, Park YS, Kim ST. The impact of primary tumor site on outcomes of treatment with etoposide and cisplatin in grade 3 gastroenteropancreatic neuroendocrine carcinoma. J Cancer. 2019;10(14):3140–4. https://doi.org/10.7150/jca.30355.

473. Delaunoit T, Ducreux M, Boige V, Dromain C, Sabourin JC, Duvillard P, Schlumberger M, Baere T, Rougier P, Ruffie P, Elias D, Lasser P, Baudin E. The doxorubicin-streptozotocin combination for the treatment of advanced well-differentiated pancreatic endocrine carcinoma: a judicious option? Eur J Cancer. 2004;40(4):515–20. https://doi.org/10.1016/j.ejca.2003.09.035.

474. Thorn CF, Oshiro C, Marsh S, Hernandez-Boussard T, McLeod H, Klein TE, Altman RB. Doxorubicin pathways: pharmacodynamics and adverse effects. Pharmacogenet Genomics. 2011;21(7):440–6. https://doi.org/10.1097/FPC.0b013e32833ffb56.

475. Edwardson DW, Narendrula R, Chewchuk S, Mispel-Beyer K, Mapletoft JPJ, Parissenti AM. Role of drug metabolism in the cytotoxicity and clinical efficacy of anthracyclines. Curr Drug Metab. 2015;16(6):412–26. https://doi.org/10.2174/1389200216888150915112039.

476. Krug S, Boch M, Daniel H, Nimphius W, Muller D, Michl P, Rinke A, Gress TM. Streptozocin-based chemotherapy in patients with advanced neuroendocrine neoplasms—predictive and

prognostic markers for treatment stratification. PLoS One. 2015;10(12):e0143822. https://doi.org/10.1371/journal.pone.0143822.

477. Al Nahdi AMT, John A, Raza H. Elucidation of molecular mechanisms of Streptozotocin-induced oxidative stress, apoptosis, and mitochondrial dysfunction in Rin-5F pancreatic β-cells. Oxidative Med Cell Longev. 2017;2017:7054272. https://doi.org/10.1155/2017/7054272.

478. Palmieri LJ, Dermine S, Barré A, Dhooge M, Brezault C, Cottereau AS, Coriat R. Medical treatment of advanced pancreatic neuroendocrine neoplasms. J Clin Med. 2020;9(6):1860. https://doi.org/10.3390/jcm9061860.

479. Pavel ME, Baum U, Hahn EG, Hensen J. Doxorubicin and streptozotocin after failed biotherapy of neuroendocrine tumors. Int J Gastrointest Cancer. 2005;35:179–85. https://doi.org/10.1385/IJGC:35:3:179.

480. Fjallskog MLH, Janson ET, Falkmer UG, Vatn MH, Oberg KE, Eriksson BK. Treatment with combined Streptozotocin and liposomal doxorubicin in metastatic endocrine pancreatic tumors. Neuroendocrinology. 2008;88:53–8. https://doi.org/10.1159/000117575.

481. Eriksson B, Annibale B, Bajetta E, Mitry E, Pavel M, Platania M, Salazar R, Plockinger U. ENETS consensus guidelines for the standards of care in neuroendocrine tumors: chemotherapy in patients with neuroendocrine tumors. Neuroendocrinology. 2009;90:214–9. https://doi.org/10.1159/000225950.

482. BC Cancer (2019) BC Cancer Protocol Summary for Palliative Therapy for Pancreatic Endocrine Tumours using Streptozocin and DOXOrubicin. BC Cancer. British Columbia. Available in: http://www.bccancer.bc.ca/chemotherapy-protocols-site/Documents/Gastrointestinal/GIENDO2_Protocol.pdf. Accessed Sep 2 2021.

483. Moscicki AB, Darragh TM, Berry-Lawhorn JM, Roberts JM, Khan MJ, Boardman LA, Chiao E, Einstein MH, Goldstone SE, Jay N, Likes WM, Stier EA, Welton ML, Wiley DJ, Palefsky JM. Screening for anal cancer in women. J Low Genit Tract Dis. 2015;19(3):S26–41. https://doi.org/10.1097/LGT.0000000000000117.

484. American Cancer Society (2021) Key statistics for anal cancer. The American Cancer Society. Georgia. USA. Available in: https://www.cancer.org/cancer/anal-cancer/about/what-is-key-statistics.html. Accessed Sep 2 2021.

485. Nelson VM, Benson AB. Epidemiology of Anal Canal cancer. Surg Oncol Clin N Am. 2017;26:9–15. https://doi.org/10.1016/j.soc.2016.07.001.

486. Gautier M, Brochard C, Lion A, Henno S, Mallet AL, Bodere A, Bouguen G, Lièvre A, Siproudhis L. High-grade anal intraepithelial neoplasia: progression to invasive cancer is not a certainty. Dig Liver Dis. 2016;48(7):806–11. https://doi.org/10.1016/j.dld.2016.03.011.

487. Roberts JR, Siekas LL, Kaz AM. Anal intraepithelial neoplasia: a review of diagnosis and management. World J Gastrointest Oncol. 2017;9(2):50–61. https://doi.org/10.4251/wjgo.v9.i2.50.

488. Stewart DB, Gaertner WB, Glasgow SC, Herzig DO, Feingold D, Steele SR. The American Society of Colon and Rectal Surgeons clinical practice guidelines for anal squamous cell cancers (revised 2018). Dis Colon Rectum. 2018;61:755–74. https://doi.org/10.1097/DCR.0000000000001114.

489. Babiker HM, Kashyap S, Mehta SR, Lekkala MR, Cagir B. Anal Cancer. Treasure Island USA: StatPearls Publishing; 2021.

490. Wietfeldt ED, Thiele J. Malignancies of the anal margin and perianal skin. Clin Colon Rectal Surg. 2009;22(2):127–35. https://doi.org/10.1055/s-0029-1223845.

491. American Cancer Society (2020) Treatment of Anal Cancer, by Stage. The American Cancer Society. Georgia. USA. Available in: https://www.cancer.org/cancer/anal-cancer/treating/by-stage.html. Accessed Sep 3 2021.

492. Pawlowski J, Jones WE. Radiation therapy for anal cancer. Treasure Island USA: StatPearls Publishing; 2020.

493. Doci R, Zucali R, La Monica G, Meroni E, Kanda R, Eboli M, Lozza L. Primary chemoradiation therapy with fluorouracil and cisplatin for cancer of the anus: results in 35 consecutive patients. J Clin Oncol. 1996;14(12):3121–5. https://doi.org/10.1200/JCO.1996.14.12.3121.

494. Eng C, Chang GJ, You YN, Das P, Rodriguez-Bigas M, Xing Y, Vauthey JN, Rogers JE, Ohinata A, Pathak P, Sethi S, Phillips JK, Crane CH, Wolff RA. The role of systemic chemotherapy and multidisciplinary management in improving the overall survival of patients with metastatic squamous cell carcinoma of the anal canal. Oncotarget. 2014;5:11133–42. https://doi.org/10.18632/oncotarget.2563.

495. Zampino MG, Magni E, Leonardi MC, Santoro L, Petazzi E, Fodor C, Petralia G, Trovato C, Nolè F, Orecchia R. Concurrent cisplatin, continuous infusion fluorouracil and radiotherapy followed by tailored consolidation treatment in non metastatic anal squamous cell carcinoma. BMC Cancer. 2011;11:55. https://doi.org/10.1186/1471-2407-11-55.

496. Kim R, Byer J, Fulp WJ, Mahipal A, Dinwoodie W, Shibata D. Carboplatin and paclitaxel treatment is effective in advanced anal cancer. Oncology. 2014;87(2):125–32. https://doi.org/10.1159/000361051.

497. Rotundo MS, Zampino MG, Ravenda OS, Bagnardi V, Peveri G, Dell'Acqua V, Surgo A, Trovato C, Bottiglieri L, Bertani E, Petz WL, Romario UF, Fazio N. Cisplatin plus capecitabine concomitant with intensity-modulated radiation therapy in non-metastatic anal squamous cell carcinoma: the experience of a single research cancer center. Ther Adv Med Oncol. 2020;12:1–14. https://doi.org/10.1177/1758835920940945.

498. Ajani JA, Winter KA, Gunderson LL, Pedersen J, Benson AB, Thomas CR, Mayer RJ, Haddock MG, Rich TA, Willett C. Fluorouracil, Mitomycin, and radiotherapy vs fluorouracil, cisplatin, and radiotherapy for carcinoma of the Anal Canal: a randomized controlled trial. JAMA. 2008;299(16):1914–21. https://doi.org/10.1001/jama.299.16.1914.

499. NCT01858025 (2019) Concurrent chemoradiation + 5-FU + Mitomycin-C in Anal Carcinoma. Clinical Trials. Available in: https://clinicaltrials.gov/ct2/show/NCT01858025. Accessed Sep 3 2021.

500. Snodgrass RG, Collier AC, Coon AE, Pritsos CA. Mitomycin C inhibits ribosomal RNA: a novel cytotoxic mechanism for bioreductive drugs. J Biol Chem. 2010;285(25):19068–75. https://doi.org/10.1074/jbc.M109.040477.

501. Gao Y, Shang Q, Li W, Guo W, Stojadinovic A, Mannion C, Man YG, Chen T. Antibiotics for cancer treatment: a double-edged sword. J Cancer. 2020;11(17):5135–49. https://doi.org/10.7150/jca.47470.

502. Hofheinz RD, Hartmann JT, Willer A, Oechsle K, Hartung G, Gnad U, Saussele S, Kreil S, Bokemeyer C, Hehlmann R, Hochhaus A. Capecitabine in combination with mitomycin C in patients with gastrointestinal cancer: results of an extended multicentre phase-I trial. Br J Cancer. 2004;91(5):834–8. https://doi.org/10.1038/sj.bjc.6602025.

503. Saint A, Evesque L, Falk AT, Cavaglione G, Montagne L, Benezery K, Francois E. Mitomycin and 5-fluorouracil for second-line treatment of metastatic squamous cell carcinomas of the anal canal. Cancer Med. 2019;8(16):6853–9. https://doi.org/10.1002/cam4.2558.

504. NHS (2020) Chemotherapy Protocol. Colorectal Cancer. Fluorouracil-mitomycin-radiotherapy. NHS. University Hospital Southampton. NHS Foundation Trust. England. Available in: https://www.uhs.nhs.uk/Media/SUHTExtranet/Services/Chemotherapy-SOPs/Colorectal/Fluorouracil-Mitomycin-Radiotherapy.pdf. Accessed Sep 3 2021.

505. Thind G, Johal B, Follwell M, Kennecke HF. Chemoradiation with capecitabine and mitomycin-C for stage I-III anal squamous cell carcinoma. Radiat Oncol. 2014;9:124. https://doi.org/10.1186/1748-717X-9-124.

506. Goodman KA, Julie D, Cercek A, Cambridge L, Woo KM, Zhang Z, Wu AJ, Reidy DL, Segal NH, Stadler ZK, Saltz LB. Capecitabine with Mitomycin reduces acute hematologic toxicity and treatment delays in patients undergoing definitive Chemoradiation using intensity modulated radiation therapy for anal cancer. Int J Radiat Oncol Biol Phys. 2017;98(5):1087–95. https://doi.org/10.1016/j.ijrobp.2017.03.022.

507. Meulendijks D, Dewit L, Tomasoa NB, van Tinteren H, Beijnen JH, Schellens JHM, Cats A. Chemoradiotherapy with capecitabine for locally advanced anal carcinoma: an alternative treatment option. Br J Cancer. 2014;111:1726–33. https://doi.org/10.1038/bjc.2014.467.
508. Peixoto RD, Wan DD, Schellenberg D, Lim HJ. A comparison between 5-fluorouracil/mitomycin and capecitabine/mitomycin in combination with radiation for anal cancer. J Gastrointest Oncol. 2016;7(4):665–72. https://doi.org/10.21037/jgo.2016.06.04.
509. NHS (2020) Chemotherapy Protocol. Anal Cancer. Capecitabine-mitomycin-radiotherapy. NHS. University Hospital Southampton. NHS Foundation Trust. England. Available in: https://www.uhs.nhs.uk/Media/SUHTExtranet/Services/Chemotherapy-SOPs/Colorectal/Capecitabine-Mitomycin-Radiotherpy.pdf. Accessed Sep 3 2021.

Chapter 6
Chemotherapeutic Protocols for the Treatment of Genitourinary Cancer

6.1 Epidemiological Profile of Genitourinary Cancers

Genitourinary cancers involve the genitals and urinary organs in men and the urinary organs in women. Cancers such as those in the penis, testicle, scrotum and adrenal cortex, prostate, bladder, kidney, renal pelvis, ureter, and urethra are part of genitourinary cancers. Among genitourinary cancers, prostate cancer is the most incident where 1.41 million cases were reported worldwide in 2020 according to the World Health Organization (WHO), followed by bladder cancer with 573,000 cases in 2020. As for the mortality rate, prostate cancer is also in the first place with 375,000 deaths and bladder cancer in second with 213,000 deaths [1–5]. Figure 6.1 presents the estimated data for 2040 of incidence of cases and mortality of genitourinary cancers.

Genitourinary cancers can occur at any age and in both sexes, accounting for about 42% of cancers in men and 4% in women. In men, prostate cancer has the highest estimated incidence and mortality, while penile cancer affects a small portion of the population, despite being more aggressive. While prostate and penile tumors have a higher incidence in patients over 50 years old, testicular cancer is usually present in men between 15 and 39 years old, being one of the most curable cancers [5, 6].

In women, kidney cancer was the most frequent in 2020, with 160,000 cases, followed by bladder cancer with 132,000 cases. The mortality rate is also higher for kidney cancer in women with 63,800 deaths, and bladder cancer was responsible for 53,800 deaths [5].

I. D. Lima Cavalcanti, *Chemotherapy Protocols and Infusion Sequence*,
https://doi.org/10.1007/978-3-031-10839-6_6

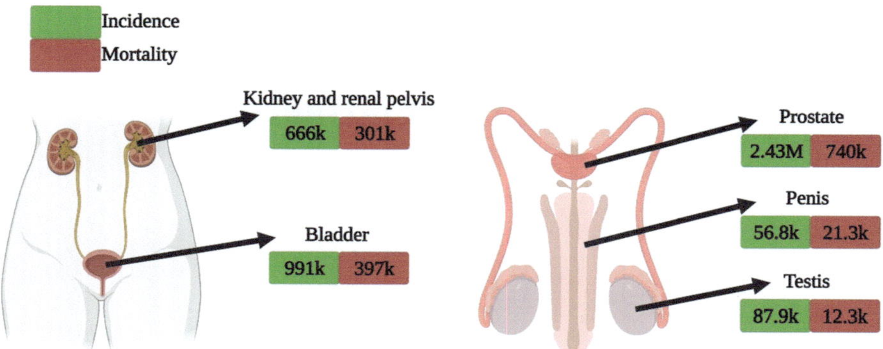

Fig. 6.1 Estimate data for the year 2040 of incidence of cases and mortality of genitourinary cancers. (Source: Created with BioRender.com. and data were extracted from [5])

6.2 Pathophysiology of Bladder Cancer

Bladder cancer is more common in men than in women worldwide, with an incidence in 2020 in men of 441,000 cases and women of 132,000 cases [5]. It is believed that the main risk factor for bladder cancer is tobacco consumption. Bladder cancer is the tenth most common cancer worldwide and the 13th deadliest, accounting for 2.1% of all cancer deaths. The 5-year survival rate in the USA is 77.1%, with a 5-year survival rate in cases diagnosed in situ at 95.8%, falling to 69.5% for localized disease, 36.3% for regional disease, and 4.6% in metastatic disease [7–9].

Cumberbatch et al. [10] found some evidence on gene-environment interactions in the development of bladder cancer, especially in smoking and occupational exposure to chemicals. The authors note that incidence rates in some populations are likely to be declining as a result of decreasing smoking. Wong et al. [11] believe that the global incidence of bladder cancer was increasing, being positively correlated with the country's socioeconomic development, but the mortality rate seems to decrease.

The development of bladder cancer is related to two pathways, the invasive pathway and the non-invasive papillary pathway, where the urothelium is the epithelial layer that gives rise to the papillary pathway, which is composed of basal, intermediate, and umbrella cells which are responsible for the lining of the bladder tissue. In the urothelium stem cells are present that have a capacity for self-renewal, thus being more susceptible to the development of cancer. Genetic alterations, such as mutations in the fibroblast growth factor receptor 3 (FGFR3) and the Harvey rat sarcoma viral oncogene (HRAS), can induce the development of cancer with the growth of the hyperplastic urothelium toward the bladder lumen [12–17].

Among the types of bladder cancer, urothelial carcinoma is the most common, which originates in the urothelial cells that border the interior of the bladder, as well as part of the kidney, ureters, and urethra. Other less frequent bladder cancers are

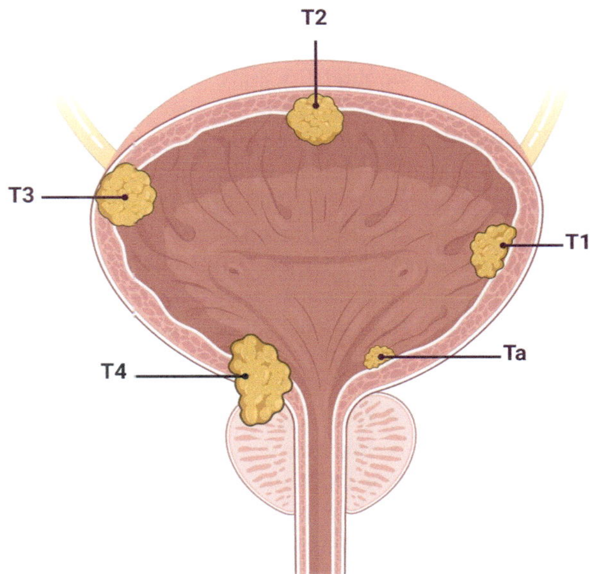

Fig. 6.2 Bladder tumor classification according to size. (Source: Created with BioRender.com)

squamous cell carcinoma, adenocarcinoma, small cell carcinoma, and sarcoma. Bladder cancers are classified as invasive that grow in the lamina propria or deeper muscle layer, which are more likely to spread to other organs and/or tissues, and noninvasive tumors that are located in the inner layer of cells of the bladder transitional epithelium but do not invade the deeper layers [18–22].

Regarding the tumor size, noninvasive papillary tumors (Ta) are tumors contained in the inner layer of the bladder, whereas stage I bladder cancer are tumors that grew in the connective tissue layer of the bladder wall, being classified as T1. When the tumor invades the muscle layer of the bladder wall, they are classified as T2, while T3 are tumors that have reached the outside of the bladder and can grow in adjacent tissues and/or lymph nodes and spread to other organs, being classified as T4 [23–24]. Figure 6.2 presents the tumor classification according to size.

6.2.1   Chemotherapy for the Treatment of Bladder Cancer

The treatment of bladder cancer is based on the stage of the disease, in which stages 0 and 1, noninvasive papillary carcinoma and carcinoma in situ, can be treated with transurethral resection, and partial or radical cystectomy may also be indicated. Chemotherapy can also be indicated in stages 0 and 1, with intravesical chemotherapy after a surgical procedure [25–28]. Intravesical chemotherapy is based on administering the antineoplastic agent directly into the bladder, through a catheter. Intravesical administration is indicated in cancers that line the inside of the bladder, without inducing major side effects in other regions of the body [29–30].

In stages 2 and 3 of bladder cancer, radical or partial cystectomy and transurethral resection may also be indicated. External radiotherapy and combined chemotherapy are also two modality that can be used in stages 2 and 3 [31–34]. In stage 4, without the spread of the tumor to other organs, treatment modalities include chemotherapy, radical cystectomy, and external radiotherapy, and urinary diversion can also be indicated as palliative therapy for symptom relief. In metastatic bladder cancer, in addition to the treatment modalities already mentioned in the other stages of the disease, it may also include immunotherapy [28, 32, 35].

As isolated therapy, pembrolizumab, which is a monoclonal antibody, may be indicated for the treatment of locally advanced or metastatic urothelial carcinoma [36], and BCG as a treatment for high-risk superficial transitional cell bladder cancer [37–38] and cisplatin in the treatment of locally advanced bladder cancer with associated radiotherapy [32, 39]. Gemcitabine and mitomycin can be used as intravesical therapy in non-muscle invasive bladder cancer [40–41].

Combination chemotherapy may also be indicated, where some protocols used in the treatment of cancers of the gastrointestinal tract, such as the combination of cisplatin and gemcitabine (Chap. 5, Sect. 5.4.1.1) have been indicated as neoadjuvant, adjuvant, and palliative therapy of urothelial carcinoma [42–47].

6.2.1.1 BCGIFN Protocol (BCG and Interferon)

As palliative therapy for refractory high-grade superficial transitional cell carcinoma of the bladder, one option is a combination of BCG and interferon [48–51]. BCG is composed of the bacillus Calmette-Guérin which is a bacterium that causes tuberculosis, but this bacillus is attenuated. In bladder cancer, BCG is administered directly into the bladder, where it will stimulate the immune system, which will be attracted to the bladder and activated by BCG, thereby affecting cancer cells in the bladder [52–53].

Interferon, like BCG, also stimulates the immune system, intending to increase the ability of immune cells to attack cancer cells, as well as retarding their growth. Interferons are glycoproteins that are part of the class of cytokines to which they are secreted by immune system cells, acting as immune response modulators by stimulating the proliferation and anticellular toxicity of other immune system cells such as macrophages and NK cells (natural killer) [54–58].

The combination of BCG with interferon has brought positive results in the treatment of non-muscle invasive bladder cancer refractory to BCG. Correa et al. [51] highlight that the combination promoted a recurrence-free survival of 38.6% at 12 months and 18.2% at 24 months, showing that the combination appears to be a reasonable alternative in the treatment of bladder cancer. The inclusion of interferon seems to enhance the effects of BCG, contributing to its therapeutic efficacy [49, 59].

O'Donnell, Lilli, and Leopold [48] performed a phase II study combining BCG and interferon in the treatment of superficial bladder cancer. As a result, the authors observed a simple tumor recurrence rate of 52%, with progression to muscle invasion of 4.3% and serious adverse events less prevalent than treatment with BCG as

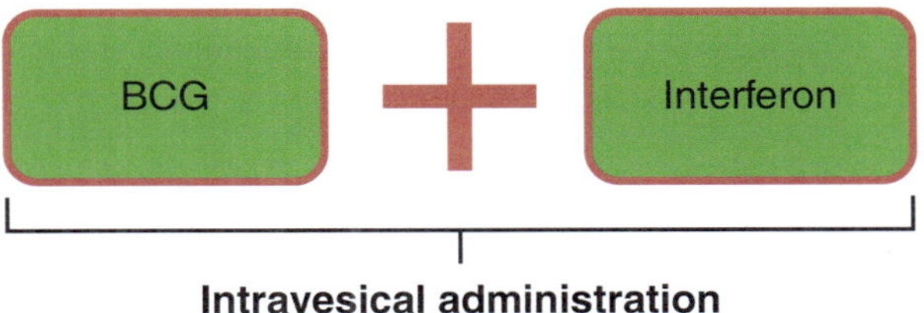

Fig. 6.3 BCGIFN protocol administration schedule

monotherapy. The combination has been shown to be safe and effective as initial and rescue therapy for superficial bladder cancer.

Downs, Szilvasi, and O'Donnell [60] observed the compatibility of the concomitant administration of interferon and BCG via the intravesical route. The authors observed that the combined administration did not inhibit the pharmacological activity of any of the drugs, nor did it induce the formation of clusters, showing that the drugs are compatible.

Administration of the BCGIFN protocol occurs intravesically of both drugs concurrently through an empty bladder catheter with a 2-h bladder residence time (Fig. 6.3) [61].

6.2.1.2   GEMDOC Protocol (Gemcitabine and Docetaxel)

Another combination that can be used as intravesical therapy for non-muscle invasive bladder cancer is gemcitabine plus docetaxel [62–64]. Steinberg et al. [62] evaluated the combination of sequential intravesical gemcitabine and docetaxel as intravesical therapy in the treatment of non-muscle invasive bladder cancer. Results were promising with treatment success of 66% at first surveillance, 54% at 1 year, and 34% at 2 years.

Milbar et al. [63], as well as Steinberg et al. [62], also evaluated the effectiveness of the combination in non-muscle invasive bladder cancer. The authors did not observe serious adverse effects, proving to be a well-tolerated protocol, with median disease-free survival of 6.5 months and median high-grade recurrence-free survival of 17.1 months.

Thomas et al. [65] evaluated the GEMDOC protocol in BCG-naive non-muscle invasive bladder cancer patients. The authors noted that the protocol promoted treatment success of 96% at 3 months, 89% at 1 year, and 89% at 2 years. In addition, the protocol was well tolerated with side effects that included urinary urgency/frequency, dysuria, and hematuria.

In a more recent study, Steinberg et al. [66] evaluated the effectiveness of the combination of gemcitabine and docetaxel in the salvage treatment for non-muscle invasive bladder cancer in several institutions. The protocol promoted a 1-year recurrence-free survival rate of 60% and 2 years of 46% and a high-grade 1-year recurrence-free survival rate of 65% and 2 years of 52%, proving to be a therapy

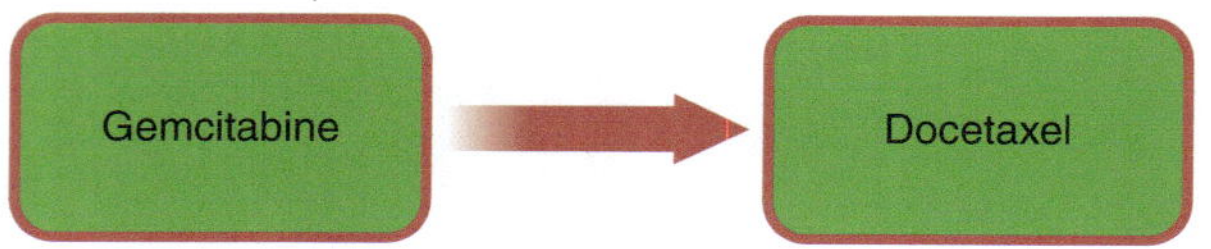

Fig. 6.4 Intravesical administration schedule of the GEMDOC protocol

well-tolerated and effective for the treatment of recurrent non-muscle invasive bladder cancer, providing a durable response.

As for the sequence of administration, it starts with the intravesical administration of gemcitabine with a residence time of 1 to 2 h followed by the administration of docetaxel also by intravesical route with a residence time of 1 to 2 h (Fig. 6.4) [67].

6.2.1.3 MVAC Protocol (Methotrexate, Vinblastine, Doxorubicin, and Cisplatin)

The MVAC protocol combines methotrexate, vinblastine, doxorubicin, and cisplatin in the treatment of transitional cell urothelium cancer [68–70]. Methotrexate, doxorubicin, and cisplatin are three antineoplastics widely used in cancer treatment, as we saw in Chapters 4 and 5, the inclusion of these drugs in protocols for the treatment of breast cancer and cancers of the gastrointestinal tract. Vinblastine, on the other hand, is a natural compound that is part of the vinca alkaloids class; it acts by inhibiting the polymerization of mitotic spindle proteins, preventing the formation of microtubules and thus interrupting cell division in metaphase [71–72].

Sternberg et al. [73] observed that the MVAC protocol in advanced transitional cell carcinoma of the urothelium, promoting complete remission in 37 ± 10% of patients, with an estimated 2-year survival probability of 71% and a 3-year survival probability of 55%. According to another study by Sternberg et al. [74], the combination induced significant tumor regression of 72%, with complete remission of 36%; of those patients who achieved complete remission, 68% relapsed, but the median survival will exceed 38 months compared to patients who responded partial (11 months of median survival).

In advanced urothelial cancer, Ueki et al. [75] found that the combination promoted complete remission in 14% of patients and partial remission in 48% of patients. As for the toxicity profile, the authors observed moderate to severe myelosuppression, mild nausea and vomiting, and moderate renal toxicity and mucositis.

Han et al. [69] evaluated the efficacy and safety of the MVAC protocol in advanced or metastatic transitional cell carcinoma after failure of the combination of gemcitabine and cisplatin. Patients presented neutropenia and thrombocytopenia as the main toxic effects of the protocol. The protocol provided an overall response of 30%, an overall disease control rate of 50%, overall survival of 10.9 months, and progression-free survival of 5.3 months.

Kim et al. [76] also evaluated the efficacy of the MVAC protocol after gemcitabine and platinum failure in advanced urothelial cancer. The protocol promoted

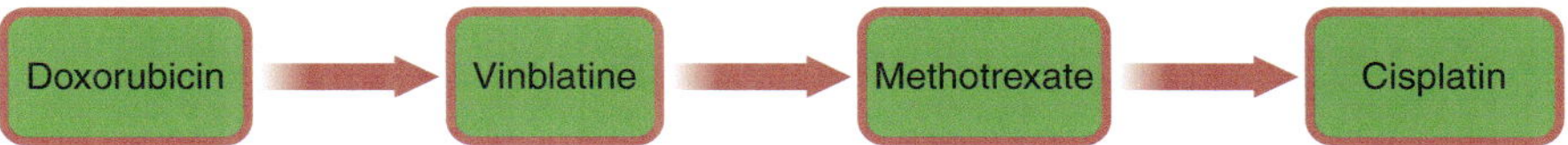

Fig. 6.5 MVAC protocol infusion sequence

a progression-free survival of 6.5 months and overall survival of 14.5 months, with an overall response rate of 57.8%. Choueiri et al. [70] evaluated the efficacy of a combination of methotrexate, vinblastine, doxorubicin, and cisplatin in muscle-invasive urothelial cancer. The protocol promoted a disease-free survival of 89% at 1 year and pathological response in 49% of patients.

The infusion sequence of the MVAC protocol is based on the initial infusion of vesicant drugs, doxorubicin followed by vinblastine since vinblastine can increase the metabolism of doxorubicin; in addition, care must be taken as the association of vinblastine with doxorubicin can increase the risk of thromboembolism [77–79].

After the infusion of vinblastine, the infusion of methotrexate follows; the association of these drugs can increase myelosuppression, as well as the combination with doxorubicin. Finally, cisplatin is infused, when associated with vinblastine, it can increase the risk of ototoxicity. The combination of methotrexate may increase the risk of myelosuppression, as well as may increase the risk of nephrotoxicity, and the patient's renal function should be evaluated [80–84]. Figure 6.5 shows the MVAC protocol infusion sequence.

6.3   Pathophysiology of Prostate Cancer

Prostate cancer is the second most frequent malignant disease in men, second only to lung cancer, and is responsible for the fifth leading cause of death worldwide. The incidence rate appears to be higher in African-American men than in White men, but mortality in White men is higher [85–87]. The incidence rate of prostate cancer has greatly increased since the 1980s/early 1990s due to the inclusion of prostate-specific antigen (PSA) testing in the asymptomatic detection of prostate cancer [88–90].

Prostate cancer can be asymptomatic in its early stage and may require minimal treatment or even no treatment, just medical follow-up. As for symptoms, one of the complaints is the difficulty to urinate, where the more advanced stage of the disease can induce urinary retention and back pain since one of the most common sites of prostate cancer metastasis is in the bones [86, 91].

The inclusion of the PSA test in the diagnosis of prostate cancer allows the assessment of plasma levels of the prostate-specific antigen, where above 4 ng/mL may be an indication of prostate cancer and should be evaluated with other parameters, such as the biopsy of the prostate tissue needed in confirming the presence of cancer [91–93].

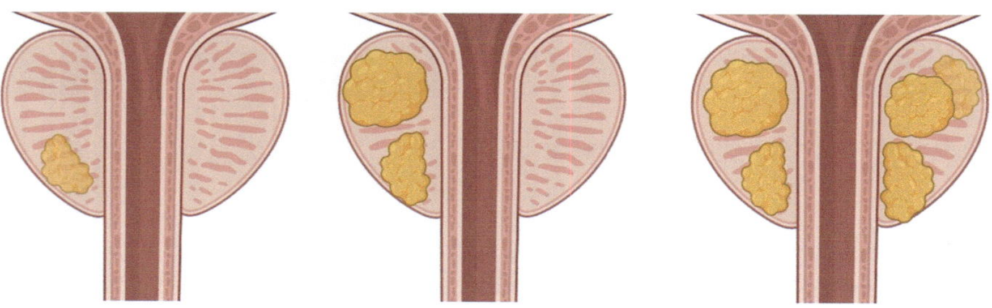

Fig. 6.6 Evolution in the development of prostate cancer. (Source: Created with BioRender.com)

Prostate cancer starts from a mutation in normal prostate gland cells, usually starting in peripheral basal cells. The peripheral zone is the most common region in the development of prostate cancer. Because it develops in the glandular part, prostate cancer is an adenocarcinoma that initially spreads to the prostate tissue forming a tumor nodule, which can grow outside the prostate or remain in the prostate for decades. When it metastasis, prostate cancer can invade bones and lymph nodes [91, 94–95]. Figure 6.6 shows the progression of prostate cancer.

6.3.1   Chemotherapy for the Treatment of Prostate Cancer

The treatment option for prostate cancer will depend on the stage of cancer, the age of the patient, and the patient's clinical condition [96–97]. The treatment modality includes surgery, radiotherapy, hormonal therapy, chemotherapy, and immunotherapy, among others [91, 98–99]. In stage 1 cancer is found only in the prostate, not being felt by rectal examination, being found by biopsy, and due to high levels of PSA. Stage 1 treatment can be based on medical monitoring and observing whether cancer will grow; if yes, hormone therapy may be indicated; radiotherapy and radical prostatectomy may also be indicated [100–104].

In stage 2 the cancer is more advanced than in stage 1, but it has not spread outside the prostate. The medical approach in stage 2 is similar to that in stage 1, and hormone therapy, radiotherapy, and surgery may be indicated. In stage 3 cancer can be found on both sides of the prostate and may have spread to the seminal vesicles or nearby tissues or organs such as the rectum, bladder, or pelvic wall. The treatment of stage 3 prostate cancer is based on external radiotherapy, hormone therapy, and radical prostatectomy where radiotherapy can be indicated after the surgical procedure [104–106].

In stage 4 cancer has already spread to other organs such as bones or distant lymph nodes, where treatment can be based on hormonal therapy combined with chemotherapy—the use of bisphosphonate drugs and radiotherapy are the main treatment modalities [96, 104].

The ease of treatment for prostate cancer is that most drugs are given orally, including abiraterone in the treatment of metastatic castration-sensitive prostate cancer and as palliative therapy for metastatic castration-resistant prostate cancer, darolutamide, apalutamide, and enzalutamide in the treatment of nonmetastatic castration-resistant prostate cancer [107–109].

A group of drugs used in the treatment of prostate cancer is luteinizing hormone-releasing hormone (LHRH) receptor agonists whose function is to reduce testosterone levels, such as goserelin, leuprolide, or buserelin. LHRH antagonists such as degarelix are used in the treatment of advanced prostate cancer [110–113].

Some indicated anticancer drugs include cabazitaxel, which is given intravenously and indicated as palliative therapy for metastatic castration-resistant prostate cancer [114, 115]. Docetaxel which is widely used in cancer treatment is indicated as palliative monotherapy for metastatic hormone-refractory prostate cancer and as first-line in castration-sensitive metastatic prostate cancer and mitoxantrone in palliative therapy for hormone-refractory prostate cancer [116, 117].

6.4   Testicular Cancer

Of all cancers that affect men, testicular cancer is responsible for 1 to 2% of cases. Although rare, testicular cancers are the most common in young people between 15 and 35 years old. The incidence rate in young White men is ten times higher than Black and Asian men. The most common type is testicular germ cell cancers, of which there are two main types, seminomas and non-seminomatous germ cell tumors [118–121]. Figure 6.7 shows testicular cancer.

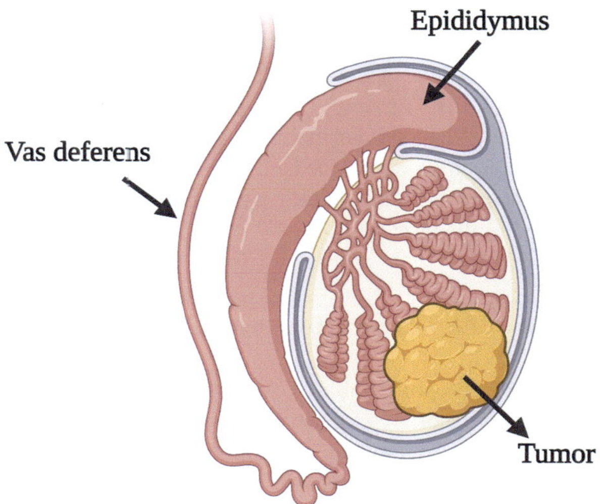

Fig. 6.7 Testicular cancer. (Source: Created with BioRender.com)

Seminomas are more incidents in men aged 20 to 35 years, which mostly tend to grow and spread more slowly than non-seminomas and can secrete human chorionic gonadotropin (HCG), presenting less aggressive behavior and are sensitive radiotherapy [122–124]. On the other hand, non-seminomatous testicular cancers present variations in appearance and prognosis, affect young people between 15 and 35 years of age, are more aggressive, thermosensitive, and have little radiosensitive. Non-seminomatous tumors are classified as embryonic carcinoma (rapid growing and potentially aggressive, may secrete HCG or alpha-fetoprotein (AFP)), yolk sac carcinoma (but common in children, almost always secrete AFP), choriocarcinoma (rare and aggressive, may secreting HCG), and teratoma [122, 124, 125].

Metastases are more common in non-seminomatous tumors, in which the main dissemination is via the lymphatic route, and may reach cord vessels, with the appearance of periaortic lymphadenopathy at the level of the renal vessels. The spread of testicular cancer can affect organs such as the lungs, liver, and brain [126–128].

6.4.1 Chemotherapy for the Treatment of Testicular Cancer

Concerning the treatment of testicular cancer, radical orchiectomy is a primary treatment method. Post-surgical treatment will depend on the histological type of tumor, serum marker levels, and disease stage, in addition to the presence of residual retroperitoneal masses. Some testicular tumors respond well to chemotherapy, such as yolk sac carcinoma, while other tumors, such as teratoma, are resistant to chemotherapy and radiotherapy, the best approach being surgical removal [129–132].

Monotherapy may be indicated as adjuvant treatment in stage 1 high-risk seminoma using carboplatin, but combined chemotherapy is more common in disseminated tumors and may be associated with radiotherapy [133–135]. Some protocols indicated for the treatment of other cancers may also be indicated for the treatment of testicular cancer; an example is the ETCIS protocol (Chap. 5, Sect. 5.6.1.1) which combines etoposide and cisplatin in the treatment of non-seminoma germ cell cancer [136–138]. Other protocols [45–47] used in testicular cancer will be covered in the next topics.

6.4.1.1 BEP Protocol (Bleomycin, Etoposide, and Cisplatin)

The BEP protocol combines bleomycin, etoposide, and cisplatin and has been used as a curative therapy in germ cell cancer [139–142]. As we saw in Chap. 5, cisplatin is an alkylating agent that interconnects to DNA, while etoposide is a semi-synthetic derivative of podophyllotoxin that acts by inhibiting topoisomerase II, with both

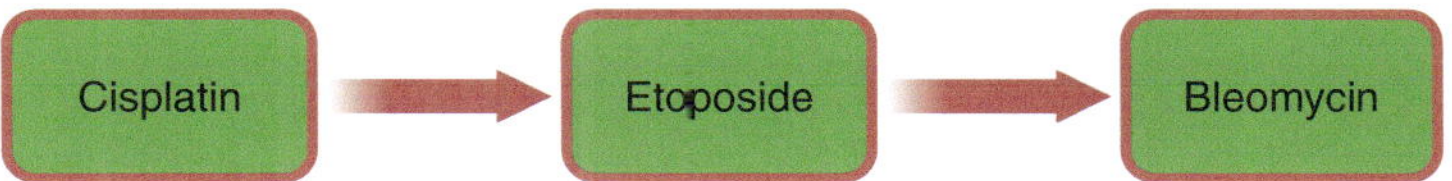

Fig. 6.8 BEP protocol infusion sequence

drugs inhibiting DNA synthesis. Bleomycin is an antineoplastic antibiotic, whose action is also at the DNA level, in which bleomycin binds to the DNA of tumor cells, inducing the breaking of the DNA strands and preventing cell division [143, 144].

Behnia et al. [140] evaluated the effectiveness of the BEP protocol in the treatment of non-seminomatous testicular cancer. The protocol proved to be effective in preventing recurrence after two cycles of the BEP protocol in fully resected stage II patients. As for toxicity, 10% of patients developed granulocytopenic fever. Horwich et al. [139] also observed the efficacy of the BEP protocol in the treatment of metastatic non-seminoma testis cancer with a good prognosis, in which 94.4% of patients achieved a complete response.

Kier et al. [145] evaluated the effectiveness of the BEP protocol in germ cell cancer. As a result, the authors evidenced a 5-year progression-free survival of 87%, a disease-specific 5-year survival of 95%, and a 5-year overall survival of 93% in patients with testicular cancer of seminomatous germ cells. Patients with non-seminomatous cancer with a good prognosis had a 5-year progression-free survival of 90%, a diseasespecific 5-year survival of 97%, and 5-year overall survival of 95%.

As for the infusion sequence of the BEP protocol (Fig. 6.8), it starts with the infusion of cisplatin, which is the vesicant or irritant agent, followed by the etoposide, which is irritant, and finally, the infusion of bleomycin, which is non-vesicant. There are no studies that demonstrate a possible interaction between drugs depending on the infusion schedule [146, 147].

6.4.1.2 VIP Protocol (Etoposide, Cisplatin, Ifosfamide, and Mesna)

In the VIP protocol, instead of combining etoposide and cisplatin with bleomycin (BEP protocol), it replaces bleomycin with ifosfamide and mesna. The VIP protocol is indicated in the treatment of consolidation and recovery for non-seminoma [148, 149]. Ifosfamide is nitrogen mustard, which, like cyclophosphamide, is part of the class of alkylating agents, acting through binding with nucleic acids, through the alkylation of DNA. Mesna is a drug used to prevent urothelial toxicity, such as hemorrhagic cystitis, microhematuria, and ifosfamide-induced macrohematuria [150–152].

Hinton et al. [153] compared the effectiveness of the BEP protocol with the VIP protocol in treating disseminated germ cell tumors, showing that both protocols had comparable results with modestly greater hematologic toxicity in the VIP protocol

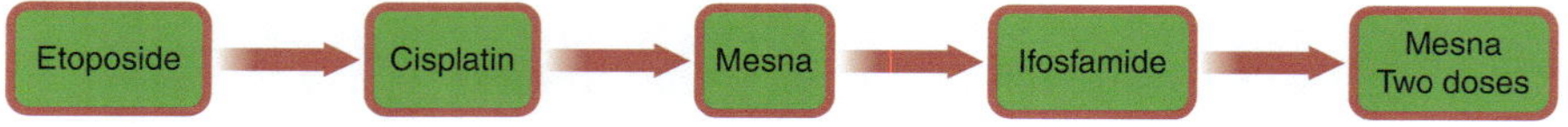

Fig. 6.9 VIP protocol infusion sequence

group. The VIP protocol promoted a progression-free survival of 64% and an overall survival rate of 69%.

Schmoll et al. [149] evaluated the effectiveness of the VIP protocol in the treatment of advanced metastatic germ cell cancer. The protocol presented as toxicity the mucositis, neurological toxicity, renal, and granulocytopenia. As for efficacy, the protocol promoted a progression-free survival rate in 2 years of 69% and disease-specific survival in 2 years of 79%.

Bokemeyer et al. [148] evaluated the use of the VIP protocol of sequential high-dose as a first-line treatment in patients with non-seminomatous germ cell tumors. The protocol promoted a 2-year progression-free survival rate of 64% and an overall survival rate of 68%. The VIP protocol infusion sequence (Fig. 6.9) is based on the initial infusion of etoposide followed by cisplatin, then the first dose of mesna followed by the infusion of ifosfamide with a subsequent infusion of two more doses of mesna [154].

6.4.1.3   TAXGEM Protocol (Paclitaxel and Gemcitabine)

The combination of paclitaxel with gemcitabine has been indicated in palliative therapy for germ cell cancer [155, 156]. Einhorn et al. [155] evaluated the effectiveness of the combination of paclitaxel and gemcitabine in treating germ cell tumors. The combination promoted an objective response in 31% of patients, of which four achieved partial remissions and six had complete responses, showing that it may be possible to achieve long-term disease-free survival with the combination.

Mulherin, Brames, and Einhorn [157] confirmed that the combination of paclitaxel and gemcitabine may offer long-term survival in patients with relapsed/refractory germ cell tumors, with three disease-free patients for 64, 94, and 122 months.

Hinton et al. [158], in a phase II study, evaluated the efficacy of the combination of paclitaxel and gemcitabine in refractory germ cell tumors. As a result, the authors observed that 21.4% of patients responded to treatment, with three patients achieving a complete response, with two patients free of disease for more than 15 and 25 months. Regarding the infusion sequence, the protocol starts with the infusion of paclitaxel followed by gemcitabine (Fig. 6.10) [155, 157, 158].

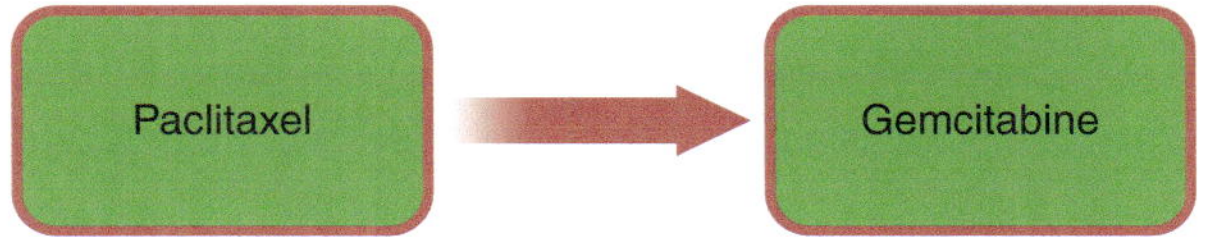

Fig. 6.10 TAXGEM protocol infusion sequence

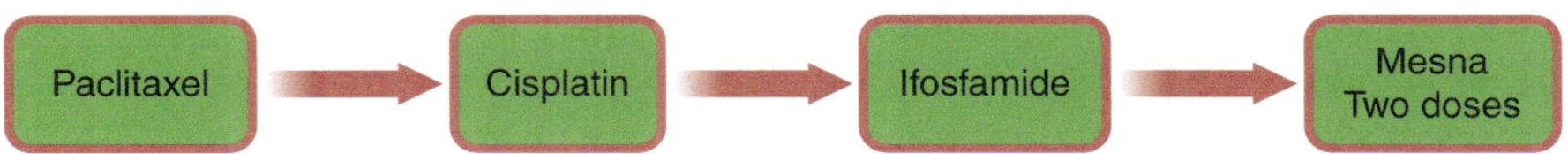

Fig. 6.11 TIP protocol infusion sequence

6.4.1.4   TIP Protocol (Paclitaxel, Cisplatin, Ifosfamide, and Mesna)

The TIP protocol combines paclitaxel, ifosfamide, and cisplatin for the treatment of recurrent testicular germ cell cancer [159–162]. In patients with recurrent testicular germ cell cancer, Motzer et al. [159] evaluated the effectiveness of the TIP protocol. The authors noted that 77% of patients achieved a complete response, and 73% of patients who had favorable responses remained durable with an average duration of 33 months. As protocol toxicity, patients had myelosuppression and neurotoxicity.

As well as the study by Motzer et al. [159], Kondagunta et al. [160] also looked at the efficacy of the TIP protocol as second-line therapy in recurrent testicular germ cell tumors. The combination promoted a complete response in 70% of patients, of which 3% relapsed after chemotherapy with the TIP protocol. The durable complete protocol response rate was 63% and 2-year progression-free survival 65%.

The results were also promising in the study by Kawai et al. [163], promoting disease-free status in 62% of patients, in which 60% of these patients remained free from disease progression for an average duration of 24 months. As for the toxicity profile, the patients had leukocytopenia, thrombocytopenia, and sensory neuropathy.

Mead et al. [161], in a phase II study, evaluated the efficacy of the TIP protocol as a second-line after treatment with the BEP protocol in the treatment of metastatic germ cell cancer. The favorable response rate for the combination was 60%, with a 1-year survival of 70% and failure-free survival of 36%.

The infusion sequence of the TIP protocol (Fig. 6.11) is based on the initial infusion of paclitaxel, which is the vesicant drug and specific cycle, followed by the infusion of cisplatin, which can be irritating or vesicant, and nonspecific cycle, and finally the infusion of ifosfamide, which it is a drug-irritating and nonspecific cycle with a dose of concomitant mesna followed by another dose of mesna [147, 164, 165].

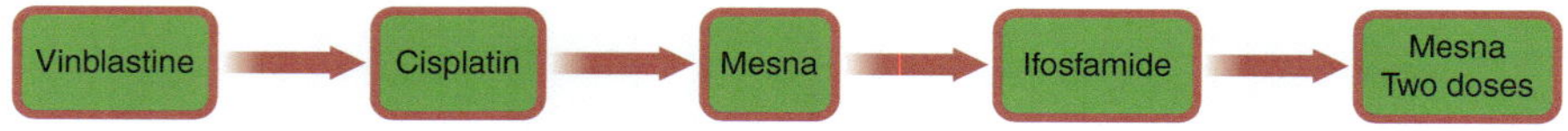

Fig. 6.12 VEIP protocol infusion sequence

6.4.1.5 VEIP Protocol (Vinblastine, Cisplatin, Ifosfamide, and Mesna)

The VEIP protocol is a combination of the antineoplastics vinblastine, cisplatin, and ifosfamide for the treatment of consolidation/recovery in germ cell cancer [166–168]. Loehrer Sr et al. [167] evaluated the use of the VEIP protocol as initial rescue therapy in patients with recurrent germ cell tumors. As a result, 49.6% of patients have achieved disease-free status, of which 23.7% are disease-free, showing that the protocol can promote lasting complete remissions in patients with disseminated germ cell cancer.

Farhat et al. [166] highlight that combined therapy for refractory or relapsing germ cell cancer, with VEIP or VIP protocols, can increase the effectiveness of treatment as rescue therapy, promoting complete remission in 31% of patients, partial response in 19%, and relapse-free survival in 63%. As the main toxicity, patients had severe myelotoxicity.

As for the infusion sequence of the VEIP protocol (Fig. 6.12), the initial vinblastine protocol followed by cisplatin, then the first dose of mesna followed by ifosfamide, and finally two more doses of mesna in sequence to reduce the risks of urological toxicity induced by ifosfamide [169].

6.5 Pathophysiology of Kidney Cancer

Renal cell cancer accounts for 2% of global diagnoses and deaths of all cancers and is the ninth most common neoplasm in the USA. North America and Western Europe have the highest incidence of kidney cancer, but it is believed that Latin America, Asia, and Africa will have an increase in incidence due to the nation's transition to a Western lifestyle. The diagnosis of kidney cancer usually occurs in people aged 65 to 74 years, being very uncommon in people under 45 years [170–172].

Regarding gender, kidney cancer is more common in men than in women, being more common in African Americans and American Indians/Alaska natives. Survival is dependent on the stage of cancer at diagnosis, with the metastatic disease having a 5-year survival rate of 12% [172–174].

Renal cell carcinoma originates from renal tubular epithelial cells, accounting for 85% of primary renal neoplasms. Other types of renal tumors include transitional cell carcinoma, nephroblastoma or Wilms' tumor, renal sarcomas, medullary renal carcinoma, and collecting duct cancer. Some risk factors include old age, treatment for kidney failure, smoking, high blood pressure, and obesity. Genetic

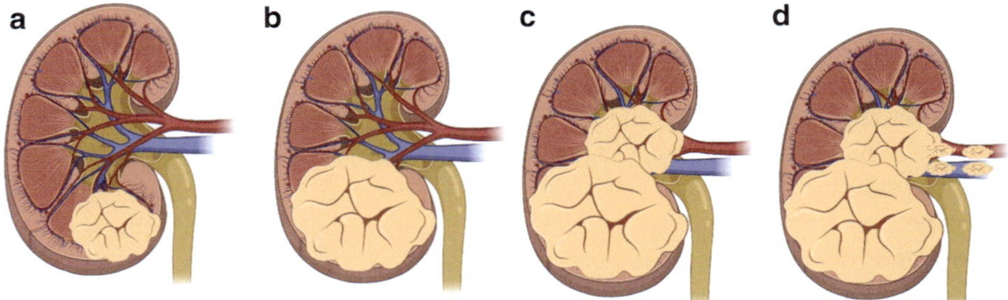

Fig. 6.13 Stages of kidney cancer. (**a**) Stage 1; (**b**) stage 2; (**c**) stage 3; and (**d**) stage 4. (Source: Created with BioRender.com)

alterations are also associated with the development of renal cell carcinoma, such as loss of the short arm of chromosome 3, seen in 95% of cases. Some genes involved in renal cancer pathogenesis include *VHL*, *mTOR*, *SETD2*, *PBRM-1*, *KDM5C*, and *BAP-1* [174–180].

The stages of kidney cancer range from 1 to 4 (Fig. 6.13) according to the extent of the tumor and its spread to other organs and/or tissues. In stage 1, the tumor is less than or equal to 7 cm, being located only in the kidney. In stage 2 the tumor is above 7 cm, but it is still located in the kidney with no invasion of lymph nodes or distant organs. In stage 3, the tumor grows in a major vein, such as a renal vein or vena cava, or in the tissue around the kidney, whether or not the tumor has spread to nearby lymph nodes. In stage 4, however, the tumor may be of any size, may have grown outside the kidney, and may or may not have spread to nearby lymph nodes and/or distant lymph nodes and/or organs [177, 181, 182].

6.5.1 Chemotherapy for the Treatment of Kidney Cancer

The choice of therapeutic approach will depend on the stage of the kidney cancer, where the main approaches include surgery to remove part or all of the affected kidney, ablation therapy, embolization, radiotherapy, and targeted therapy [183, 184]. In stages 1 and 2, as the tumor is located in the kidney, usually the chosen approach is surgery, which can be partial nephrectomy (usually indicated in stage 1, with tumors smaller than 7 cm) and radical nephrectomy, which may involve the lymph nodes near the kidney being removed if they are enlarged [185, 186]. In stage 3, nearby veins may present a tumor, in which, during surgery, the veins need to be opened to remove the tumor; when there is a high risk of cancer recurrence, targeted therapy may be indicated to reduce the risk [187, 188].

In stage 4, when you know cancer has spread to other parts of the body, in some cases surgery may be indicated, while radiation may be a treatment option in the area of cancer spread. But when cancer has spread to other places and there is no possibility of removal by surgery in the metastatic organ and kidney, systemic therapy is the first choice of treatment [189–191].

Targeted therapy is the therapeutic option, and some monoclonal antibodies such as nivolumab may be indicated as monotherapy in the treatment of metastatic or advanced renal cell carcinoma [192, 193]. mTOR inhibitors such as everolimus and temsirolimus are indicated for the treatment of advanced kidney cancer [194, 195]. Tyrosine kinase inhibitors are also indicated as axitinib and cabozantinib in the treatment of metastatic renal cell carcinoma, pazopanib, sorafenib, and sunitinib in palliative therapy for renal cell carcinoma [196–198].

In addition to monotherapy, some combinations may also be indicated, such as the combination between the monoclonal antibodies nivolumab and ipilimumab, which is also indicated in the treatment of cancers of the gastrointestinal tract (see Chap. 5), which is indicated in the treatment of carcinoma of the metastatic or advanced kidney cells [199, 200]. Other protocols [45–47] will be covered in the next topics.

6.5.1.1 PEMAX Protocol (Pembrolizumab and Axitinib)

The PEMAX protocol combines pembrolizumab with axitinib for the treatment of metastatic renal cell carcinoma [201–203]. Pembrolizumab is a humanized monoclonal antibody acting like a programmed death protein (PD-1) anti-receptor. Pembrolizumab has the function of blocking the interaction of PD-1 with PD-L1 and PD-L2, being involved in the control of the immune response of T lymphocytes [204–206]. On the other hand, axitinib is a potent and selective inhibitor of vascular endothelial growth factor receptor (VEGFR) tyrosine kinase, acting on VEGFR-1, VEGFR-2, and VEGFR-3. Inhibition of these receptors reduces pathological angiogenesis, tumor growth, and metastatic progression of cancer [207–209].

The combination of pembrolizumab and axitinib has been shown to be effective in the treatment of advanced kidney cancer. According to Rini et al. [201], the combination promoted a median progression-free survival of 15.1 months, with an objective response rate of 59.3%, being superior to sunitinib monotherapy.

In a phase III study, Powles et al. [210] also compared the effectiveness of the PEMAX protocol with sunitinib monotherapy. As in the study by Rini et al. [201], Powles et al. [210] also observed clinical results of the protocol superior to sunitinib. The results showed an overall survival of 30.6 months with a progression-free survival of 15.4 months. As for toxicity, the most frequent adverse events included hypertension, increased alanine aminotransferase, and diarrhea.

Watson et al. [211] compared the PEMAX protocol with the combination of nivolumab plus ipilimumab in the first-line treatment of advanced renal cell carcinoma, regarding the cost-effectiveness of each protocol. The PEMAX protocol was associated with longer quality-adjusted life compared to the other protocol in patients with advanced renal cell carcinoma, but it may not be cost-effective.

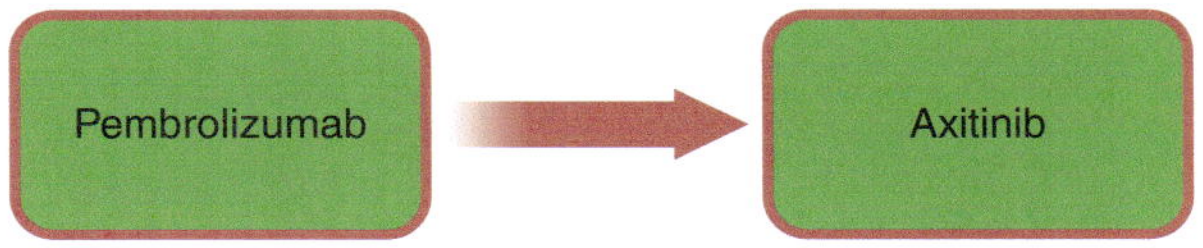

Fig. 6.14 PEMAX protocol administration schedule with oral administration of axitinib

Plimack et al. [212] evaluated patients who received the PEMAX protocol for 2 years. About 29.9% of patients have completed 2 years of treatment with the combination, with overall 36-month survival rates of 93.8%, 24-month progression-free survival rates of 72.1%, and 36-month of 57.7%, and an objective response rate of 85.3%. Regarding the administration schedule, pembrolizumab is infused intravenously, and axitinib is given orally twice daily (Fig. 6.14) [213].

6.5.1.2 Avelumab and Axitinib Protocol

The combination of avelumab with axitinib has been indicated for the treatment of unresectable locally advanced or metastatic renal cell carcinoma [214–217]. Avelumab is a fully human monoclonal antibody, acting against the PD-L1 ligand, blocking its interaction with programmed cell death receptors (PD-1 and B7.1), thereby removing the suppressive effects of PD-L1 on the cytotoxic CD8 T cells [218, 219].

Motzer et al. [214] compared the effectiveness of combining avelumab and axitinib with sunitinib in the treatment of advanced renal cell carcinoma. As a result, the authors noted that the combination increased progression-free survival from 7.2 months (sunitinib alone) to 13.8 months (combination); it also increased overall survival from 10.7 months to 11.6 months and response rate from 25.5% to 55.2%. In a phase III study, Motzer et al. [216] continued to observe that the combination promoted a prolonged progression-free survival in patients with advanced renal cell carcinoma compared with sunitinib monotherapy.

Choueiri et al. [215] evaluated the efficacy of the combination in first-line treatment of patients with advanced renal cell carcinoma, also showing that the combination promoted an increase in progression-free survival (from 7 months to 13.8 months) compared to patients who received only sunitinib.

Tomita et al. [220] looked at the efficacy and safety of the combination of avelumab and axitinib versus sunitinib in elderly patients with advanced renal cell carcinoma. The combination provided an overall survival of 19.3 months and progression-free survival of 16.8 months. As for adverse events, the patients had diarrhea, hypertension, palmoplantar erythrodysesthesia syndrome, and nausea. Regarding the administration schedule, avelumab is administered intravenously, and the patient takes axitinib orally twice a day (Fig. 6.15) [217].

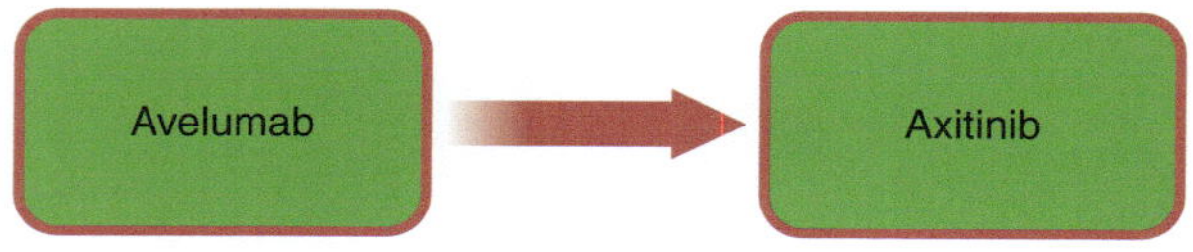

Fig. 6.15 Infusion schedule for the combination of avelumab and axitinib, with oral administration of axitinib

References

1. Pack R. Descriptive epidemiology of genitourinary cancers. Semin Oncol Nurs. 1993;9(4):218–23. https://doi.org/10.1016/S0749-2081(05)80050-6.
2. Darre T, Folligan K, Kpatcha TM, Kanassouwa K, Sewa E, Dare S, Tengue K, Amegbor K, Napo Koura G. Evolution of the histo-epidemiological profile of urological cancers in Togo. Asian Pac J Cancer Prev. 2017;18(2):491–4.
3. Kockelbergh R, Hounsome L, Mayer E. The epidemiology of urological cancer 2001–2013. J Clin Urol. 2017;10(1S):3–8. https://doi.org/10.1177/2051415816674103.
4. Turcatto IM, Ferreira PMP, Takahashi AAR, Alcantara SSA, Paiva LS, Sousa LVA. Análise epidemiológica de câncer de trato geniturinário na região do ABC paulista. Clin Oncol Lett. 2020; https://doi.org/10.4322/col.2019.002.
5. WHO—World Health Organization (2020) Estimated number of incident cases from 2018 to 2040. International Agency for Research on Cancer. Available in: https://gco.iarc.fr/tomorrow/graphic-isotype?type=0&type_sex=0&mode=population&sex=0&populations=900&cancers=36&age_group=value&apc_male=0&apc_female=0&single_unit=100000&print=0. Access on: Sep 4, 2021.
6. Porto LTR, Pedrosa ACMF, Alves MRB, Santos GA, Werner HL, Silva MHS, Muniz E, Paula AJF, Pujatti PB. Sobrevida Global dos Pacientes com Cânceres do Sistema Geniturinário Atendidos em Barbacena-MG. Revista Médica de Minas Gerais. 2019;29(Supl 8):S71–8. https://doi.org/10.5935/2238-3182.20190047.
7. Korkes F, Juliano CAB, Bunduky MAP, Costa ACDM, Castro MG. Amount of tobacco consumption is associated with superficial bladder cancer progression. Einstein. 2010;8(4 Pt 1):473–6. https://doi.org/10.1590/S1679-45082010AO1751.
8. Antoni S, Ferlay J, Soerjomataram I, Znaor A, Jemal A, Bray F. Bladder cancer incidence and mortality: a global overview and recent trends. Eur Urol. 2017;71(1):96–108. https://doi.org/10.1016/j.eururo.2016.06.010.
9. Saginala K, Barsouk A, Aluru JS, Rawla P, Padala AS, Barsouk A. Epidemiology of bladder cancer. Med Sci. 2020;8(1):15. https://doi.org/10.3390/medsci8010015.
10. Cumberbatch MGK, Jubber I, Black PC, Esperto F, Figueroa JD, Kamat AM, Kiemeney L, Lotan Y, Pang K, Silverman DT, Znaor A, Catto JWF. Epidemiology of bladder cancer: a systematic review and contemporary update of risk factors in 2018. Eur Urol. 2018;74(6):784–95. https://doi.org/10.1016/j.eururo.2018.09.001.
11. Wong MCS, Fung FDH, Leung C, Cheung WWL, Goggins WB, Ng CF. The global epidemiology of bladder cancer: a joinpoint regression analysis of its incidence and mortality trends and projection. Sci Rep. 2018;8:1129. https://doi.org/10.1038/s41598-018-19199-z.
12. Panov S, Roganovic-Zafirova D, Stavric G, Yashar G, Popov Z. High frequency of the HRAS oncogene codon 12 mutation in Macedonian patients with urinary bladder cancer. Genet Mol Biol. 2004;27(1):9–14. https://doi.org/10.1590/S1415-47572004000100002.
13. Reuter VE. The pathology of bladder cancer. Urology. 2006;67(3 Suppl 1):11–7. https://doi.org/10.1016/j.urology.2006.01.037.
14. Otto W, Denzinger S, Bertz S, Gaumann A, Wild PJ, Hartmann A, Stoehr R. No mutations of FGFR3 in normal urothelium in the vicinity of urothelial carcinoma of the blad-

der harbouring activating FGFR3 mutations in patients with bladder cancer. Int J Cancer. 2009;125(9):2205–8. https://doi.org/10.1002/ijc.24598.

15. McConkey DJ, Lee S, Choi W, Tran M, Majewski T, Lee S, Siefker-Radtke A, Dinney C, Czerniak B. Molecular genetics of bladder cancer: emerging mechanisms of tumor initiation and progression. Urol Oncol. 2010;28(4):429–40. https://doi.org/10.1016/j.urolonc.2010.04.008.

16. Thompson DB, Siref LE, Feloney MP, Hauke RJ, Agrawal DK. Immunological basis in the pathogenesis and treatment of bladder cancer. Expert Rev Clin Immunol. 2015;11(2):265–79. https://doi.org/10.1586/1744666X.2015.983082.

17. Yang L, Shi P, Zhao G, Xu J, Peng W, Zhang J, Zhang G, Wang X, Dong Z, Chen F, Cui H. Targeting cancer stem cell pathways for cancer therapy. Signal Transduct Target Ther. 2020;5:8. https://doi.org/10.1038/s41392-020-0110-5.

18. Cheong JJWY, Woodward PJ, Manning MA, Sesterhenn IA. Neoplasms of the urinary bladder: radiologic-pathologic correlation. Radiographics. 2006;26(2):553–80. https://doi.org/10.1148/rg.262055172.

19. Amin MB. Histological variants of urothelial carcinoma: diagnostic, therapeutic and prognostic implications. Mod Pathol. 2009;22:S96–S118. https://doi.org/10.1038/modpathol.2009.26.

20. Cheng L, Montironi R, Davidson DD, Lopez-Beltran A. Staging and reporting of urothelial carcinoma of the urinary bladder. Mod Pathol. 2009;22:S70–95. https://doi.org/10.1038/modpathol.2009.1.

21. Le O, Roy A, Silverman PM, Kundra V. Common and uncommon adult unilateral renal masses other than renal cell carcinoma. Cancer Imaging. 2012;12(1):194–204. https://doi.org/10.1102/1470-7330.2012.0019.

22. Kaseb H, Aeddula NR. Bladder Cancer. Treasure Island, USA: StatPearls Publishing; 2021.

23. Verma S, Rajesh A, Prasad SR, Gaitonde K, Lall CG, Mouraviev V, Aeron G, Bracken RB, Sandrasegaran K. Urinary bladder cancer: role of MR imaging. Radiographics. 2012;32(2):371–87. https://doi.org/10.1148/rg.322115125.

24. Lee CH, Tan CH, Faria SC, Kundra V. Role of imaging in the local staging of urothelial carcinoma of the bladder. Am J Roentgenol. 2017;208(6):1193–205. https://doi.org/10.2214/AJR.16.17114.

25. Sharma S, Ksheersagar P, Sharma P. Diagnosis and treatment of bladder cancer. Am Fam Physician. 2009;80(7):717–23.

26. Anastasiadis A, Reijke TM. Best practice in the treatment of nonmuscle invasive bladder cancer. Ther Adv Urol. 2012;4(1):13–32. https://doi.org/10.1177/1756287211431976.

27. Porten SP, Leapman MS, Greene KL. Intravesical chemotherapy in non-muscle-invasive bladder cancer. Indian J Urol. 2015;31(4):297–303. https://doi.org/10.4103/0970-1591.166446.

28. NIH – National Cancer Institute. Bladder cancer treatment (PDQ®)-patient version. USA: National Cancer Institute at the National Institutes of Health; 2021.

29. Shen Z, Shen T, Wientjes MG, O'Donnell MA, Au JLS. Intravesical treatments of bladder cancer: review. Pharm Res. 2008;25(7):1500–10. https://doi.org/10.1007/s11095-008-9566-7.

30. Chade DC, Shariat SF, Dalbagni G. Intravesical therapy for urothelial carcinoma of the urinary bladder: a critical review. Int Braz J Urol. 2009;35(6):640–51. https://doi.org/10.1590/S1677-55382009000600002.

31. Balar A, Bajorin DF, Milowsky MI. Management of invasive bladder cancer in patients who are not candidates for or decline cystectomy. Ther Adv Urol. 2011;3(3):107–17. https://doi.org/10.1177/1756287211407543.

32. Marta GN, Hanna SA, Gadia R, Correa SFM, Silva JLF, Carvalho HA. The role of radiotherapy in urinary bladder cancer: current status. Int Braz J Urol. 2012;38(2):144–54. https://doi.org/10.1590/S1677-55382012000200002.

33. Russell CM, Lebastchi AH, Borza T, Spratt DE, Morgan TM. The role of transurethral resection in trimodal therapy for muscle-invasive bladder cancer. Bladder Cancer (Amsterdam, Netherlands). 2016;2(4):381–94. https://doi.org/10.3233/BLC-160076.

34. Hamad J, McCloskey H, Milowsky MI, Royce T, Smith A. Bladder preservation in muscle-invasive bladder cancer: a comprehensive review. Int Braz J Urol. 2020;46(2):169–84. https://doi.org/10.1590/S1677-5538.IBJU.2020.99.01.

35. Witjes JA, Compérat E, Cowan NC, De Santis M, Gakis G, Lebrét T, van der Heijden AG, Ribal MJ. EAU guidelines on muscle-invasive and metastatic bladder cancer. Netherlands: European Association of Urology; 2016.

36. Bellmunt J, Wit R, Vaughn DJ, Fradet Y, Lee JL, Fong L, Vogelzang NJ, Climent MA, Petrylak DP, Choueiri TK, Necchi A, Gerritsen W, Gurney H, Quinn DI, Culine S, Sternberg CN, Mai Y, Poehlein CH, Perini RF, Bajorin DF. Pembrolizumab as second-line therapy for advanced urothelial carcinoma. N Engl J Med. 2017;376:1015–26. https://doi.org/10.1056/NEJMoa1613683.

37. Bassi PF. BCG (bacillus of Calmette Guerin) therapy of high-risk superficial bladder cancer. Surg Oncol. 2002;11(1–2):77–83. https://doi.org/10.1016/s0960-7404(02)00008-7.

38. Taylor JH, Davis J, Schellhammer P. Long-term follow-up of intravesical bacillus Calmette-Guérin treatment for superficial transitional-cell carcinoma of the bladder involving the prostatic urethra. Clin Genitourin Cancer. 2007;5(6):386–9. https://doi.org/10.3816/CGC.2007.n.021.

39. Jouhadi H Sr, Sahraoui S, Benider A. Concurrent weekly cisplatin during radiation treatment of locally advanced bladder carcinoma in elderly patients. J Clin Oncol. 2008;26(15_suppl):16109. https://doi.org/10.1200/jco.2008.26.15_suppl.16109.

40. Jones G, Cleves A, Wilt TJ, Mason M, Kynaston HG, Shelley M. Intravesical gemcitabine for non-muscle invasive bladder cancer. Cochrane. Library. 2012;1:CD009294. https://doi.org/10.1002/14651858.CD009294.pub2.

41. Li R, Li Y, Song J, Gao K, Chen K, Yang X, Ding Y, Ma X, Wang Y, Li W, Wang Y, Wang Z, Dong Z. Intravesical gemcitabine versus mitomycin for non-muscle invasive bladder cancer: a systematic review and meta-analysis of randomized controlled trial. BMC Urol. 2020;20:97. https://doi.org/10.1186/s12894-020-00610-9.

42. Moore MJ, Winquist EW, Murray N, Tannock IF, Huan S, Bennett K, Walsh W, Seymour L. Gemcitabine plus cisplatin, an active regimen in advanced urothelial cancer: a phase II trial of the National Cancer Institute of Canada clinical trials group. J Clin Oncol. 1999;17(9):2876. https://doi.org/10.1200/JCO.1999.17.9.2876.

43. Bae KS, Ahn KI, Jeon SH, Huh JS, Chang SG. Efficacy of combined gemcitabine/cisplatin chemotherapy for locally advanced or metastatic urothelial cancer. Cancer Res Treat. 2006;38(2):78–83. https://doi.org/10.4143/crt.2006.38.2.78.

44. Dash A, Pettus JA 4th, Herr HW, Bochner BH, Dalbagni G, Donat SM, Russo P, Boyle MG, Milowsky MI, Bajorin DF. A role for neoadjuvant gemcitabine plus cisplatin in muscle-invasive urothelial carcinoma of the bladder: a retrospective experience. Cancer. 2008;113(9):2471–7. https://doi.org/10.1002/cncr.23848.

45. Kuehr T, Thaler J, Woell E (2017) Chemotherapy protocols 2017: current protocols and "targeted therapies". Klinikum Wels-Grieskirchen and Caritas Christi URGET NOS. Austria. www.chemoprotocols.eu.

46. BC Cancer (2021) Supportive care protocols. BC Cancer. British Columbia. Available in: http://www.bccancer.bc.ca/health-professionals/clinical-resources/chemotherapy-protocols/supportive-care. Accessed July 2 2021.

47. NHS (2021) Chemotherapy Protocols. NHS. University Hospital Southampton. NHS Foundation Trust. England. Available in: https://www.uhs.nhs.uk/HealthProfessionals/Chemotherapy-protocols/Chemotherapy-protocols.aspx. Accessed July 2 2021.

48. O'Donnell MA, Lilli K, Leopold C. Interim results from a national multicenter phase II trial of combination bacillus Calmette-Guerin plus interferon alfa-2b for superficial bladder cancer. J Urol. 2004;172(3):888–93. https://doi.org/10.1097/01.ju.0000136446.37840.0a.

49. Witjes JA. Management of BCG failures in superficial bladder cancer: a review. Eur Urol. 2006;49:790–7. https://doi.org/10.1016/j.eururo.2006.01.017.

50. Askeland EJ, Newton MR, O'Donnelll MA, Luo Y. Bladder cancer immunotherapy: BCG and beyond. Adv Urol. 2012;2012:181987. https://doi.org/10.1155/2012/181987.
51. Correa AF, Theisen K, Ferroni M, Maranchie JK, Hrebinko R, Davies BJ, Gingrich JR. The role of interferon in the management of BCG refractory nonmuscle invasive bladder cancer. Adv Urol. 2015;2015:656918. https://doi.org/10.1155/2015/656918.
52. Guallar-Garrido S, Julián E. Bacillus Calmette-Guérin (BCG) therapy for bladder cancer: an update. Immunotargets Ther. 2020;9:1–11. https://doi.org/10.2147/ITT.S202006.
53. Klinger D, Hill BL, Barda N, Halperin E, Gofrit ON, Greenblatt CL, Rappoport N, Linial M, Bercovier H. Bladder cancer immunotherapy by BCG is associated with a significantly reduced risk of Alzheimer's disease and Parkinson's disease. Vaccine. 2021;9:491. https://doi.org/10.3390/vaccines9050491.
54. Le Page C, Génin P, Baines MG, Hiscott J. Interferon activation and innate immunity. Rev Immunogenet. 2000;2(3):374–86.
55. Minn AJ. Interferons and the immunogenic effects of cancer therapy. Trends Immunol. 2015;36(11):725–37. https://doi.org/10.1016/j.it.2015.09.007.
56. Musella M, Manic G, Maria RD, Vitale I, Sistigu A. Type-I-interferons in infection and cancer: unanticipated dynamics with therapeutic implications. OncoImmunology. 2017;6(5):e1314424. https://doi.org/10.1080/2162402X.2017.1314424.
57. Ferreira VL, Borba HHL, Bonetti AF, Leonart LP, Pontarolo R. Cytokines and interferons: types and functions. London, United Kingdom: Intechopen; 2018.
58. Borden EC. Interferons α and β in cancer: therapeutic opportunities from new insights. Nat Rev Drug Discov. 2019;18:219–34. https://doi.org/10.1038/s41573-018-0011-2.
59. Zlotta AR, Fleshner NE, Jewett MA. The management of BCG failure in non-muscle-invasive bladder cancer: an update. Can Urol Assoc J. 2009;3(6 Suppl 4):S199–205. https://doi.org/10.5489/cuaj.1196.
60. Downs TM, Szilvasi A, O'Donnell MA. Pharmacological biocompatibility between intravesical preparations of BCG and interferon-alpha 2B. J Urol. 1997;158(6):2311–5. https://doi.org/10.1016/s0022-5347(01)68241-7.
61. Chair GUTG (2009) BCCA protocol summary for palliative therapy for BCG-refractory superficial high-grade transitional cell carcinoma bladder with BCG and interferon. BC cancer. British Columbia. Available in: http://www.bccancer.bc.ca/chemotherapy-protocols-site/Documents/Genitourinary/GUBCGIFN_Protocol.pdf. Accessed Sep 5 2021.
62. Steinberg RL, Thomas LJ, O'Donnell MA, Nepple KG. Sequential intravesical gemcitabine and docetaxel for the salvage treatment of non-muscle invasive bladder cancer. Bladder Cancer. 2015;1(1):65–72. https://doi.org/10.3233/BLC-150008.
63. Milbar N, Kates M, Chappidi MR, Pederzoli F, Yoshida T, Sankin A, Pierorazio PM, Schoenberg MP, Bivalacqua TJ. Oncological outcomes of sequential intravesical gemcitabine and docetaxel in patients with non-muscle invasive bladder cancer. Bladder Cancer. 2017;3(4):293–303. https://doi.org/10.3233/BLC-170126.
64. NCT04386746 (2020) Intravesical Gemcitabine and Docetaxel for BCG naïve Non-muscle Invasive Bladder Cancer (GEMDOCE). Clinical Trials. Available in: https://clinicaltrials.gov/ct2/show/NCT04386746. Accessed Sep 6 2021.
65. Thomas L, Steinberg R, Nepple KG, O'Donnell MA. Sequential intravesical gemcitabine and docetaxel in the treatment of BCG-naive patients with non-muscle invasive bladder cancer. J Clin Oncol. 2019;37(7_suppl):469. https://doi.org/10.1200/JCO.2019.37.7_suppl.469.
66. Steinberg RL, Thomas LJ, Brooks N, Mott SL, Vitale A, Crump T, Rao MY, Daniels MJ, Wang J, Nagaraju S, DeWolf WC, Lamm DL, Kates M, Hyndman ME, Kamat AM, Bivalacqua TJ, Nepple KG, O'Donnell MA. Multi-institution evaluation of sequential gemcitabine and docetaxel as rescue therapy for nonmuscle invasive bladder cancer. J Urol. 2020;203(5):902–9. https://doi.org/10.1097/JU.0000000000000688.
67. Black P (2021) BC cancer protocol summary for intravesical therapy for non-muscle invasive bladder cancer using gemcitabine and docetaxel. BC cancer. British Columbia. Available

in: http://www.bccancer.bc.ca/chemotherapy-protocols-site/Documents/Genitourinary/GUBGEMDOC_Protocol.pdf. Accessed Sep 9 2021.

68. Sternberg CN, Mulder PH, Schornagel JH, Théodore C, Fossa SD, van Oosterom AT, Witjes F, Spina M, van Groeningen CJ, Balincourt C, Collette L. Randomized phase III trial of high-dose-intensity methotrexate, vinblastine, doxorubicin, and cisplatin (MVAC) chemotherapy and recombinant human granulocyte colony-stimulating factor versus classic MVAC in advanced urothelial tract tumors: European Organization for Research and Treatment of Cancer Protocol no. 30924. J Clin Oncol. 2001;19(10):2638–46. https://doi.org/10.1200/JCO.2001.19.10.2638.

69. Han KS, Joung JY, Kim TS, Jeong IG, Seo HK, Chung J, Lee KH. Methotrexate, vinblastine, doxorubicin and cisplatin combination regimen as salvage chemotherapy for patients with advanced or metastatic transitional cell carcinoma after failure of gemcitabine and cisplatin chemotherapy. Br J Cancer. 2008;98:86–90. https://doi.org/10.1038/sj.bjc.6604113.

70. Choueiri TK, Jacobus S, Bellmunt J, Qu A, Appleman LJ, Tretter C, Bucley GJ, Stack EC, Signoretti S, Walsh M, Steele G, Hirsch M, Sweeney CJ, Taplin ME, Kibel AS, Krajewski KM, Kantoff PW, Ross RW, Rosenberg JE. Neoadjuvant dose-dense methotrexate, vinblastine, doxorubicin, and cisplatin with Pegfilgrastim support in muscle-invasive urothelial cancer: pathologic, radiologic, and biomarker correlates. J Clin Oncol. 2014;32(18):1889–94. https://doi.org/10.1200/JCO.2013.52.4785.

71. Mukhtar E, Adhami VM, Mukhtar H. Targeting microtubules by natural agents for cancer therapy. Mol Cancer Ther. 2014;13(2):275–84. https://doi.org/10.1158/1535-7163.MCT-13-0791.

72. Bates D, Eastman A. Microtubule destabilising agents: far more than just antimitotic anticancer drugs. Br J Clin Pharmacol. 2017;83:255–68. https://doi.org/10.1111/bcp.13126.

73. Sternberg CN, Yagoda A, Scher HI, Watson RC, Herr HW, Morse MJ, Sogani PC, Vaughan ED Jr, Bander N, Weiselberg LR, Geller N, Hollander PS, Lipperman R, Fair WR, Whitmore WF Jr. M-vac (methotrexate, vinblastine, doxorubicin and cisplatin) for advanced transitional cell carcinoma of the urothelium. J Urol. 1988;139(3):461–9.

74. Sternberg CN, Yagoda A, Scher HI, Watson RC, Geller N, Herr HW, Morse MJ, Sogani PC, Vaughan ED, Bander N, Weiselberg L, Rosado K, Smart T, Lin SY, Penenberg D, Fair WR, Whitmore WF Jr. Methotrexate, vinblastine, doxorubicin, and cisplatin for advanced transitional cell carcinoma of the urothelium. Efficacy and patterns of response and relapse. Cancer. 1989;64(12):2448–58.

75. Ueki O, Hisazumi H, Uchibayashi T, Naito K, Tajiri S, Takemae K, Kawaguchi K, Kameda K, Nishino A, Nango C, Tsukahara K, Sugata T. Methotrexate, vinblastine, doxorubicin, and cisplatin for advanced urothelial cancer. Cancer Chemother Pharmacol. 1992;30:S72–6. https://doi.org/10.1007/BF00686947.

76. Kim KH, Hong SJ, Han KS. Predicting the response of patients with advanced urothelial cancer to methotrexate, vinblastine, Adriamycin, and cisplatin (MVAC) after the failure of gemcitabine and platinum (GP). BMC Cancer. 2015;15:812. https://doi.org/10.1186/s12885-015-1825-5.

77. Dorr RT. Antidotes to vesicant chemotherapy extravasations. Blood Rev. 1990;4(1):41–60. https://doi.org/10.1016/0268-960x(90)90015-k.

78. DrugBank (2021) Vinblastine. DrugBank online. Available in: https://go.drugbank.com/about. Accessed Sep 6 2021.

79. Borchmann S, Muller H, Hude I, Fuchs M, Borchmann P, Engert A. Thrombosis as a treatment complication in Hodgkin lymphoma patients: a comprehensive analysis of three prospective randomized German Hodgkin study group (GHSG) trials. Ann Oncol. 2019;30:1329–34. https://doi.org/10.1093/annonc/mdz168.

80. Moss PE, Hickman S, Harrison BR. Ototoxicity associated with vinblastine. Ann Pharmacother. 1999;33(4):423–5. https://doi.org/10.1345/aph.18288.

81. NHS (2015a) Chemotherapy Protocol. Bladder. Cisplatin-doxorubicin-methotrexate-vinblastine (Accelerated MVAC). NHS. University Hospital Southampton. NHS Foundation Trust. England. Available in: https://www.uhs.nhs.uk/Media/SUHTExtranet/Services/

Chemotherapy-SOPs/Bladdercancer/Cisplatin-Doxorubicin-Methotrexate-Vinblastine-(accelerated)-ver1.1.pdf. Accessed Sep 6 2021.

82. Sheth S, Mukherjea D, Rybak LP, Ramkumar V. Mechanisms of cisplatin-induced ototoxicity and otoprotection. Front Cell Neurosci. 2017;11:338. https://doi.org/10.3389/fncel.2017.00338.

83. Sales GTM, Foresto RD. Drug-induced nephrotoxicity. Rev Assoc Med Bras. 2020;66(Suppl 1):82–90. https://doi.org/10.1590/1806-9282.66.S1.82.

84. Hannoodee M, Mittal M. Methotrexate. Treasure Island USA: StatPearls Publishing; 2021.

85. Dess RT, Hartman HE, Mahal BA, Soni PD, Jackson WC, Cooperberg MR, Amling CL, Aronson WJ, Kane CJ, Terris MK, Zumsteg ZS, Butler S, Osborne JR, Morgan TM, Mehra R, Salami SS, Kishan AU, Wang C, Schaeffer EM, Roach M, Pisansky TM, Shipley WU, Freedland SJ, Sandler HM, Halabi S, Feng FY, Dignam JJ, Nguyen PL, Schipper MJ, Spratt DE. Association of black race with prostate cancer-specific and other-cause mortality. JAMA Oncol. 2019;5(7):975–83. https://doi.org/10.1001/jamaoncol.2019.0826.

86. Rawla P. Epidemiology of prostate cancer. World J Oncol. 2019;10(2):63–89. https://doi.org/10.14740/wjon1191.

87. Sung H, Ferlay J, Siegel RL, Laversanne M, Soerjomataram I, Jemal A, Bray F. Global cancer statistics 2020: GLOBOCAN estimates of incidence and mortality worldwide for 36 cancers in 185 countries. CA Cancer J Clin. 2021 71(3):209–49. https://doi.org/10.3322/caac.21660.

88. Potosky AL, Miller BA, Albertsen PC, Kramer BS. The role of increasing detection in the rising incidence of prostate cancer. JAMA. 1995;273(7):548–52.

89. Zhou CK, Check DP, Lortet-Tieulent J, Laversanne M, Jemal A, Ferlay J, Bray F, Cook MB, Devesa SS. Prostate cancer incidence in 43 populations worldwide: an analysis of time trends overall and by age group. Int J Cancer. 2016;138(6):1388–400. https://doi.org/10.1002/ijc.29894.

90. Kearns JT, Holt SK, Wright JL, Lin DW, Lange PH, Gore JL. PSA screening, prostate biopsy, and treatment of prostate cancer in the years surrounding the USPSTF recommendation against prostate cancer screening. Cancer. 2018;124(13):2733–9. https://doi.org/10.1002/cncr.31337.

91. Leslie SW, Soon-Sutton TL, Sajjad H, Siref LE. Prostate cancer. Treasure Island USA: StatPearls Publishing; 2021.

92. Constantinou J, Feneley MR. PSA testing: an evolving relationship with prostate cancer screening. Prostate Cancer Prostatic Dis. 2006;9:6–13. https://doi.org/10.1038/sj.pcan.4500838.

93. Shtricker A, Shefi S, Ringel A, Gillon G. PSA levels of 4.0–10 ng/mL and negative digital rectal examination: antibiotic therapy versus immediate prostate biopsy. Int Braz J Urol. 2009;35(5):551–8. https://doi.org/10.1590/S1677-55382009000500006.

94. Li Y, Mongan J, Behr SC, Sud S, Coakley FV, Simko J, Westphalen AC. Beyond prostate adenocarcinoma: expanding the differential diagnosis in prostate pathologic conditions. Radiographics. 2016;36(4):1055–75. https://doi.org/10.1148/rg.2016150226.

95. Wang G, Zhao D, Spring DJ, DePinho RA. Genetics and biology of prostate cancer. Genes Dev. 2018;32(17–18):1105–40. https://doi.org/10.1101/gad.315739.118.

96. Kaliks RA, Giglio AD. Management of advanced prostate cancer. Rev Assoc Med Bras. 2008;54(2):178–82. https://doi.org/10.1590/S0104-42302008000200025.

97. Stangelberger A, Waldert M, Djavan B. Prostate cancer in elderly men. Rev Urol. 2008;10(2):111–9.

98. Santos-Filho SD, Missailids S, Fonseca AS, Bernardo-Filho M. Prostate cancer, treatment modalities and complications: an evaluation of the scientific literature. Braz Arch Biol Technol. 2008;51:51–6. https://doi.org/10.1590/S1516-89132008000700009.

99. Janiczek M, Szylberg L, Kasperka A, Kowalewski A, Parol M, Antosik P, Radecka B, Marszalek A. Immunotherapy as a promising treatment for prostate cancer: a systematic review. J Immunol Res. 2017;2017:4861570. https://doi.org/10.1155/2017/4861570.

100. Sciarra A, Cardi A, Salvatori G, D'Eramo G, Mariotti G, Silverio FD. Which patients with prostate cancer are actually candidates for hormone therapy? Int Braz J Urol. 2004;30(6):455–65. https://doi.org/10.1590/S1677-55382004000600002.

101. Trock BJ, Han M, Freedland SJ, Humphreys EB, TL DW, Partin AW, Walsh PC. Prostate Cancer–Specific Survival Following Salvage Radiotherapy vs Observation in Men With Biochemical Recurrence After Radical Prostatectomy. JAMA. 2008;299(23):2760–9. https://doi.org/10.1001/jama.299.23.2760.
102. Borley N, Feneley MR. Prostate cancer: diagnosis and staging. Asian J Androl. 2009;11(1):74–80. https://doi.org/10.1038/aja.2008.19.
103. Nogueira L, Corradi R, Eastham JA. Prostatic specific antigen for prostate cancer detection. Int Braz J Urol. 2009;35(5):521–31. https://doi.org/10.1590/S1677-55382009000500003.
104. NIH—National Cancer Institute. Prostate cancer treatment (PDQ®)–patient version. USA: National Cancer Institute at the National Institutes of Health; 2021.
105. Novaes PERS, Motta RT, Lundgren MSFS. Treatment of prostate cancer with intensity modulated radiation therapy (IMRT). Rev Assoc Med Bras. 2013;61(1):8–16. https://doi.org/10.1590/1806-9282.61.01.008.
106. Bohmer D, Wirth M, Miller K, Budach V, Heidenreich A, Wiegel T. Radiotherapy and hormone treatment in prostate cancer: the use of combined external beam radiotherapy and hormonal therapy in the Management of Localized and Locally Advanced Prostate Cancer. Dtsch Arztebl Int. 2016;113(14):235–41. https://doi.org/10.3238/arztebl.2016.0235.
107. Mostaghel E. Abiraterone in the treatment of metastatic castration-resistant prostate cancer. Cancer Manag Res. 2014;2014(6):39–51. https://doi.org/10.2147/CMAR.S39318.
108. Fizazi K, Tran N, Fein L, Matsubara N, Rodriguez-Antolin A, Alekseev BY, Ozguroglu M, Ye D, Feyerabend S, Protheroe A, Porre PD, Kheoh T, Park YC, Todd MB, Chi KN. Abiraterone plus prednisone in metastatic, castration-sensitive prostate cancer. N Engl J Med. 2017;377:352–60. https://doi.org/10.1056/NEJMoa1704174.
109. Barata PC, Sartor AO. Metastatic castration-sensitive prostate cancer: abiraterone, docetaxel, or…. Cancer. 2019;125(11):1777–88. https://doi.org/10.1002/cncr.32039.
110. Chodak GW. Luteinizing hormone-releasing hormone (LHRH) agonists for treatment of advanced prostatic carcinoma. Urology. 1989;33(5 Suppl):42–4. https://doi.org/10.1016/0090-4295(89)90105-2.
111. Hall MC, Fritzsch RJ, Sagalowsky AI, Ahrens A, Petty B, Roehrborn CG. Prospective determination of the hormonal response after cessation of luteinizing hormone-releasing hormone agonist treatment in patients with prostate cancer. Urology. 1999;53(5):898–902. https://doi.org/10.1016/s0090-4295(99)00061-8.
112. Kovacs M, Schally AV. Comparison of mechanisms of action of luteinizing hormone-releasing hormone (LHRH) antagonist cetrorelix and LHRH agonist triptorelin on the gene expression of pituitary LHRH receptors in rats. Proc Natl Acad Sci U S A. 2001;98(21):12197–202. https://doi.org/10.1073/pnas.211442598.
113. Crawford ED, Hou AH. The role of LHRH antagonists in the treatment of prostate cancer. Oncology (Williston Park). 2009;23(7):626–30.
114. Paller CJ, Antonarakis ES. Cabazitaxel: a novel second-line treatment for metastatic castration-resistant prostate cancer. Drug Des Devel Ther. 2011;5:117–24. https://doi.org/10.2147/DDDT.S13029.
115. Abidi A. Cabazitaxel: a novel taxane for metastatic castration-resistant prostate cancer-current implications and future prospects. J Pharmacol Pharmacother. 2013;4(4):230–7. https://doi.org/10.4103/0976-500X.119704.
116. Antonarakis ES, Armstrong AJ. Evolving standards in the treatment of docetaxel-refractory castration-resistant prostate cancer. Prostate Cancer Prostatic Dis. 2011;14(3):192–205. https://doi.org/10.1038/pcan.2011.23.
117. Nader R, El Amm J, Aragon-Ching JB. Role of chemotherapy in prostate cancer. Asian J Androl. 2018;20(3):221–9. https://doi.org/10.4103/aja.aja_40_17.
118. Manecksha RP, Fitzpatrick JM. Epidemiology of testicular cancer. BJU Int. 2009;104(9 Pt B):1329–33. https://doi.org/10.1111/j.1464-410X.2009.08854.x.
119. McGlynn KA, Cook MB. Etiologic factors in testicular germ cell tumors. Future Oncol. 2009;5(9):1389–402. https://doi.org/10.2217/fon.09.116.

120. Park JS, Kim J, Elghiaty A, Ham WS. Recent global trends in testicular cancer incidence and mortality. Medicine (Baltimore). 2018;97(37):e12390. https://doi.org/10.1097/MD.0000000000012390.

121. Li Y, Lu Q, Wang Y, Ma S. Racial differences in testicular cancer in the United States: descriptive epidemiology. BMC Cancer. 2020;20:284. https://doi.org/10.1186/s12885-020-06789-2.

122. Woodward PJ, Sohaey R, O'Donoghue MJ, Green DE. From the archives of the AFIP: tumors and tumorlike lesions of the testis radiologic-pathologic correlation. Radiographics. 2002;22(1):189–216. https://doi.org/10.1148/radiographics.22.1.g02ja14189.

123. Hayes-Lattin B, Nichols CR. Testicular cancer: a prototypic tumor of young adults. Semin Oncol. 2009;36(5):432–8. https://doi.org/10.1053/j.seminoncol.2009.07.006.

124. Nauman M, Leslie SW. Nonseminomatous testicular tumors. Treasure Island USA: StatPearls Publishing; 2021.

125. Salvati M, Piccirilli M, Raco A, Santoro A, Frati R, Lenzi J, Lanzetta G, Agrillo A, Frati A. Brain metastasis from non-seminomatous germ cell tumors of the testis: indications for aggressive treatment. Neurosurg Rev. 2006;29(2):130–7.

126. Hale GR, Teplitsky S, Truong H, Gold SA, Bloom JB, Agarwal PK. Lymph node imaging in testicular cancer. Transl Androl Urol. 2018;7(5):864–74. https://doi.org/10.21037/tau.2018.07.18.

127. Syu SH, Chang CL, Shih HJ. Testicular mixed germ cell tumor presenting with seizure as the initial symptom: a case report and literature review. Int Braz J Urol. 2019;45(3):629–33. https://doi.org/10.1590/S1677-5538.IBJU.2018.0523.

128. Park S, Moon SK, Lim JW. Mechanism of metastasis to the spermatic cord and testis from advanced gastric cancer: a case report. BMC Gastroenterol. 2020;20:119. https://doi.org/10.1186/s12876-020-01269-0.

129. Shaw J. Diagnosis and treatment of testicular cancer. Am Fam Physician. 2008;77(4):469–74.

130. Daneshmand S. Management of residual mass in nonseminomatous germ cell tumors following chemotherapy. Ther Adv Urol. 2011;3(4):163–71. https://doi.org/10.1177/1756287211418721.

131. Meyts ER, Skakkebaek NE, Toppari J (2018) Testicular cancer pathogenesis, diagnosis and endocrine aspects. MDText.com Inc. South Dartmouth. Canada.

132. Farci F, Shamsudeen S. Testicular teratoma. Treasure Island USA: StatPearls Publishing; 2021.

133. Einhorn LH, Williams SD. Chemotherapy of disseminated testicular cancer. West J Med. 1979;131(1):1–3.

134. Willemse PM, Hamdy NAT, Kam ML, Burggraaf J, Osanto S. Changes in bone mineral density in newly diagnosed testicular cancer patients after anticancer treatment. J Clin Endocrinol Metabol. 2014;99(11):4101–8. https://doi.org/10.1210/jc.2014-1722.

135. Tandstad T, Stahl O, Dahl O, Haugnes HS, Hakansson U, Karlsdottir A, Kjellman A, Langberg CW, Laurell A, Oldenburg J, Solberg A, Soderstrom K, Stierner U, Cavallin-Stahl E, Wahlqvist R, Wall N, Cohn-Cedermark G. Treatment of stage I seminoma, with one course of adjuvant carboplatin or surveillance, risk-adapted recommendations implementing patient autonomy: a report from the Swedish and Norwegian testicular cancer group (SWENOTECA). Ann Oncol. 2016;27(7):1299–304. https://doi.org/10.1093/annonc/mdw164.

136. Kondagunta GV, Bacik J, Bajorin D, Dobrzynski D, Sheinfeld J, Motzer RJ, Bosl GJ. Etoposide and cisplatin chemotherapy for metastatic good-risk germ cell tumors. J Clin Oncol. 2005;23(36):9290–4. https://doi.org/10.1200/JCO.2005.03.6616.

137. McHugh DJ, Funt SA, Silber D, Knezevic A, Patil S, O'Donnell D, Tsai S, Reuter VE, Sheinfeld J, Carver BS, Motzer RJ, Bajorin DF, Bosl GJ, Feldman DR. Adjuvant chemotherapy with etoposide plus cisplatin for patients with pathologic stage II Nonseminomatous germ cell tumors. J Clin Oncol. 2020;38(12):1332–7. https://doi.org/10.1200/JCO.19.02712.

138. Funt SA, McHugh DJ, Tsai S, Knezevic A, O'Donnell D, Patil S, Silber D, Bromberg M, Carousso M, Reuter VE, Carver BS, Sheinfeld J, Motzer RJ, Bajorin DF, Bosl GJ, Feldman DR. Four cycles of etoposide plus cisplatin for patients with good-risk advanced germ cell tumors. Oncologist. 2021;26(6):483–91. https://doi.org/10.1002/onco.13719.

139. Horwich A, Sleijfer DT, Fossa SD, Kaye SB, Oliver RT, Cullen MH, Mead GM, Wit R, Mulder PH, Dearnaley DP, Pa C, Sylvester RJ, Stenning SP. Randomized trial of bleomycin, etoposide, and cisplatin compared with bleomycin, etoposide, and carboplatin in good-prognosis metastatic nonseminomatous germ cell cancer: a multiinstitutional Medical Research Council/European Organization for Research and Treatment of cancer trial. J Clin Oncol. 1997;15(5):1844–52. https://doi.org/10.1200/JCO.1997.15.5.1844.

140. Behnia M, Foster R, Einhorn LH, Donohue J, Nichols CR. Adjuvant bleomycin, etoposide and cisplatin in pathological stage II non-seminomatous testicular cancer. The Indiana University experience. Eur J Cancer. 2000;36(4):472–5. https://doi.org/10.1016/s0959-8049(99)00316-0.

141. NCT00324298 (2013) Bleomycin, Etoposide, and Cisplatin in Treating Patients With Metastatic Germ Cell Cancer of the Testicles. Clinical Trials. Available in: https://www.clinicaltrials.gov/ct2/show/NCT00324298. Accessed Sep 11 2021.

142. Aurilio G, Verri E, Frassoni S, Bagnardi V, Rocca MC, Cullurà D, Milani M, Mascia R, Curigliano G, Orsi F, Jereczek-Fossa BA, Musi G, Salè EO, Cobelli OD, Nolè F. Modified-BEP chemotherapy in patients with germ-cell tumors treated at a comprehensive cancer center. Am J Clin Oncol. 2020;43(6):381–7.

143. Hecht SM. Bleomycin: new perspectives on the mechanism of action. J Nat Prod. 2000;63(1):158–68. https://doi.org/10.1021/np990549f.

144. Brandt JP, Gerriets V. Bleomycin. Treasure Island USA: StatPearls Publishing; 2021.

145. Kier MG, Lauritsen J, Mortensen MS, Bandak M, Andersen KK, Hansen MK, Agerbaek M, Holm NV, Dalton SO, Johansen C, Daugaard G. Prognostic factors and treatment results after bleomycin, etoposide, and cisplatin in germ cell cancer: a population-based study. Eur Urol. 2017;71(2):290–8. https://doi.org/10.1016/j.eururo.2016.09.015.

146. NHS (2015) Chemotherapy Protocol. Germ Cell. Bleomycin-cisplatin-etoposide. NHS. University Hospital Southampton. NHS Foundation Trust. England. Available in: https://www.uhs.nhs.uk/Media/SUHTExtranet/Services/Chemotherapy-SOPs/Germcell/Bleomycin-Cisplatin-Etoposide%20(3%20day%20BEP)%20Ver1.2.pdf. Accessed Sep 11 2021.

147. Gama CS, Nobre SMPC, Neusquen LPDG (2016) Extravasamento de medicamentos antineoplásicos. Eurofarma. São Paulo. Brazil. Available in: https://cdn.eurofarma.com.br//wp-content/uploads/2019/11/530382..pdf. Accessed Sep 11 2021.

148. Bokemeyer C, Schleucher N, Metzner B, Thomas M, Rick O, Schmoll HJ, Kollmannsberger C, Boehlke I, Kanz L, Hartmann JT. First-line sequential high-dose VIP chemotherapy with autologous transplantation for patients with primary mediastinal nonseminomatous germ cell tumours: a prospective trial. Br J Cancer. 2003;89:29–35. https://doi.org/10.1038/sj.bjc.6600999.

149. Schmoll HJ, Kollmannsberger C, Metzner B, Hartmann JT, Schleucher N, Schoffski P, Schleicher J, Rick O, Beyer J, Hossfeld D, Kanz L, Berdel WE, Andreesen R, Bokemeyer C. Long-term results of first-line sequential high-dose etoposide, Ifosfamide, and cisplatin chemotherapy plus autologous stem cell support for patients with advanced metastatic germ cell cancer: an extended phase I/II study of the German testicular cancer study group. J Clin Oncol. 2003;21(22):4083–91. https://doi.org/10.1200/JCO.2003.09.035.

150. Colvin M (2003) Alkylating agents. In: Kufe DW, Pollock RE, Weichselbaum RR et al. Holland-Frei cancer medicine. 6th ed. Hamilton Canada, BC Decker.

151. Manikandan R, Kumar S, Dorairajan LN. Hemorrhagic cystitis: a challenge to the urologist. Indian J Urol. 2010;26(2):159–66. https://doi.org/10.4103/0970-1591.65380.

152. Monach PA, Arnold LM, Merkel PA. Incidence and prevention of bladder toxicity from cyclophosphamide in the treatment of rheumatic diseases. Arthritis Rheum. 2010;62(1):9–21. https://doi.org/10.1002/art.25061.

153. Hinton S, Catalano PJ, Einhorn LH, Nichols CR, Crawford ED, Vogelzang N, Trump D, Loehrer PJ Sr. Cisplatin, etoposide and either bleomycin or ifosfamide in the treatment of dis-

seminated germ cell tumors: final analysis of an intergroup trial. Cancer. 2003;97(8):1869–75. https://doi.org/10.1002/cncr.11271.

154. Kollmannsberger C, Eigl B (2021) BC cancer protocol summary for consolidation and salvage therapy for nonseminoma using etoposide, CISplatin, Ifosfamide, Mesna. BC cancer. British Columbia. Available in: http://www.bccancer.bc.ca/chemotherapy-protocols-site/Documents/Genitourinary/GUVIP2_Protocol.pdf. Accessed Sep 11 2021.

155. Einhorn LH, Brames MJ, Juliar B, Williams SD. Phase II study of paclitaxel plus gemcitabine salvage chemotherapy for germ cell tumors after progression following high-dose chemotherapy with tandem transplant. J Clin Oncol. 2007;25(5):513–6. https://doi.org/10.1200/JCO.2006.07.7271.

156. NCT00003518 (2010) Paclitaxel Plus Gemcitabine in Treating Patients With Refractory Metastatic Germ Cell Tumors. Clinical Trials. Available in: https://clinicaltrials.gov/ct2/show/NCT00003518. Accessed Sep 11 2021.

157. Mulherin BP, Brames MJ, Einhorn LH. Long-term survival with paclitaxel and gemcitabine for germ cell tumors after progression following high-dose chemotherapy with tandem transplant. Am J Clin Oncol. 2015;38(4):373–6. https://doi.org/10.1097/COC.0b013e31829e19e0.

158. Hinton S, Catalano PJ, Einhorn LH, Loehrer PJ Sr, Kuzel T, Vaughn D, Wilding G. Phase II study of paclitaxel plus gemcitabine in refractory germ cell tumors (E9897): a trial of the eastern cooperative oncology group. J Clin Oncol. 2002;20(7):1859–63. https://doi.org/10.1200/JCO.2002.07.158.

159. Motzer RJ, Sheinfeld J, Mazumdar M, Bains M, Mariani T, Bacik J, Bajorin D, Bosl GJ. Paclitaxel, ifosfamide, and cisplatin second-line therapy for patients with relapsed testicular germ cell cancer. J Clin Oncol. 2000;18(12):2413–8. https://doi.org/10.1200/JCO.2000.18.12.2413.

160. Kondagunta GV, Bacik J, Donadio A, Bajorin D, Marion S, Sheinfeld J, Bosl GJ, Motzer RJ. Combination of paclitaxel, ifosfamide, and cisplatin is an effective second-line therapy for patients with relapsed testicular germ cell tumors. J Clin Oncol. 2005;23(27):6549–55. https://doi.org/10.1200/JCO.2005.19.638.

161. Mead GM, Cullen MH, Huddart R, Harper P, Rustin GJS, Cook PA, Stenning SP, Mason M. A phase II trial of TIP (paclitaxel, ifosfamide and cisplatin) given as second-line (post-BEP) salvage chemotherapy for patients with metastatic germ cell cancer: a medical research council trial. Br J Cancer. 2005;93:178–84. https://doi.org/10.1038/sj.bjc.6602682.

162. NCT00004077 (2013) Paclitaxel, Ifosfamide, and Cisplatin in Treating Patients With Metastatic Testicular Cancer. Clinical Trials. Available in: https://clinicaltrials.gov/ct2/show/NCT00004077. Accessed Sep 12 2021.

163. Kawai K, Miyazaki J, Tsukamoto S, Hinotsu S, Hattori K, Shimazui T, Akaza H. Paclitaxel, Ifosfamide and cisplatin regimen is feasible for Japanese patients with advanced germ cell cancer. Jpn J Clin Oncol. 2003;33(3):127–31.

164. Almeida VL, Leitão A, Reina LCB, Montanari CA, Donnici CL, Lopes MTP. Câncer e agentes antineoplásicos não específicos do ciclo celular que interagem com o DNA: uma introdução. Química Nova. 2005;28(1):118–29. https://doi.org/10.1590/S0100-40422005000100021.

165. NHS (2015c) Chemotherapy Protocol. Germ Cell. Cisplatin-ifosfamide-paclitaxel (TIP). NHS. University Hospital Southampton. NHS Foundation Trust. England. Available in: https://www.uhs.nhs.uk/Media/SUHTExtranet/Services/Chemotherapy-SOPs/Germcell/InP-Cisplatin-Ifosfamide-Paclitaxel%20(TIP)%20Ver1.2.pdf. Accessed Sep 12 2021.

166. Farhat F, Culine S, Théodore C, Békradda M, Terrier-Lacombe MJ, Droz JP. Cisplatin and ifosfamide with either vinblastine or etoposide as salvage therapy for refractory or relapsing germ cell tumor patients: the Institut Gustave Roussy experience. Cancer. 1996;77(6):1193–7. https://doi.org/10.1002/(sici)1097-0142(19960315)77:6<1193::aid-cncr28>3.0.co;2-w.

167. Loehrer PJ Sr, Gonin R, Nichols CR, Weathers T, Einhorn LH. Vinblastine plus ifosfamide plus cisplatin as initial salvage therapy in recurrent germ cell tumor. J Clin Oncol. 1998;16(7):2500–4. https://doi.org/10.1200/JCO.1998.16.7.2500.

168. Sydnor BK, Sano HS, Waddell JA, Solimando DA. Cisplatin and ifosfamide with either vinblastine or etoposide (VIP) regimen for testicular cancer. Hosp Pharm. 2003;38(11):1016–22. https://doi.org/10.1177/001857870303801102.

169. Kollmannsberger C, Eigl B (2021b) BC cancer protocol summary for consolidation and salvage treatment for germ cell cancer using vinBLAStine, CISplatin, Ifosfamide and Mesna. BC cancer. British Columbia. Available in: http://www.bccancer.bc.ca/chemotherapy-protocols-site/Documents/Genitourinary/GUVEIP_Protocol.pdf. Accessed Sep 12 2021.

170. Ornellas AA, Andrade DM, Ornellas P, Wisnescky A, Schwindt ABS. Prognostic factors in renal cell carcinoma: analysis of 227 patients treated at the Brazilian National Cancer Institute. Int Braz J Urol. 2012;38(2):185–94. https://doi.org/10.1590/S1677-55382012000200006.

171. Quivy A, Daste A, Harbaoui A, Duc S, Bernhard JC, Gross-Goupil M, Ravaud A. Optimal management of renal cell carcinoma in the elderly: a review. Clin Interv Aging. 2013;8:433–42. https://doi.org/10.2147/CIA.S30765.

172. Padala SA, Barsouk A, Thandra KC, Saginala K, Mohammed A, Vakiti A, Rawla P, Barsouk A. Epidemiology of renal cell carcinoma. World J Oncol. 2020;11(3):79–87. https://doi.org/10.14740/wjon1279.

173. White MC, Espey DK, Swan J, Wiggins CL, Eheman C, Kaur JS. Disparities in cancer mortality and incidence among American Indians and Alaska natives in the United States. Am J Public Health. 2014;104(Suppl 3):S377–87. https://doi.org/10.2105/AJPH.2013.301673.

174. Nabi S, Kessler ER, Bernard B, Flaig TW, Lam ET. Renal cell carcinoma: a review of biology and pathophysiology. F1000Res. 2018;7:307. https://doi.org/10.12688/f1000research.13179.1.

175. Srigley JR, Delahunt B. Uncommon and recently described renal carcinomas. Mod Pathol. 2009;22:S2–S23. https://doi.org/10.1038/modpathol.2009.70.

176. Sanfilippo KM, McTigue KM, Fidler CJ, Neaton JD, Chang Y, Fried LF, Liu S, Kuller LH. Hypertension and obesity and the risk of kidney cancer in two large cohorts of us men and women. Hypertension. 2014;63(5):934–41. https://doi.org/10.1161/HYPERTENSIONAHA.113.02953.

177. Hsieh JJ, Purdue MP, Signoretti S, Swanton C, Albiges L, Schmidinger M, Heng DY, Larkin J, Ficarra V. Renal cell carcinoma. Nat Rev Dis Primers. 2017;3:17009. https://doi.org/10.1038/nrdp.2017.9.

178. Lopez-Beltran A, Henriques V, Cimadamore A, Santoni M, Cheng L, Gevaert T, Blanca A, Massari F, Scarpelli M, Montironi R. The identification of immunological biomarkers in kidney cancers. Front Oncol. 2018;8:456. https://doi.org/10.3389/fonc.2018.00456.

179. Testa U, Pelosi E, Castelli G. Genetic alterations in renal cancers: identification of the mechanisms underlying cancer initiation and progression and of therapeutic targets. Medicines (Basel). 2020;7(8):44. https://doi.org/10.3390/medicines7080044.

180. Garfield K, LaGrange CA. Renal cell cancer. Treasure Island USA: StatPearls Publishing; 2021.

181. Reznek RH. CT/MRI in staging renal cell carcinoma. Cancer Imaging. 2004;4:S35-S32. https://doi.org/10.1102/1470-7330.2004.0012.

182. Ng CS, Wood CG, Silverman PM, Tannir NM, Tamboli P, Sandler CM. Renal cell carcinoma: diagnosis, staging, and surveillance. AJR Am J Roentgenol. 2008;191(4):1220–32. https://doi.org/10.2214/AJR.07.3568.

183. Ljungberg B, Bensalah K, Bex A, Canfield S, Dabestani S, Giles RH, Hofmann F, Hora M, Kuczyk MA, Lam T, Marconi L, Merseburger AS, Powles T, Staehler M, Volpe A. Guidelines on Renal Cell Carcinoma. Netherlands: European Association of Urology; 2015.

184. Zequi SC, Abreu D. Consideration in the management of renal cell carcinoma during the COVID-19 pandemic. Int Braz J Urol. 2020;46(Suppl 1):68–78. https://doi.org/10.1590/S1677-5538.IBJU.2020.S108.

185. Heldwein FL, Mccullough TC, Souto CAV, Galiano M, Barret E. Localized renal cell carcinoma management: an update. Int Braz J Urol. 2008;34(6):676–90. https://doi.org/10.1590/S1677-55382008000600002.

186. Finelli A, Ismaila N, Bro B, Durack J, Eggener S, Evans A, Gill I, Graham D, Huang W, Jewett MAS, Latcha S, Lowrance W, Rosner M, Shayegan B, Thompson RH, Uzzo R, Russo

P. Management of Small Renal Masses: American Society of Clinical Oncology clinical practice guideline. J Clin Oncol. 2017;35(6):668–80. https://doi.org/10.1200/JCO.2016.69.9645.

187. Hassan F, Lambe S, Sharma K, Kapoor A. Current role of adjuvant therapy in high risk for recurrence resected kidney cancer. London, United Kingdom: Intechopen; 2018.

188. Sharma T, Tajzler C, Kapoor A. Is there a role for adjuvant therapy after surgery in "high risk for recurrence" kidney cancer? An update on current concepts. Curr Oncol. 2018;25(5):e444–53. https://doi.org/10.3747/co.25.3865.

189. Chin AI, Lam JS, Figlin RA, Belldegrun AS. Surveillance strategies for renal cell carcinoma patients following nephrectomy. Rev Urol. 2006;8(1):1–7.

190. Bhat S. Role of surgery in advanced/metastatic renal cell carcinoma. Indian J Urol. 2010;26(2):167–76. https://doi.org/10.4103/0970-1591.65381.

191. Logan JE, Rampersaud EN, Sonn GA, Chamie K, Belldegrun AS, Pantuck AJ, Slamon DJ, Kabbinavar FF. Systemic therapy for metastatic renal cell carcinoma: a review and update. Rev Urol. 2012;14(3–4):65–78.

192. Mennitto A, Grassi P, Ratta R, Verzoni E, Prisciandaro M, Procopio G. Nivolumab in the treatment of advanced renal cell carcinoma: clinical trial evidence and experience. Ther Adv Urol. 2016;8(5):319–26. https://doi.org/10.1177/1756287216656811.

193. Arasaratnam M, Gurney H. Nivolumab in the treatment of advanced renal cell carcinoma. Future Oncol. 2018;14(17):1679–89. https://doi.org/10.2217/fon-2017-0533.

194. Battelli C, Cho DC. mTOR inhibitors in renal cell carcinoma. Therapy. 2011;8(4):359–67. https://doi.org/10.2217/thy.11.32.

195. Pal SK, Quinn DI. Differentiating mTOR inhibitors in renal cell carcinoma. Cancer Treat Rev. 2013;39(7):709–19. https://doi.org/10.1016/j.ctrv.2012.12.015.

196. Santoni M, Conti A, Porta C, Procopio G, Sternberg CN, Basso U, Giorgi UD, Bracarda S, Rizzo M, Ortega C, Massari F, Iacovelli R, Derosa L, Masini C, Milella M, Lorenzo GD, Atzori F, Pagano M, Buti S, Vivo RD, Mosca A, Rossi M, Paglino C, Verzoni E, Cerbone L, Muzzonigro G, Falconi M, Montironi R, Burattini L, Santini D, Cascinu S. Sunitinib, pazopanib or sorafenib for the treatment of patients with late relapsing metastatic renal cell carcinoma. J Urol. 2015;193(1):41–7. https://doi.org/10.1016/j.juro.2014.07.011.

197. Bellesoeur A, Carton E, Alexandre J, Goldwasser F, Huillard O. Axitinib in the treatment of renal cell carcinoma: design, development, and place in therapy. Drug Des Devel Ther. 2017;11:2801–11. https://doi.org/10.2147/DDDT.S109640.

198. Campbell MT, Bilen MA, Shah AY, Lemke E, Jonasch E, Venkatesan AM, Altinmakas E, Duran C, Msaouel P, Tannir NM. Cabozantinib for the treatment of patients with metastatic non-clear cell renal cell carcinoma: a retrospective analysis. Eur J Cancer. 2018;104:188–94. https://doi.org/10.1016/j.ejca.2018.08.014.

199. Cancel-Treviño LA, López-Chuken Y, Hernández-Barajas D, Velázquez-Pacheco A. Nivolumab and ipilimumab in the treatment of metastatic renal cell carcinoma. Report of two patients Medicina Universitaria. 2017;19(74):22–6. https://doi.org/10.1016/j.rmu.2017.02.003.

200. Gao X, McDermott DF. Ipilimumab in combination with nivolumab for the treatment of renal cell carcinoma. Expert Opin Biol Ther. 2018;18(9):947–57. https://doi.org/10.1080/14712598.2018.1513485.

201. Rini BI, Plimack ER, Stus V, Gafanov R, Hawkins R, Nosov D, Pouliot F, Alekseev B, Soulières D, Melichar B, Vynnychenko I, Kryzhanivska A, Bondarenko I, Azevedo SJ, Borchiellini D, Szczylik C, Markus M, McDermott RS, Bedke J, Tartas S, Chang YH, Tamada S, Shou Q, Perini RF, Chen M, Atkins MB, Powles T. Pembrolizumab plus Axitinib versus sunitinib for advanced renal-cell carcinoma. N Engl J Med. 2019;380:1116–27. https://doi.org/10.1056/NEJMoa1816714.

202. Chau V, Bilusic M. pembrolizumab in combination with Axitinib as first-line treatment for patients with renal cell carcinoma (RCC): evidence to date. Cancer Manag Res. 2020;12:7321–30. https://doi.org/10.2147/CMAR.S216605.

203. Spisarová M, Melichar B, Vitásková D, Studentová H. Pembrolizumab plus axitinib for the treatment of advanced renal cell carcinoma. Expert Rev Anticancer Ther. 2021;21(7):693–703. https://doi.org/10.1080/14737140.2021.1903321.

204. Jiang Y, Chen M, Nie H, Yuan Y. PD-1 and PD-L1 in cancer immunotherapy: clinical implications and future considerations. Hum Vaccin Immunother. 2019;15(5):1111–22. https://doi.org/10.1080/21645515.2019.1571892.

205. Wu X, Gu Z, Chen Y, Chen B, Chen W, Weng L, Liu X. Application of PD-1 blockade in cancer immunotherapy. Comput Struct Biotechnol J. 2019;17:661–74. https://doi.org/10.1016/j.csbj.2019.03.006.

206. Han Y, Liu D, Li L. PD-1/PD-L1 pathway: current researches in cancer. Am J Cancer Res. 2020;10(3):727–42.

207. Kelly RJ, Rixe O. Axitinib--a selective inhibitor of the vascular endothelial growth factor (VEGF) receptor. Target Oncol. 2009;4(4):297–305. https://doi.org/10.1007/s11523-009-0126-9.

208. Gross-Goupil M, François L, Quivy A, Ravaud A. Axitinib: a review of its safety and efficacy in the treatment of adults with advanced renal cell carcinoma. Clin Med Insights Oncol. 2013;7:269–77. https://doi.org/10.4137/CMO.S10594.

209. Shaik F, Cuthbert GA, Homer-Vanniasinkam S, Muench SP, Ponnambalam S, Harrison MA. Structural basis for vascular endothelial growth factor receptor activation and implications for disease therapy. Biomol Ther. 2020;10:1673. https://doi.org/10.3390/biom10121673.

210. Powles T, Plimack ER, Soulières D, Waddell T, Stus V, Gafanov R, Nosov D, Pouliot F, Melichar B, Vynnychenko I, Azevedo SJ, Borchiellini D, McDermott RS, Bedke J, Tamada S, Yin L, Chen M, Molife LR, Atkins MB, Rini B. Pembrolizumab plus axitinib versus sunitinib monotherapy as first-line treatment of advanced renal cell carcinoma (KEYNOTE-426): extended follow-up from a randomised, open-label, phase 3 trial. Lancet Oncol. 2020;21(12):1563–73. https://doi.org/10.1016/S1470-2045(20)30436-8.

211. Watson TR, Gao X, Reynolds KL, Kong CY. Cost-effectiveness of pembrolizumab plus Axitinib vs nivolumab plus ipilimumab as first-line treatment of advanced renal cell carcinoma in the US. JAMA Netw Open. 2020;3(10):e2016144. https://doi.org/10.1001/jamanetworkopen.2020.16144.

212. Plimack ER, Powles T, Bedke J, Pouliot F, Stus V, Waddell T, Gafanov R, Nosov D, Alekseev B, McDermott RS, Markus M, Tartas S, Kryzhanivska A, Bondarenko I, Szczylik C, Lin J, Perini RF, Molife LR, Atkins MB, Rini BI. Outcomes for patients in the pembrolizumab+axitinib arm with advanced renal cell carcinoma (RCC) who completed two years of treatment in the phase III KEYNOTE-426 study. J Clin Oncol. 2021;39(6_suppl):327. https://doi.org/10.1200/JCO.2021.39.6_suppl.327.

213. Kollmannsberger C (2021) BC cancer protocol summary for the treatment of metastatic renal cell carcinoma using pembrolizumab and aXitinib. BC cancer. British Columbia. Available in: http://www.bccancer.bc.ca/chemotherapy-protocols-site/Documents/Genitourinary/GUAVPEMAX_Protocol.pdf. Accessed Sep 15 2021.

214. Motzer RJ, Penkov K, Haanen J, Rini B, Albiges L, Campbell MT, Venugopal B, Kollmannsberger C, Negrier S, Uemura M, Lee JL, Vasiliev A, Miller WH, Gurney H, Schmidinger M, Larkin J, Atkins MB, Bedke J, Alekseev B, Wang J, Mariani M, Robbins PB, Chudnovsky A, Fowst C, Hariharan S, Huang B, di Pietro A, Choueiri TK. Avelumab plus axitinib versus sunitinib for advanced renal-cell carcinoma. N Engl J Med. 2019;380:1103–15. https://doi.org/10.1056/NEJMoa1816047.

215. Choueiri TK, Motzer RJ, Rini BI, Haanen J, Campbell MT, Venugopal B, Kollmannsberger C, Gravis-Mescam G, Uemura M, Lee JL, Grimm MO, Gurney H, Schmidinger M, Larkin J, Atkins MB, Pal SK, Wang J, Mariani M, Krishnaswami S, Cislo P, Chudnovsky A, Fowst C, Huang B, di Pietro A, Albiges L. Updated efficacy results from the JAVELIN renal 101 trial: first-line avelumab plus axitinib versus sunitinib in patients with advanced renal cell carcinoma. Ann Oncol. 2020;31(8):1030–9. https://doi.org/10.1016/j.annonc.2020.04.010.

216. Motzer RJ, Robbins PB, Powles T, Albiges L, Haanen JB, Larkin J, Mu XJ, Ching KA, Uemura M, Pal SK, Alekseev B, Gravis G, Campbell MT, Penkov K, Lee JL, Hariharan S, Wang X, Zhang W, Wang J, Chudnovsky A, di Pietro A, Donahue AC, Choueiri TK. Avelumab plus axitinib versus sunitinib in advanced renal cell carcinoma: biomarker analysis of the

phase 3 JAVELIN renal 101 trial. Nat Med. 2020;26:1733–41. https://doi.org/10.1038/s41591-020-1044-8.

217. NHS (2020) Chemotherapy Protocol. Renal Cell. Avelumab-axitinib. NHS. University Hospital Southampton. NHS Foundation Trust. England. Available in: https://www.uhs.nhs.uk/Media/SUHTExtranet/Services/Chemotherapy-SOPs/Renal-cell/Axitinib-Avelumab.pdf. Accessed Sep 17 2021.

218. Collins JM, Gulley JL. Product review: avelumab, an anti-PD-L1 antibody. Hum Vaccin Immunother. 2019;15(4):891–908. https://doi.org/10.1080/21645515.2018.1551671.

219. Shen X, Zhang L, Li J, Li Y, Wang Y, Xu ZX. Recent findings in the regulation of programmed death ligand 1 expression. Front Immunol. 2019;10:1337. https://doi.org/10.3389/fimmu.2019.01337.

220. Tomita Y, Motzer RJ, Choueiri TK, Rini BI, Miyake H, Uemura H, Albiges L, Fujii Y, Umeyama Y, Wang J, Mariani M, Schmidinger M. Efficacy and safety of avelumab plus axitinib (a + ax) versus sunitinib (S) in elderly patients with advanced renal cell carcinoma (aRCC): extended follow-up results from JAVELIN renal 101. J Clin Oncol. 2021;39(6_suppl):301. https://doi.org/10.1200/JCO.2021.39.6_suppl.301.

Chapter 7
Chemotherapeutic Protocols
for the Treatment of Gynecological Cancer

7.1 Epidemiological Profile of Gynecological Cancers

Gynecological cancers involve cancers of the ovary, cervix, body of the uterus, vulva, vagina, and fallopian tubes. Uterine cancer stands out as the most incident worldwide, accounting for 604,000 cases and 342,000 deaths in 2020, according to WHO data. The least common is vaginal cancer with an incidence of 17,900 reported cases and 8000 deaths in 2020 [1, 2]. White women have a higher incidence rate of uterine, ovarian, and vulvar cancers, while Hispanic women had a higher incidence of cervical cancer and Black women had a higher incidence of vaginal cancer [3–5]. Figure 7.1 shows the estimated incidence and mortality cases for the year 2040.

Survival rates for gynecological cancers depend on the stage at which the cancer is diagnosed, varying according to the type of gynecological cancer. In ovarian cancers, the diagnosis tends to occur at an advanced stage, with the presence of metastases, which reduces the survival rate, while in cervical cancer the diagnosis tends to occur earlier, usually at an early stage, when the cancer is localized, thereby increasing the survival rate [6–10].

Some risk factors for the development of gynecological cancers may include increasing age, nulliparity, obesity, postmenopausal hormone replacement therapy, fertility drugs, human papillomavirus (HPV) infection, smoking, family history of breast and ovarian cancer, and cervical or colorectal. One of the main risk factors for cervical cancer is HPV infection, accounting for approximately 90% of all cervical cancers [11–15].

© The Author(s), under exclusive license to Springer Nature
Switzerland AG 2022
I. D. Lima Cavalcanti, *Chemotherapy Protocols and Infusion Sequence*,
https://doi.org/10.1007/978-3-031-10839-6_7

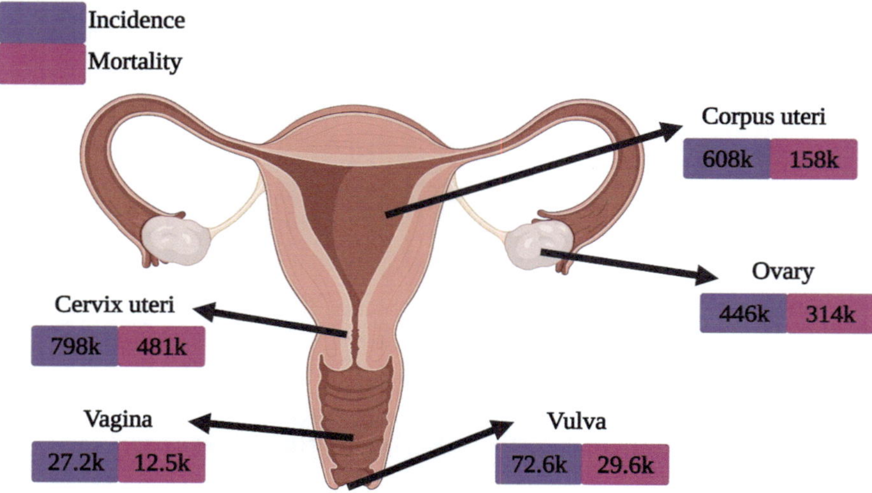

Fig. 7.1 Estimated incidence of cases and mortality for the year 2040 of gynecological cancers. (Source: Created with BioRender.com and data were extracted from [1])

7.2 Pathophysiology of Ovarian Cancer

Ovarian cancer is the third most common cancer in women, with a worse prognosis and higher mortality rate, being three times more lethal than breast cancer. One of the factors that contribute to the late diagnosis of ovarian cancer is due to its asymptomatic growth, with late onset of symptoms and lack of adequate screening, resulting in diagnosis at an advanced stage, with a 5-year survival rate of 29%, with only 15% of cases being diagnosed at an early stage [8, 13, 16–18].

The origin of the ovarian tumor can be from epithelial cells, stromal cells, and germ cells. In developed countries, there is a prevalence of epithelial cell ovarian tumors (90% of cases), followed by sex cord-stromal tumors (5–6% of cases), and then germ cell tumors (2–3% of cases). Epithelial cancers are classified as mucinous (represents 3%) and non-mucinous, where non-mucinous can be further subclassified into serous (70% of non-mucinous cases), endometrioid (represents 10% of cases), clear cells (10% of non-mucinous), and unspecified (5% of cases) [13, 19–23].

As for staging (Fig. 7.2), stage I ovarian cancers are located in the ovaries, stage II are located in the pelvis, and in stage III, they may be present on the peritoneal surface, peritoneal implants, and abdominal implants and may or may not be present in the nearby lymph nodes. In stage 4, the tumor has spread to the lung, pleura, liver parenchyma, or other extra-abdominal organs [23–25].

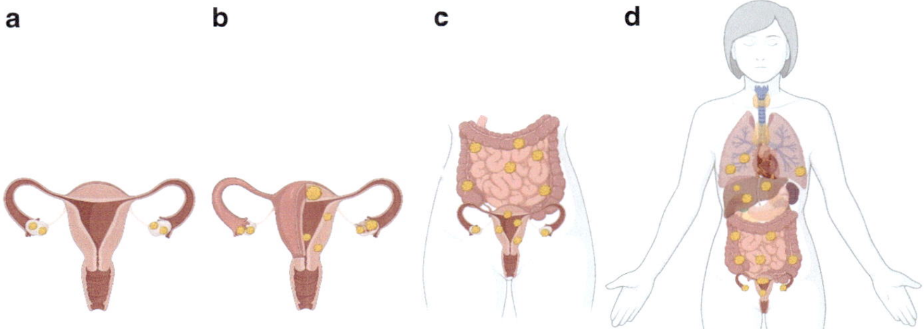

Fig. 7.2 Stages of ovarian cancer. (**a**) Stage I, (**b**) Stage II, (**c**) Stage III, (**d**) Stage IV. (Source: Created with BioRender.com)

7.2.1 Chemotherapy for the Treatment of Epithelial Ovarian Cancer

The treatment modality for epithelial ovarian cancer may include surgery, which in the early stages is an approach that can be curative, and in the advanced stage, surgical debulking followed by systemic chemotherapy may be indicated. Chemotherapy may be indicated for intravenous or intraperitoneal administration [26, 27]. As a single agent for the treatment of ovarian cancer, carboplatin or cisplatin is indicated in the treatment of invasive epithelial ovarian cancer. Cyclophosphamide can be used in palliative therapy in relapsing/progressive epithelial carcinoma, primary peritoneal, or fallopian tube carcinoma. Docetaxel, paclitaxel, gemcitabine, topotecan, or etoposide are found effective in the treatment of platinum-refractory epithelial ovarian carcinoma, primary peritoneal carcinoma, or fallopian tube carcinoma [28–37].

Pegylated liposomal doxorubicin is indicated as monotherapy in the treatment of epithelial ovarian cancer with relapse after primary treatment; vinorelbine as palliative therapy for the retreatment of ovarian, tubal, and peritoneal cancer; and olaparib as a target-directed therapy for the maintenance of responsive epithelial cancer to platinum mutated by newly diagnosed BRCA [38–42]. Hormone therapy, such as aromatase inhibitors and tamoxifen, may also be indicated in the treatment of advanced ovarian cancer [43, 44].

Combination therapy is also indicated in the treatment of epithelial ovarian cancer, such as the combination of carboplatin and paclitaxel, which is used in cancers of the gastrointestinal tract (see Chap. 5), but it is also indicated in the primary treatment of epithelial cancer invasive ovarian, fallopian tube and primary peritoneal and in the primary treatment of stage III invasive epithelial cancer or stage 1 or 2 papillary serous ovarian cancer [45–50]. More combinations used in the treatment of epithelial ovarian cancer will be covered in the next topics [51–53].

7.2.1.1 CABR Protocol (Carboplatin and Abraxane)

The CABR protocol is based on the combination of carboplatin and Abraxane (nab-paclitaxel), which is paclitaxel encapsulated in albumin nanoparticles for the alternative treatment of gynecological malignancies. Drugs of the taxane class are widely used in the treatment of gynecological cancers, due to their important therapeutic response and the discontinuation of therapy with these agents should be reconsidered with the administration of nab-paclitaxel. According to Maurer et al. [54], nab-paclitaxel is well tolerated without hypersensitivity reactions, in which complications observed with the use of nab-paclitaxel were neutropenia, thrombocytopenia, anemia, and neurotoxicity.

Benigno and Hines [55], in a phase II study, observed the efficacy of the combination of nab-paclitaxel plus carboplatin in recurrent platinum-sensitive ovarian or primary peritoneal cancer. Of the ten patients who were included in the study, two who had completed two protocol cycles and had 50% tumor reduction, and, in terms of toxicity, cases of neutropenia, thrombocytopenia, and anemia were reported.

Srinivasan, Rauthan, and Gopal [56] proposed the combination of nab-paclitaxel with carboplatin as first-line therapy in ovarian cancer. The authors looked at three cases of patients who used the combination, noting that chemotherapy was well tolerated, with all responding to chemotherapy. Pothuri et al. [57], in a phase 2 study, evaluated the effectiveness of the combination as a first line in the treatment of epithelial cancers, showing that the protocol promoted a 6-month progression-free survival of 80.5%, with adverse events that included anemia, neutropenia, and diarrhea.

Parisi et al. [58] evaluated the efficacy of the first-line combination of nab-paclitaxel and carboplatin in patients with advanced ovarian cancer after hypersensitivity reaction to solvent-based taxanes. The protocol promoted a progression-free survival of 16.7 months and overall survival of 65.4 months. As the toxicity of combination, the patients presented asthenia, hypertransaminasemia, neutropenia, thrombocytopenia, and anemia, without the occurrence of hypersensitivity reactions. The infusion sequence used is starting with nab-paclitaxel followed by carboplatin infusion (Fig. 7.3) [59, 60].

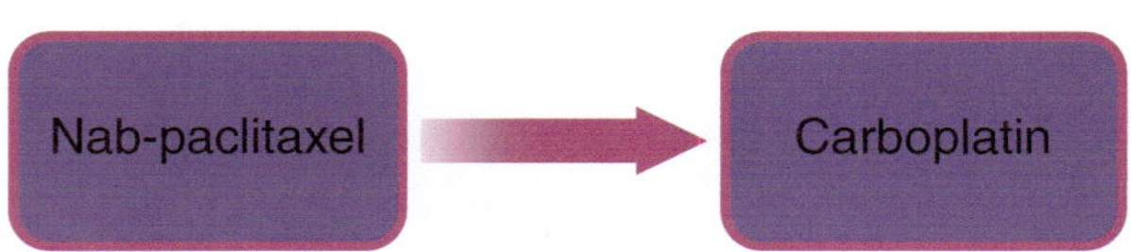

Fig. 7.3 CABR protocol infusion sequence

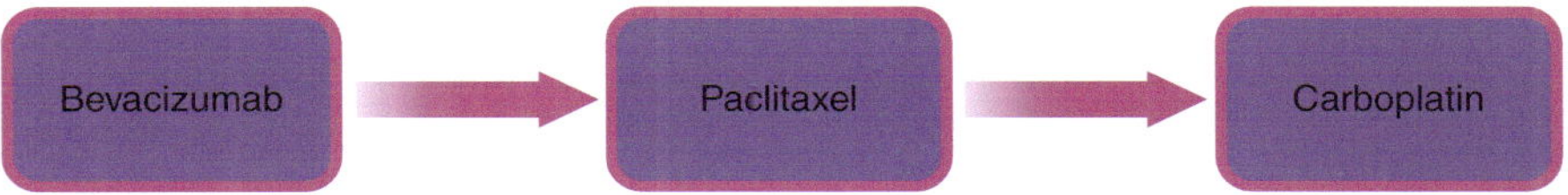

Fig. 7.4 CAPBEV protocol infusion sequence

7.2.1.2   CAPBEV Protocol (Carboplatin, Paclitaxel, and Bevacizumab)

The combination of carboplatin, paclitaxel, and bevacizumab may be indicated for the first-line treatment of patients with stage 3–4 epithelial ovarian cancer. Coleman et al. [61] evaluated the effectiveness of the combination in the treatment of platinum-sensitive recurrent ovarian cancer. The protocol promoted a median overall survival of 42.2 months, with a toxicity profile that included hypertension, fatigue, and proteinuria.

The inclusion of bevacizumab associated with carboplatin and paclitaxel brought benefits for the treatment of advanced epithelial ovarian cancer, promoting the prolongation of progression-free survival [62]. The infusion sequence of the CAPBEV protocol starts with bevacizumab followed by paclitaxel and finally carboplatin (Fig. 7.4) [63].

Despite the benefits, one of the major problems with the combination is the high rate of hypersensitivity reaction, and replacing paclitaxel with nab-paclitaxel appears to reduce the occurrence of hypersensitivity reactions [58].

The combination of nab-paclitaxel with bevacizumab appears to be effective in platinum-resistant primary recurrent epithelial carcinoma or primary peritoneal carcinoma. According to Tillmanns et al. [64], the combination promoted an overall survival of 16.5 months, with a progression-free survival of 8.3 months, and a partial response in 46.1% of patients. In another study, Tillmanns et al. [65] continued to look at the benefits of the combination, noting an overall response rate of 50%, with a progression-free survival of 8.08 months, and overall survival of 17.15 months.

As an alternative for the treatment of gynecological cancers, in patients who have experienced moderate or severe hypersensitivity reactions to paclitaxel, the combination of carboplatin, nab-paclitaxel, and bevacizumab may be a viable alternative. As for the infusion sequence, the first cycle starts with nab-paclitaxel and ends with bevacizumab (Fig. 7.5a) to prevent the patient from developing an immunogenic reaction with bevacizumab, From the second cycle, the protocol starts with bevacizumab followed by nab-paclitaxel and finally carboplatin (Fig. 7.5b) [66].

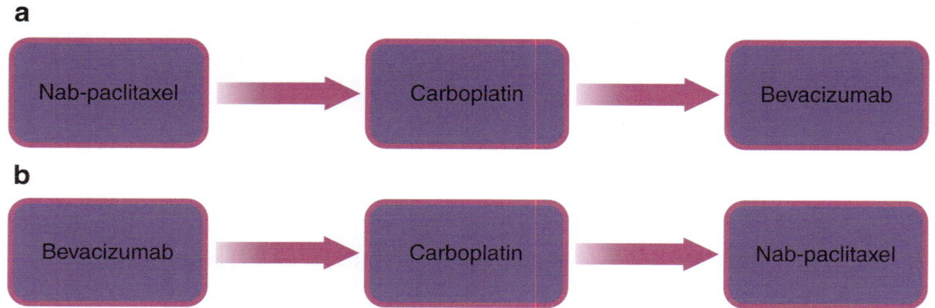

Fig. 7.5 CABRBEV infusion sequence. (**a**) First cycle infusion sequence starting with nab-paclitaxel. (**b**) Infusion sequence from the second cycle, starting with bevacizumab

7.2.1.3 CISP Protocol (Cisplatin and Paclitaxel)

The CISP protocol is another combination indicated for the alternative treatment of gynecological malignancies. Goldberg et al. [67] evaluated the combination of cisplatin and paclitaxel in recurrent epithelial ovarian cancer. The results showed a response rate of 53% and a median survival of >23 months with all complete responders alive during the median follow-up of 23 months.

Rose et al. [68] evaluated the protocol's efficacy in recurrent or advanced squamous cell cervical carcinoma. As a result, the authors observed a progression-free interval of 5.4 months and a median survival of 10 months, with adverse events that included neutropenia and thrombocytopenia, with 4.5% of deaths from neutropenic sepsis. Moore et al. [69] highlight that the combination of cisplatin and paclitaxel is superior to cisplatin monotherapy in the treatment of recurrent or persistent squamous cell cervical cancer. Patients in the study by Moore et al. [69] had progression-free survival of 4.8 months and a median survival of 9.7 months, with an objective response rate of 36%.

Bois et al. [70] found that the combination of cisplatin and paclitaxel had comparable efficacy to the combination of carboplatin and paclitaxel. The CISP protocol had progression-free survival of 19.1 months and overall survival of 44.1 months. Armstrong et al. [71] evaluated the efficacy of cisplatin plus paclitaxel given intraperitoneally, comparing the same combination given intravenously in the treatment of ovarian cancer. Intraperitoneal administration of therapy was superior, increasing progression-free survival from 18.3 to 23.8 months and overall survival from 49.7 to 65.6 months.

Moioli et al. [72] evaluated the role of the CISP protocol in the neoadjuvant treatment of locally advanced cervical cancer. The protocol induced optimal response in 21.4%, partial response in 64.3%, and no response in 14.2% of patients. As for adverse events, the authors observed a higher frequency of alopecia, asthenia, nausea and vomiting, hypersensitivity to paclitaxel, and neutropenia.

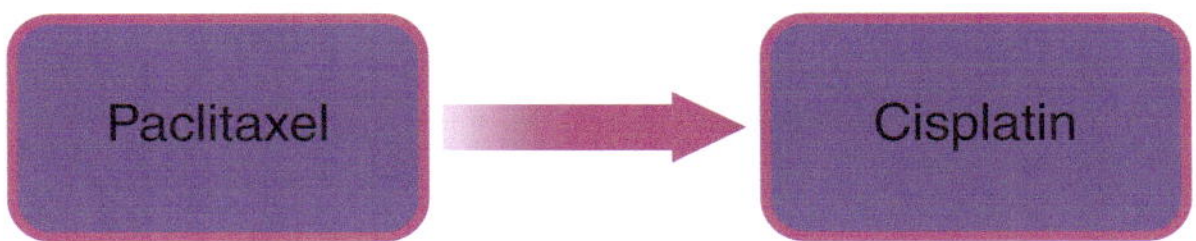

Fig. 7.6 CISP protocol infusion sequence

As for the infusion sequence of the CISP protocol (Fig. 7.6), the administration of paclitaxel must be given first, as when cisplatin is administered before it can reduce the therapeutic efficacy of paclitaxel. Jekunen et al. [73] highlight in their study that when paclitaxel is administered first, it has synergistic effects with cisplatin in the treatment of ovarian cancer, but when cisplatin is administered earlier, antagonistic effects occur, which may contribute to a possible increase in the protocol's toxicity. Thus, the authors show that the protocol's effectiveness depends on the administration schedule.

7.2.1.4   CISPBEV Protocol (Cisplatin, Paclitaxel, and Bevacizumab)

The addition of bevacizumab to the CISP protocol is also an alternative treatment for gynecological malignancies. The inclusion of bevacizumab prolongs progression-free survival as a first-line treatment in stage 4 patients [74]. Konner et al. [74] evaluated the efficacy of combining bevacizumab with intraperitoneal administration of cisplatin and paclitaxel. The protocol led to a progression-free survival of 28.6 months and adverse events that included neutropenia, vasovagal syncope, hypertension, nausea and vomiting, hypomagnesemia, and abdominal pain.

Olivia et al. [75] evaluated the combination of cisplatin plus paclitaxel with maintenance bevacizumab in ovarian carcinoma. In the study, the combination slowed tumor progression in the mouse model with epithelial ovarian cancer xenografts, in addition to prolonging survival, reducing ascites and tumor spread. In advanced cervical cancer, the CISPBEV protocol was superior to the CISP protocol without bevacizumab, in the study by Chu et al. [76], with benefits in overall survival of 16.4 months and progression-free survival of 9.2 months.

Also in the treatment of advanced cervical cancer, Sugiyama et al. [77] evaluated the efficacy of the CISPBEV protocol followed by single-agent bevacizumab. The combination promoted an overall response rate of 86%, with adverse events that included alopecia, hypertension, nausea, decreased appetite, and peripheral sensory neuropathy. Regarding the infusion schedule, start with the monoclonal antibody bevacizumab due to its target-directed action, followed by paclitaxel, and finally cisplatin to induce the synergistic effects of the association (Fig. 7.7) [73, 78].

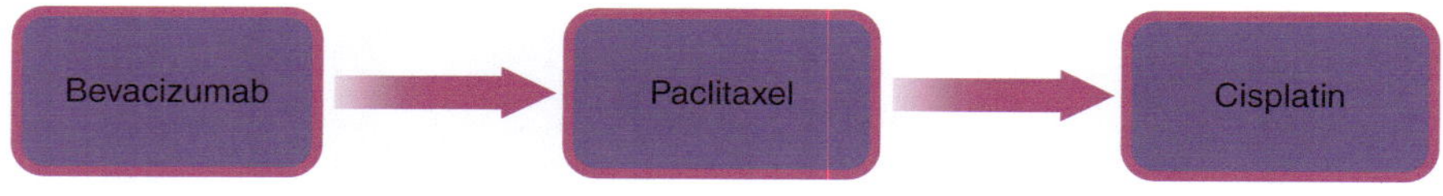

Fig. 7.7 Infusion sequence of the CISPBEV protocol

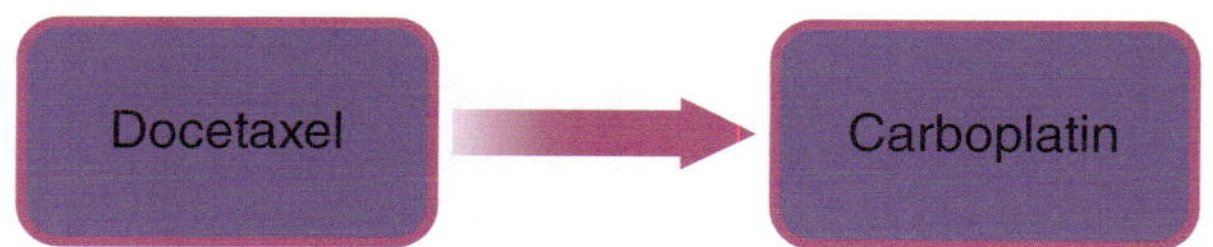

Fig. 7.8 CAD protocol infusion sequence

7.2.1.5 CAD Protocol (Carboplatin and Docetaxel)

The CAD protocol combines carboplatin and docetaxel and has been used in the treatment of invasive epithelial cancer, fallopian tube, and primary peritoneal cancer [79–81]. Vasey et al. [82] proposed the use of the CAD protocol as the first line in epithelial ovarian cancer, showing its efficacy with an overall response rate of 66% and progression-free survival of 16.6 months. In another study, Vasey et al. [83] compared the combination of carboplatin and docetaxel with the combination of paclitaxel and carboplatin as first-line chemotherapy for ovarian cancer. The authors noted that both protocols had a similar response and progression-free survival.

Markman et al. [84] evaluated the efficacy of the CAD protocol in patients with ovarian and fallopian tube cancers and primary carcinoma of the peritoneum, showing that the combination induced an objective response of 81% and the most frequent adverse events included neutropenia, hypersensitivity reactions, and peripheral neuropathy, with the greatest toxicity being bone marrow suppression.

Wang et al. [85], in a multicenter, nonrandomized, phase 3 study, evaluated the efficacy of the combination of docetaxel and carboplatin as a second line in epithelial ovarian, peritoneal, or platinum-sensitive fallopian tube cancer. The authors observed an overall response rate of 70% with 28% complete responses and progression-free survival of 12.4 months. As for toxicity, cases of neutropenia were reported in 80%, febrile neutropenia in 16%, and peripheral sensory neuropathy in 7% of the patients studied.

As for the CAD protocol infusion sequence (Fig. 7.8), it starts with docetaxel, which is a cycle-specific drug and has an irritant or vesicant characteristic, followed by carboplatin, which is a non-cell cycle specific [86].

7.2.1.6 CAG Protocol (Carboplatin and Gemcitabine)

Carboplatin combined with gemcitabine is used in the treatment of advanced ovarian cancer in patients who have progressed or recurred after first-line platinum-based treatment [87, 88]. du Bois et al. [87] evaluated the efficacy and safety of the

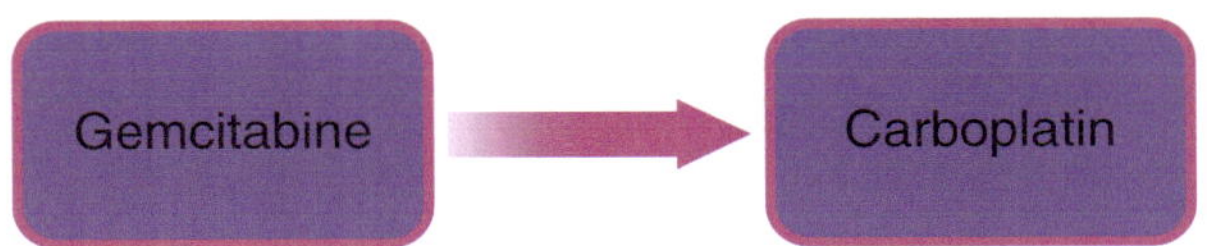

Fig. 7.9 CAG protocol infusion sequence

CAG protocol as a second line in the treatment of platinum-sensitive ovarian cancer. The authors noted that the protocol was well tolerated, with myelosuppression as dose-limiting toxicity, with thrombocytopenia being the main side effect. The objective response to treatment was 62.5% of patients and median progression of 10 months with overall survival of more than 18 months.

Pfisterer et al. [89] evaluated the effectiveness of combination therapy with gemcitabine and carboplatin in the treatment of recurrent ovarian cancer. The combination promoted a progression-free survival of 8.6 months, a response rate of 47.2%, and an overall survival hazard ratio of 0.96. In another study, Pfisterer et al. [88] compared the CAG protocol with carboplatin as monotherapy in platinum-sensitive recurrent ovarian cancer. The CAG protocol significantly improved progression-free survival (from 5.8 to 8.6 months) and response rate (from 30.9% to 47.2%) without inducing a worsening in quality of life.

Sufliarsky et al. [90] used the combination of gemcitabine and carboplatin to treat patients with relapsed ovarian cancer. The authors noted that the protocol promoted an 83% survival rate and the response rate was 67.3%. As for toxicity, the most common were leukopenia, anemia, neutropenia, and thrombocytopenia.

As for the order of infusion of the CAG protocol, Wang et al. [91] highlight in their study that the synergistic effect seems to be schedule dependent. When gemcitabine is administered first or even concomitantly with carboplatin, they seem to show the synergistic effect, but when carboplatin is administered first, it has a moderate antagonistic effect. Because gemcitabine is cell cycle specific and the findings of Wang et al. [91], perhaps the administration of gemcitabine followed by carboplatin is more appropriate (Fig. 7.9) [92, 93].

7.2.1.7 PLDC Protocol (Pegylated Liposomal Doxorubicin and Carboplatin)

The combination of pegylated liposomal doxorubicin with carboplatin is indicated in the first-line treatment of epithelial ovarian cancer [40, 41, 94, 95]. Pegylated liposomal doxorubicin (Fig. 7.10) is the drug encapsulated in liposomes, thereby reducing its toxicity and increasing its therapeutic efficacy [96–99].

Pujade-Lauraine et al. [100] compared the combination of pegylated liposomal doxorubicin and carboplatin with paclitaxel and carboplatin in the treatment of platinum-sensitive ovarian cancer in late recurrence. The protocol containing liposomal doxorubicin was superior to the protocol containing paclitaxel in terms of progression-free survival outcomes (11.3 months for the doxorubicin protocol compared to 9.4 months for the paclitaxel protocol).

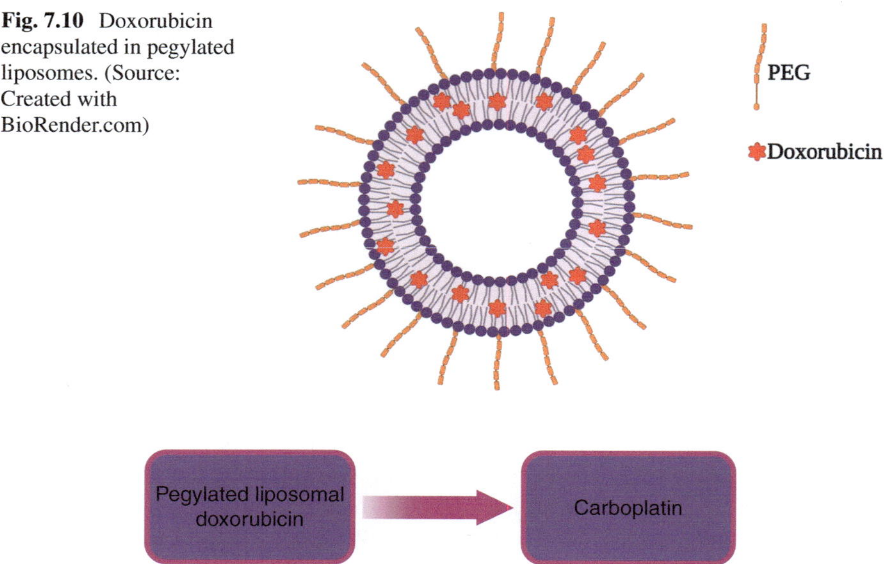

Fig. 7.10 Doxorubicin encapsulated in pegylated liposomes. (Source: Created with BioRender.com)

Fig. 7.11 PLDC protocol infusion sequence

In a phase 2 study, Weber et al. [94] evaluated the effectiveness of the PLDC protocol in late recurrence ovarian cancer. The protocol promoted an objective response rate of 65.4%, progression-free survival of 13.6 months, and overall survival of 38.9 months. No cases of cardiotoxicity were identified, thus supporting the tolerability of pegylated liposomal doxorubicin combined with carboplatin.

Ferrero et al. [101], in a phase 2 study, used the combination of the PLDC protocol in the second-line treatment of advanced ovarian cancer in late recurrence. The protocol proved to be highly effective, with an overall response of 63% with 38% of patients having a complete response. Progression-free survival was 9.4 months, and overall survival was 32 months. The most frequent toxicity was neutropenia in 51% of patients. As for the infusion sequence, the PLDC protocol starts with pegylated liposomal doxorubicin as it has a targeted action, followed by carboplatin (Fig. 7.11) [102].

7.2.1.8   BEVG Protocol (Bevacizumab and Gemcitabine)

The BEVG protocol combines bevacizumab with gemcitabine for the treatment of platinum-resistant epithelial ovarian cancer [103–105]. Kogiku et al. [104] observed the feasibility of the BEVG protocol in the treatment of platinum-resistant epithelial ovarian cancer, in which the authors observed that the protocol promoted a response rate of 66.7%, showing its efficacy and safety, with the main toxicity being neutropenia, thrombocytopenia, and hypertension.

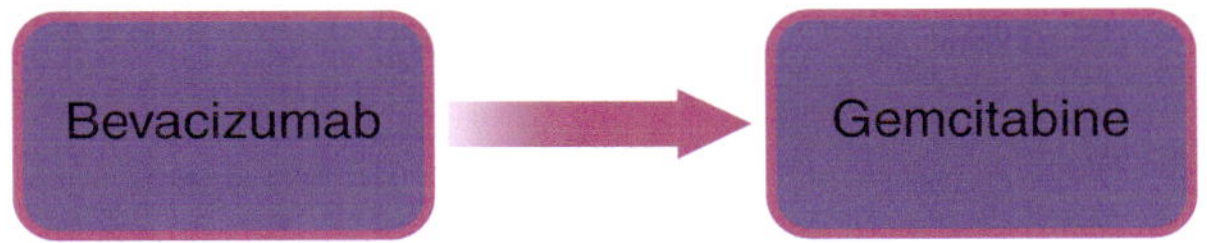

Fig. 7.12 BEVG protocol infusion sequence

Takasaki et al. [105] highlight that the addition of bevacizumab combined with gemcitabine improved progression-free survival and overall survival in patients with platinum-resistant recurrent ovarian cancer, with a response rate of 38.9%. In a phase 2 study, Nagao et al. [106] evaluated the efficacy of a combination of bevacizumab and gemcitabine in recurrent epithelial ovarian, primary peritoneal, or platinum-resistant fallopian tube cancer. The authors observed an objective response rate of 42% and a clinical control rate of 84%. Progression-free survival for the protocol was 5.1 months, and overall survival was 21.3 months. The toxicity profile was similar to other studies with cases of neutropenia, anemia, thrombocytopenia, and hypertension. As for the infusion sequence of the BEVG protocol, it might be interesting to start with bevacizumab, which is a monoclonal antibody with a target-directed action, followed by gemcitabine (Fig. 7.12) [92, 107].

7.2.1.9 BEVPLD Protocol (Bevacizumab and Pegylated Liposomal Doxorubicin)

The BEVPLD protocol combines bevacizumab with pegylated liposomal doxorubicin in the treatment of platinum-resistant epithelial ovarian cancer [108, 109]. The combination proved to be effective in the phase 2 study by Verschraegen et al. [110], in patients with platinum and taxane-resistant ovarian cancer. The protocol promoted a progression-free survival of 6.6 months and overall survival of 33.2 months. As for toxicity, mucosal and dermal erosions and asymptomatic cardiac dysfunction were observed.

The role of bevacizumab in the treatment of ovarian cancer has gained prominence because, when associated with chemotherapy, it has improved the overall survival and progression-free survival of patients with ovarian cancer [111]. According to Bamias et al. [112], the inclusion of bevacizumab in platinum-resistant ovarian cancer therapy improves overall survival and maximizes the likelihood of active treatment for this type of cancer.

As for the protocol infusion sequence, care should be taken with possible allergic reactions developed by the patients, observing whether fever, chills, skin rash, pruritus, urticaria, or angioedema during the infusion and the infusion should be interrupted. As bevacizumab is a target-directed drug, it initiates infusion followed by infusion of pegylated liposomal doxorubicin (Fig. 7.13) [113].

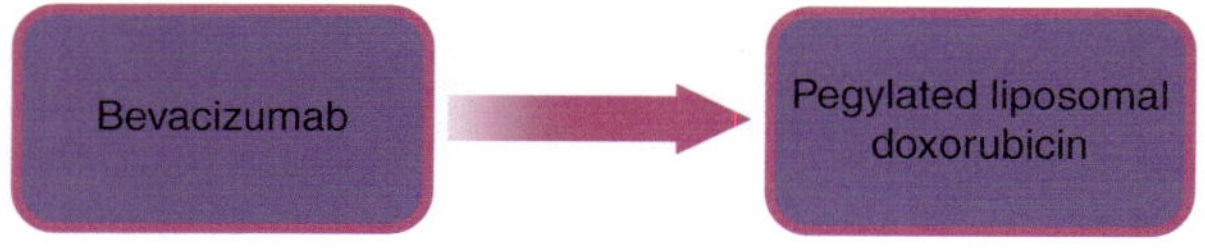

Fig. 7.13 BEVPLD protocol infusion sequence

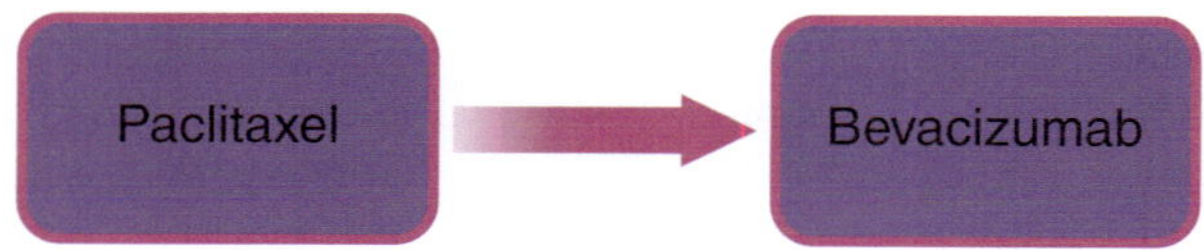

Fig. 7.14 BEVP protocol infusion sequence

7.2.1.10 BEVP Protocol (Bevacizumab and Paclitaxel)

Another protocol that includes bevacizumab is BEVP, which combines with paclitaxel in the treatment of platinum-resistant epithelial ovarian cancer [108, 114, 115]. In a phase 3 study, Perren et al. [114] evaluated the combination of bevacizumab with paclitaxel and carboplatin. The inclusion of bevacizumab resulted in an increase in overall survival to 36.6 months and progression-free survival to 18.1 months. Similar results were observed by Burger et al. [116] who also observed an increase in progression-free survival with the association of bevacizumab with chemotherapy to 14.1 months.

Lee et al. [117] highlight that the combination of bevacizumab and paclitaxel promoted a progression-free survival of 8.3 months and overall survival of 21 months. Regarding toxicity, the protocol induced the development of neutropenia, thrombocytopenia, anemia, and hypertension. As for the order of infusion, Tinker [118] recommends starting with paclitaxel followed by bevacizumab (Fig. 7.14).

7.2.2 Chemotherapy for the Treatment of Non-epithelial Ovarian Cancer

Treatment modalities for non-epithelial ovarian cancer include surgery that may or may not preserve fertility, cytoreductive, and rescue. In the initial stage, it usually opts for a conservative approach, in more advanced cases, bilateral oophorectomy, which can be combined with radiotherapy [119–121].

Adjuvant treatment with combined chemotherapy is also one of the therapeutic options, with platinum-based protocols being the standard treatment for non-epithelial ovarian cancer [120, 121]. The ETCIS protocol, discussed in Chap. 5, which combines etoposide and cisplatin in the treatment of cancers of the gastrointestinal tract, may be indicated in the treatment of non-dysgerminomatous ovarian germ cells. Another protocol also widely used is the BEP protocol, which is indicated for the treatment of genitourinary cancers, discussed in Chap. 4 and which has been indicated for the treatment of non-dysgerminomatous ovarian germ cell cancer [121–123].

7.3   Pathophysiology of Cervical Cancer

In 2020, 604,000 cases of cervical cancer and 342,000 deaths were reported worldwide [1]. More than 500,000 new cases of cervical cancer are reported annually, with approximately 250,000 deaths annually. In 2018, cervical cancer was the fourth most common in women, behind breast, colorectal, and lung cancer [124, 125].

About 99% of cases of cervical cancer are related to high-risk HPV infection, being a very common virus transmitted through sexual contact. HPV infection is mainly asymptomatic and transient, in which only 20% develop premalignant lesions, with a small portion becoming malignant [11, 126–128]. The integration of HPV into the cell genome appears to be an important step in the cancer development process, associated with genetic mutations that induce immune system failure [129–131].

Cervical cancer (Fig. 7.15) is classified based on morphological criteria such as squamous cell carcinoma, adenocarcinoma, or adenosquamous carcinoma. Most cervical cancers are squamous cell carcinomas, followed by adenocarcinomas, while sarcomas and small cell neuroendocrine tumors are rare [132–134]. Cervical cancer usually spreads either by direct extension to surrounding tissues or via the lymph node pathway to pelvic and para-aortic lymph nodes [135, 136].

As for the staging of cervical cancer, in stage 1, there is a small amount of tumor, which can be viewed under a microscope, with less than 3 mm in-depth, and in the case of stage 1B3, it can present up to 4 cm and be limited to the cervix. In stage 2,

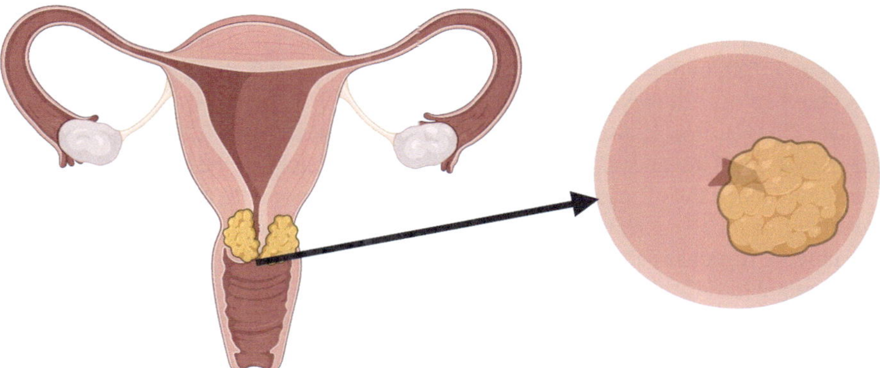

Fig. 7.15 Cervical cancer. (Source: Created with BioRender.com)

the tumor is larger, may have a size greater than 4 cm, and may have spread to nearby tissues [137, 138].

In stage 3, the tumor may have invaded the lower part of the vagina or the walls of the pelvis, blocking the ureters and spreading to nearby pelvic lymph nodes or para-aortic lymph nodes. In stage 4, the tumor has spread to other organs such as the bladder, rectum, lungs, or bones, as well as to distant lymph nodes [135, 137, 138].

7.3.1 Chemotherapy for the Treatment of Cervical Cancer

The main therapeutic options for the treatment of cervical cancer include surgery, radiotherapy, chemotherapy, targeted therapy, and immunotherapy, which can be used alone or in combination [139, 140]. The choice of therapeutic option will depend on the stage of cancer, wherein the early stages, treatment of cervical cancer can be through surgery or radiotherapy combined with chemotherapy. In the later stages, radiotherapy combined with chemotherapy has generally been the main treatment option. Chemotherapy alone is often used to treat advanced cervical cancer [141–146].

Among the chemotherapeutic agents indicated, cisplatin is widely used; as monotherapy associated with radiotherapy, it is used in the treatment of high-risk squamous cell carcinoma, adenocarcinoma, or adenosquamous carcinoma of the cervix [147–150]. Regarding combinations, the association of carboplatin with paclitaxel, used in the treatment of cancers of the gastrointestinal tract (see Chap. 5), has been indicated for the primary adjuvant treatment of adenocarcinoma/adenosquamous cancer of the cervix before or following irradiation with or without cisplatin and in the primary treatment of recurrent/advanced non-small cell cancer of the cervix [151–153].

The CAPBEV protocol (Sect. 7.2.1.2), indicated for ovarian cancer, is also indicated for the primary treatment of metastatic or recurrent cervical cancer [154–156]. The use of bevacizumab combined with carboplatin and paclitaxel promoted an overall response rate of 44%, with a progression-free survival of 5.3 months, and overall survival of 12.1 months in the study by Tinker et al. [155]. In the study by Tao et al. [157], in the treatment of advanced cervical cancer, the CAPBEV protocol promoted an overall survival of 24.52 months.

The CAD protocol, also indicated for ovarian cancer (Sect. 7.2.1.5), is used for the treatment of advanced/recurrent non-small cell cancer of the cervix. Rein et al. [158] evidenced the efficacy of the combination of carboplatin and docetaxel in the treatment of locally advanced primary and recurrent cervical cancer. The protocol promoted a response rate of 65%, with generally mild non-hematological toxicity.

Nagao et al. [159] evaluated the effectiveness of the CAD protocol in the treatment of advanced or recurrent cervical cancer, highlighting its safety and efficacy and promoting an overall response rate of 76%. The protocol induced grade 3/4 toxicity, which included neutropenia, thrombocytopenia, and anemia.

In a phase 2 study, Shimada et al. [150] used the combination of docetaxel with carboplatin in patients at stage IVB or with recurrent non-squamous cell carcinoma of the cervix. The results demonstrated the protocol's effectiveness, with a response rate of 47.9%, disease control rate of 77.1%, progression-free survival of 6.1 months, and overall survival of 15.8 months. Toxicity was similar to other studies with cases of neutropenia being the most frequent.

7.4   Pathophysiology of Endometrial Cancer

Uterine cancer is the second most common gynecological cancer in the world, second only to cervical cancer. More than 90% of uterine cancers are endometrial, originating in the epithelium [161, 162]. In Western populations, White women have a high incidence of endometrial cancer. Excess endogenous or exogenous estrogen is the main risk factor for endometrial cancer. One genetic risk factor is Lynch syndrome, which causes germ line mutation in the DNA mismatch repair gene. Other risk factors for endometrial cancer involve reproduction, such as early age at menarche, late age at menopause, and nulliparity [163–166].

Preinvasive intraepithelial lesions initiate the development of endometrial carcinomas, which progress to fully developed invasive cancers involving the endometrial stroma. With tumor growth, endometrial cancer can spread through lymphatic channels to the cervix, stroma, fallopian tubes, and ovaries [167].

Endometrial cancer (Fig. 7.16), when in stage 1, presents itself confined to the body of the uterus, limited to the endometrium or with less, equal to or greater than 50% invasion in the myometrium. In stage 2, the tumor invades the cervical stroma but does not go beyond the uterus. In stage 3, the tumor presents local or regional extension and may have vaginal or parametrial involvement, as well as the presence of regional lymph node metastases, while in stage 4, the tumor invaded other organs such as bladder, bowel mucosa, lung, bone, and liver [167–169].

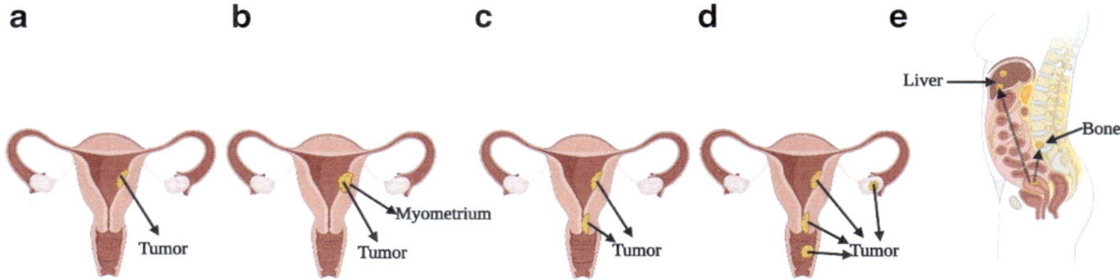

Fig. 7.16 Stages of endometrial cancer. (**a**) Stage 1A with tumor located in the endometrium; (**b**) Stage 1B with tumor invasion of the myometrium; (**c**) Stage 2 with tumor spread to the cervix; (**d**) Stage 3 with tumor spread to the ovary, cervix, and vagina; and (**e**) Stage 4 with tumor spread to bone and liver. (Source: Created with BioRender.com)

7.4.1   Chemotherapy for the Treatment of Endometrial Cancer

Treatment modalities for endometrial cancer include surgery, radiation therapy, chemotherapy, and hormone therapy [170, 171]. When the tumor is located in the body of the uterus or invades only the endometrium or myometrium, the indicated treatment is surgery, which can be combined with chemotherapy and/or radiotherapy. The surgical procedure can include the removal of the uterus, fallopian tubes, and ovaries, in which rare and aggressive tumors remove the pelvic lymph nodes and some of the abdomen [167, 172, 173].

In the treatment of stage 2 endometrial cancer, where the tumor has not yet developed outside the uterus, one treatment option is to perform surgery with radical hysterectomy first, followed by radiation therapy through vaginal brachytherapy, and external pelvic radiation therapy [174–176]. In stage 3, surgery may also be indicated if the entire tumor can be removed, if it is observed that the tumor has spread, radiotherapy may be indicated before surgery to shrink the tumor. Treatment after surgery with chemotherapy and/or radiotherapy may also be indicated [177, 178].

In stage 4, where the tumor has spread to other organs, the combination of anticancer drugs can be indicated, as well as targeted therapy, immunotherapeutic, and hormone therapy [178–180]. The use of doxorubicin as monotherapy has been indicated for the treatment of advanced endometrial cancer, as well as hormone therapy with aromatase inhibitors [181–183]. Some endometrial cancer cells may be sensitive to hormonal action, thus preventing tumor growth due to blocking or antagonistic effects of hormonal effects [184, 185].

Some combinations that are used in other tumors may also be indicated in the treatment of endometrial cancer, as in the case of the combination between carboplatin and docetaxel, which is used in ovarian cancer (Sect. 7.2.1.5), has been used in the treatment of advanced or recurrent primary endometrial cancer [186–188]. Another combination used in the treatment of advanced or recurrent primary endometrial cancer is carboplatin combined with paclitaxel (see infusion sequence in Chap. 5) [51–53, 189–191].

7.5   Pathophysiology of Gestational Trophoblastic Neoplasia

Epidemiological data for gestational trophoblastic neoplasia is unclear, due to limited information that is based on hospital data rather than population-based, and data may be based on only one hospital. The presence of hydatidiform mole may predispose to the development of gestational trophoblastic neoplasia, being associated with gametogenesis and/or abnormal fertilization. The incidence of gestational trophoblastic neoplasia is mirrored in the incidence of hydatidiform mole due to the strong association, with higher numbers in India and Indonesia and lower numbers in Southeast Asia, North America, Europe, and Oceania [192–195].

Some risk factors for the development of gestational trophoblastic neoplasia include age, age during pregnancy, genetics, ethnicity, and the use of contraceptives,

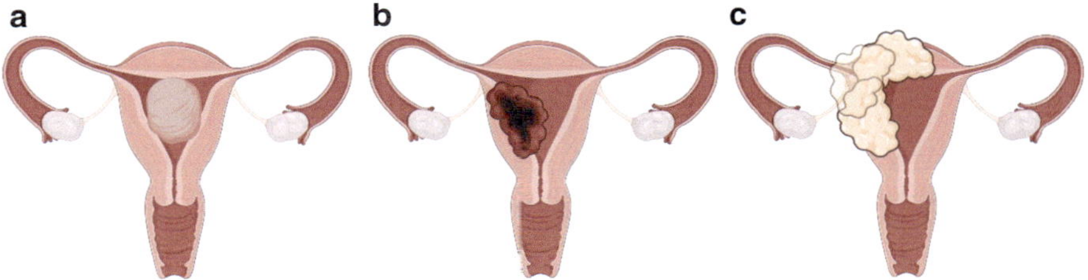

Fig. 7.17 Gestational trophoblastic neoplasm: hydatidiform spring (**a**), invasive spring (**b**), and choriocarcinoma (**c**). (Source: Created with BioRender.com)

which are involved in the risk factor for the development of hydatidiform mole [193, 196, 197].

About 50% of gestational trophoblastic neoplasms develop from a molar pregnancy, 25% due to miscarriages or tubal pregnancy, and 25% due to term or preterm pregnancy. Of the trophoblastic neoplasms that occur due to molar pregnancy, the vast majority develop as molar tissue or choriocarcinoma (Fig. 7.17), or in rarer cases as a trophoblastic tumor with a placental or epithelioid location [198–202].

As for the staging of gestational trophoblastic neoplasia, in stage 1, the disease is found only in the uterus, whereas in stage 2, the neoplasm extends outside the uterus but is limited to the genital structures. In stage 3, the trophoblastic neoplasm has spread to the lungs and may or may not involve the genital tract, and in stage 4, the tumor has already spread to distant organs and/or tissues [199].

7.5.1 Chemotherapy for the Treatment of Gestational Trophoblastic Neoplasia

The treatment of gestational trophoblastic neoplasia is based on the patient's staging, in which, in stage 1, when the tumor is located in the uterus, the use of chemotherapy is indicated, as well as surgery, through hysterectomy [203–205]. In more advanced stages, such as in stages 2 and 3, treatment is based on chemotherapy, which can be either single-agent therapy or combined therapy. In cases of placental trophoblastic tumors and epithelioid tumors that do not respond very well to chemotherapy, they are treated with surgery [206–209].

In cases of stage 4 trophoblastic tumors, in which the tumor has spread to other organs such as the liver or brain, standard treatment includes combinations of antineoplastic agents, and the tumor may be removed by surgical procedure along with chemotherapy. Radiotherapy may also be indicated in the treatment of metastases, such as in the case of brain metastases [207, 210–212].

Among the drugs used as monotherapy, they may include methotrexate, as well as dactinomycin, which has been indicated in the treatment of low-risk gestational trophoblastic cancer [213–216]. Some combinations of chemotherapy [51–53] used in the treatment of gestational trophoblastic neoplasia will be mentioned in the next topics.

7.5.1.1 EMA-CO Protocol (Etoposide, Methotrexate, Actinomycin D, Leucovorin, Cyclophosphamide, and Vincristine)

The EMA-CO protocol, indicated for the treatment of high-risk gestational trophoblastic neoplasia, combines the drugs etoposide, methotrexate, leucovorin, (calcium folinate), actinomycin D, cyclophosphamide, and vincristine [217–219]. According to Alifrangis et al. [218], the EMA-CO protocol was effective in the treatment of high-risk gestational trophoblastic neoplasia, promoting an overall survival of 94.3%, and in low-risk patients, it promoted an overall survival of 99.6%.

Lurain, Singh, and Schink [220] evaluated the efficacy of the EMA-CO protocol as primary therapy for high-risk metastatic gestational trophoblastic neoplasia, promoting an overall survival rate of 93.3%. In another study, Lu et al. [221] found an overall survival rate of 87% in patients with high-risk gestational trophoblastic neoplasia. Lybol et al. [222] observed that the EMA-CO protocol promoted a remission rate of 85.4% in the treatment of high-risk gestational trophoblastic neoplasia, with a toxicity profile that included anemia, neuropathy, and hepatotoxicity.

Despite the benefits demonstrated by the EMA-CO protocol in gestational trophoblastic neoplasia, many patients develop resistance to the protocol, and the indication of alternative protocols should be evaluated [223, 224]. The EMA-CO protocol is based on the application on day 1 of the combination of etoposide, actinomycin D, and methotrexate, followed on day 2 by the infusion of etoposide, actinomycin D, and leucovorin, and finally on day 8, the infusion of vincristine and cyclophosphamide. Figure 7.18 shows the protocol infusion sequence [225, 226].

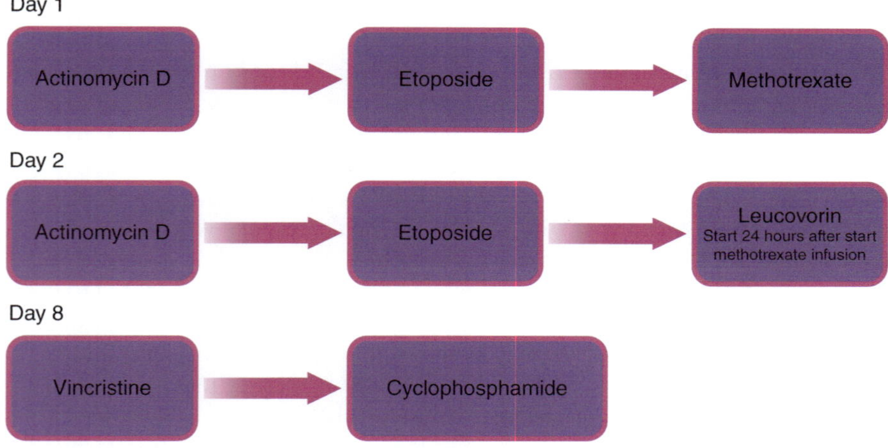

Fig. 7.18 Infusion schedule for the EMA-CO protocol

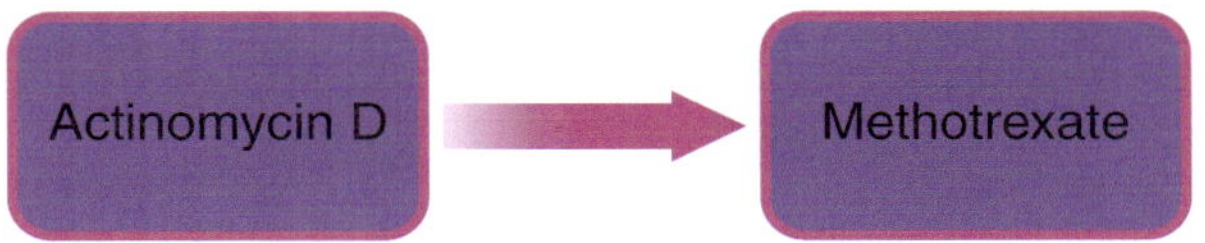

Fig. 7.19 DM protocol infusion schedule

7.5.1.2 DM Protocol (Actinomycin D and Methotrexate)

The combination of actinomycin D and methotrexate has been used in the treatment of moderate-risk gestational trophoblastic cancer [227]. Actinomycin D is an antineoplastic antibiotic, acting by inhibiting DNA-dependent RNA synthesis through complex formation with DNA due to intercalation with guanine residues. The combination of actinomycin D with methotrexate has been shown to be effective in the treatment of gestational trophoblastic neoplasia, where according to Carlson et al. [228], the combination promoted a primary cure rate of 87.2%, with an average response time of 56 days.

Eiriksson et al. [229] looked at the effectiveness of the combination in low-risk gestational trophoblastic neoplasia. The combination promoted a 98% cure rate, proving to be a reliable protocol and modest toxicity. The results were also promising in the study by Kang et al. [230], with the combination promoting a complete remission rate of 96%, showing superior results than groups of patients who received methotrexate or actinomycin D as monotherapy. Figure 7.19 shows the DM protocol infusion schedule [227, 230].

References

1. WHO—World Health Organization (2020) Estimated number of incident cases from 2018 to 2040. International Agency for Research on Cancer. Available in: https://gco.iarc.fr/tomorrow/graphic-isotype?type=0&type_sex=0&mode=population&sex=0&populations=900&cancers=36&age_group=value&apc_male=0&apc_female=0&single_unit=100000&print=0. Accessed Sep 17 2021.
2. Rosa LM, Hames ME, Dias M, Miranda GM, Bagio CB, Santos MJ, Kalinke LP. Epidemiological profile of women with gynecological cancer in brachytherapy: a cross-sectional study. Rev Bras Enferm. 2021;74(5):e20200695. https://doi.org/10.1590/0034-7167-2020-0695.
3. Watson M, Saraiya M, Wu X. Update of HPV-associated female genital cancers in the United States, 1999–2004. J Women's Health. 2009;18(11):1731–8. https://doi.org/10.1089/jwh.2009.1570.
4. Mann L, Foley KL, Tanner AE, Sun CJ, Rhodes SD. Increasing cervical cancer screening among US Hispanics/Latinas: a qualitative systematic review. J Cancer Educ. 2015;30(2):374–87. https://doi.org/10.1007/s13187-014-0716-9.
5. CDCP—Centers for Disease Control and Prevention (2019) gynecologic cancer incidence, United States—2012–2016. USCS data brief, no 11. Centers for Disease Control and Prevention, US Department of Health and Human Services. Atlanta, Georgia.

6. Son H, Khan SM, Rahaman J, Cameron KL, Prasad-Hayes M, Chuang L, Machac J, Heiba S, Kostakoglu L. Role of FDG PET/CT in staging of recurrent ovarian cancer. Radiographics. 2011;31(2):569–83. https://doi.org/10.1148/rg.312105713.

7. Singh GK, Azuine RE, Siahpush M. Global inequalities in cervical cancer incidence and mortality are linked to deprivation, low socioeconomic status, and human development. Int J MCH AIDS. 2012;1(1):17–30.

8. Doubeni CA, Doubeni ARB, Myers AE. Diagnosis and management of ovarian cancer. Am Fam Physician. 2016;93(11):937–44.

9. Matulonis UA, Sood AK, Fallowfield L, Howitt BE, Sehouli J, Karlan BY. Ovarian cancer. Nat Rev Dis Primers. 2016;2:16061. https://doi.org/10.1038/nrdp.2016.61.

10. Costa AM, Hashim D, Fregnani JHTG, Weiderpass E. Overall survival and time trends in breast and cervical cancer incidence and mortality in the regional Health District (RHD) of Barretos, São Paulo. Brazil BMC Cancer. 2018;18:1079. https://doi.org/10.1186/s12885-018-4956-7.

11. Burd EM. Human papillomavirus and cervical cancer. Clin Microbiol Rev. 2003;16(1):1–17. https://doi.org/10.1128/CMR.16.1.1-17.2003.

12. Braaten KP, Laufer MR. Human papillomavirus (HPV), HPV-related disease, and the HPV vaccine. Rev Obstet Gynecol. 2008;1(1):2–10.

13. Reid BM, Permuth JB, Sellers TA. Epidemiology of ovarian cancer: a review. Cancer Biol Med. 2017;14(1):9–32. https://doi.org/10.20892/j.issn.2095-3941.2016.0084.

14. Torre LA, Islami F, Siegel RL, Ward EM, Jemal A. Global cancer in women: burden and trends. Cancer Epidemiol Biomark Prev. 2017;26(4):444–57. https://doi.org/10.1158/1055-9965.EPI-16-0858.

15. D'Alonzo M, Bounous VE, Villa M, Biglia N. Current evidence of the oncological benefit-risk profile of hormone replacement therapy. Medicina (Kaunas). 2019;55(9):573. https://doi.org/10.3390/medicina55090573.

16. Jammal MP, Lima CA, Murta EFC, Nomelini RS. Is ovarian cancer prevention currently still a recommendation of our grandparents? Rev Bras Ginecol Obstet. 2017;39(12):676–85. https://doi.org/10.1055/s-0037-1608867.

17. Park HK, Ruterbusch JJ, Cote ML. Recent trends in ovarian cancer incidence and relative survival in the United States by race/ethnicity and histologic subtypes. Cancer Epidemiol Biomark Prev. 2017;26(10):1511–8. https://doi.org/10.1158/1055-9965.EPI-17-0290.

18. Momenimovahed Z, Tiznobaik A, Taheri S, Salehiniya H. Ovarian cancer in the world: epidemiology and risk factors. Int J Women's Health. 2019;11:287–99. https://doi.org/10.2147/IJWH.S197604.

19. Oosterkamp HM, Scheiner L, Stefanova MC, Lloyd KO, Finstad CL. Comparison of MUC-1 mucin expression in epithelial and non-epithelial cancer cell lines and demonstration of a new short variant form (MUC-1/Z). Int J Cancer. 1997;72(1):87–94. https://doi.org/10.1002/(sici)1097-0215(19970703)72:1<87::aid-ijc13>3.0.co;2-7.

20. Kim SI, Lim MC, Lim J, Won YJ, Seo SS, Kang S, Park SY. Incidence of epithelial ovarian cancer according to histologic subtypes in Korea, 1999 to 2012. J Gynecol Oncol. 2016;27(1):e5. https://doi.org/10.3802/jgo.2016.27.e5.

21. Ricci F, Affatato R, Carrassa L, Damia G. Recent insights into mucinous ovarian carcinoma. Int J Mol Sci. 2018;19(6):1569. https://doi.org/10.3390/ijms19061569.

22. Gomes TA, Campos EA, Yoshida A, Sarian LO, Andrade LALA, Derchain SF. Preoperative differentiation of benign and malignant non-epithelial ovarian tumors: clinical features and tumor markers. Rev Bras Ginecol Obstet. 2020;42(9):555–61. https://doi.org/10.1055/s-0040-1712993.

23. Shabir S, Gill PK. Global scenario on ovarian cancer—its dynamic, relative survival treatment, and epidemiology. Adesh Univer J Med Sci Res. 2020;2(1):17–25.

24. Pannu HK, Bristow RE, Montz FJ, Fishman EK. Multidetector CT of peritoneal carcinomatosis from ovarian cancer. Radiographics. 2003;23(3):687–701. https://doi.org/10.1148/rg.233025105.

25. Nougaret S, Addley HC, Colombo PE, Fujii S, Sharif SSA, Tirumani SH, Jardon K, Sala E, Reinhold C. Ovarian carcinomatosis: how the radiologist can help plan the surgical approach. Radiographics. 2012;32(6):1800–3. https //doi.org/10.1148/rg.326125511.
26. Kim A, Ueda Y, Naka T, Enomoto T. Therapeutic strategies in epithelial ovarian cancer. J Exp Clin Cancer Res. 2012;31:14. https://doi.org/10.1186/1756-9966-31-14.
27. Kuroki L, Guntupalli SR. Treatment of epithelial ovarian cancer. BMJ. 2020;371:m3773. https://doi.org/10.1136/bmj.m3773.
28. Palmer MC, Shepert E, Schepansky A, MacLean GD. Novel, dose intensive, single-agent cisplatin in the first-line management of advanced stage ovarian cancer. Int J Gynecol Cancer. 1992;2(6):301–6. https://doi.org/10.1046/j.1525-1438.1992.02060301.x.
29. ICON – The International Collaborative Ovarian Neoplasm Group. Paclitaxel plus carboplatin versus standard chemotherapy with either single-agent carboplatin or cyclophosphamide, doxorubicin, and cisplatin in women with ovarian cancer: the ICON3 randomised trial. Lancet. 2002;360(9332):505–15. https://doi.org/10.1016/S0140-6736(02)09738-6.
30. Berkenblit A, Seiden MV, Matulonis UA, Penson RT, Krasner CN, Roche M, Mezzetti L, Atkinson T, Cannistra SA. A phase II trial of weekly docetaxel in patients with platinum-resistant epithelial ovarian, primary peritoneal serous cancer, or fallopian tube cancer. Gynecol Oncol. 2004;95(3):624–31. https://doi.org/10.1016/j.ygyno.2004.08.028.
31. Lorusso D, Di Stefano A, Fanfani F, Scambia G. Role of gemcitabine in ovarian cancer treatment. Ann Oncol. 2006;17(Supplement 5):188–94. https://doi.org/10.1093/annonc/mdj979.
32. Safra T, Berman T, Yachnin A, Bruchim I, Meirovitz M, Barak F, Atlas I, Levy T, Rosengarten OS. Weekly topotecan for recurrent ovarian, fallopian tube and primary peritoneal carcinoma: tolerability and efficacy study--the Israeli experience. Int J Gynecol Cancer. 2013;23(3):475–80. https://doi.org/10.1097/IGC.0b013e3182866944.
33. Kwon JS, McGahan C, Dehaeck U, Santos J, Swenerton K, Carey MS. The significance of combination chemotherapy in epithelial ovarian cancer. Int J Gynecol Cancer. 2014;24(2):226–32. https://doi.org/10.1097/IGC.0000000000000055.
34. Wong CN, Wong CN, Liu FS. Continuous oral cyclophosphamide as salvage or maintenance therapy in ovarian, primary peritoneal, and fallopian tube cancers: a retrospective, single institute study. Taiwan J Obstet Gynecol. 2017;56(3):302–5. https://doi.org/10.1016/j.tjog.2017.04.006.
35. Gupta R, Cristea M, Frankel P, Ruel C, Chen C, Wang Y, Morgan R, Leong L, Chow W, Koczywas M, Koehler S, Lim D, Luu T, Martel C, McNamara M, Somlo G, Twardowski P, Yen Y, Idorenyi A, Raechelle T, Carroll M, Chung V. Randomized trial of oral cyclophosphamide versus oral cyclophosphamide with celecoxib for recurrent epithelial ovarian, fallopian tube, and primary peritoneal cancer. Cancer Treat Res Commun. 2019;21:100155. https://doi.org/10.1016/j.ctarc.2019.100155.
36. Okunade K, Akinsete AM, Salako O, Afolabi BB, Neal RD. Oral etoposide for treatment and/or maintenance treatment of recurrent epithelial ovarian cancer. Cochrane Library. 2020;2020(2):CD013537. https://doi.org/10.1002/14651858.CD013537.
37. NCT04055649 (2021) ONC201 Plus Weekly Paclitaxel in Patients With Platinum Refractory or Resistant Ovarian Cancer. Clinical Trials. Available in: https://clinicaltrials.gov/ct2/show/NCT04055649. Accessed Sep 18 2021.
38. Burger RA, DiSaia PJ, Roberts JA, O'rourke M, Gershenson DM, Homesley HD, Lichtman SM, Barnes W, Moore DH, Monk BJ. Phase II trial of vinorelbine in recurrent and progressive epithelial ovarian cancer. Gynecol Oncol. 1999;72(2):148–53. https://doi.org/10.1006/gyno.1998.5243.
39. Ledermann J, Harter P, Gourley C, Friedlander M, Vergote I, Rustin G, Scott C, Meier W, Shapira-Frommer R, Safra T, Matei D, Macpherson E, Watkins C, Carmichael J, Matulonis U. Olaparib maintenance therapy in platinum-sensitive relapsed ovarian cancer. N Engl J Med. 2012;366:1382–92. https://doi.org/10.1056/NEJMoa1105535.
40. Lawrie TA, Bryant A, Cameron A, Gray E, Morrison J. Pegylated liposomal doxorubicin for relapsed epithelial ovarian cancer. Cochrane. Library. 2013;2013(7):CD006910. https://doi.org/10.1002/14651858.CD006910.pub2.

41. Staropoli N, Ciliberto D, Botta C, Fiorillo L, Grimaldi A, Lama S, Caraglia M, Salvino A, Tassone P, Tagliaferri P. Pegylated liposomal doxorubicin in the management of ovarian cancer: a systematic review and metaanalysis of randomized trials. Cancer Biol Ther. 2014;15(6):707–20. https://doi.org/10.4161/cbt.28557.
42. Lorusso D, Tripodi E, Maltese G, Lepori S, Sabatucci I, Bogani G, Raspagliesi F. Spotlight on olaparib in the treatment of BRCA-mutated ovarian cancer: design, development and place in therapy. Drug Des Devel Ther. 2018;12:1501–9. https://doi.org/10.2147/DDDT.S124447.
43. Simpkins F, Garcia-Soto A, Slingerland J. New insights on the role of hormonal therapy in ovarian cancer. Steroids. 2013;78(6):530–7. https://doi.org/10.1016/j.steroids.2013.01.008.
44. George A, McLachlan J, Tunariu N, Pepa CD, Migali C, Gore M, Kaye S, Banerjee S. The role of hormonal therapy in patients with relapsed high-grade ovarian carcinoma: a retrospective series of tamoxifen and letrozole. BMC Cancer. 2017;17:456. https://doi.org/10.1186/s12885-017-3440-0.
45. Hoskind PJ, Swenerton KD, Pike JA, Wong F, Lim P, Acquino-Parsons C, Lee N. Paclitaxel and carboplatin, alone or with irradiation, in advanced or recurrent endometrial cancer: a phase II study. J Clin Oncol. 2001;19(20):4048–53. https://doi.org/10.1200/JCO.2001.19.20.4048.
46. Ozols RF, Bundy BN, Greer BE, Fowler JM, Clarke-Pearson D, Burger RA, Mannel RS, DeGeest K, Hartenbach EM, Baergen R. Phase III trial of carboplatin and paclitaxel compared with cisplatin and paclitaxel in patients with optimally resected stage III ovarian cancer: a gynecologic oncology group study. J Clin Oncol. 2003;21(17):3194–200. https://doi.org/10.1200/JCO.2003.02.153.
47. Alektiar KM, Makker V, Abu-Rustum NR, Soslow RA, Chi DS, Barakat RR, Aghajanian CA. Concurrent carboplatin/paclitaxel and intravaginal radiation in surgical stage I-II serous endometrial cancer. Gynecol Oncol. 2009;112(1):142–5. https://doi.org/10.1016/j.ygyno.2008.10.006.
48. Clamp AR, James EC, McNeish IA, Dean A, Kim JW, O'Donnell DM, Hook J, Coyle C, Blagden S, Brenton JD, Naik R, Perren T, Sundar S, Cook AD, Gopalakrishnan GS, Gabra H, Lord R, Dark G, Earl HM, Hall M, Banerjee S, Glasspool RM, Jones R, Williams S, Swart AM, Stenning S, Parmar M, Kaplan R, Ledermann JA. Weekly dose-dense chemotherapy in first-line epithelial ovarian, fallopian tube, or primary peritoneal carcinoma treatment (ICON8): primary progression free survival analysis results from a GCIG phase 3 randomised controlled trial. Lancet. 2019;394(10214):2084–95. https://doi.org/10.1016/S0140-6736(19)32259-7.
49. Fader AN, Roque DM, Siegel E, Buza N, Hui P, Abdelghany O, Chambers S, Secord AA, Havrilesky L, O'Malley DM, Backes FJ, Nevadunsky N, Edraki B, Pikaart D, Lowery W, ElSahwi K, Celano P, Bellone S, Azodi M, Litkouhi B, Ratner E, Silisi DA, Schwartz PE, Santin AD. Randomized Phase II Trial of Carboplatin–Paclitaxel Compared with Carboplatin–Paclitaxel–Trastuzumab in Advanced (Stage III–IV) or Recurrent Uterine Serous Carcinomas that Overexpress Her2/Neu (NCT01367002): Updated Overall Survival Analysis. Clin Cancer Res. 2020;26(15):3928–35. https://doi.org/10.1158/1078-0432.CCR-20-0953.
50. Shibutani T, Nagao S, Suzuki K, Kaneda M, Yamamoto K, Jimi T, Yano H, Kitai M, Shiozaki T, Matsuoka K, Sudo T, Yamaguchi S. Dose-dense paclitaxel and carboplatin vs. conventional paclitaxel and carboplatin as neoadjuvant chemotherapy for advanced epithelial ovarian, fallopian tube, or primary peritoneal cancer: a retrospective study. Int J Clin Oncol. 2020;25:502–7. https://doi.org/10.1007/s10147-019-01567-y.
51. Kuehr T, Thaler J, Woell E (2017) Chemotherapy protocols 2017: current protocols and "targeted therapies". Klinikum Wels-Grieskirchen and Caritas Christi URGET NOS. Austria. www.chemoprotocols.eu.
52. BC Cancer (2021) Supportive care protocols. BC Cancer. British Columbia. Available in: http://www.bccancer.bc.ca/health-professionals/clinical-resources/chemotherapy-protocols/supportive-care. Accessed July 2 2021.
53. NHS (2021) Chemotherapy Protocols. NHS. University Hospital Southampton. NHS Foundation Trust. England. Available in: https://www.uhs.nhs.uk/HealthProfessionals/Chemotherapy-protocols/Chemotherapy-protocols.aspx. Accessed July 2 2021.

54. Maurer K, Michener C, Mahdi H, Rose PG. Universal tolerance of nab-paclitaxel for gynecologic malignancies in patients with prior taxane hypersensitivity reactions. J Gynecol Oncol. 2017;28(4):e38. https://doi.org/10.3802/jgo.2017.28.e38.

55. Benigno BB, Hines JF. Phase II study of nab-paclitaxel plus carboplatin in patients with recurrent platinum-sensitive ovarian or primary peritoneal cancer. J Clin Oncol. 2006;24(18_suppl):15033. https://doi.org/10.1200/jco 2006.24.18_suppl.15033.

56. Srinivasan KN, Rauthan A, Gopal R. Combination therapy of albumin-bound paclitaxel and carboplatin as first line therapy in a patient with ovarian cancer. Case Rep Oncol Med. 2014;2014:940591. https://doi.org/10.1155/2014/940591.

57. Pothuri B, Sawaged Z, Lee J, Musa F, Lutz K, Reese E, Blank SV, Boyd LR, Curtin JP, Li X, Goldberg JD, Muggia FM. A phase II feasibility study of nab-paclitaxel and carboplatin in chemotherapy naïve epithelial neoplasms of the uterus. Gynecol Oncol. 2019;154(Supplement 1):247–8. https://doi.org/10.1016/j.ygyno.2019.04.571.

58. Parisi A, Palluzzi E, Cortellini A, Sidoni T, Cocciolone V, Lanfiuti Baldi P, Porzio G, Ficorella C, Cannita K. First-line carboplatin/nab-paclitaxel in advanced ovarian cancer patients, after hypersensitivity reaction to solvent-based taxanes: a single-institution experience. Clin Transl Oncol. 2020;22:158–62. https://doi.org/10.1007/s12094-019-02122-x.

59. Muggia F, Pothuri B, Gildberg JD (2017) A Phase 2 Feasibility Study of Abraxane and Carboplatin in Epithelial Neoplasms of the Uterus. NYU Langone Medical Center Cancer Institute. New York. Available in: https://clinicaltrials.gov/ProvidedDocs/98/NCT02744898/Prot_SAP_000.pdf. Accessed Sep 18 2021.

60. Chan T (2021) BC cancer protocol summary for alternative treatment of gynecological malignancies using CARBOplatin and PACLitaxel NAB (ABRAXANE). BC cancer. British Columbia. Available in: http://www.Bccancer.Bc.Ca/chemotherapy-protocols-site/documents/gynecology/GOCABR_Protocol.Pdf. Accessed Sep 18 2021.

61. Coleman RL, Brady MF, Herzog TJ, Sabbatini P, Armstrong DK, Walker JL, Kim BG, Fujiwara K, Tewari KS, O'Malley DM, Davidson SA, Rubin SC, DiSilvestro P, Basen-Engquist K, Huang H, Chan JK, Spirtos NM, Ashfaq R, Mannel RS. Bevacizumab and paclitaxel–carboplatin chemotherapy and secondary cytoreduction in recurrent, platinum-sensitive ovarian cancer (NRG oncology/gynecologic oncology group study GOG-0213): a multicentre, open-label, randomised, phase 3 trial. Lancet Oncol. 2017;18(6):779–91. https://doi.org/10.1016/S1470-2045(17)30279-6.

62. Marth C, Reimer D, Zeimet AG. Front-line therapy of advanced epithelial ovarian cancer: standard treatment. Ann Oncol. 2017;28(Supplement 8):viii36–9. https://doi.org/10.1093/annonc/mdx450.

63. NHS (2020) Chemotherapy protocol. Gynaecological cancer. Bevacizumab (7.5)-carboplatin (AUC5)-paclitaxel (21 day). NHS. University Hospital Southampton. NHS Foundation Trust. England. Available in: https://www.uhs.nhs.uk/Media/SUHTExtranet/Services/Chemotherapy-SOPs/Ovarian-cancer/Bevacizumab7.5mgkgCarboplatinandPaclitaxel21day.pdf. Accessed Sep 19 2021.

64. Tillmanns TD, Lowe MP, Schwartzberg LS, Walker MS, Stepanski EJ. A phase II study of bevacizumab with nab-paclitaxel in patients with recurrent, platinum-resistant primary epithelial ovarian or primary peritoneal carcinoma. J Clin Oncol. 2010;28(15_suppl):5009. https://doi.org/10.1200/jco.2010.28.15_suppl.5009.

65. Tillmanns TD, Lowe MP, Walker MS, Stepanski EJ, Schwartzberg LS. Phase II clinical trial of bevacizumab with albumin-bound paclitaxel in patients with recurrent, platinum-resistant primary epithelial ovarian or primary peritoneal carcinoma. Gynecol Oncol. 2013;128(2):221–8. https://doi.org/10.1016/j.ygyno.2012.08.039.

66. Chan T (2021) BC cancer protocol summary for alternative treatment of gynecological malignancies using bevacizumab, CARBOplatin and PACLitaxel NAB (ABRAXANE). BC cancer. British Columbia. Available in: http://www.Bccancer.Bc.Ca/chemotherapy-protocols-site/documents/gynecology/GOCABRBEV_Protocol.Pdf. Accessed Sep 19 2021.

67. Goldberg JM, Piver MS, Hempling RE, Recio FO. Paclitaxel and cisplatin combination chemotherapy in recurrent epithelial ovarian cancer. Gynecol Oncol. 1996;63(3):312–7. https://doi.org/10.1006/gyno.1996.0328.

68. Rose PG, Blessing JA, Gershenson DM, McGehee R. Paclitaxel and cisplatin as first-line therapy in recurrent or advanced squamous cell carcinoma of the cervix: a gynecologic oncology group study. J Clin Oncol. 1999;17(9):2676–80. https://doi.org/10.1200/JCO.1999.17.9.2676.

69. Moore DH, Blessing JA, McQuellon RP, Thaler HT, Cella D, Benda J, Miller DS, Olt G, King S, Boggess JF, Rocereto TF. Phase III study of cisplatin with or without paclitaxel in stage IVB, recurrent, or persistent squamous cell carcinoma of the cervix: a gynecologic oncology group study. J Clin Oncol. 2004;22(15):3113–9. https://doi.org/10.1200/JCO.2004.04.170.

70. Bois AD, Luck HJ, Meier W, Adams HP, Mobus V, Costa S, Bauknecht T, Richter B, Warm M, Schroder W, Olbricht S, Nitz U, Jackisch C, Emons G, Wagner U, Kuhn W. A randomized clinical trial of cisplatin/paclitaxel versus carboplatin/paclitaxel as first-line treatment of ovarian cancer. J Natl Cancer Inst. 2003;95(17):1320–9. https://doi.org/10.1093/jnci/djg036.

71. Armstrong DK, Bundy B, Wenzel L, Huang HQ, Baergen R, Lele S, Copeland LJ, Walker JL, Burger RA. Intraperitoneal cisplatin and paclitaxel in ovarian cancer. N Engl J Med. 2006;354:34–43. https://doi.org/10.1056/NEJMoa052985.

72. Moioli M, Papadia A, Mammoliti S, Pacella E, Menoni S, Menada MV, Ragni N. Chemotherapy with cisplatin and paclitaxel in locally advanced cervical cancer: has this regimen still a role as neoadjuvant setting? Minerva Ginecol. 2012;64(2):95–107.

73. Jekunen AP, Christen RD, Shalinsky DR, Howell SB. Synergistic interaction between cisplatin and taxol in human ovarian carcinoma cells in vitro. Br J Cancer. 1994;69:299–306. https://doi.org/10.1038/bjc.1994.55.

74. Konner JA, Grabon DM, Gerst SR, Iasonos A, Thaler H, Pezzulli SD, Sabbatini PJ, Bell-McGuinn KM, Tew WP, Hensley ML, Spriggs DR, Aghajanian CA. Phase II study of intraperitoneal paclitaxel plus cisplatin and intravenous paclitaxel plus bevacizumab as adjuvant treatment of optimal stage II/III epithelial ovarian cancer. J Clin Oncol. 2011;29(35):4662–8. https://doi.org/10.1200/JCO.2011.36.1352.

75. Oliva P, Decio A, Castiglioni V, Bassi A, Pesenti E, Cesca M, Scanziani E, Belotti D, Giavazzi R. Cisplatin plus paclitaxel and maintenance of bevacizumab on tumour progression, dissemination, and survival of ovarian carcinoma xenograft models. Br J Cancer. 2012;107(2):360–9. https://doi.org/10.1038/bjc.2012.261.

76. Chu G, Liu X, Yu W, Chen M, Dong L. Cisplatin plus paclitaxel chemotherapy with or without bevacizumab in postmenopausal women with previously untreated advanced cervical cancer: a retrospective study. BMC Cancer. 2021;21:133. https://doi.org/10.1186/s12885-021-07869-7.

77. Sugiyama T, Mizuno M, Aoki Y, Sakurai M, Nishikawa T, Ueda E, Tajima K, Takeshima N. A single-arm study evaluating bevacizumab, cisplatin, and paclitaxel followed by single-agent bevacizumab in Japanese patients with advanced cervical cancer. Jpn J Clin Oncol. 2017;47(1):39–46. https://doi.org/10.1093/jjco/hyw143.

78. Kumar A (2021) BC cancer protocol summary for alternative treatment of gynecological malignancies using bevacizumab, CISplatin and PACLitaxel. BC cancer. British Columbia. Available in: http://www.Bccancer.Bc.Ca/chemotherapy-protocols-site/documents/gynecology/GOCISPBEV_Protocol.Pdf. Accessed Sep 19 2021.

79. NCT00138242 (2013) Docetaxel and Carboplatin in Treating Patients With Ovarian Epithelial, Fallopian Tube, or Peritoneal Cavity Cancer. Clinical Trials. Available in: https://www.clinicaltrials.gov/ct2/show/NCT00138242. Accessed Sep 19 2021.

80. NCT00003560 (2014) Docetaxel Plus Carboplatin in Treating Patients With Stage III or Stage IV Ovarian, Fallopian Tube, or Primary Peritoneal Cancer. Clinical Trials. Available in: https://clinicaltrials.gov/ct2/show/NCT00003560. Accessed Sep 19 2021.

81. NCT00214058 (2019) Weekly Carboplatin/Docetaxel for Recurrent Ovarian/Peritoneal Cancer. Clinical Trials. Available in: https://clinicaltrials.gov/ct2/show/NCT00214058. Access on: Sep 19, 2021.

82. Vasey PA, Atkinson R, Coleman R, Crawford M, Cruickshank M, Eggleton P, Fleming D, Graham J, Parkin D, Paul J, Reed NS, Kaye SB. Docetaxel-carboplatin as first line chemo-

therapy for epithelial ovarian cancer. Br J Cancer. 2001;84(2):170–8. https://doi.org/10.1054/bjoc.2000.1572.

83. Vasey Pa, Jayson GC, Gordon A, Gabra H, Coleman R, Atkinson R, Parkin D, Paul J, Hay A, Kaye SB (2004) Phase III Randomized Trial of Docetaxel–Carboplatin Versus Paclitaxel–Carboplatin as First-line Chemotherapy for Ovarian Carcinoma. J Natl Cancer Inst 96(22):1682–1691. doi: https://doi.org/10.1093/jnci/djh323.

84. Markman M, Kennedy A, Webster K, Peterson G, Kulp B, Belinson J. Combination chemotherapy with carboplatin and docetaxel in the treatment of cancers of the ovary and fallopian tube and primary carcinoma of the peritoneum. J Clin Oncol. 2001;19(7):1901–5. https://doi.org/10.1200/JCO.2001.19.7.1901.

85. Wang Y, Herrstedt J, Havsteen H, Christensen RD, Mirza MR, Lund B, Maenpaa J, Kristensen G. A multicenter, non-randomized, phase II study of docetaxel and carboplatin administered every 3 weeks as second line chemotherapy in patients with first relapse of platinum sensitive epithelial ovarian, peritoneal or fallopian tube cancer. BMC Cancer. 2014;14:937. https://doi.org/10.1186/1471-2407-14-937.

86. Ko J (2021) BC cancer protocol summary for primary treatment with visible or no visible residual tumour (moderate, high, or extreme risk) or treatment at relapse of invasive epithelial ovarian, fallopian tube, and primary peritoneal cancer, using CARBOplatin and DOCEtaxel. BC cancer. British Columbia. Available in: http://www.Bccancer.Bc.Ca/chemotherapy-protocols-site/documents/gynecology/GOOVCAD_Protocol.Pdf. Accessed Sep 19 2021.

87. du Bois A, Luck HJ, Pfisterer J, Schroeder W, Blohmer JU, Kimmig R, Moebus V, Quaas J. Second-line carboplatin and gemcitabine in platinum sensitive ovarian cancer - a dose-finding study by the Arbeitsgemeinschaft Gynakologische Onkologie (AGO) ovarian cancer study group. Ann Oncol. 2001;12:1115–20.

88. Pfisterer J, Plante M, Vergote I, du Bois A, Hirte H, Lacave AJ, Wagner U, Stahle A, Stuart G, Kimmig R, Olbricht S, Le T, Emerich J, Kuhn W, Bentley J, Jackisch C, Luck HJ, Rochon J, Zimmermann AH, Eisenhauer E. Gemcitabine plus carboplatin compared with carboplatin in patients with platinum-sensitive recurrent ovarian cancer: an intergroup trial of the AGO-OVAR, the NCIC CTG, and the EORTC GCG. J Clin Oncol. 2006;24(29):4699–707. https://doi.org/10.1200/JCO.2006.06.0913.

89. Pfisterer J, Vergote I, Du Bois A, Eisenhauer E. Combination therapy with gemcitabine and carboplatin in recurrent ovarian cancer. Int J Gynecol Cancer. 2005;15(Suppl 1):36–41. https://doi.org/10.1111/j.1525-1438.2005.15355.x.

90. Sufliarsky J, Chovanec J, Svetlovska D, Minarik T, Packan T, Kroslakova D, Lalabova R, Helpianska L, Horvathova D, Sevcik L, Spacek J, Laluha A, Tkacova V, Malec V, Rakicka G, Magdin D, Jancokova I, Dorr A, Stresko M, Habetinek V, Koza I. Gemcitabine and carboplatin treatment in patients with relapsing ovarian cancer. Neoplasma. 2009;56(4):291–7. https://doi.org/10.4149/neo_2009_04_291.

91. Wang S, Zhang H, Cheng L, Evans C, Pan CX. Analysis of the cytotoxic activity of carboplatin and gemcitabine combination. Anticancer Res. 2010;30:4573–8.

92. Silva AA, Carlotto J, Rotta I. Padronização da ordem de infusão de medicamentos antineoplásicos utilizados no tratamento dos cânceres de mama e colorretal. Einstein. 2018;16(2):1–9.

93. NHS (2020) Chemotherapy protocol. Gynaecological cancer. Carboplatin (AUC4)-Gemcitabine (day 1) retreat. NHS. University Hospital Southampton. NHS Foundation Trust. England. Available in: https://www.uhs.nhs.uk/Media/SUHTExtranet/Services/Chemotherapy-SOPs/Ovarian-cancer/CarboplatinAUC4-Gemcitabineday1Retreat.pdf. Accessed Sep 23 2021.

94. Weber B, Lortholary A, Mayer F, Bourgeois H, Orfeuvre H, Combe M, Platini C, Cretin J, Fric D, Paraiso D, Pujade-Lauraine E. Pegylated liposomal doxorubicin and carboplatin in late-relapsing ovarian cancer: a GINECO group phase II trial. Anticancer Res. 2009;29(10):4195–200.

95. Pisano C, Cecere SC, Napoli MD, Cavaliere C, Tambaro R, Facchini G, Scaffa C, Losito S, Pizzolorusso A, Pignata S. Clinical trials with pegylated liposomal doxoru-

bicin in the treatment of ovarian cancer. J Drug Deliv. 2013;2013:898146. https://doi.org/10.1155/2013/898146.

96. Gabizon A, Tzemach D, Mak L, Bronstein M, Horowitz AT. Dose dependency of pharmacokinetics and therapeutic efficacy of pegylated liposomal doxorubicin (DOXIL) in murine models. J Drug Target. 2002;10(7):539–48. https://doi.org/10.1080/1061186021000072447.

97. Allen TM, Martin FJ. Advantages of liposomal delivery systems for anthracyclines. Semin Oncol. 2004;31(Suppl 13):5–15. https://doi.org/10.1053/j.seminoncol.2004.08.001.

98. Andreopoulou E, Gaiotti D, Kim E, Downey A, Mirchandani D, Hamilton A, Jacobs A, Curtin J, Muggia F. Pegylated liposomal doxorubicin HCL (PLD; Caelyx/Doxil®): experience with long-term maintenance in responding patients with recurrent epithelial ovarian cancer. Ann Oncol. 2007;18(4):716–21.

99. Sercombe L, Veerati T, Moheimani F, Wu SY, Sood AK, Hua S. Advances and challenges of liposome assisted drug delivery. Front Pharmacol. 2015;6:286. https://doi.org/10.3389/fphar.2015.00286.

100. Pujade-Lauraine E, Wagner U, Aavall-Lundqvist E, Gebski V, Heywood M, Vasey PA, Volgger B, Vergote I, Pignata S, Ferrero A, Sehouli J, Lortholary A, Kristensen G, Jackisch C, Joly F, Brown C, Fur NL, du Bois A. Pegylated liposomal doxorubicin and carboplatin compared with paclitaxel and carboplatin for patients with platinum-sensitive ovarian cancer in late relapse. J Clin Oncol. 2010;28(20):3323–9. https://doi.org/10.1200/JCO.2009.25.7519.

101. Ferrero JM, Weber B, Geay JF, Lepille D, Orfeuvre H, Combe M, Mayer F, Leduc B, Bourgeois H, Paraiso D, Pujade-Lauraine E. Second-line chemotherapy with pegylated liposomal doxorubicin and carboplatin is highly effective in patients with advanced ovarian cancer in late relapse: a GINECO phase II trial. Ann Oncol. 2007;18(2):263–8. https://doi.org/10.1093/annonc/mdl376.

102. NHS (2020) Chemotherapy protocol. Gynaecological cancer. Carboplatin (AUC5)-Pegylated liposomal doxorubicin (Caelyx) retreat. NHS. University Hospital Southampton. NHS Foundation Trust. England. Available in: https://www.uhs.nhs.uk/Media/SUHTExtranet/Services/Chemotherapy-SOPs/Ovarian-cancer/Carboplatin-Pegylated-Liposomal-Doxorubicin-Retreat.pdf. Accessed Sep 25 2021.

103. NCT01131039 (2013) Safety and Efficacy Study of Gemcitabine Plus Bevacizumab in Patients With Platinum-Resistant Ovarian, Primary Peritoneal or Fallopian Tube Cancer. Clinical Trials. Available in: https://clinicaltrials.gov/ct2/show/NCT01131039. Accessed Sep 25 2021.

104. Kogiku A, Nagao S, Suzuki K, Yamamoto K, Senda T, Kitai M, Shiozaki T, Matsuoka K, Sudo T, Yamaguchi S. Feasibility of bevacizumab combined with gemcitabine in treatment of platinum-resistant epithelial ovarian cancer. J Clin Oncol. 2017;35(15_suppl):e17064. https://doi.org/10.1200/JCO.2017.35.15_suppl.e17064.

105. Takasaki K, Miyamoto M, Takano M, Soyama H, Aoyama T, Matsuura H, Kato K, Sakamoto T, Kuwahara M, Iwahashi H, Ishibashi H, Yoshikawa T, Furuya K. Addition of bevacizumab to gemcitabine for platinum-resistant recurrent ovarian cancer: a retrospective analysis. Cancer Chemother Pharmacol. 2018;81(5):809–14. https://doi.org/10.1007/s00280-018-3552-5.

106. Nagao S, Kogiku A, Suzuki K, Shibutani T, Yamamoto K, Jimi T, Kitai M, Shiozaki T, Matsuoka K, Yamaguchi S. A phase II study of the combination chemotherapy of bevacizumab and gemcitabine in women with platinum-resistant recurrent epithelial ovarian, primary peritoneal, or fallopian tube cancer. J Ovarian Res. 2020;13(1):14. https://doi.org/10.1186/s13048-020-0617-y.

107. Ko J (2021) BC cancer protocol for treatment of platinum resistant epithelial ovarian cancer with bevacizumab and gemcitabine. BC cancer. British Columbia. Available in: http://www.Bccancer.Bc.Ca/chemotherapy-protocols-site/documents/gynecology/GOOVBEVG_Protocol.Pdf. Accessed Sep 25 2021.

108. McClung E, Wenham R. Profile of bevacizumab in the treatment of platinum-resistant ovarian cancer: current perspectives. Int J Women's Health. 2016;8:59–75. https://doi.org/10.2147/IJWH.S78101.

109. NCT02839707 (2021) Pegylated Liposomal Doxorubicin Hydrochloride With Atezolizumab and/or Bevacizumab in Treating Patients With Recurrent Ovarian, Fallopian Tube, or Primary Peritoneal Cancer. Clinical Trials. Available in: https://clinicaltrials.gov/ct2/show/NCT02839707. Accessed Sep 26 2021.

110. Verschraegen CF, Czok S, Muller CY, Boyd L, Lee SJ, Rutledge T, Blank S, Pothuri B, Eberhardt S, Muggia F. Phase II study of bevacizumab with liposomal doxorubicin for patients with platinum- and taxane-resistant ovarian cancer. Ann Oncol. 2012;23(12):3104–10. https://doi.org/10.1093/annonc/mds172.

111. Pujade-Lauraine E, Hilpert F, Weber B, Reuss A, Poveda A, Kristensen G, Sorio R, Vergote I, Witteveen P, Bamias A, Pereira D, Wimberger P, Oaknin A, Mirza MR, Follana P, Bollag D, Ray-Coquard I. Bevacizumab combined with chemotherapy for platinum-resistant recurrent ovarian cancer: the AURELIA open-label randomized phase III trial. J Clin Oncol. 2014;32(13):1302–8. https://doi.org/10.1200/JCO.2013.51.4489.

112. Bamias A, Gibbs E, Lee CK, Davies L, Dimopoulos M, Zagouri F, Veillard AS, Kosse J, Santaballa A, Mirza MR, Tabaro G, Vergote I, Bloemendal H, Lykka M, Floquet A, Gebski V, Pujade-Lauraine E. Bevacizumab with or after chemotherapy for platinum-resistant recurrent ovarian cancer: exploratory analyses of the AURELIA trial. Ann Oncol. 2017;28(8):1842–8. https://doi.org/10.1093/annonc/mdx228.

113. Tinker A (2021) BC cancer protocol for treatment of platinum resistant epithelial ovarian cancer with bevacizumab and DOXOrubicin pegylated liposomal. BC cancer. British Columbia. Available in: http://www.Bccancer.Bc.Ca/chemotherapy-protocols-site/documents/gynecology/GOOVBEVLD_Protocol.Pdf. Accessed Sep 26 2021.

114. Perren TJ, Swat AM, Pfisterer J, Ledermann JA, Pujade-Lauraine E, Kristensen G, Carey MS, Beale P, Cervantes A, Kurzeder C, du Bois A, Sehouli J, Kimmig R, Stahle A, Collinson F, Essapen S, Gourley C, Lortholary A, Selle F, Mirza MR, Leminen A, Plante M, Stark D, Qian W, Parmar MKB, Oza AM. A phase 33 trial of bevacizumab in ovarian cancer. N Engl J Med. 2011;365(26):2484–96. https://doi.org/10.1056/NEJMoa1103799.

115. Lyon KA, Huang JH. Bevacizumab combined with chemotherapy in platinum-resistant ovarian cancer: beyond the AURELIA trial. Transl Cancer Res. 2020;9(4):2164–7. https://doi.org/10.21037/tcr.2020.02.42.

116. Burger RA, Brady MF, Bookman MA, Fleming GF, Monk BJ, Huang H, Mannel RS, Homesley HD, Fowler J, Greer BE, Boente M, Birrer MJ, Liang SX. Incorporation of bevacizumab in the primary treatment of ovarian cancer. N Engl J Med. 2011;365(26):2473–83. https://doi.org/10.1056/NEJMoa1104390.

117. Lee JY, Jeong-Yeol P, Yoon PS, Lee JW, Kim JW, Kim YB, Jeong DH, Lee KB, Kim TH, Lee EH, Choi MC, Kim KH, Kim YM, Lee YJ, Kang S, Pujade-Lauraine E. Real-world effectiveness of bevacizumab based on AURELIA in platinum-resistant recurrent ovarian cancer (REBECA): a Korean gynecologic oncology group study (KGOG 3041). Gynecol Oncol. 2019;152(1):61–7. https://doi.org/10.1016/j.ygyno.2018.10.031.

118. Tinker A (2021) BC cancer protocol for treatment of platinum resistant epithelial ovarian cancer with bevacizumab and PACLitaxel. BC cancer. British Columbia. Available in: http://www.Bccancer.Bc.Ca/chemotherapy-protocols-site/documents/gynecology/GOOVBEVP_Protocol.Pdf. Accessed Sep 26 2021.

119. Berek JS, Bast RC. Nonepithelial ovarian cancer. In: Kufe DW, Pollock RE, Weichselbaum RR, et al., editors. Holland-Frei cancer medicine. 6th ed. Hamilton. Canada: BC Decker; 2003.

120. Boussios S, Zarkavelis G, Seraj E, Zerdes I, Tatsi K, Pentheroudakis G. Non-epithelial ovarian cancer: elucidating uncommon gynaecological malignancies. Anticancer Res. 2016;36(10):5031–42.

121. Ray-Coquard I, Morice P, Lorusso D, Prat J, Oaknin A, Pautier P, Colombo N. Non-epithelial ovarian cancer: ESMO clinical practice guidelines for diagnosis, treatment and follow-up. Ann Oncol. 2018;29(Suppl 4):IV1–IV18. https://doi.org/10.1093/annonc/mdy001.

122. Simone CG, Markham MJ, Dizon DS. Chemotherapy in ovarian germ cell tumors: a systematic review. Gynecol Oncol. 2016;141(3):602–7. https://doi.org/10.1016/j.ygyno.2016.02.007.

123. Uccello M, Boussios S, Samartzis EP, Moschetta M. Systemic anti-cancer treatment in malignant ovarian germ cell tumours (MOGCTs): current management and promising approaches. Ann Transl Med. 2020;8(24):1713. https://doi.org/10.21037/atm.2020.04.15.

124. Arbyn M, Weiderpass E, Bruni L, Sanjosé S, Saraiya M, Ferlay J, Bray F. Estimates of incidence and mortality of cervical cancer in 2018: a worldwide analysis. Lancet Glob Health. 2019;8(2):E191–203. https://doi.org/10.1016/S2214-109X(19)30482-6.

125. Fowler JR, Maani EV, Jack BW. Cervical cancer. Treasure Island USA: StatPearls Publishing; 2021.

126. Castellsagué X. Natural history and epidemiology of HPV infection and cervical cancer. Gynecol Oncol. 2008;110:S4–7. https://doi.org/10.1016/j.ygyno.2008.07.045.

127. Juckett G, Hartman-Adams H. Human papillomavirus: clinical manifestations and prevention. Am Fam Physician. 2010;82(10):1209–14.

128. Tulay P, Serakinci N. The role of human papillomaviruses in cancer progression. J Cancer Metastasis Treat. 2016;2:201–13. https://doi.org/10.20517/2394-4722.2015.67.

129. Munger K, Baldwin A, Edwards KM, Hayakawa H, Nguyen CL, Owens M, Grace M, Huh KW. Mechanisms of human papillomavirus-induced oncogenesis. J Virol. 2004;78(21):11451–60. https://doi.org/10.1128/JVI.78.21.11451-11460.2004.

130. Williams VM, Fillippova M, Soto U, Duerksen-Hughes PJ. HPV-DNA integration and carcinogenesis: putative roles for inflammation and oxidative stress. Futur Virol. 2011;6(1):45–57. https://doi.org/10.2217/fvl.10.73.

131. Prati B, Marangoni B, Boccardo E. Human papillomavirus and genome instability: from productive infection to cancer. Clinics. 2018;73(suppl 1):e539s. https://doi.org/10.6061/clinics/2018/e539s.

132. Spaans VM, Trietsch MD, Peters AAW, Osse M, ter Haar N, Fleuren GJ, Jordanova ES. Precise classification of cervical carcinomas combined with somatic mutation profiling contributes to predicting disease outcome. PLoS One. 2015;10(7):e0133670. https://doi.org/10.1371/journal.pone.0133670.

133. Tempfer CB, Tischoff I, Dogan A, Hilal Z, Schultheis B, Kern P, Rezniczek GA. Neuroendocrine carcinoma of the cervix: a systematic review of the literature. BMC Cancer. 2018;18:530. https://doi.org/10.1186/s12885-018-4447-x.

134. Wipperman J, Neil T, Williams T. Cervical cancer: evaluation and management. Am Fam Physician. 2018;97(7):449–54.

135. Paño B, Sebastià C, Ripoll E, Paredes P, Salvador R, Buñesch L, Nicolau C. Pathways of lymphatic spread in gynecologic malignancies. Radiographics. 2015;35(3):916–45. https://doi.org/10.1148/rg.2015140086.

136. Šarenac T, Mikov M. Cervical cancer, different treatments and importance of bile acids as therapeutic agents in this disease. Front Pharmacol. 2019;10:484. https://doi.org/10.3389/fphar.2019.00484.

137. Nicolet V, Carignan L, Bourdon F, Prosmanne O. MR imaging of cervical carcinoma: a practical staging approach. Radiographics. 2000;20(6):1539–49. https://doi.org/10.1148/radiographics.20.6.g00nv111539.

138. Bhatla N, Berek JS, Fredes MC, Denny LA, Grenman S, Karunaratne K, Kehoe ST, Konishi I, Olawaiye AB, Prat J, Sankaranarayanan R. Revised FIGO staging for carcinoma of the cervix uteri. Int J Gynaecol Obstet. 2019;145(10):129–35. https://doi.org/10.1002/ijgo.12749.

139. Odiase O, Noah-Vermillion L, Simone BA, Aridgides PD. The incorporation of immunotherapy and targeted therapy into chemoradiation for cervical cancer: a focused review. Front Oncol. 2021;11:663749. https://doi.org/10.3389/fonc.2021.663749.

140. Randall LM, Walker AJ, Jia AY, Miller DT, Zamarin D. Expanding our impact in cervical cancer treatment: novel immunotherapies, radiation innovations, and consideration of rare Histologies. Am Soc Clin Oncol Educ Book. 2021;41:252–63. https://doi.org/10.1200/EDBK_320411.

141. Kokka F, Bryant A, Brockbank E, Powell M, Oram D. Hysterectomy with radiotherapy or chemotherapy or both for women with locally advanced cervical cancer. Cochrane Library. 2015;4:CD010260. https://doi.org/10.1002/14651858.CD010260.pub2.

142. Sadalla JC, Andrade JM, Genta MLND, Baracat EC. Cervical cancer: what's new? Rev Assoc Med Bras. 2015;61(6):536–42. https://doi.org/10.1590/1806-9282.61.06.536.

143. Somashekhar SP, Ashwin KR. Management of early stage cervical cancer. Rev Recent Clin Trials. 2015;10(4):302–8. https://doi.org/10.2174/1574887110666150923113629.

144. Chuang LT, Temin S, Camacho R, Dueñas-Gonzalez A, Feldman S, Gultekin M, Gupta V, Horton S, Jacob G, Kidd EA, Lishimpi K, Nakisige C, Nam JH, Ngan HYS, Small W, Thomas G, Berek JS. Management and Care of Women with Invasive Cervical Cancer: American Society of Clinical Oncology resource-stratified clinical practice guideline. J Glob Oncol. 2016;2(5):311–40. https://doi.org/10.1200/JGO.2016.003954.

145. Kumar L, Gupta S. Integrating chemotherapy in the management of cervical cancer: a critical appraisal. Oncology. 2016;91(Suppl 1):8–17. https://doi.org/10.1159/000447576.

146. Costa SCS, Bonadio RC, Gabrielli FCG, Aranha AS, Genta MLND, Miranda VC, Freitas D, Abdo Filho E, Ferreira PAO, Machado KK, Scaranti M, Carvalho HÁ, Estevez-Diz MDP. Neoadjuvant chemotherapy with cisplatin and gemcitabine followed by chemoradiation versus chemoradiation for locally advanced cervical cancer: a randomized phase II trial. J Clin Oncol. 2019;37(33):3124–31. https://doi.org/10.1200/JCO.19.00674.

147. Colombo N, Carinelli S, Colombo A, Marini C, Rollo D, Sessa C. Cervical cancer: ESMO clinical practice guidelines for diagnosis, treatment and follow-up. Ann Oncol. 2012;23(Suppl 7):VII27–32. https://doi.org/10.1093/annonc/mds268.

148. Scatchard K, Forrest JL, Flubacher M, Cornes P, Williams C. Chemotherapy for metastatic and recurrent cervical cancer. Cochrane Library. 2012;2012(10):CD006469. https://doi.org/10.1002/14651858.CD006469.pub2.

149. Serkies K, Jassem J. Systemic therapy for cervical carcinoma—current status. Chin J Cancer Res. 2018;30(2):209–21. https://doi.org/10.21147/j.issn.1000-9604.2018.02.04.

150. Gennigens C, Cuypere MD, Hermesse J, Kridelka F, Jerusalem G. Optimal treatment in locally advanced cervical cancer. Expert Rev Anticancer Ther. 2021;21(6):657–71. https://doi.org/10.1080/14737140.2021.1879646.

151. Dueñas-Gonzalez A, López-Graniel C, González-Enciso A, Cetina L, Rivera L, Mariscal I, Montalvo G, Gómez E, la Garza J, Chanona G, Mohar A. A phase II study of multimodality treatment for locally advanced cervical cancer: neoadjuvant carboplatin and paclitaxel followed by radical hysterectomy and adjuvant cisplatin chemoradiation. Ann Oncol. 2003;14(8):1278–84. https://doi.org/10.1093/annonc/mdg333.

152. Yavas G, Yavas C, Sen E, Oner I, Celik C, Ata O. Adjuvant carboplatin and paclitaxel after concurrent cisplatin and radiotherapy in patients with locally advanced cervical cancer. Int J Gynecol Cancer. 2019;29(1):42–7. https://doi.org/10.1136/ijgc-2018-000022.

153. NCT01414608 (2021) Cisplatin and Radiation Therapy With or Without Carboplatin and Paclitaxel in Patients With Locally Advanced Cervical Cancer. Clinical Trials. Available in: https://clinicaltrials.gov/ct2/show/NCT01414608. Accessed Sep 30 2021.

154. Martin AG. Will the carboplatin-paclitaxel-bevacizumab combination become the preferred option as the first line in advanced cervical cancer? A small experience from a single oncologic center. Cancer Breaking News. 2017;5(1):21–4. https://doi.org/10.19156/cbn.2017.0035.

155. Tinker AV, Fiorino L, O'Dwyer H, Kumar A. Bevacizumab in metastatic, recurrent, or persistent cervical cancer: the BC cancer experience. Int J Gynecol Cancer. 2018;28(8):1592–9. https://doi.org/10.1097/IGC.0000000000001351.

156. NCT02467907 (2019) Safety and Efficacy of Bevacizumab in Combination With Carboplatin and Paclitaxel for Metastatic, Recurrent or Persistent Cervical Cancer. Clinical Trials. Available in: https://clinicaltrials.gov/ct2/show/NCT02467907. Accessed Sep 30 2021.

157. Tao W, Yang J, Jiang Y, Chen W, Wang Y. Paclitaxel, carboplatin, and bevacizumab in advanced cervical cancer: a treatment response and safety analysis. Dose-response: an. Int J. 2020;18(3):155932582094135. https://doi.org/10.1177/1559325820941351.

158. Rein DT, Kurbacher CM, Breidenbach M, Schondorf T, Schmidt T, Konig E, Gohring UJ, Blohmer JU, Mallmann P. Weekly carboplatin and docetaxel for locally advanced primary and recurrent cervical cancer: a phase I study. Gynecol Oncol. 2002;87(1):98–103. https://doi.org/10.1006/gyno.2002.6786.

159. Nagao S, Fujiwara K, Oda T, Ishikawa H, Koike H, Tanaka H, Kohno I. Combination chemotherapy of docetaxel and carboplatin in advanced or recurrent cervix cancer. A pilot study. Gynecol Oncol. 2005;96(3):805–9. https://doi.org/10.1016/j.ygyno.2004.11.044.

160. Shimada M, Sato S, Shoji T, Nagao S, Tokunaga H, Sueoka K, Takehara K, Nakamura K, Yamaguchi S, Kigawa J. Docetaxel and carboplatin chemotherapy for treating patients with stage IVB or recurrent non-squamous cell carcinoma of the uterine cervix: a phase II study. Int J Clin Oncol. 2021;26:1314–21. https://doi.org/10.1007/s10147-021-01903-1.

161. Cancer.Net Editorial Board (2021) Uterine Cancer: Statistics. American Society of Clinical Oncology (ASCO). Available in: https://www.cancer.net/cancer-types/uterine-cancer/statistics. Accessed Sep 30 2021.

162. Sung H, Ferlay J, Siegel RL, Laversanne M, Soerjomataram I, Jemal A, Bray F. Global cancer statistics 2020: GLOBOCAN estimates of incidence and mortality worldwide for 36 cancers in 185 countries. CA Cancer J Clin. 2021;71(3):209–49. https://doi.org/10.3322/caac.21660.

163. Purdie DM, Green AC. Epidemiology of endometrial cancer. Best Pract Res Clin Obstet Gynaecol. 2001;15(3):341–54. https://doi.org/10.1053/beog.2000.0180.

164. Kaaks R, Lukanova A, Kurzer MS. Obesity, endogenous hormones, and endometrial cancer risk: a synthetic review. Cancer Epidemiol Biomark Prev. 2002;11(12):1531–43.

165. Mills AM, Liou S, Ford JM, Berek JS, Pai RK, Longacre TA. Lynch syndrome screening should be considered for all patients with newly diagnosed endometrial cancer. Am J Surg Pathol. 2014;38(11):1501–9. https://doi.org/10.1097/PAS.0000000000000321.

166. Passarello K, Kurian S, Villanueva V. Endometrial cancer: na overview of pathophysiology, management, and care. Semin Oncol Nurs. 2019;35(2):157–65. https://doi.org/10.1016/j.soncn.2019.02.002.

167. Mahdy H, Casey MJ, Crotzer D. Endometrial Cancer. Treasure Island USA: StatPearls Publishing; 2021.

168. May K, Bryant A, Dickinson HO, Kehoe S, Morrison J. Lymphadenectomy for the management of endometrial cancer. Cochrane Library. 2010;1:CD007585. https://doi.org/10.1002/14651858.CD007585.pub2.

169. Otero-García MM, Mesa-Álvarez A, Nikolic O, Blanco-Lobato P, Basta-Nikolic M, Llano-Ortega RM, Paredes-Velázquez L, Nikolic N, Szewczyk-Bieda M. Role of MRI in staging and follow-up of endometrial and cervical cancer: pitfalls and mimickers. Insights Imaging. 2019;10:19. https://doi.org/10.1186/s13244-019-0696-8.

170. Amant F, Moerman P, Neven P, Timmerman D, Limbergen EV, Vergote I. Treatment modalities in endometrial cancer. Curr Opin Oncol. 2007;19(5):479–85. https://doi.org/10.1097/CCO.0b013e32827853c0.

171. Tucci CD, Capone C, Galati G, Iacobelli V, Schiavi MC, Donato VD, Muzii L, Panici PB. Immunotherapy in endometrial cancer: new scenarios on the horizon. J Gynecol Oncol. 2019;30(3):e46. https://doi.org/10.3802/jgo.2019.30.e46.

172. Amant F, Mirza MR, Koskas M, Creutzberg CL. Cancer of the corpus uteri. Gynecol Obstet. 2018;143(S2):37–50. https://doi.org/10.1002/ijgo.12612.

173. Bakir MS. Brachytherapy in endometrial cancer. London, United Kingdom: Intechopen; 2020.

174. Rauh-Hain JA, del Carmen MG. Treatment for advanced and recurrent endometrial carcinoma: combined modalities. Oncologist. 2010;15(8):852–61. https://doi.org/10.1634/theoncologist.2010-0091.

175. Denschlag D, Ulrich U, Emons G. The diagnosis and treatment of endometrial cancer: progress and controversies. Dtsch Arztebl Int. 2011;108(34–35):571–7. https://doi.org/10.3238/arztebl.2011.0571.

176. Concin N, Matias-Guiu X, Vergote I, Cibula D, Mirza MR, Marnitz S, Ledermann J, Bosse T, Chargari C, Fagotti A, Fotopoulou C, Martin AG, Lax S, Lorusso D, Marth C, Morice P, Nout RA, O'Donnell D, Querleu D, Raspollini MR, Sehouli J, Sturdza A, Taylor A, Westermann A, Wimberger P, Colombo N, Planchamp F, Creutzberg CL. ESGO/ESTRO/ESP guidelines for the management of patients with endometrial carcinoma. Int J Gynecol Cancer. 2020;31:12–39. https://doi.org/10.1136/ijgc-2020-002230.

177. Lachance JA, Darus CJ, Rice LW. Surgical management and postoperative treatment of endometrial carcinoma. Rev Obstet Gynecol. 2008;1(3):97–105.

178. Bestvina CM, Fleming GF. Chemotherapy for endometrial cancer in adjuvant and advanced disease settings. Oncologist. 2016;21(10):1250–9. https://doi.org/10.1634/theoncologist.2016-0062.

179. Kurra V, Krajewski KM, Jagannathan J, Giardino A, Berlin S, Ramaiya N. Typical and atypical metastatic sites of recurrent endometrial carcinoma. Cancer Imaging. 2013;13(1):113–22. https://doi.org/10.1102/1470-7330.2013.0011.

180. MacKay HJ, Freixinos VR, Fleming GF. Therapeutic targets and opportunities in endometrial cancer: update on endocrine therapy and nonimmunotherapy targeted options. Am Soc Clin Oncol Educ Book. 2020;40:245–55. https://doi.org/10.1200/EDBK_280495.

181. Aapro MS, van Wijk FH, Bolis G, Chevallier B, van der Burg MEL, Poveda A, Oliveira CF, Tumolo S, Scotto di Palumbo V, Piccart M, Franchi M, Zanaboni F, Lacave AJ, Fontanelli R, Favalli G, Zola P, Guastalla JP, Rosso R, Marth C, Nooij M, Presti M, Scarabelli C, Splinter TAW, Ploch E, Beex LVA, ten Bokkel Huinink W, Forni M, Melpignano M, Blake P, Kerbrat P, Mendiola C, Cervantes A, Goupil A, Harper PG, Madronal C, Namer M, Scarfone G, Stoot JE, Teodorovic I, Coens C, Vergote I, Vermorken JB. Doxorubicin versus doxorubicin and cisplatin in endometrial carcinoma: definitive results of a randomised study (55872) by the EORTC Gynaecological cancer group. Ann Oncol. 2003;14(3):441–8. https://doi.org/10.1093/annonc/mdg112.

182. van Wijk FH, Aapro MS, Bolis G, Chevallier B, van der Burg MEL, Poveda A, Oliveira CF, Tumolo S, Scotto di Palumbo V, Piccart M, Franchi M, Zanaboni F, Lacave AJ, Fontanelli R, Favalli G, Zola P, Guastalla JP, Rosso R, Marth C, Nooij M, Presti M, Scarabelli C, Splinter TAW, Ploch E, Beex LVA, ten Bokkel HW, Forni M, Melpignano M, Blake P, Kerbrat P, Mendiola C, Cervantes A, Goupil A, Harper PG, Madronal C, Namer M, Scarfone G, Stoot JEGM, Teodorovic I, Coens C, Vergote I, Vermorken JB. Doxorubicin versus doxorubicin and cisplatin in endometrial carcinoma: definitive results of a randomised study (55872) by the EORTC Gynaecological cancer group. Ann Oncol. 2003;14(3):441–8. https://doi.org/10.1093/annonc/mdg112.

183. van Weelden WJ, Massuger LFAG, ENITEC, JMA P, Romano A. Anti-estrogen treatmen in endometrial cancer: a systematic review. Front Oncol. 2019;9:359. https://doi.org/10.3389/fonc.2019.00359.

184. Yang S, Thiel KW, Leslie KK. Progesterone: the ultimate endometrial tumor suppressor. Trends Endocrinol Metab. 2011;22(4):145–52. https://doi.org/10.1016/j.tem.2011.01.005.

185. Kim JJ, Kurita T, Bulun SE. Progesterone action in endometrial cancer, endometriosis, uterine fibroids, and breast cancer. Endocr Rev. 2013;34(1):130–62. https://doi.org/10.1210/er.2012-1043.

186. Nomura H, Aoki D, Takahashi F, Katsumata N, Watanabe Y, Konishi I, Jobo T, Hatae M, Hiura M, Yaegashi N. Randomized phase II study comparing docetaxel plus cisplatin, docetaxel plus carboplatin, and paclitaxel plus carboplatin in patients with advanced or recurrent endometrial carcinoma: a Japanese gynecologic oncology group study (JGOG2041). Ann Oncol. 2011;22(3):636–42. https://doi.org/10.1093/annonc/mdq401.

187. Yoshida H, Imai Y, Fujiwara K. Combination chemotherapy with docetaxel and carboplatin for elderly patients with endometrial cancer. Mol Clin Oncol. 2016;4(5):783–8. https://doi.org/10.3892/mco.2016.781.

188. NCT00258362 (2017) Carboplatin, Docetaxel, and Radiation Therapy in Treating Patients With Stage III/IV, or Recurrent Endometrial Cancer. Clinical Trials. Available in: https://clinicaltrials.gov/ct2/show/NCT00258362. Accessed Oct 1 2021.

189. Sovak MA, Dupont J, Hensley ML, Ishill N, Gerst S, Abu-Rustum N, Anderson S, Barakat R, Konner J, Poyner E, Sabbatini P, Spriggs DR, Aghajanian C. Paclitaxel and carboplatin in the treatment of advanced or recurrent endometrial cancer: a large retrospective study. Int J Gynecol Cancer. 2007;17(1):197–203. https://doi.org/10.1111/j.1525-1438.2006.00746.x.

190. Sorbe B, Andersson H, Boman K, Rosenberg P, Kalling M. Treatment of primary advanced and recurrent endometrial carcinoma with a combination of carboplatin and paclitaxel-long-term follow-up. Int J Gynecol Cancer. 2008;18(4):803–8. https://doi.org/10.1111/j.1525-1438.2007.01094.x.

191. Miller DS, Filiaci VL, Mannel RS, Cohn DE, Matsumoto T, Tewari KS, DiSilvestro P, Pearl ML, Argenta PA, Powell MA, Zweizig SL, Warshal DP, Hanjani P, Carney ME, Huang H, Cella D, Zaino R, Fleming GF. Carboplatin and paclitaxel for advanced endometrial cancer: final overall survival and adverse event analysis of a phase III trial (NRG oncology/GOG0209). J Clin Oncol. 2020;38(33):3841–50. https://doi.org/10.1200/JCO.20.01076.

192. Cintio ED, Parazzini F, Rosa C, Chatenoud L, Benzi G. The epidemiology of gestational trophoblastic disease. Gen Diagn Pathol. 1997;143(2–3):103–8.

193. Steigrad SJ. Epidemiology of gestational trophoblastic diseases. Best Pract Res Clin Obstet Gynaecol. 2003;17(6):837–47. https://doi.org/10.1016/S1521-6934(03)00049-X.

194. Garner EIO, Goldstein DP, Feltmate CM, Berkowitz RS. Gestational trophoblastic disease. Clin Obstet Gynecol. 2007;50(1):112–22. https://doi.org/10.1097/GRF.0b013e31802f17fc.

195. Candelier JJ. The hydatidiform mole. Cell Adhes Migr. 2016;10(1–2):226–35. https://doi.org/10.1080/19336918.2015.1093275.

196. La Vecchia C, Franceschi S, Parazzini F, Fasoli M, Decarli A, Gallus G, Tognoni G. Risk factors for gestational trophoblastic disease in Italy. Am J Epidemiol. 1985;121(3):457–64. https://doi.org/10.1093/oxfordjournals.aje.a114018.

197. Lima LLA, Parente RCM, Maestá I, Junior JÁ, Filho JFR, Montenegro CAB, Braga A. Clinical and radiological correlations in patients with gestational trophoblastic disease. Radiol Bras. 2016;49(4):241–50. https://doi.org/10.1590/0100-3984.2015.0073.

198. Shih IM, Mazur MT, Kurman RJ. Gestational trophoblastic tumors and related tumor-like lesions. In: Kurman RJ, Ellenson LH, Ronnett BM, editors. Blaustein's pathology of the female genital tract. Boston, MA: Springer; 2011. https://doi.org/10.1007/978-1-4419-0489-8_20.

199. Goldstein DP, Berkowitz RS. Current management of gestational trophoblastic neoplasia. Hematol Oncol Clin North Am. 2012;26:111–31. https://doi.org/10.1016/j.hoc.2011.10.007.

200. Begum SA, Bhuiyan ZR, Akther R, Afroz R, Chowdhury A, Keya KA. A review on gestational trophoblastic disease. Bangladesh Med J. 2015;44(1):51–6.

201. Shaaban AM, Rezvani M, Haroun RR, Kennedy AM, Elsayes KM, Olpin JD, Salama ME, Foster BR, Menias CO. Gestational trophoblastic disease: clinical and imaging features. Radiographics. 2017;37:681–700. https://doi.org/10.1148/rg.2017160140.

202. López CL, Lopes VGS, Resende FR, Steim JL, Padrón L, Sun SY, Jpunior EA, Braga A. Gestational trophoblastic neoplasia after ectopic molar pregnancy: clinical, diagnostic, and therapeutic aspects. Rev Bras Ginecol Obstet. 2018;40(05):294–9. https://doi.org/10.1055/s-0038-1653976.

203. Lertkhachonsuk AA, Israngura N, Wilailak S, Tangtrakul S. Actinomycin d versus methotrexate-folinic acid as the treatment of stage I, low-risk gestational trophoblastic neoplasia: a randomized controlled trial. Int J Gynecol Cancer. 2009;19(5):985–8. https://doi.org/10.1111/IGC.0b013e3181a8333d.

204. Lima LLA, Padron L, Câmara R, Sun SY, Filho JR, Braga A. The role of surgery in the management of women with gestational trophoblastic disease. Rev Col Bras Cir. 2017;44(1):94–101. https://doi.org/10.1590/0100-69912017001009.

205. Biscaro A, Braga A, Berkowitz RS. Diagnosis, classification and treatment of gestational trophoblastic neoplasia. Rev Bras Ginecol Obstet. 2015;37(1):42–51. https://doi.org/10.1590/SO100-720320140005198.

206. Vencken PMLH, Ewing PC, Zweemer RP. Epithelioid trophoblastic tumour: a case report and review of the literature. J Clin Pathol. 2006;59(12):1307–8. https://doi.org/10.1136/jcp.2005.030734.

207. May T, Goldstein DP, Berkowitz RS. Current chemotherapeutic management of patients with gestational trophoblastic neoplasia. Chemother Res Pract. 2011;2011:806256. https://doi.org/10.1155/2011/806256.

208. Alazzam M, Tidy J, Hancock BW, Osborne R, Lawrie TA. First-line chemotherapy in low-risk gestational trophoblastic neoplasia. Cochrane Library. 2012;7:CD007102. https://doi.org/10.1002/14651858.CD007102.pub3.

209. Froeling FEM, Ramaswami R, Papanastasopoulos P, Kaur B, Sebire NJ, Short D, Fisher RA, Sarwar N, Wells M, Singh K, Ellis L, Horsman JM, Winter MC, Tidy J, Hancock BW, Seckl MJ. Intensified therapies improve survival and identification of novel prognostic factors for placental-site and epithelioid trophoblastic tumours. Br J Cancer. 2019;120:587–94. https://doi.org/10.1038/s41416-019-0402-0.

210. Xiao C, Yang J, Zhao J, Ren T, Feng F, Wan X, Xiang Y. Management and prognosis of patients with brain metastasis from gestational trophoblastic neoplasia: a 24-year experience in Peking union medical college hospital. BMC Cancer. 2015;15:318. https://doi.org/10.1186/s12885-015-1325-7.

211. Ngan HYS, Secki MJ, Berkowitz RS, Xiang Y, Golfier F, Sekharan PK, Lurain JR, Massuger L. Update on the diagnosis and management of gestational trophoblastic disease. Int J Gynecol Obstet. 2018;143(S2):79–85. https://doi.org/10.1002/ijgo.12615.

212. Masocatto NO, Carmignani LO, Lisboa NS. Epithelioid trophoblastic tumor: diagnosis and treatment. Relatos de Casos Cirúrgicos. 2021;7(2):e2956. https://doi.org/10.30928/2527-2039e-20212956.

213. Wong LC, Ngan HY, Cheng DK, Ng TY. Methotrexate infusion in low-risk gestational trophoblastic disease. Am J Obstet Gynecol. 2000;183(6):1579–82. https://doi.org/10.1067/mob.2000.108077.

214. Maestá I, Nitecki R, Horowitz NS, Goldstein DP, Moreira MFS, Elias KM, Berkowitz RS. Effectiveness and toxicity of first-line methotrexate chemotherapy in low-risk postmolar gestational trophoblastic neoplasia: the New England trophoblastic disease center experience. Gynecol Oncol. 2017;148(1):161–7. https://doi.org/10.1016/j.ygyno.2017.10.028.

215. NCT01535053 (2019) Dactinomycin or Methotrexate in Treating Patients With Low-Risk Gestational Trophoblastic Neoplasia. Clinical Trials. Available in: https://clinicaltrials.gov/ct2/show/NCT01535053. Accessed Oct 1 2021.

216. Hoeijmakers YM, Sweep FCGJ, Lok CAR, Ottevanger PB. Risk factors for second-line dactinomycin failure after methotrexate treatment for low-risk gestational trophoblastic neoplasia: a retrospective study. BJOG. 2020;127(9):1139–45. https://doi.org/10.1111/1471-0528.16198.

217. Lurain JR, Schink JC. Importance of salvage therapy in the management of high-risk gestational trophoblastic neoplasia. J Reprod Med. 2012;57(5–6):219–24.

218. Alifrangis C, Agarwal R, Short D, Fisher RA, Sebire NJ, Harvey R, Savage PM, Seckl MJ. EMA/CO for high-risk gestational trophoblastic neoplasia: good outcomes with induction low-dose etoposide-cisplatin and genetic analysis. J Clin Oncol. 2013;31(2):280–6. https://doi.org/10.1200/JCO.2012.43.1817.

219. Silva ACB, Passos JP, Filho RCS, Braga A, Mattar R, Sun SY. Uterine Rescue in High-Risk Gestational Trophoblastic Neoplasia Treated with EMA-CO by uterine arteries embolization due to arteriovenous malformations. Rev Bras Ginecol Obstet. 2021;43(4):323–8. https://doi.org/10.1055/s-0041-1725054.

220. Lurain JR, Singh DK, Schink JC. Primary treatment of metastatic high-risk gestational trophoblastic neoplasia with EMA-CO chemotherapy. J Reprod Med. 2006;51(10):767–72.

221. Lu WG, Ye F, Shen YM, Fu YF, Chen HZ, Wan XY, Xie X. EMA-CO chemotherapy for high-risk gestational trophoblastic neoplasia: a clinical analysis of 54 patients. Int J Gynecol Cancer. 2008;18(2):357–62. https://doi.org/10.1111/j.1525-1438.2007.00999.x.

222. Lybol C, Thomas CMG, Blanken EA, Sweep FCGJ, Verheijen RH, Westermann AM, Boere IA, Reyners AKL, Massuger LFAG, van Hoesel RQGCM, Ottevanger PB. Comparing cisplatin-based combination chemotherapy with EMA/CO chemotherapy for the treatment of high risk gestational trophoblastic neoplasia. Eur J Cancer. 2013;49:860–7. https://doi.org/10.1016/j.ejca.2012.09.015.

223. Patel SM, Desai A. Management of drug resistant gestational trophoblastic neoplasia. J Reprod Med. 2010;55(7–8):296–300.

224. Babaier A, Jim B, Ghatage P. Management of EMA-CO resistant/refractory gestational trophoblastic neoplasia. Cancer Rep Rev. 2019;3:1–8. https://doi.org/10.15761/CRR.1000179.
225. Cancer Institute NSW (2017) Gestational trophoblastic disease high risk EMA-CO (etoposide methotrexate daCTINomycin (actinomycin D) CYCLOPHOSPHamide vinCRISTine). Cancer Institute NSW. Australia. Available in: https://www.Eviq.Org.Au/medical-oncology/gynaecological/gestational-trophoblastic-disease/599-gestational-trophoblastic-disease-high-risk-em#interactions. Accessed Oct 2 2021.
226. Tinker A (2021) BC cancer protocol summary for therapy for high risk gestational trophoblastic neoplasia (GTN) using etoposide, methotrexate, leucovorin (Folinic acid), DACTINomycin, cyclophosphamide and vincristine. BC cancer. British Columbia. Available in: http://www.Bccancer.Bc.Ca/chemotherapy-protocols-site/documents/gynecology/GOTDEMACO_Protocol.Pdf. Accessed Oct 2 2021.
227. Tinker A (2021) BC cancer protocol summary for therapy for moderate risk gestational trophoblastic cancer using DACTINomycin and methotrexate. BC cancer. British Columbia. Available in: http://www.Bccancer.Bc.Ca/chemotherapy-protocols-site/documents/gynecology/GOTDMR_Protocol.Pdf. Accessed Oct 2 2021.
228. Carlson V, Walters L, Lambert P, Dean E, Lotocki R, Altman AD. Low-risk gestational trophoblastic neoplasia in Manitoba: experience with alternating methotrexate and dactinomycin. Int J Gynecol Cancer. 2018;28:1448–52. https://doi.org/10.1097/IGC.0000000000001347.
229. Eiriksson L, Wells T, Steed H, Schepansky A, Capstick V, Hoskins P, Pike J, Swenerton K. Combined methotrexate-dactinomycin: an effective therapy for low-risk gestational trophoblastic neoplasia. Gynecol Oncol. 2012;124(3):553–7. https://doi.org/10.1016/j.ygyno.2011.10.036.
230. Kang HL, Zhao Q, Yang SL, Duan W. Efficacy of combination therapy with actinomycin D and methotrexate in the treatment of low-risk gestational trophoblastic neoplasia. Chemotherapy. 2019;64:42–7. https://doi.org/10.1159/000500165.

Chapter 8
Chemotherapeutic Protocols for the Treatment of Head and Neck Cancer

8.1 Epidemiological Profile of Head and Neck Cancers

Head and neck cancers are the fifth most common type of cancer worldwide, with more than 550,000 new cases reported each year. Head and neck tumors, in addition to their high incidence, also have high mortality and morbidity. According to WHO data, in 2020, 932,000 cases and 467,000 deaths from head and neck cancers were reported [1, 2]. Men are more affected than women, with the number of cases in 2020 being 700,000 for men compared with 232,000 cases for women [2]. Figure 8.1 presents the estimate for the year 2040 of the incidence of cases and deaths from head and neck cancers.

Head and neck cancers comprise cancers that affect the oral cavity, pharynx, larynx, salivary glands, and among others [1, 3]. These tumors usually start in the squamous cells that line the surfaces of mucosal of the head and neck such as inside the mouth, throat, and voice box. Although less frequent, cancers can also start in the salivary glands, sinuses, or muscles or nerves in the head and neck. Generally not classified as head and neck cancers are the cancers of the brain, eyes, esophagus, thyroid gland, and skin of the head and neck [4–7].

Some risk factors for the development of head and neck cancer include alcohol and tobacco use, infections especially with human papillomavirus (HPV) type 16 and Epstein-Barr virus, genetic disorders, occupational exposure to chemicals, and radiation [3, 7, 8].

© The Author(s), under exclusive license to Springer Nature
Switzerland AG 2022
I. D. Lima Cavalcanti, *Chemotherapy Protocols and Infusion Sequence*,
https://doi.org/10.1007/978-3-031-10839-6_8

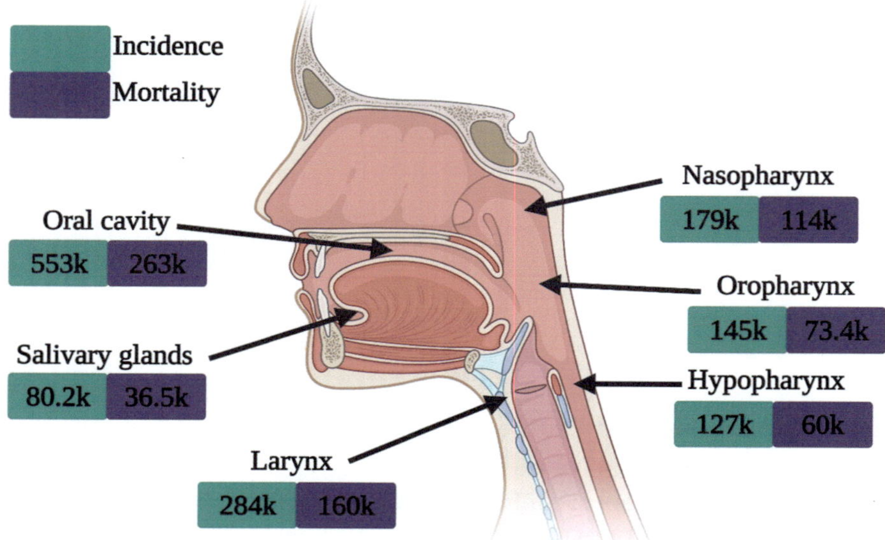

Fig. 8.1 Estimated incidence of cases and mortality of head and neck cancers for the year 2040. (Source: Created with BioRender.com and data were extracted from [2])

8.2   Pathophysiology of Nasopharyngeal Carcinoma

Nasopharyngeal cancers (Fig. 8.2) are rare in many countries, but in regions such as southern China, Southeast Asia, and Africa Notch, the incidence is exceptionally high. According to the WHO, in 2020, 133,000 cases were reported, of which the predominance of cases are in men with 96,400 cases and 37,000 in women. As for mortality, 80 thousand deaths from nasopharyngeal cancer were reported [2, 9].

Most nasopharyngeal cancers originate from squamous cells that line the nasopharynx, which is why squamous cell carcinomas are most common in adults [10–12]. Nasopharyngeal carcinoma can be classified as differentiated and keratinizing squamous cell carcinoma, differentiated and nonkeratinizing, and undifferentiated and nonkeratinizing [10, 13–15].

Epstein-Barr virus infection is associated with the development of differentiated, nonkeratinizing, or undifferentiated, nonkeratinizing squamous cell carcinoma. Other factors that can contribute to the development of nasopharyngeal carcinoma are the consumption of salty, smoked, and preserved foods and genetic susceptibility [14, 16–19].

As for staging, in stage 1, the tumor is located in the nasopharynx, while in stage 2, it extends to the nasal cavity and oropharynx and may present homolateral adenopathy smaller than 6 cm. In stage 3, the tumor invades bone structures or the paranasal sinuses and may present contralateral or bilateral adenopathy smaller than

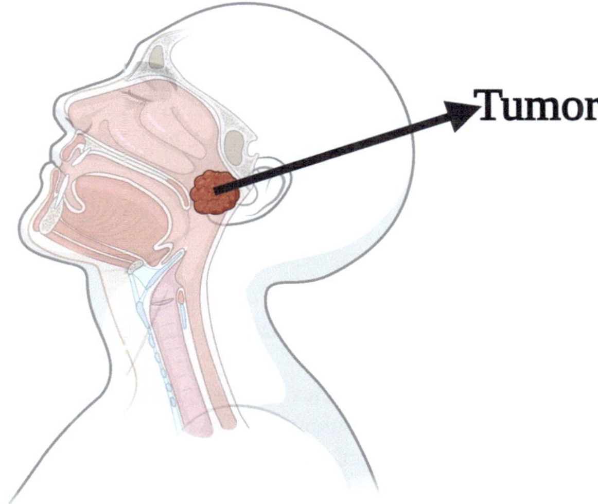

Fig. 8.2 Nasopharyngeal carcinoma. (Source: Created with BioRender.com)

6 cm; in stage 4A, the tumor spreads to the intracranial region and/or in the involvement of the cranial nerves, hypopharynx, infratemporal fossa, and orbits and may present adenopathy smaller or larger than 6 cm; and in stage 4B, in addition to the characteristics mentioned in stage 4A, it presents metastases [20–23].

8.2.1 Chemotherapy for the Treatment of Nasopharyngeal Carcinoma

Treatment of nasopharyngeal carcinoma in early stages may be based on radiotherapy to the tumor and lymph nodes of the neck in stage 1 patients, or chemotherapy-associated with radiotherapy in stage 2 patients may also be indicated [24–27]. In stage 3, the treatment of nasopharyngeal carcinoma can be based on chemotherapy combined with radiotherapy, as well as radiotherapy followed by surgery to remove the lymph nodes, and can be indicated. The treatment modalities for stage 4 are similar to stage 3, with only the possibility of specific chemotherapy being indicated for metastatic cancer [28–32].

Some antineoplastic agents may be indicated as monotherapy, such as capecitabine or fluorouracil in the treatment of recurrent or metastatic nasopharyngeal cancer [33, 34], gemcitabine in the treatment of locoregionally recurrent/metastatic non-amenable nasopharyngeal cancer for local curative therapy [35, 36], and cisplatin as palliative therapy in advanced nasopharyngeal carcinoma [37, 38]. Cisplatin may also be indicated in combination with radiotherapy in the treatment of locally advanced nasopharyngeal cancer [39, 40].

As a combination therapy, some protocols used in other cancers may also be indicated, such as the combination of cisplatin and gemcitabine (see Chap. 5), which is indicated in the treatment of cancers of the gastrointestinal tract and genitourinary tract and has been used in the treatment of locally advanced nasopharyngeal cancer induction [41–43]. Another combination indicated for the treatment of recurrent or metastatic nasopharyngeal carcinoma is carboplatin combined with paclitaxel (see infusion sequence in Chap. 5), which is also indicated for the treatment of gastrointestinal and gynecological cancers [44–46]. Other protocols [47–49] indicated for the treatment of nasopharyngeal cancers will be mentioned in the next topics.

8.2.1.1 FUP Protocol (5-Fluorouracil and Platinum)

The FUP protocol combines 5-fluorouracil with a platinum compound (carboplatin or cisplatin) in the treatment of advanced nasopharyngeal cancer [50]. Au and Ang [51] evaluated the efficacy of the combination of 5-fluorouracil and cisplatin in the treatment of recurrent or metastatic nasopharyngeal carcinoma. The protocol induced an overall response rate in 66% of patients, with a median time to progression of 8 months and median survival of 11 months. In the study by Jin et al. [52], the combination between 5-fluorouracil and cisplatin showed greater tolerance than the combination of 5-fluorouracil, cisplatin, and docetaxel, but the efficacy was lower in the treatment of advanced locoregional nasopharyngeal carcinoma.

The infusion sequence of the combination of 5-fluorouracil and cisplatin (Fig. 8.3) starts with the infusion of cisplatin because 5-fluorouracil is administered by continuous infusion using the infusion pump [50, 53].

The association between carboplatin and 5-fluorouracil had similar efficacy when compared with the combination of cisplatin and 5-fluorouracil [54]. Kua et al. [54] observed in patients with metastatic and recurrent squamous cell carcinoma and nasopharyngeal carcinoma a progression-free survival of 7 months in the group of patients who received cisplatin/5-fluorouracil and 9 months in patients who received carboplatin/5-fluorouracil and 10-month overall survival for cisplatin/5-fluorouracil and 12 months in the cisplatin/5-fluorouracil group.

Dechaphunkul et al. [55] evaluated the efficacy of concomitant chemoradiotherapy with carboplatin followed by the combination of carboplatin and 5-fluorouracil in locally advanced nasopharyngeal carcinoma. The therapeutic regimen promoted

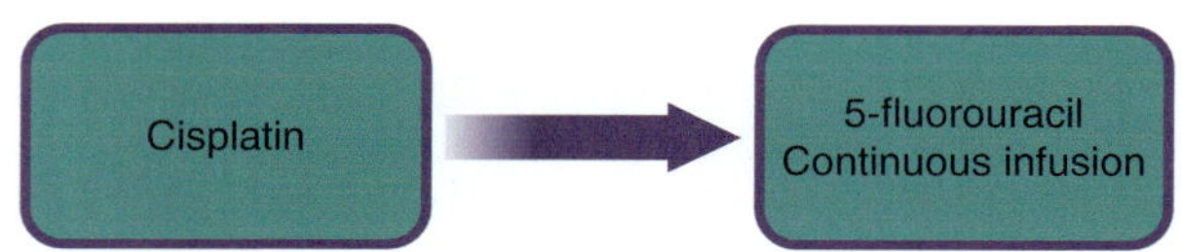

Fig. 8.3 Infusion sequence of the combination of cisplatin and 5-fluorouracil

Fig. 8.4 Infusion sequence of the combination between carboplatin and 5-fluorouracil

Fig. 8.5 EP protocol infusion sequence

a complete objective response rate of 64%, an overall 3-year survival rate of 89.7%, and a progression-free survival rate of 72.7%. The main acute toxicity of the regimen was weight loss and mucositis. In locally advanced squamous cell carcinoma of the head and neck, Hanemaaijer et al. [56] found that the combination of carboplatin and 5-fluorouracil promoted an overall 3-year survival of 65.4% and 3-year disease-free survival of 70%. The infusion sequence of the combination of carboplatin and 5-fluorouracil (Fig. 8.4) starts with the infusion of carboplatin followed by the continuous infusion of 5-fluorouracil [50].

8.2.1.2 EP Protocol (Etoposide and Platinum)

The combination of etoposide and platinum (carboplatin or cisplatin) is indicated in the treatment of recurrent and/or metastatic nasopharyngeal cancer [57]. The study by Osoba et al. [58] evaluated the use of cisplatin as monotherapy or in combination in the treatment of recurrent and metastatic head and neck cancer. The combination of cisplatin and etoposide promoted a response rate of 47%, with a progression time of 12 weeks and a response duration of 12 weeks. The authors believe that the combination of etoposide and cisplatin has synergistic effects in the treatment of recurrent head and neck cancer.

In a phase 2 study, Chi et al. [59] evaluated the efficacy of carboplatin in the treatment of nasopharyngeal carcinoma, promoting a partial response rate of 44%, with 47% with stable disease and 9% with progressive disease. The toxicity was tolerable and carboplatin proved to be effective for the treatment of nasopharyngeal carcinoma.

The use of carboplatin may be an alternative to replace cisplatin in combination with etoposide. As for the infusion sequence of the EP protocol, cisplatin or carboplatin is administered initially followed by the administration of etoposide (Fig. 8.5) [57].

8.2.1.3   PG Protocol (Gemcitabine and Platinum)

Platinum compounds (carboplatin and cisplatin) can also be combined with gemcitabine in the treatment of locoregionally recurrent and/or metastatic nasopharyngeal cancer [60]. Ngan et al. [61] combined gemcitabine plus cisplatin in the treatment of metastatic or recurrent nasopharyngeal carcinoma. As a result, the authors found that the combination promoted an overall response rate of 73% and mean duration of response of 5.3 months. Protocol toxicity was mainly hematologic with induction of anemia, granulocytopenia, and thrombocytopenia.

According to Hsieh et al. [62], in Taiwanese patients with recurrent or metastatic nasopharyngeal carcinoma, the combination of gemcitabine and cisplatin promoted an overall response rate of 51.9%, overall survival of 14.6 months, and progression-free survival of 9.8 months. The main toxicity was leukopenia, proving to be a tolerable protocol.

Zhang et al. [43] found that the combination of gemcitabine and cisplatin promoted a 3-year recurrence-free survival of 85.3%, 3-year overall survival of 94.6%, and an incidence of adverse events of 75.7% in patients with carcinoma of the nasopharynx. Major adverse events included neutropenia, thrombocytopenia, anemia, nausea, and vomiting.

Beldjilali et al. [63] evaluated the efficacy of carboplatin with gemcitabine in the treatment of recurrent nasopharyngeal carcinoma. The combination promoted a median overall survival of 8.2 months and a partial response rate of 32%. The toxicity profile was similar to the combination of cisplatin with gemcitabine, inducing anemia, granulocytopenia, and thrombocytopenia. Lim et al. [64], in a phase 2 study, evaluated the treatment of locally advanced nasopharyngeal carcinoma with a combination of carboplatin and gemcitabine followed by chemoradiotherapy. The protocol promoted an overall 3-year survival rate of 89.3%, proving to be a tolerable combination.

The combination of gemcitabine plus platinum promoted a progression-free survival of 10.3 months and overall survival of 42.8 months, in the study by Chen et al. [65] in patients with recurrent or metastatic nasopharyngeal carcinoma. The protocol also promoted an objective response rate of 67.9% and a disease control rate of 92.9%. As for the infusion sequence, the PG protocol starts with the infusion of gemcitabine followed by platinum (carboplatin or cisplatin) (Fig. 8.6) [60].

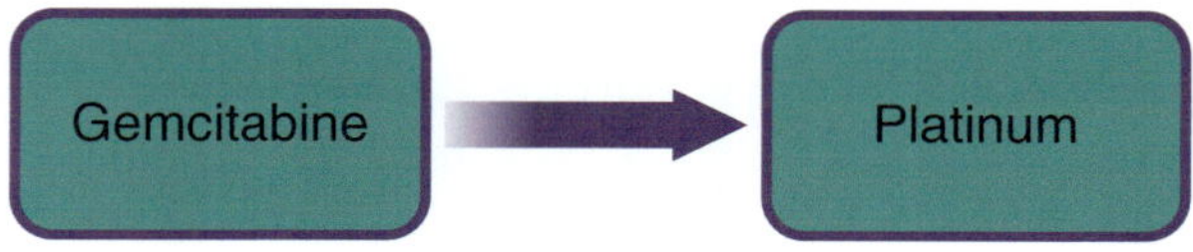

Fig. 8.6 PG protocol infusion sequence

8.3 Pathophysiology of Squamous Cell Carcinoma

Of all head and neck cancers, about 90% are squamous cell carcinomas, being the sixth most incident cancer worldwide, with an estimated increase in incidence for 2030 of 30% [5, 66]. Head and neck squamous cell cancer originates from the mucosal epithelium in the oral cavity, pharynx, and larynx and is associated with several risk factors such as tobacco and alcohol consumption and HPV infections. In Southeast Asia and Australia, the high prevalence of squamous cell carcinoma of the head and neck seems to be associated with the consumption of products containing carcinogens; on the other hand, in the United States and Europe, oropharyngeal infections by HPV are responsible for the high prevalence. As for gender, men are more probability, with a risk two to four times greater than women [5, 67–70].

The development of squamous cell carcinoma (Fig. 8.7) starts with epithelial cell hyperplasia followed by dysplasia (mild, moderate, and severe), then carcinoma in situ, and finally invasive carcinoma [5, 71, 72]. Due to the heterogeneity of squamous cell carcinoma, the cell of origin will depend on the anatomical location and the etiological agent and may also develop from adult stem cells or progenitor cells, giving rise to cancer stem cells with self-renewal and pluripotency [5].

8.3.1 Chemotherapy for the Treatment of Head and Neck Squamous Cell Carcinoma

The treatment of early-stage squamous cell carcinoma of the head and neck may be based on a surgical procedure in cases of tumors in the oral cavity and may be associated with the removal of lymph nodes in the neck. Postoperative radiotherapy may

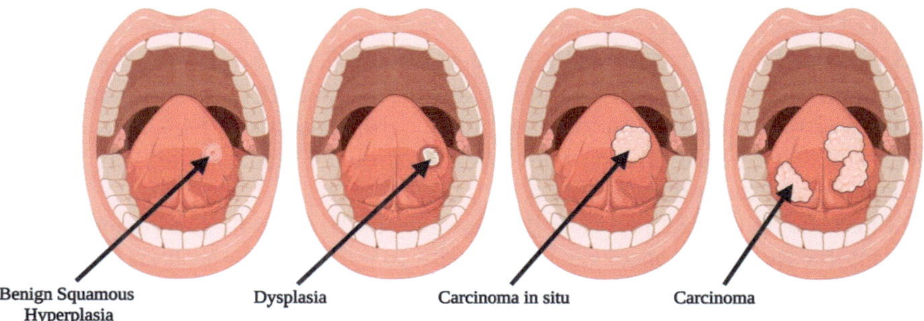

Fig. 8.7 Development of head and neck squamous cell carcinoma. (Source: Created with BioRender.com)

also be indicated in patients with compromised resection margins. Surgery and radiotherapy can also be used in HPV negative oropharyngeal tumors, whereas in HPV positive, radiotherapy with or without chemotherapy is indicated [5, 73, 74].

In patients with advanced squamous cell carcinoma of the oral cavity, surgery may be indicated to remove the lymph nodes followed by radiotherapy with or without chemotherapy. As for oropharyngeal, hypopharyngeal, and laryngeal tumors, the treatment of choice may be radiotherapy associated with chemotherapy. In patients who present distant metastases, multidrug therapy may be indicated [5, 75, 76].

As monotherapy, cisplatin may be indicated in the treatment of locally advanced squamous cell carcinoma and advanced squamous cell carcinoma of the head and neck, carboplatin, and cetuximab in the treatment of locally advanced squamous cell carcinoma of the head and neck associated with radiotherapy [77–79]. Capecitabine or 5-fluorouracil is indicated in the treatment of recurrent or metastatic squamous cells of the head and neck, docetaxel in recurrent or metastatic squamous cell carcinoma, nivolumab as palliative therapy in squamous cell cancer, and pembrolizumab as the first line in squamous cell carcinoma advanced [48, 80–83].

Some protocols used in the treatment of nasopharyngeal carcinomas, such as the FUP protocol (topic 8.2.1.1) and the EP (topic 8.2.1.2), may also be indicated in the treatment of advanced squamous cell carcinoma and recurrent and metastatic squamous cell carcinoma, respectively [48, 56, 84–86]. Other protocols [47–49] used in the treatment of squamous cell carcinoma of the head and neck will be covered in the next topics.

8.3.1.1   DCF Protocol (Docetaxel, Cisplatin, and 5-Fluorouracil)

The combination of docetaxel, cisplatin, and 5-fluorouracil is indicated in the treatment of locally advanced squamous cell carcinoma of the head and neck [87, 88]. Schrijvers et al. [89] performed a phase 1–2 study using the DCF protocol in the treatment of locally advanced non-resectable head and neck cancer. As a result, the authors observed that the protocol promoted a response rate of 64% at level 1 and 78.3% at level 2. The limiting toxicity of the protocol was renal toxicity, nausea, stomatitis, and thrombocytopenia.

In another study, Haddad et al. [90] used the DCF protocol as induction chemotherapy for locally advanced squamous cell carcinoma of the head and neck. The protocol induced an overall response rate of 67%, leading the authors to conclude that the inclusion of docetaxel in the combination of cisplatin and 5-fluorouracil incrementally increased the effectiveness of the combination.

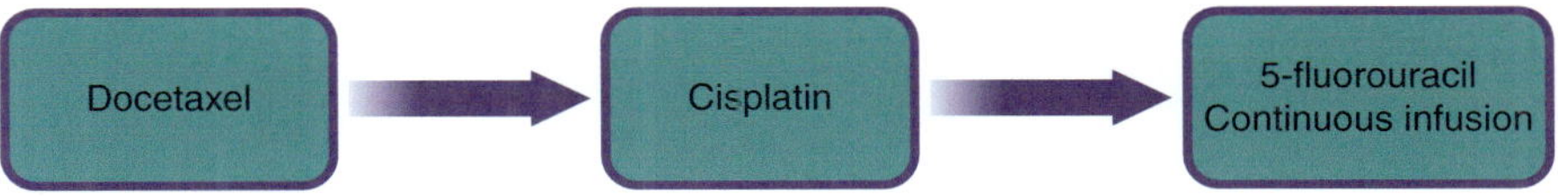

Fig. 8.8 DCF protocol infusion sequence

Komatsu et al. [91] evaluated chemoradiotherapy concomitantly with the DCF protocol in patients with locally advanced squamous cell carcinoma of the head and neck. The regimen promoted an overall response rate of 97.1%, with an overall 3- and 5-year survival rate of 83.3% and 79.2%, respectively. Regarding the infusion sequence of the DCF protocol (Fig. 8.8), it starts with the infusion of docetaxel as it is a specific cycle, followed by cisplatin, and finally the administration of 5-fluorouracil by continuous infusion [92, 93].

8.3.1.2 PC Protocol (Paclitaxel and Carboplatin or Cisplatin)

The PC protocol combines paclitaxel with carboplatin or cisplatin for the treatment of unresectable, locoregionally recurrent, or metastatic head and neck squamous cell carcinoma. The combination of paclitaxel with carboplatin in the treatment of recurrent or metastatic head and neck cancer was studied by Fountzilas et al. [94] who observed the effectiveness of the PC protocol. The overall protocol response rate was 20%, with a toxicity profile that included anemia, leukopenia, thrombocytopenia, vomiting, stomatitis, and infection.

In another study, Fountzilas et al. [95] evaluated the combination with a 3-hour infusion of paclitaxel plus carboplatin in advanced nasopharyngeal carcinoma and other head and neck tumors. The protocol proved to be effective, promoting an overall response rate of 57%, with a toxicity profile similar to the previous study with the development of anemia, leukopenia, thrombocytopenia, stomatitis, nausea/vomiting, and diarrhea.

Pergolizzi et al. [96] evaluated the combination of paclitaxel and cisplatin as induction chemotherapy in the treatment of locoregional advanced squamous cell carcinoma. Induction therapy led to an overall response in 74.4% of the patients studied, with a 3- and 5-year disease progression rate of 33% and 23%, respectively, and overall survival of 24 months.

Langer et al. [97] also evaluated the efficacy of the combination of paclitaxel and cisplatin in recurrent squamous cell carcinoma of the head and neck. The authors obtained as a result a median survival time of 12.1 months and overall survival at 1 and 2 years of 50.2% and 25.9%, respectively. Regarding the infusion sequence, the PC protocol starts with the infusion of paclitaxel as it is a specific cycle followed by the infusion of cisplatin or carboplatin (Fig. 8.9) [98].

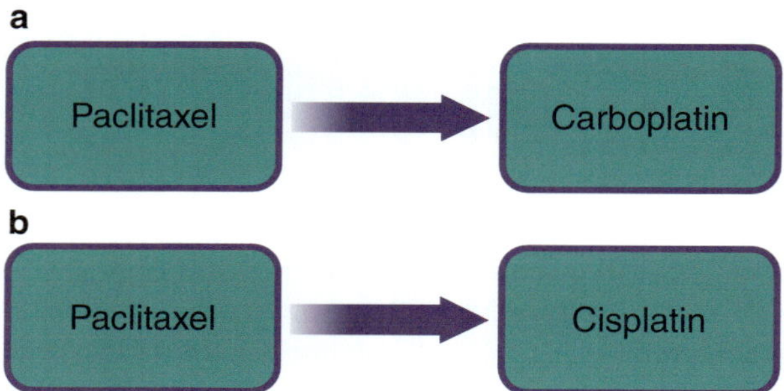

Fig. 8.9 PC protocol infusion sequence combining paclitaxel with carboplatin (**a**) or paclitaxel with cisplatin (**b**)

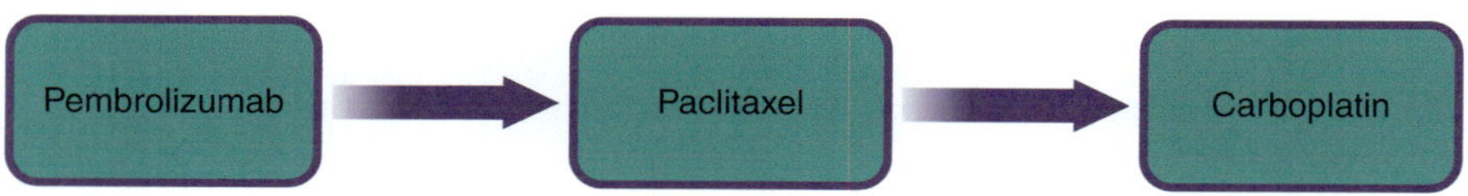

Fig. 8.10 PCP protocol infusion sequence

8.3.1.3   PCP Protocol (Paclitaxel, Carboplatin, and Pembrolizumab)

Pembrolizumab, which is a monoclonal antibody that acts on PD-L1 overexpressing tumors, may be indicated for the first-line treatment of advanced head and neck squamous cell carcinoma combined with paclitaxel and carboplatin [99, 100]. Valadez et al. [101] evaluated the combination of carboplatin, paclitaxel, and pembrolizumab in the first-line treatment of recurrent and/or metastatic squamous cell carcinoma of the head and neck. The authors noted that the combination induced an overall response rate of 78%, proving to be an active protocol for squamous cell carcinoma.

Cabezas-Camarero et al. [102] evaluated the efficacy of the PCP protocol as a second line in oral cavity cancer, in a case report. As a result, the authors observed that the second-line protocol induced a deep and lasting response in oral cavity cancer. As for the infusion sequence of the PCP protocol (Fig. 8.10), starting with the administration of pembrolizumab, only in cases where the patient has presented reactions before the infusion of pembrolizumab is it indicated to start with paclitaxel, after the administration of pembrolizumab followed with the infusion of paclitaxel and finally carboplatin [103].

8.3.1.4   PFP Protocol (Platinum, 5-Fluorouracil, and Pembrolizumab)

Pembrolizumab can also be combined with a platinum compound (carboplatin or cisplatin) and 5-fluorouracil in the first-line treatment of advanced squamous cell carcinoma of the head and neck [104]. Rischin et al. [105] evaluated the efficacy of

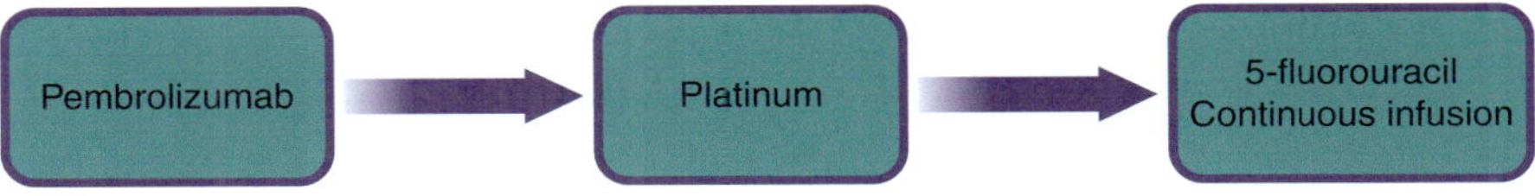

Fig. 8.11 PFP protocol infusion sequence

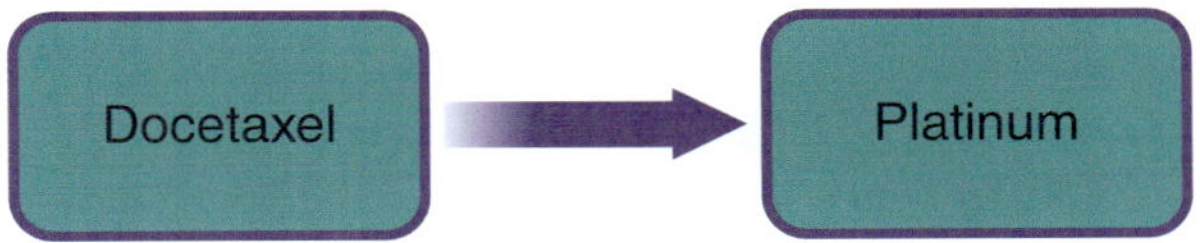

Fig. 8.12 PD protocol infusion sequence

the PFP protocol as a first line in recurrent/metastatic squamous cell carcinoma of the head and neck. The results showed an objective response rate of 42.9% and overall survival of 14.7 months.

Burtness et al. [82] evaluated the efficacy of pembrolizumab alone or in combination with 5-fluorouracil and platinum. The PFP protocol improved overall survival to 13 months compared with the protocol containing cetuximab instead of pembrolizumab, but the inclusion of pembrolizumab did not improve progression-free survival. As for the infusion sequence, the PFP protocol starts with pembrolizumab as it is a target-directed drug followed by platinum (carboplatin or cisplatin) and finally the continuous infusion of 5-fluorouracil (Fig. 8.11) [106].

8.3.1.5 PD Protocol (Platinum and Docetaxel)

The PD protocol combines platinum (carboplatin or cisplatin) and docetaxel in the treatment of recurrent or metastatic squamous cell carcinoma of the head and neck [48, 107]. Kucukzeybek et al. [107] demonstrate the effectiveness of the PD protocol in the treatment of locally advanced or metastatic head and neck cancer. The protocol promoted an overall response rate of 33%, with a disease control rate of 83% and overall survival of 19 months. Hematological toxicity was the most frequent, affecting about 54% of patients.

The combination of docetaxel and cisplatin was evaluated by Gedlicka et al. [108] in the treatment of recurrent and/or metastatic squamous cell carcinoma of the head and neck. As a result, the overall response rate was 52.5%, and the overall survival was 11 months. As for toxicity, myelosuppression was more frequent. Schoffski et al. [109] report the efficacy of the combination of cisplatin and docetaxel in locally advanced, recurrent, or metastatic squamous cell carcinoma of the head and neck, showing an overall response rate of 53.7%. Regarding the infusion sequence, the PD protocol starts with the infusion of docetaxel as it is a specific cycle followed by platinum (carboplatin or cisplatin) (Fig. 8.12) [110].

8.4   Pathophysiology of Salivary Tumors

Salivary tumors (Fig. 8.13) are uncommon, corresponding to about 3–10% of head and neck neoplasms. The incidence rate ranges from 0.4 to 13.5 cases per 100,000 population, most of which are benign salivary gland tumors [111–113]. Mucoepidermoid carcinoma is the most common neoplasm of the salivary gland in adults and children, with 89% in the parotid gland, while 8.4% are tumors in the submandibular gland. Although less common, submandibular gland tumors have a higher frequency of malignancy than that of the parotid gland [114–117].

Mucoepidermoid carcinoma starts from the epithelium of the interlobular and intralobular salivary ducts. Some genetic factors are associated with the development of salivary cancers, the most common being chromosomal translocation, being present in 50–70% of patients with mucoepidermoid carcinoma and more than 50% of patients with adenoid cystic carcinoma tumors [6, 118].

The presence of biological receptors has been identified, such as the epidermal growth factor receptor (EGFR) in 71% of salivary gland cancers and the human epidermal growth factor receptor 2 (HER2) present in cancers derived from the intercalated ducts of the salivary glands, as in adenoid cystic carcinoma. Hormone

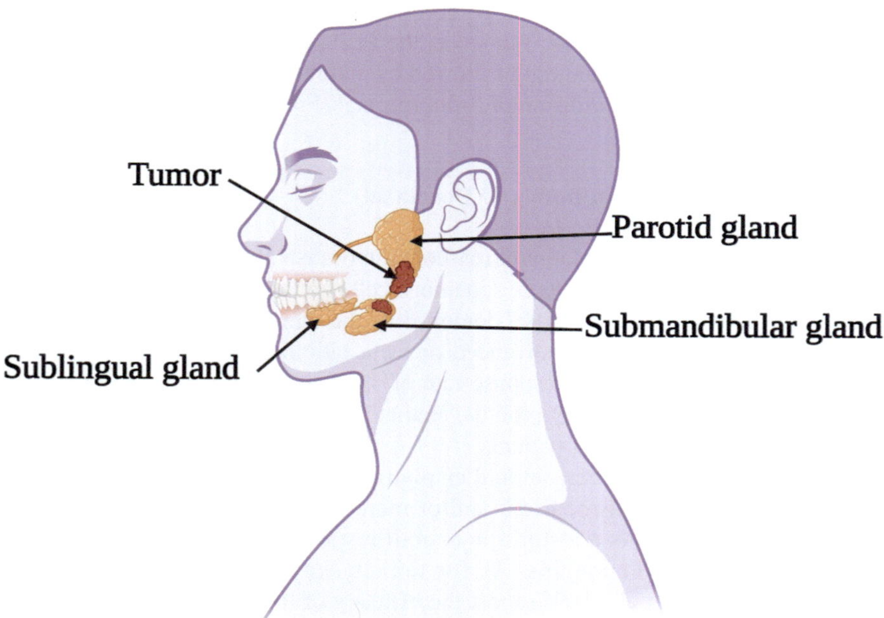

Fig. 8.13 Salivary tumors located in the parotid and submandibular glands. (Source: Created with BioRender.com)

receptors have also been found in benign and malignant salivary gland neoplasms [6, 119, 120].

8.4.1 Chemotherapy for the Treatment of Salivary Tumors

The treatment of benign tumors is performed through a surgical procedure. In the case of malignant tumors of the salivary glands, surgery may be indicated followed by radiotherapy [121–123]. In more advanced cases, when there is the dissemination of the tumor to the lymph nodes, extensive surgery is indicated, with the removal of the salivary gland and adjacent tissues and lymph nodes in the neck, and radiotherapy with or without chemotherapy may be indicated [123–127].

In stage 4 tumors, when distant metastases are present, surgery may be indicated as long as it is possible to remove the tumor, followed by radiotherapy and chemotherapy. In most cases, radiotherapy can be used to reduce the size of the tumor and to relieve pain, bleeding, or other symptoms caused by cancer [124, 127–129].

Hormone therapy may be indicated in the treatment of salivary tumors; an example is tamoxifen, which may be indicated in the treatment of recurrent/metastatic salivary gland cancers of the head and neck [130]. The combination of chemotherapy is also indicated, for example, the FAC protocol, used in the treatment of breast cancer (see Chap. 4), being indicated as palliative therapy for advanced salivary gland cancer, and the FUP protocol, indicated in the treatment of nasopharyngeal cancer (see topic 8.2.1.1), used in the treatment of advanced head and neck cancer [131–133]. Other protocols will be covered in the following topics [47–49].

8.4.1.1 VNC Protocol (Vinorelbine and Cisplatin)

The VNC protocol combines vinorelbine and cisplatin in the treatment of advanced salivary gland cancers. Airoldi et al. [134] performed a phase 2 study comparing vinorelbine as monotherapy and combined with cisplatin in the treatment of patients with recurrent salivary gland neoplasia. The combination of vinorelbine and cisplatin proved to be more effective than vinorelbine alone.

Hong et al. [135] evaluated the efficacy and safety of vinorelbine combined with cisplatin in the treatment of recurrent and/or metastatic head and neck salivary gland cancer. The protocol promoted an objective response rate of 35%, progression-free survival of 6.3 months, and overall survival of 16.9 months. As for the infusion sequence of the VNC protocol, according to Ho [136], the infusion can be in any sequence, in which Levêque et al. [137] report that the observed activity of the drug combination appears not to be related to pharmacokinetic interactions. Perhaps starting the protocol with vinorelbine is interesting because of its vesicant action, followed by infusion of cisplatin (Fig. 8.14) [138].

Fig. 8.14 VNC protocol infusion sequence

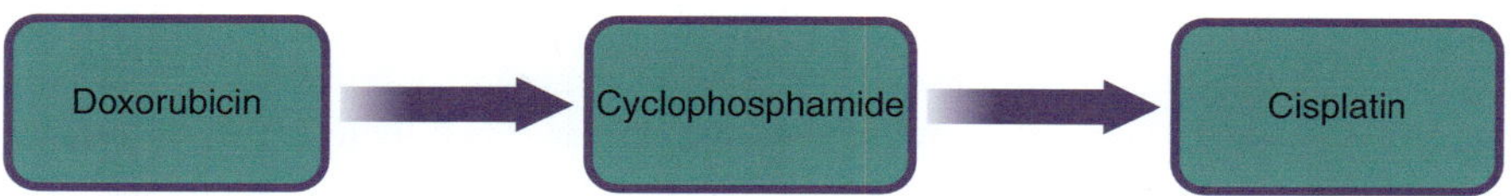

Fig. 8.15 Infusion sequence of the PAC protocol

8.4.1.2   PAC Protocol (Cisplatin, Doxorubicin, and Cyclophosphamide)

The combination of a platinum compound (carboplatin or cisplatin), doxorubicin, and cyclophosphamide has been indicated for the treatment of advanced salivary gland cancer. Alberts et al. [139] evaluated the efficacy of the combination of doxorubicin, cisplatin, and cyclophosphamide in the treatment of advanced parotid gland carcinoma. The authors observed that the protocol promoted complete remission in 40% of patients and partial remission in 60%, proving to be a well-tolerated protocol.

In a phase 2 study, Licitra et al. [140] evaluated the protocol's efficacy in the treatment of advanced salivary gland carcinoma, showing that the protocol promoted a partial response in 27% of patients, with a response duration ranging from 3 to 13 months and a mean survival time of 21 months. Regarding the infusion sequence of the PAC protocol (Fig. 8.15), it starts with the infusion of doxorubicin, which is a vesicant, followed by cyclophosphamide and finally by cisplatin [140].

References

1. Campana IG, Goiato MC. Tumores de cabeça e pescoço: epidemiologia, fatores de risco, diagnóstico e tratamento. Revista Odontológica de Araçatuba. 2013;34(1):20–6.
2. WHO – World Health Organization. Estimated number of incident cases from 2018 to 2040. International Agency for Research on Cancer. 2020. Available in: https://gco.iarc.fr/tomorrow/graphic-isotype?type=0&type_sex=0&mode=population&sex=0&populations=900&cancers=36&age_group=value&apc_male=0&apc_female=0&single_unit=100000&print=0. Accessed 2 Oct 2021.
3. Silva FA, Roussenq SC, Tavares MGS, Souza CPF, Mozzini CB, Benetti M, Dias M. Epidemiological profile of patients with head and neck cancer at a cancer center in Southern Brazil. Revista Brasileira de Cancerologia. 2020;66(1):e-08455. https://doi.org/10.32635/2176-9745.RBC.2020v66n1.455.
4. Vigneswaran N, Williams MD. Epidemiological trends in head and neck cancer and Aids in diagnosis. Oral Maxillofac Surg Clin North Am. 2014;26(2):123–41. https://doi.org/10.1016/j.coms.2014.01.001.

5. Johnson DE, Burtness B, Leemans CR, Lui VWY, Bauman JE, Grandis JR. Head and neck squamous cell carcinoma. Nat Rev Dis Primers. 2020;6:92. https://doi.org/10.1038/s41572-020-00224-3.

6. Young A, Okuyemi OT. Malignant salivary gland tumors. Treasure Island: StatPearls Publishing; 2020.

7. NIH – National Cancer Institute. Head and neck cancers. National Cancer Institute at the National Institutes of Health; 2021.

8. Mody MD, Rocco JW, Yom SS, Haddad RI, Saba NF. Head and neck cancer. Lancet. 2021;398(10318):2289–99. https://doi.org/10.1016/S0140-6736(21)01550-6.

9. Arslan N, Tuzuner A, Koycu A, Dursun S, Hucumenoglu S. The role of nasopharyngeal examination and biopsy in the diagnosis of malignant diseases. Braz J Otorhinolaryngol. 2019;85(4):481–5. https://doi.org/10.1016/j.bjorl.2018.04.006.

10. Thompson LDR. Update on nasopharyngeal carcinoma. Head Neck Pathol. 2007;1(1):81–6. https://doi.org/10.1007/s12105-007-0012-7.

11. Yamashiro I, Souza RP. Imaging diagnosis of nasopharyngeal tumors. Radiol Bras. 2007;40(1):45–52. https://doi.org/10.1590/S0100-39842007000100011.

12. Chou J, Lin YC, Kim J, You L, Xu Z, He B, Jablons DM. Nasopharyngeal carcinoma-review of the molecular mechanisms of tumorigenesis. Head Neck. 2008;30(7):946–63. https://doi.org/10.1002/hed.20833.

13. Ou SHI, Zell JA, Ziogas A, Anton-Culver H. Epidemiology of nasopharyngeal carcinoma in the United States: improved survival of Chinese patients within the keratinizing squamous cell carcinoma histology. Ann Oncol. 2007;18(1):29–35. https://doi.org/10.1093/annonc/mdl320.

14. He JQ, Sun L, He J, Zhu C, Li P, Lei J, He Q, Mackey V, Lin Z, Cheng P, Coy DH. The pathogenesis and therapeutics of nasopharyngeal carcinoma. Health Sci J. 2019;13(2):642. https://doi.org/10.36648/1791-809X.1000642.

15. Pontoriero F, Silverman AM, Pascasio JM, Bajaj R. Nonkeratinizing nasopharyngeal carcinoma, undifferentiated type with trisomy 2: a case report and short review of cytogenetic and molecular literature. Pediatr Dev Pathol. 2020;23(6):448–52. https://doi.org/10.1177/1093526620945861.

16. Pathmanathan R, Prasad U, Chandrika G, Sadler R, Flynn K, Raab-Traub N. Undifferentiated, nonkeratinizing, and squamous cell carcinoma of the nasopharynx. Variants of Epstein-Barr virus-infected neoplasia. Am J Pathol. 1995;146(6):1355–67.

17. Yong SK, Ha TC, Yeo MCR, Gaborieau V, McKay JD, Wee J. Associations of lifestyle and diet with the risk of nasopharyngeal carcinoma in Singapore: a case–control study. Chin J Cancer. 2017;36:3. https://doi.org/10.1186/s40880-016-0174-3.

18. Okekpa SI, Mydin RBSMN, Mangantig E, Azmi NSA, Zahari SNS, Kaur G, Musa Y. Nasopharyngeal carcinoma (NPC) risk factors: a systematic review and meta-analysis of the association with lifestyle, diets, socioeconomic and sociodemographic in Asian region. Asian Pac J Cancer Prev. 2019;20(11):3505–14. https://doi.org/10.31557/APJCP.2019.20.11.3505.

19. Salano VE, Mwakigonja AR, Abdulshakcor A, Kahinga AA, Richard EM. Epstein-Barr vírus latente membrane protein-1 expression in nasopharyngeal carcinoma. JCO Global Oncol. 2021;7:1406–12. https://doi.org/10.1200/GO.21.00120.

20. Hsu WM, Wang AG. Nasopharyngeal carcinoma with orbital invasion. Eye. 2004;18:833–8. https://doi.org/10.1038/sj.eye.6701358.

21. Vogel DWT, Zbaeren P, Thoeny HC. Cancer of the oral cavity and oropharynx. Cancer Imaging. 2010;10(1):62–72. https://doi.org/10.1102/1470-7330.2010.0008.

22. Razek AAKA, King A. MRI and CT of nasopharyngeal carcinoma. Am J Roentgenol. 2012;198:11–8. https://doi.org/10.2214/AJR.11.6954.

23. OuYang PY, Xiao Y, You KY, Zhang LN, Lan XW, Zhang XM, Xie FY. Validation and comparison of the 7th and 8th edition of AJCC staging systems for non-metastatic nasopharyngeal carcinoma, and proposed staging systems from Hong Kong, Guangzhou, and Guangxi. Oral Oncol. 2017;72:65–72. https://doi.org/10.1016/j.oraloncology.2017.07.011.

24. Chen QY, Wen YF, Guo L, Liu H, Huang PY, Mo HY, Li NW, Xiang YQ, Luo DH, Qiu F, Sun R, Deng MQ, Chen MY, Hua YJ, Guo X, Cao KJ, Hong MH, Qian CN, Mai HQ. Concurrent chemoradiotherapy vs radiotherapy alone in stage II nasopharyngeal carcinoma: phase III randomized trial. JNCI: J Nat Cancer Inst. 2011;103(23):1761–70. https://doi.org/10.1093/jnci/djr432.

25. Chen YP, Ismaila N, Chua MLK, Colevas AD, Haddad R, Huang SH, Wee JTS, Whitley AC, Yi JL, Yom SS, Chan ATC, Hu CS, Lang JY, Le QT, Lee AWM, Lee N, Lin JC, Ma B, Morgan TJ, Shah J, Sun Y, Ma J. Chemotherapy in combination with radiotherapy for definitive-intent treatment of stage II-IVA nasopharyngeal carcinoma: CSCO and ASCO guideline. J Clin Oncol. 2021;39(7):840–59. https://doi.org/10.1200/JCO.20.03237.

26. Zheng Y, Han F, Xiao W, Xiang Y, Lu L, Deng X, Cui N, Zhao C. Analysis of late toxicity in nasopharyngeal carcinoma patients treated with intensity modulated radiation therapy. Radiat Oncol. 2015;10:17. https://doi.org/10.1186/s13014-014-0326-z.

27. Simo R, Robinson M, Lei M, Sibtain A, Hickey S. Nasopharyngeal carcinoma: United Kingdom national multidisciplinary guidelines. J Laryngol Otol. 2016;130(Suppl 2):S97–S103. https://doi.org/10.1017/S0022215116000517.

28. Yeh SA. Radiotherapy for head and neck cancer. Semin Plast Surg. 2010;24(2):127–36. https://doi.org/10.1055/s-0030-1255330.

29. Zhang Y, Li WF, Chen L, Mao YP, Guo R, Zhang F, Peng H, Liu LZ, Li L, Liu Q, Ma J. Prognostic value of parotid lymph node metastasis in patients with nasopharyngeal carcinoma receiving intensity-modulated radiotherapy. Sci Rep. 2015;5:13919. https://doi.org/10.1038/srep13919.

30. Chua GWY, Chua ET. Long-term disease-free survival of a patient with oligometastatic nasopharyngeal carcinoma treated with radiotherapy alone. Case Rep Oncol. 2018;11:392–8. https://doi.org/10.1159/000490236.

31. Weng JJ, Wei JZ, Li M, Zhang SJ, Wei YZ, Wang HW, Qin DX, Lu JL, Jiang H, Qu SH. Effects of surgery combined with chemoradiotherapy on short- and long-term outcomes of early-stage nasopharyngeal carcinoma. Cancer Manag Res. 2020;12:7813–26. https://doi.org/10.2147/CMAR.S262567.

32. You R, Liu YP, Huang PY, Zou X, Sun R, He YX, Wu YS, Shen GP, Zhang HD, Duan CY, Tan SH, Cao JY, Li JB, Xie YL, Zhang YN, Wang ZQ, Yang Q, Lin M, Jiang R, Zhang MX, Hua J, Tang LQ, Zhuang AH, Chen QY, Guo L, Mo HY, Chen Y, Mai HQ, Ling L, Liu Q, Chua MLK, Chen MY. Efficacy and safety of locoregional radiotherapy with chemotherapy vs chemotherapy alone in de novo metastatic nasopharyngeal carcinoma: a multicenter phase 3 randomized clinical trial. JAMA Oncol. 2020;6(9):1345–52. https://doi.org/10.1001/jamaoncol.2020.1808.

33. Chua D, Wei WI, Sham JST, Au GKH. Capecitabine monotherapy for recurrent and metastatic nasopharyngeal cancer. Jpn J Clin Oncol. 2008;38(4):244–9. https://doi.org/10.1093/jjco/hyn022.

34. Prawira A, Oosting SF, Chen TW, delos Santos KA, Saluja R, Wang L, Siu LL, Chan KKW, Hansen AR. Systemic therapies for recurrent or metastatic nasopharyngeal carcinoma: a systematic review. Br J Cancer. 2017;117:1743–52. https://doi.org/10.1038/bjc.2017.357.

35. Foo KF, Tan EH, Leong SS, Wee JTS, Tan T, Fong KW, Koh L, Tai BC, Lian LG, Machin D. Gemcitabine in metastatic nasopharyngeal carcinoma of the undifferentiated type. Ann Oncol. 2002;13(1):150–6. https://doi.org/10.1093/annonc/mdf002.

36. Zhang L, Zhang Y, Huang PY, Xu F, Peng PJ, Guan ZZ. Phase II clinical study of gemcitabine in the treatment of patients with advanced nasopharyngeal carcinoma after the failure of platinum-based chemotherapy. Cancer Chemother Pharmacol. 2008;61(1):33–8. https://doi.org/10.1007/s00280-007-0441-8.

37. Tan WL, Tan EH, Lim DWT, Ng QS, Tan DSW, Jain A, Ang MK. Advances in systemic treatment for nasopharyngeal carcinoma. Chin Clin Oncol. 2016;5(2):21. https://doi.org/10.21037/cco.2016.03.03.

38. Patil VM, Joshi A, Noronha V, Talreja V, Simha V, Dhumal S, Bandekar B, Chandrasekharan A, Prabhash K. Palliative chemotherapy in carcinoma nasopharynx. South Asian J Cancer. 2019;8(3):173–7. https://doi.org/10.4103/sajc.sajc_230_18.

39. Marcu L, van Doorn T, Olver I. Cisplatin and radiotherapy in the treatment of locally advanced head and neck cancer. Acta Oncol. 2003;42(4):315–25. https://doi.org/10.1080/02841860310004364.

40. Hui EP, Ma BB, Leung SF, King AD, Mo F, Kam MK, Yu BK, Chiu SK, Kwan WH, Ho R, Chan I, Ahuja AT, Zee BC, Chan AT. Randomized phase II trial of concurrent cisplatin-radiotherapy with or without neoadjuvant docetaxel and cisplatin in advanced nasopharyngeal carcinoma. J Clin Oncol. 2009;27(2):242–9. https://doi.org/10.1200/JCO.2008.18.1545.

41. Jamshed A, Hussain R, Iqbal H. Gemcitabine and cisplatin followed by chemo-radiation for advanced nasopharyngeal carcinoma. Asian Pac J Cancer Prev. 2014;15(2):899–904. https://doi.org/10.7314/apjcp.2014.15.2.899.

42. NCT01872962. Induction gemcitabine and cisplatin in patients with locoregionally advanced nasopharyngeal carcinoma. Clinical Trials. 2018. Available in: https://clinicaltrials.gov/ct2/show/NCT01872962. Accessed 3 Oct 2021.

43. Zhang Y, Chen L, Hu GQ, Zhang N, Zhu XD, Yang KY, Jin F, Shi M, Chen YP, Hu WH, Cheng ZB, Wang SY, Tian Y, Wang XC, Sun Y, Li JG, Li WF, Li YH, Tang LL, Mao YP, Zhou GQ, Sun R, Liu X, Guo R, Long GX, Liang SQ, Li L, Huang J, Long JH, Zang J, Liu QD, Zou L, Su QF, Zheng BM, Xiao Y, Guo Y, Han F, Mo HY, Lv JW, Du XJ, Xu C, Liu N, Li YQ, Chua MLK, Xie FY, Sun Y, Ma J. Gemcitabine and cisplatin induction chemotherapy in nasopharyngeal carcinoma. N Engl J Med. 2019;381(12):1124–35. https://doi.org/10.1056/NEJMoa1905287.

44. Yeo W, Leung TW, Chan AT, Chiu SK, Yu P, Mok TS, Johnson PJ. A phase II study of combination paclitaxel and carboplatin in advanced nasopharyngeal carcinoma. Eur J Cancer. 1998;34(13):2027–31. https://doi.org/10.1016/s0959-8049(98)00280-9.

45. NCT00003206. Carboplatin and paclitaxel in treating patients with locally recurrent or metastatic nasopharyngeal cancer. Clinical Trials. 2013. Available in: https://clinicaltrials.gov/ct2/show/NCT00003206. Accessed 3 Oct 2021.

46. Zhang L, Huang Y, Yang Y, Ma S, Lin X, Lin L, Zhou T, Deng Y, Zhang C, Ding X, Wang S, Wang R, Feng G, Chen Y, Xu R. First-line paclitaxel plus carboplatin with/without bevacizumab in recurrent or metastatic nasopharyngeal carcinoma: a multicenter, randomized, open-label, phase II trial. Ann Oncol. 2017;28(Suppl 5):376–7. https://doi.org/10.1093/annonc/mdx374.009.

47. Kuehr T, Thaler J, Woell E. Chemotherapy protocols 2017: current protocols and "Targeted therapies". Klinikum Wels-Grieskirchen and Caritas Christi URGET NOS. Austria. 2017. www.chemoprotocols.eu.

48. BC Cancer. Supportive care protocols. BC Cancer. British Columbia. 2021. Available in: http://www.bccancer.bc.ca/health-professionals/clinical-resources/chemotherapy-protocols/supportive-care. Accessed 2 July 2021.

49. NHS. Chemotherapy protocols. NHS. University Hospital Southampton. NHS Foundation Trust. England. 2021. Available in: https://www.uhs.nhs.uk/HealthProfessionals/Chemotherapy-protocols/Chemotherapy-protocols.aspx. Accessed 2 July 2021.

50. Ho C. BC cancer protocol summary for advanced nasopharyngeal cancer of the head and neck using platinum and fluorouracil. BC Cancer. British Columbia. 2021. Available in: http://www.bccancer.bc.ca/chemotherapy-protocols-site/Documents/Head%20and%20Neck/HNNAVFUP_Protocol.pdf. Accessed 3 Oct 2021.

51. Au E, Ang PT. A phase II trial of 5-fluorouracil and cisplatinum in recurrent or metastatic nasopharyngeal carcinoma. Ann Oncol. 1994;5:87–9.

52. Jin T, Qin WF, Jiang F, Jin QF, Wei QC, Jia YS, Sun XN, Li WF, Chen XZ. Cisplatin and fluorouracil induction chemotherapy with or without docetaxel in locoregionally advanced nasopharyngeal carcinoma. Transl Oncol. 2019;12(4):633–9. https://doi.org/10.1016/j.tranon.2019.01.002.

53. NHS. Chemotherapy protocols. Head and neck cancer. Cisplatin-fluorouracil. NHS. University Hospital Southampton. NHS Foundation Trust. England. 2020. Available in: https://www.uhs.nhs.uk/Media/SUHTExtranet/Services/Chemotherapy-SOPs/Headandneckcancer/Cisplatin-Fluorouracil.pdf. Accessed 3 Oct 2021.

54. Kua VF, Ismail F, Phua VCE, Aslan NM. Carboplatin/5-fluorouracil as an alternative to cisplatin/5-fluorouracil for metastatic and recurrent head and neck squamous cell carcinoma and nasopharyngeal carcinoma. Asian Pac J Cancer Prev. 2013;14(2):1121–6. https://doi.org/10.7314/APJCP.2013.14.2.1121.

55. Dechaphunkul T, Pruegsanusak K, Sangthawan D, Sunpaweravong P. Concurrent chemoradiotherapy with carboplatin followed by carboplatin and 5-fluorouracil in locally advanced nasopharyngeal carcinoma. Head Neck Oncol. 2011;3:30. https://doi.org/10.1186/1758-3284-3-30.

56. Hanemaaijer SH, Kok IC, Fehrmann RSN, van der Vegt B, Gietema JA, Plaat BEC, van Vugt MATM, Vergeer MR, Leemans CR, Langendijk JA, Voortman J, Buter J, Oosting SF. Comparison of carboplatin with 5-fluorouracil vs. cisplatin as concomitant chemoradiotherapy for locally advanced head and neck squamous cell carcinoma. Front Oncol. 2020;10:761. https://doi.org/10.3389/fonc.2020.00761.

57. Ho C. BC cancer protocol summary for treatment of recurrent and/or metastatic nasopharyngeal cancer with platinum and etoposide. BC Cancer. British Columbia. 2021. Available in: http://www.bccancer.bc.ca/chemotherapy-protocols-site/Documents/Head%20and%20Neck/HNNAVPE_Protocol.pdf. Accessed 11 Oct 2021.

58. Osoba D, Band PR, Goldine JH, Connors JM, Gelmon K, Knowling MA, Fetherstonhaugh EM. Efficacy of weekly cisplatin-based chemotherapy in recurrent and metastatic head and neck cancer. Ann Oncol. 1992;3(Suppl 3):S57–62. https://doi.org/10.1093/annonc/3.suppl_3.S57.

59. Chi KH, Chang YC, Chan WK, Liu JM, Law CK, Lo SS, Shu CH, Yen SH, Whang-Peng J, Chen KY. A phase II study of carboplatin in nasopharyngeal carcinoma. Oncology. 1997;54(3):203–7. https://doi.org/10.1159/000227689.

60. Ho C. BC cancer protocol summary for treatment of locoregionally recurrent and/or metastatic nasopharyngeal cancer with platinum and gemcitabine. BC Cancer. British Columbia. 2021. Available in: http://www.bccancer.bc.ca/chemotherapy-protocols-site/Documents/Head%20and%20Neck/HNNAVPG_Protocol.pdf. Accessed 11 Oct 2021.

61. Ngan RKC, Yiu HHY, Lau WH, Yau S, Cheung FY, Chan TM, Kwok CH, Chiu CY, Au SK, Foo W, Law CK, Tse KC. Combination gemcitabine and cisplatin chemotherapy for metastatic or recurrent nasopharyngeal carcinoma: report of a phase II study. Ann Oncol. 2002;13:1252–8. https://doi.org/10.1093/annonc/mdf200.

62. Hsieh JCH, Hsu CL, Ng SH, Wang CH, Lee KD, Lu CH, Chang YF, Hsieh RK, Yeh KH, Hsiao CH, Chen SY, Shiau CY, Wang HM. Gemcitabine plus cisplatin for patients with recurrent or metastatic nasopharyngeal carcinoma in Taiwan: a multicenter prospective phase II trial. Jpn J Clin Oncol. 2015;45(9):819–27. https://doi.org/10.1093/jjco/hyv083.

63. Beldjilali Y, Yamouni M, Benhadji KA, Khellafi H, Abdelaoui A, Betkaoui F, Kaid A, Daim FZ, Benchlef L, Djellali L. Combination of gemcitabine and carboplatin chemotherapy for recurrent nasopharyngeal carcinoma. J Clin Oncol. 2010;28(15_suppl) https://doi.org/10.1200/jco.2010.28.15_suppl.e16006.

64. Lim AM, Corry J, Collins M, Peters L, Hicks RJ, D'Costa L, Coleman A, Chua M, Solomon B, Rischin D. A phase II study of induction carboplatin and gemcitabine followed by chemoradiotherapy for the treatment of locally advanced nasopharyngeal carcinoma. Oral Oncol. 2013;49(5):468–74. https://doi.org/10.1016/j.oraloncology.2012.12.012.

65. Chen C, Zhang X, Zhou Y, Fu S, Lin Z, Hong S, Zhang L. Treatment of recurrent or metastatic nasopharyngeal carcinoma by targeting the epidermal growth factor receptor combined with gemcitabine plus platinum. Cancer Manag Res. 2020;12:10353–60. https://doi.org/10.2147/CMAR.S275947.

66. Alvarenga LM, Ruiz MT, Pavarino-Bertelli EC, Ruback MJC, Maniglia JV, Goloni-Bertollo M. Epidemiologic evaluation of head and neck patients in a university hospital of Northwestern São Paulo state. Rev Bras Otorrinolaringol. 2008;74(1):68–73. https://doi.org/10.1590/S0034-72992008000100011.

67. Scheidt JHG, Yurgel LS, Cherubini K, Figueiredo MAS, Salum FG. Characteristics of oral squamous cell carcinoma in users or non users of tobacco and alcohol. Revista Odonto Ciência. 2012;27(1):69–73. https://doi.org/10.1590/S1980-65232012000100013.

68. Betiol J, Villa LL, Sichero L. Impacto f HPV infection on the development of head and neck cancer. Braz J Med Biol Res. 2013;46(3):217–26. https://doi.org/10.1590/1414-431X20132703.

69. Woods RSR, O'Regan EM, Kennedy S. Martin C, O'Leary JJ, Timon C. Role of human papillomavirus in oropharyngeal squamous cell carcinoma: a review. World J Clin Cases. 2014;2(6):172–93. https://doi.org/10.12998/wjcc.v2.i6.172.

70. Canning M, Guo G, Yu M, Myint C, Groves MW, Byrd JK, Cui Y. Heterogeneity of the head and neck squamous cell carcinoma immune landscape and its impact on immunotherapy. Front Cell Develop Biol. 2019;7:52. https://doi.org/10.3389/fcell.2019.00052.

71. Lumerman H, Freedman P, Kerpel S. Oral epithelial dysplasia and the development of invasive squamous cell carcinoma. Oral Surg Oral Med Oral Pathol Oral Radiol. 1995;79(3):321–9. https://doi.org/10.1016/s1079-2104(05)80226-4.

72. Reibel J. Prognosis of oral pre-malignant lesions: significance of clinical, histopathological, and molecular biological characteristics. Crit Rev Oral Biol Med. 2003;14(1):47–32. https://doi.org/10.1177/154411130301400105.

73. d'Alessandro AF, Pinto FR, Lin CS, Kulcsar MAV, Cernea CR, Brandão LG, Matos LL. Oral cavity squamous cell carcinoma: factors related to occult lymph node metastasis. Braz J Otorhinolaryngol. 2015;81(3):248–54. https://doi.org/10.1016/j.bjorl.2015.03.004.

74. Parvathaneni U, Lavertu P, Gibson MK, Glastonbury CM. Advances in diagnosis and multidisciplinary management of oropharyngeal squamous cell carcinoma: state of the art. Radiographics. 2019;39(7):2055–68. https://doi.org/10.1148/rg.2019190007.

75. Chedid HM, Lehn CN, Rapoport A, Amar A, Franzi SA. Assessment of disease-free survival in patients with laryngeal squamous cell carcinoma treated with radiotherapy associated or not with chemotherapy. Braz J Otorhinolaryngol. 2010;76(2):225–30. https://doi.org/10.1590/S1808-86942010000200013.

76. Ionna F, Bossi P, Guida A, Alberti A, Muto P, Salzano G, Ottaiano A, Maglitto F, Leopardo D, Felice MD, Longo F, Tafuto S, Scarpati GDV, Perri F. Recurrent/metastatic squamous cell carcinoma of the head and neck: a big and intriguing challenge which may be resolved by integrated treatments combining locoregional and systemic therapies. Cancers. 2021;13(10):2371. https://doi.org/10.3390/cancers13102371.

77. Griffin S, Walker S, Sculpher M, White S, Erhorn S, Brent S, Dyker A, Ferrie L, Gilfillan C, Horsley W, Macfarlane K, Thomas S. Cetuximab plus radiotherapy for the treatment of locally advanced squamous cell carcinoma of the head and neck. Health Technol Assess. 2009;13(Suppl 1):49–54. https://doi.org/10.3310/hta13suppl1/08.

78. Sautois B, Schroeder H, Martin M, Piret P, Demez P, Bouchain O, Mutijima E, Moreau P. Weekly cisplatin with radiotherapy for locally advanced head and neck squamous cell carcinoma. J BUON. 2016;21(4):979–88.

79. Hamauchi S, Yokota T, Mizumachi T, Onozawa Y, Ogawa H, Onoe T, Kamijo T, Iida Y, Nishimura T, Onitsuka T, Yasui H, Homma A. Safety and efficacy of concurrent carboplatin or cetuximab plus radiotherapy for locally advanced head and neck cancer patients ineligible for treatment with cisplatin. Int J Clin Oncol. 2019;24(5):468–75. https://doi.org/10.1007/s10147-018-01392-9.

80. Martinez-Trufero J, Isla D, Adansa JC, Irigoyen A, Hitt R, Gil-Arnaiz I, Lambea J, Lecumberri MJ, Cruz JJ. Phase II study of capecitabine as palliative treatment for patients with recurrent and metastatic squamous head and neck cancer after previous platinum-based treatment. Br J Cancer. 2010;102:1687–91. https://doi.org/10.1038/sj.bjc.6605697.

81. Specenier P, Rasschaert M, Vroman P, den Brande JV, Dyck J, Schrijvers D, Huizing MT, Vermorken JB. Weekly docetaxel in patients with recurrent and/or metastatic squamous cell carcinoma of the head and neck. Am J Clin Oncol. 2011;34(5):472–7. https://doi.org/10.1097/COC.0b013e3181ec5f16.

82. Burtness B, Harrington KJ, Greil R, Soulières D, Tahara M, Castro G Jr, Psyrri A, Basté N, Neupane P, Bratland A, Fuereder T, Hughes BGM, Mesía R, Ngamphaiboon N, Rordorf T, Ishak WZW, Hong RL, Mendoza RG, Roy A, Zhang Y, Gumuscu B, Cheng JD, Jin F, Rischin D. Pembrolizumab alone or with chemotherapy versus cetuximab with chemotherapy for recurrent or metastatic squamous cell carcinoma of the head and neck (KEYNOTE-048):

a randomised, open-label, phase 3 study. Lancet. 2019;394(10212):1915–28. https://doi. org/10.1016/S0140-6736(19)32591-7.

83. Vasiliadou I, Breik O, Baker H, Leslie I, Sim VR, Hegarty G, Michaelidou A, Nathan K, Hartley A, Good J, Sanghera P, Fong C, Urbano TG, Lei M, Petkar I, Ferreira MR, Nutting C, Wong KH, Newbold K, Harrington K, Bhide S, Kong A. Safety and treatment outcomes of nivolumab for the treatment of recurrent or metastatic head and neck squamous cell carcinoma: retrospective multicenter cohort study. Cancers (Basel). 2021;13(6):1413. https://doi. org/10.3390/cancers13061413.

84. Junor E, Canney P, Yosef H. Carboplatin and 5-fluorouracil in advanced and recurrent squamous carcinoma of the head and neck. Clin Oncol. 1993;5(1):43–5. https://doi.org/10.1016/ S0936-6555(05)80697-1.

85. Hatton MQF, Junor EJ, Paul J, Canney PA, Yosef H, Robertson AG, McGurk FM, Symonds RP. Carboplatin, 5-fluorouracil and folinic acid: a 48-hour chemotherapy regimen in advanced and recurrent squamous carcinoma of the head and neck. Clin Oncol. 1996;8(6):380–3. https://doi.org/10.1016/S0936-6555(96)80085-9.

86. Krengli M, Masini L, Gambaro G, Turri L, Loi G, Aluffi P, Pia F. Concurrent chemotherapy with carboplatin + 5-fluorouracil and radiotherapy in advanced squamous cell head and neck carcinoma: a retrospective single institution's study. Tumori. 2001;87(5):312–6.

87. NCT00139269. Study of docetaxel in combination with cisplatin and 5-fluorouracil in locally advanced squamous cell carcinoma of the head and neck. Clinical Trials. 2008. Available in: https://clinicaltrials.gov/ct2/show/NCT00139269. Accessed 11 Oct 2021.

88. NCT00273546. Induction chemotherapy comparing Taxotere® cisplatin and 5-fluorouracil (TPF) with standard cisplatin and 5-fluorouracil (PF) followed by chemoradiation in locally advanced head and neck cancer. Clinical Trials. 2009. Available in: https://clinicaltrials.gov/ ct2/show/NCT00273546. Accessed 11 Oct 2021.

89. Schrijvers D, Van Herpen C, Kerger J, Joosens E, Van Laer C, Awada A, Van den Weyngaert D, Nguyen H, Le Bouder C, Castelijns JA, Kaanders J, De Mulder P, Vermorken JB. Docetaxel, cisplatin and 5-fluorouracil in patients with locally advanced unresectable head and neck cancer: a phase I–II feasibility study. Ann Oncol. 2004;15(4):638–45. https://doi.org/10.1093/ annonc/mdh145.

90. Haddad R, Colevas AD, Tishler R, Busse P, Goguen L, Sullivan C, Norris CM, Lake-Willcutt B, Case MA, Costello R, Posner M. Docetaxel, cisplatin, and 5-fluorouracil-based induction chemotherapy in patients with locally advanced squamous cell carcinoma of the head and neck: the Dana Farber cancer institute experience. Cancer. 2003;97(2):412–8. https://doi. org/10.1002/cncr.11063.

91. Komatsu M, Shiono O, Taguchi T, Sakuma Y, Nishimura G, Sano D, Sakuma N, Yabuki K, Arai Y, Takahashi M, Isitoya J, Oridate N. Concurrent chemoradiotherapy with docetaxel, cisplatin and 5-fluorouracil (TPF) in patients with locally advanced squamous cell carcinoma of the head and neck. Jpn J Clin Oncol. 2014;44(5):416–21. https://doi.org/10.1093/ jjco/hyu026.

92. NHS. Chemotherapy protocols. Head and neck cancer. Cisplatin (75)-docetaxel(75)-fluorouracil(4000). NHS. University Hospital Southampton. NHS Foundation Trust. England. 2020. Available in: https://www.uhs.nhs.uk/Media/SUHTExtranet/Services/Chemotherapy-SOPs/Headandneckcancer/Cisplatin-(75)-Docetaxel(75)-Fluorouracil(4000).pdf. Access 11 Oct 2021.

93. Ho C. BC cancer protocol summary for treatment of locally advanced squamous cell carcinoma of the head and neck with DOCEtaxel, CISplatin and infusional fluorouracil. BC Cancer. British Columbia. 2021. Available in: http://www.bccancer.bc.ca/chemotherapy-protocols-site/Documents/Head%20and%20Neck/HNLADCF_Protocol.pdf. Accessed 11 Oct 2021.

94. Fountzilas G, Athanassiadis A, Samantas E, Skarlos D, Kalogera-Fountzila A, Nikolaou A, Bacoyiannis H, Stathopoulos G, Kosmidis P, Daniilidis J. Paclitaxel and carboplatin in recurrent or metastatic head and neck cancer: a phase II study. Semin Oncol. 1997;24(1 suppl 2):S2-65-S2-67.

95. Fountzilas G, Skarlos D, Athanassiades A, Kalogera-Fountzila A, Samantas E, Bacoyiannis C, Nicolaou A, Dombros N, Briasoulis E, Dinopoulou M, Stathopoulos G, Pavlidis N, Kosmidis P, Daniilidis N. Paclitaxel by three-hour infusion and carboplatin in advanced carcinoma of nasopharynx and other sites of the head and neck: a phase II study conducted by the Hellenic Cooperative Oncology Group. Ann Oncol. 1997;8(5):451–5. https://doi.org/10.1023/A:1008279503428.

96. Pergolizzi S, Santacaterina A, Adamo B, Franchina T, Denaro N, Ferraro P, Ricciardi GRR, Settineri N, Adamo V. Induction chemotherapy with paclitaxel and cisplatin to concurrent radiotherapy and weekly paclitaxel in the treatment of loco-regionally advanced, stage IV (M0), head and neck squamous cell carcinoma. Mature results of a prospective study. Radiat Oncol. 2011;6:162. https://doi.org/10.1186/1748-717X-6-162.

97. Langer CJ, Harris J, Horwitz EM, Nicolaou N, Kies M, Curran W, Wong S, Ang K. Phase II study of low-dose paclitaxel and cisplatin in combination with split-course concomitant twice-daily reirradiation in recurrent squamous cell carcinoma of the head and neck: results of radiation therapy oncology group protocol 9911. J Clin Oncol. 2016;25(30):4800–5. https://doi.org/10.1200/JCO.2006.07.9194.

98. Ho C. BC cancer protocol summary of treatment for unresectable, locoregionally recurrent or metastatic squamous cell carcinoma of the head and neck using PACLitaxel and CISplatin or CARBOplatin. BC Cancer. British Columbia. 2021. Available in: http://www.bccancer.bc.ca/chemotherapy-protocols-site/Documents/Head%20and%20Neck/HNAVPC_Protocol.pdf. Accessed 12 Oct 2021.

99. Han Y, Liu D, Li L. PD-1/PD-L1 pathway: current researches in cancer. Am J Cancer Res. 2020;10(3):727–42.

100. NCT04489888. A study of pembrolizumab (MK-3475) plus carboplatin and paclitaxel as first-line treatment of recurrent/metastatic head and neck squamous cell carcinoma (MK-3475-B10/KEYNOTE B10). Clinical Trials. 2021. Available in: https://clinicaltrials.gov/ct2/show/NCT04489888. Accessed 12 Oct 2021.

101. Valadez A, Welsh M, Kim C, Johns A, Algazi A, Kang H, Kang H. 201 Carboplatin, paclitaxel and pembrolizumab for the first line treatment of recurrent and/or metastatic head and neck squamous cell carcinoma. J ImmunoTherapy Cancer. 2020;8(Suppl 3):A1–A559. https://doi.org/10.1136/jitc-2020-SITC2020.0201.

102. Cabezas-Camarero S, Cabrera-Martin MN, Sanz MSP, Perez-Segura P. Major and durable response to second-line pembrolizumab-carboplatin-paclitaxel in an oral cavity cancer patient. Anti-Cancer Drugs. 2021;32(5):580–4. https://doi.org/10.1097/CAD.0000000000001040.

103. Ho C. BC cancer protocol summary for first-line treatment of advanced squamous cell carcinoma of the head and neck with PACLitaxel, CARBOplatin and pembrolizumab. BC Cancer. British Columbia. 2021. Available in: http://www.bccancer.bc.ca/chemotherapy-protocols-site/Documents/Head%20and%20Neck/UHNAVPCPMB_Protocol.pdf. Accessed 12 Oct 2021.

104. NCT04428333. Study of GSK3359609 with pembrolizumab and 5-fluorouracil (5-FU)-platinum chemotherapy in participants with recurrent or metastatic head and neck squamous cell carcinoma (INDUCE-4). Clinical Trials. 2021. Available in: https://clinicaltrials.gov/ct2/show/NCT04428333. Accessed 12 Oct 2021.

105. Rischin D, Harrington KJ, Greil R, Soulieres D, Tahara M, Castro G, Psyrri A, Baste N, Neupane PC, Bratland A, Fuereder T, Hughes BGM, Mesia R, Ngamphaiboon N, Rordorf T, Ishak WZW, Zhang Y, Jin F, Gumuscu B, Burtness B. Protocol-specified final analysis of the phase 3 KEYNOTE-048 trial of pembrolizumab (pembro) as first-line therapy for recurrent/metastatic head and neck squamous cell carcinoma (R/M HNSCC). J Clin Oncol. 2019;37(15_suppl):6000. https://doi.org/10.1200/JCO.2019.37.15_suppl.6000.

106. Ho C. BC cancer protocol summary for first-line treatment of advanced squamous cell carcinoma of the head and neck using platinum, fluorouracil and pembrolizumab. BC Cancer. British Columbia. 2021. Available in: http://www.bccancer.bc.ca/chemotherapy-protocols-site/Documents/Head%20and%20Neck/UHNAVPFPMB_Protocol.pdf. Accessed 12 Oct 2021.

107. Kucukzeybek Y, Gorumlu G, Karaca B, Erten C, Cengiz E, Kemal Gul M, Karabulut B, Uslu R, Sanli UA, Goker E. Docetaxel and platinum combination chemotherapy in locally advanced or metastatic head and neck cancer. J BUON. 2008;13(2):199–203.
108. Gedlicka C, Formanek M, Selzer E, Burian M, Kornfehl J, Fiebiger W, Cartellieri M, Marks B, Kornek GV. Phase II study with docetaxel and cisplatin in the treatment of recurrent and/ or metastatic squamous cell carcinoma of the head and neck. Oncology. 2002;63(2):145–50. https://doi.org/10.1159/000063809.
109. Schoffski P, Catimel G, Planting AS, Droz JP, Verweij J, Schrijvers D, Gras L, Schrijvers A, Wanders J, Hanauske AR. Docetaxel and cisplatin: an active regimen in patients with locally advanced, recurrent or metastatic squamous cell carcinoma of the head and neck. Results of a phase II study of the EORTC Early Clinical Studies Group. Ann Oncol. 1999;10(1):119–22. https://doi.org/10.1023/a:1008360323986.
110. Ho C. BC cancer protocol summary for the treatment of recurrent or metastatic squamous cell carcinoma of the head and neck with platinum and DOCEtaxel. BC Cancer. British Columbia. 2021. Available in: http://www.bccancer.bc.ca/chemotherapy-protocols-site/ Documents/Head%20and%20Neck/HNAVPD_Protocol.pdf. Accessed 12 Oct 2021.
111. Vargas PA, Gerhard R, Araújo Filho VJF, Castro IV. Salivary gland tumors in a Brazilian population: a retrospective study of 124 cases. Revista do Hospital das Clínicas. 2002;57(6):271–6. https://doi.org/10.1590/S0041-87812002000600005.
112. Araya J, Martinez R, Niklander S, Marshall M, Esguep A. Incidence and prevalence of salivar gland tumours in Valparaiso, Chile. Medicina Oral Patologia Oral y Cirugia Bucal. 2015;20(5):e532–9. https://doi.org/10.4317/medoral.20337.
113. Gontarz M, Bargiel J, Gasiorowski K, Marecik T, Szczurowski P, Zapala J, Wyszynska-Pawelec G. Epidemiology of primary epithelial salivary gland tumors in Southern Poland—A 26-year, clinicopathologic, retrospective analysis. J Clin Med. 2021;10:1663. https://doi.org/10.3390/jcm10081663.
114. Bentz BG, Hughes CA, Ludemann JP, Maddalozzo J. Masses of the salivary gland region in children. Arch Otolaryngol Head Neck Surg. 2000;126(12):1435–9. https://doi.org/10.1001/archotol.126.12.1435.
115. Junior AT, Almeida OP, Kowalski LP. Parotid neoplasms: analysis of 600 patients attended at a single institution. Braz J Otorhinolaryngol. 2009;75(4):497–501. https://doi.org/10.1590/S1808-86942009000400005.
116. Lee RJ, Tan AP, Tong EL, Satyadev N, Christensen RE. Epidemiology, prognostic factors, and treatment of malignant submandibular gland tumors: a population-based cohort analysis. JAMA Otolaryngol Head Neck Surg. 2015;141(10):905–12. https://doi.org/10.1001/jamaoto.2015.1745.
117. Son E, Panwar A, Mosher CH, Lydiatt D. Cancers of the major salivary gland. J Oncol Pract. 2018;14(2):99–108. https://doi.org/10.1200/JOP.2017.026856.
118. Gomes DQC, Silva MFA, Pereira JV, Bento PM, Figueiredo RLQ, Miguel MCC. Mucoepidermoid carcinoma of the retromolar region: reporto f a clinical case. RGO – Revista Gaúcha de. Odontologia. 2015;63(1):103–8. https://doi.org/10.1590/1981-863720150001000152576.
119. Glisson B, Colevas AD, Haddad R, Krane J, El-Naggar A, Kies M, Costello R, Summey C, Arquette M, Langer C, Amrein PC, Posner M. HER2 expression in salivary gland carcinomas: dependence on histological subtype. Clin Cancer Res. 2004;10(3):944–6. https://doi.org/10.1158/1078-0432.ccr-03-0253.
120. Porcheri C, Meisel CT, Mitsiadis TA. Molecular and cellular modelling of salivary gland tumors open new landscapes in diagnosis and treatment. Cancers (Basel). 2020;12(11):3107. https://doi.org/10.3390/cancers12113107.
121. Garden AS, Weber RS, Ang KK, Morrison WH, Matre J, Peters LJ. Postoperative radiation therapy for malignant tumors of minor salivary glands. Outcome and patterns of failure. Cancer. 1994;73(10):2563–9. https://doi.org/10.1002/1097-0142(19940515)73:10<2563::aid-cncr2820731018>3.0.co;2-x.

122. Soares ECS, Costa FWG, Bezerra TP, Nogueira CBP, Medeiros JR, Neto ICP. Surgical approach to pleomorphic adenomas arising in the palate: a 10-year retrospective study in a Brazilian population. J Oral Diagn. 2016;01:e1. https://doi.org/10.18762/2525-5711.20160001.

123. Melo GM, Cervantes O, Abrahao M, Covolan L, Ferreira ES, Baptista HA. A brief history of salivary gland surgery. Rev Col Bras Cir. 2017;44(4):403–12. https://doi.org/10.1590/0100-69912017004004.

124. Bussu F, Parrilla C, Rizzo D, Almadori G, Paludetti G, Galli J. Clinical approach and treatment of benign and malignant parotid masses, personal experience. Acta Otorhinolaryngol Ital. 2011;31(3):135–43.

125. Dispenza F, Cicero G, Mortellaro G, Marchese D, Kulamarva G, Dispenza C. Primary non-hodgkins lymphoma of the parotid gland. Braz J Otorhinolaryngol. 2011;77(5):639–44. https://doi.org/10.1590/S1808-86942011000500017.

126. López F, Rodrigo JP, Silver CE, Haigentz M Jr, Bishop JÁ, Strojan P, Hartl DM, Bradley PJ, Mendenhall WM, Suárez C, Takes RP, Hamoir M, Robbins KT, Shaha AR, Werner JA, Rinaldo A, Ferlito A. Cervical lymph node metastases from remote primary tumor sites. Head Neck. 2016;38(Suppl 1):E2374–85. https://doi.org/10.1002/hed.24344.

127. Geiger JL, Ismaila N, Beadle B, Caudell JJ, Chau N, Deschler D, Glastonbury C, Kaufman M, Lamarre E, Lau HY, Licitra L, Moore MG, Rodriguez C, Roshal A, Seethala R, Swiecicki P, Ha P. Management of salivary gland malignancy: ASCO guideline. J Clin Oncol. 2021;39(17):1909–41. https://doi.org/10.1200/JCO.21.00449.

128. Andreoli MT, Andreoli SM, Shrime MG, Devaiah AK. Radiotherapy in parotid acinic cell carcinoma: does it have an impact on survival? Arch Otolaryngol Head Neck Surg. 2012;138(5):463–6. https://doi.org/10.1001/archoto.2012.226.

129. Wang X, Luo Y, Li M, Yan H, Sun M, Fan T. Management of salivary gland carcinomas – a review. Oncotarget. 2017;8(3):3946–56. https://doi.org/10.18632/oncotarget.13952.

130. Lagha A, Chraiet N, Ayadi M, Krimi S, Allani B, Rifi H, Raies H, Mezlini A. Systemic therapy in the management of metastatic or advanced salivary gland cancers. Head Neck Oncol. 2012;4:19. https://doi.org/10.1186/1758-3284-4-19.

131. Hill ME, Constenla DO, A'Hern RP, Henk JM, Rhys-Evans P, Breach N, Archer D, Gore ME. Cisplatin and 5-fluorouracil for symptom control in advanced salivary adenoid cystic carcinoma. Oral Oncol. 1997;33(4):275–8. https://doi.org/10.1016/s0964-1955(97)00026-2.

132. Debaere D, Poorten VV, Nuyts S, Hauben E, Schoenaers J, Schoffski P, Clement PMJ. Cyclophosphamide, doxorubicin, and cisplatin in advanced salivary gland cancer. B-ENT. 2011;7(1):1–6.

133. Ha H, Keam B, Ock CY, Heo DS. Efficacy of cyclophosphamide, doxorubicin, and cisplatin for adenoid cystic carcinoma, and their relationship with the pre-chemotherapy tumor growth rate. Chin Clin Oncol. 2020;9(2):15. https://doi.org/10.21037/cco.2020.03.07.

134. Airoldi M, Pedani F, Succo G, Gabriele AM, Ragona R, Marchionatti S, Bumma C. Phase II randomized trial comparing vinorelbine versus vinorelbine plus cisplatin in patients with recurrent salivary gland malignancies. Cancer. 2001;91(3):541–7. https://doi.org/10.1002/1097-0142(20010201)91:3<541::aid-cncr1032>3.0.co;2-y.

135. Hong MH, Kim CG, Koh YW, Choi EC. Kim J, Yoon SO, Kim HR, Cho BC. Efficacy and safety of vinorelbine plus cisplatin chemotherapy for patients with recurrent and/or metastatic salivary gland cancer of the head and neck. J Sci Specialt Head Neck. 2017;40(1):55–62. https://doi.org/10.1002/hed.24933.

136. Ho C. BC cancer protocol summary for palliative treatment of advanced salivary gland cancers with CISplatin and vinorelbine. BC Cancer. British Columbia. 2021. Available in: http://www.bccancer.bc.ca/chemotherapy-protocols-site/Documents/Head%20and%20Neck/HNSAVNP_Protocol.pdf. Accessed 12 Oct 2021.

137. Levêque D, Jehl F, Quoix E, Breillout F. Clinical pharmacokinetics of vinorelbine alone and combined with cisplatin. J Clin Pharmacol. 1992;32(12):1096–8. https://doi.org/10.1177/009127009203201206.

138. Gama CS, Nobre SMPC, Neusquen LPDG. Extravasamento de medicamentos antineoplásicos. Eurofarma. São Paulo. Brazil. 2016. Available in: https://cdn.eurofarma.com.br//wp-
content/uploads/2019/11/530382..pdf. Accessed 12 Oct 2021.
139. Alberts DS, Manning MR, Coulthard SW, Koopmann CF Jr, Herman TS. Adriamycin/cis-
platinum/cyclophosphamide combination chemotherapy for advanced carcinoma of the
parotid gland. Cancer. 1981;47(4):645–8. https://doi.org/10.1002/1097-0142(19810215)47:
4<645::aid-cncr2820470404>3.0.co;2-a.
140. Licitra L, Cavina R, Grandi C, Palma SD, Guzzo M, Demicheli R, Molinari R. Cisplatin,
doxorubicin and cyclophosphamide in advanced salivary gland carcinoma. A phase II trial
of 22 patients. Ann Oncol. 1996;7(6):640–2. https://doi.org/10.1093/oxfordjournals.annonc.
a010684.

Chapter 9
Chemotherapeutic Protocols for the Treatment of Lung Cancer

9.1 Epidemiological Profile of Lung Cancers

Until the beginning of the twentieth century, lung cancer was considered rare, but its occurrence increased rapidly and is currently one of the most prevalent cancers in the world and with a high mortality rate [1–3]. According to WHO [4], in 2020, approximately 2.21 million cases and 1.8 billion deaths were reported worldwide. The incidence was higher in men (1.44 million cases) than in women (771 thousand cases). Figure 9.1 provides the estimated incidence and mortality from lung cancer for the year 2040.

Among the risk factors for the development of lung cancer, in addition to genetic and environmental factors, smoking is one of the main factors responsible for most cases [5–7]. According to Cruz et al. [8], the average age for diagnosis of lung and bronchial cancer in the period 2004–2008 was 71 years. In 2008, lung cancer was the most diagnosed and the leading cause of death in men and women and was the fourth most diagnosed type and the second leading cause of death worldwide [8–10].

Among the types of cancers that affect the lungs, the main ones are squamous cell carcinoma, adenocarcinoma, small-cell carcinoma, and extensive cell carcinoma. There has been an increase in the number of adenocarcinomas in recent decades with a reduction in the number of squamous cell carcinomas, probably due to changes in the composition of tobacco products [3, 8, 11, 12].

Lung cancer is classified as either non-small-cell lung cancer or small-cell lung cancer. Non-small-cell lung cancer can be subclassified into adenocarcinoma (cancer starts in the cells that line the alveoli and produce substances), squamous cell carcinoma (starts in the epidermoid cells that line the interior of the airways), and extensive cell carcinoma (may start anywhere in the lung and tend to grow rapidly).

I. D. Lima Cavalcanti, *Chemotherapy Protocols and Infusion Sequence*,
https://doi.org/10.1007/978-3-031-10839-6_9

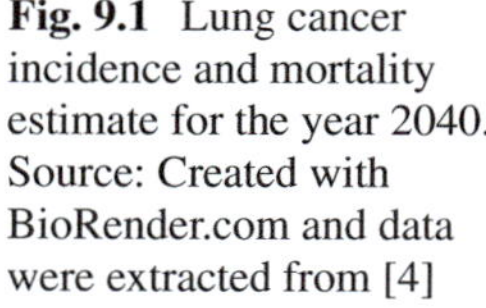

Fig. 9.1 Lung cancer incidence and mortality estimate for the year 2040. Source: Created with BioRender.com and data were extracted from [4]

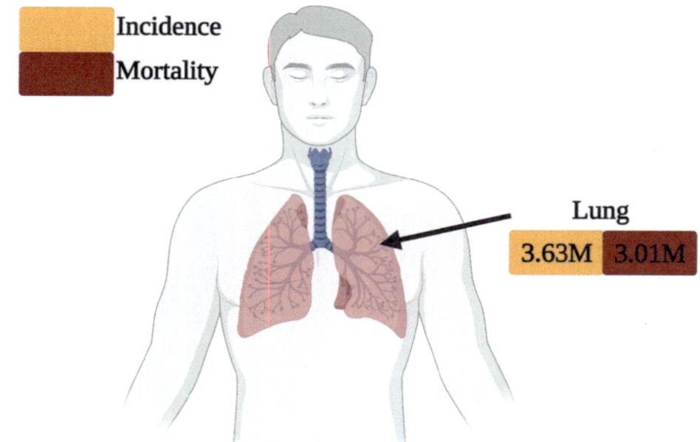

Small-cell lung cancer, on the other hand, proliferates and spreads faster than non-small-cell lung cancer [12–14].

9.2   Pathophysiology of Lung Cancer

The pathophysiology of lung cancer is complex and poorly understood, where it is believed that repeated exposure to carcinogens can induce dysplasia of the pulmonary epithelium, thereby leading to genetic mutations and affecting protein synthesis. Exposure to these agents consequently leads to cell cycle disruption and promotes carcinogenesis. Among the genetic mutations, the most common are MYC, BCL2, and p53 in small-cell lung cancer and EGFR, KRAS, and p16 in non-small-cell lung cancer [15–19].

Lung tumors usually start in the bronchi and invade the adjacent parenchyma as well as the pleura and chest wall. The parenchymal lymph nodes are responsible for the spread of the tumor to other regions, such as the homolateral hilum and mediastinal lymph nodes, and may subsequently spread to other organs and tissues [20–22].

Regarding the staging of lung cancer (Fig. 9.2), in stage 1, the tumor is restricted to the lung with a size smaller or larger than 3 cm without dissemination to the lymph nodes. In stage 2, the tumor size is also smaller or larger than 3 cm, but it has the invasion of lymph nodes in the peribronchial region and/or ipsilateral hilar lymph nodes [22–26].

Stage 3 in lung cancer is defined as tumors with direct invasion of the chest wall, diaphragm, pericardium, or mediastinal pleura, without invasion of visceral structures, with invasion also in lymph nodes in the peribronchial, ipsilateral hilar, ipsilateral mediastinal or subcarinal regions, among others. Finally, in stage 4, the tumor can present in any size with the invasion of the mediastinum, affecting the

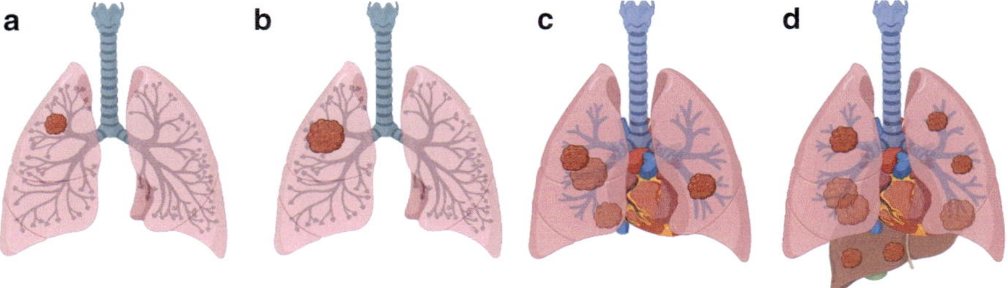

Fig. 9.2 Staging of lung cancer. (**a**) Stage 1. (**b**) Stage 2, (**c**) Stage 3, and (**d**) Stage 4. Source: Created with BioRender.com

heart, great vessels, trachea, esophagus, vertebral body, or carina, and the presence of metastases in lymph nodes and distant organs [22–24, 27].

9.3 Lung Cancer Treatment

The treatment of lung cancer will depend on the stage of the tumor, in which at an early stage, because the tumor is located, the surgical procedure is the first choice and radiotherapy or chemotherapy may be indicated in patients who cannot undergo surgery. In stage 2, when the tumor has already spread to nearby tissues or lymph nodes, radiotherapy combined with another therapeutic modality that may include radiotherapy is indicated [28–31].

In stage 3, the tumor has already spread to lymph nodes or nearby structures, where the indication for treatment involves surgery, radiotherapy, or chemotherapy. Finally, in stage 4, treatment options include radiotherapy, chemotherapy, and immunotherapy, with a focus on tumor shrinkage and symptom relief [29, 32, 33].

9.3.1 Chemotherapy for the Treatment of Non-Small-Cell Lung Cancer

Adjuvant chemotherapy for the treatment of non-small-cell lung cancer can be based on the use of monotherapy, with the administration of drugs such as durvalumab in the treatment of locally advanced non-small-cell lung cancer [34, 35]. Regarding the combinations, the use of cisplatin plus vinorelbine, also used in head and neck cancers (see Chap. 8), has been indicated in the adjuvant treatment of non-small-cell lung cancer, as well as the combination of carboplatin and paclitaxel that also indicated for the treatment of other cancers (see Chaps. 5 and 8) [36–38].

In the treatment of advanced non-small-cell lung cancer, docetaxel monotherapy has been indicated as a second line, as has vinorelbine which is indicated for elderly patients with advanced non-small-cell lung cancer. The use of tyrosine kinase inhibitors such as afatinib, alectinib, ceritinib, crizotinib, erlotinib, gefitinib, and osimertinib has been indicated in the treatment of non-small-cell lung cancer that overexpresses receptors or target genes such as EGFR, ALK, or ROS1 [39–45].

Some monoclonal antibodies, checkpoint inhibitors, are also indicated in advanced non-small-cell lung cancer, such as atezolizumab, nivolumab, and pembrolizumab, and may also be associated with chemotherapeutic agents, for example, pembrolizumab combined with carboplatin and paclitaxel, which is used in head and neck cancers (see Chap. 8) and is indicated in the first-line treatment of advanced squamous non-small-cell lung cancer [46, 47]. Other combinations already mentioned in Chap. 8, such as the combination of cisplatin and docetaxel, cisplatin combined with etoposide, and the combination of gemcitabine and platinum, are also indicated in the treatment of non-small-cell lung cancer [48–53]. Other protocols for the treatment of non-small-cell lung cancer will be covered in the next topics [54–56].

9.3.1.1 PPMB Protocol (Pemetrexed and Pembrolizumab)

The combination of pemetrexed and pembrolizumab is indicated as maintenance therapy for advanced non-squamous non-small-cell lung cancer. Pemetrexed is an antifolate antineoplastic agent whose function occurs through the disruption of folate-dependent metabolic processes that are essential for cell replication [57, 58].

Garon et al. [59] evaluated maintenance treatment of non-squamous non-small-cell lung cancer with pemetrexed with or without pembrolizumab. According to the authors, the combination of pemetrexed and pembrolizumab was well tolerated by patients, improving overall survival, progression-free survival, and objective response rate.

The infusion sequence of the PPMB protocol can start with the monoclonal antibody pembrolizumab due to its target-directed action followed by the infusion of pemetrexed (Fig. 9.3) [60].

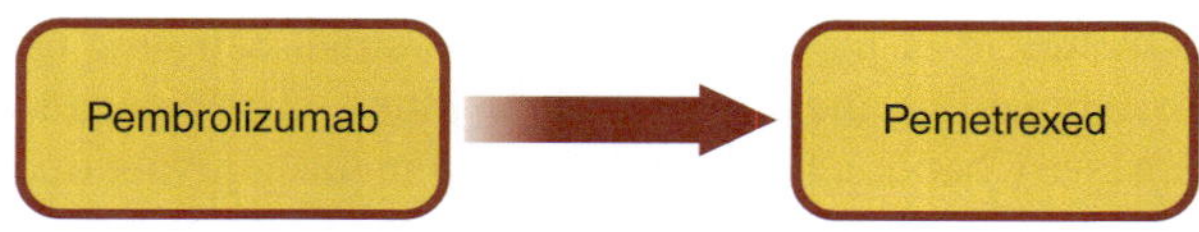

Fig. 9.3 PPMB protocol infusion sequence

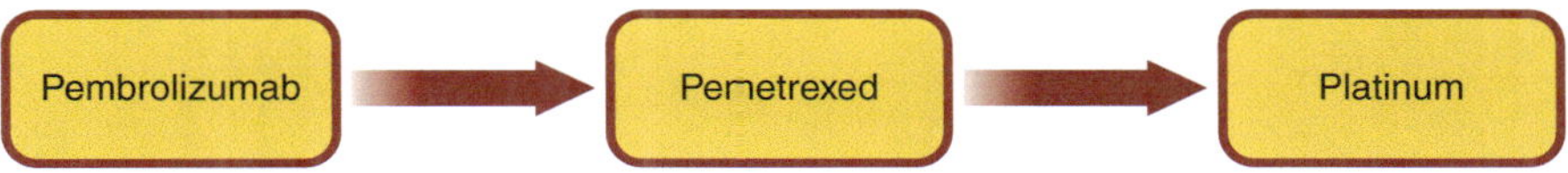

Fig. 9.4 PPPMB protocol infusion sequence

9.3.1.2 PPPMB Protocol (Platinum, Pemetrexed, and Pembrolizumab)

Platinum compounds (carboplatin or cisplatin) can also be combined with pemetrexed and pembrolizumab in the first-line treatment of advanced non-squamous non-small-cell lung cancer. In the study by Gandhi et al. [61], they found that the PPPMB protocol promoted an estimated 12-month overall survival rate of 69.2% and progression-free survival of 8.8 months. Gadgeel et al. [62] found that the combination of pembrolizumab, pemetrexed, and platinum promoted 22-month overall survival and 9-month progression-free survival.

Langer et al. [63] evaluated the efficacy of the combination of carboplatin, pemetrexed, and pembrolizumab in the treatment of advanced non-squamous cell lung cancer. The combination proved to be effective and tolerable, with the most frequent adverse events including anemia, neutropenia, fatigue, and thrombocytopenia.

Real-world results in the study by Velcheti et al. [64], who used the PPPMB protocol in patients with advanced-stage non-small-cell lung cancer, showed that the combination promoted an overall survival of 16.5 months, a progression-free survival of 6.4 months, and a response rate of tumor of 56.6%. As for the infusion sequence, the PPPMB protocol starts with the infusion of pembrolizumab followed by pemetrexed, and finally the infusion of platinum (Fig. 9.4) [65, 66].

9.3.1.3 PP Protocol (Platinum and Pemetrexed)

Pemetrexed combined with platinum (carboplatin or cisplatin) is indicated in the first-line treatment of advanced non-small-cell lung cancer [67]. Socinski et al. [68] evaluated the efficacy of the PP protocol in untreated extensive-stage small-cell lung cancer. The results showed that the combination of cisplatin and pemetrexed promoted a survival time of 7.6 months, with a 1-year survival of 33.4% and a response rate of 35%, while the combination of carboplatin and pemetrexed promoted time to the survival of 10.4 months, with a 1-year survival of 39% and response rate of 39.5%.

Xiao et al. [69] evaluated the efficacy of the combination of pemetrexed plus platinum doublet as a first-line treatment in advanced non-squamous cell lung cancer. The authors highlight the protocol's effectiveness, with an objective response rate of 37.8%, progression-free survival of 5.7 months, and overall survival of 16.05 months.

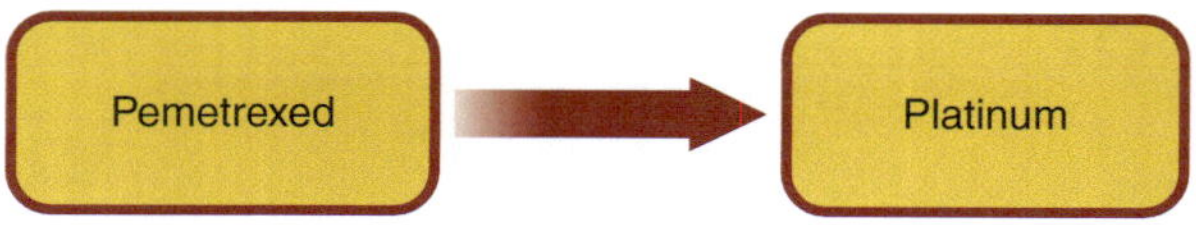

Fig. 9.5 PP protocol infusion sequence

In the study by Fujita et al. [70], the combination of pemetrexed with platinum led to a progression-free survival of 4.7 months and a mean overall survival time of 9.5 months, but the protocol has a high risk of interstitial lung disease. Li et al. [71] proposed the use of the PP protocol as a first-line treatment for advanced non-small-cell lung cancer. As a result, the authors observed an improvement in patient survival compared to other regimens, particularly in patients with non-squamous histology. The PP protocol infusion sequence is based on pemetrexed infusion first followed by platinum infusion (Fig. 9.5) [72, 73].

9.3.2 Chemotherapy for the Treatment of Small-Cell Lung Cancer

The treatment of small-cell lung cancer is based on tumor staging [74–76]. In the limited stage, when the tumor is restricted to the lung, with no evidence of the disease has spread to the lymph nodes or other organs, one of the treatment options is surgery, which may be followed by chemotherapy and radiotherapy. In cases where the patient has a tumor in a limited but very large stage, surgery is not an option, and chemotherapy associated with radiotherapy is indicated [75, 77–79].

In extensive-stage small-cell lung cancer, the first treatment option is based on chemotherapy-associated with immunotherapy or chemotherapy combined with other chemotherapy drugs [80, 81]. Among the antineoplastics that may be indicated as monotherapy, etoposide may be indicated in the palliative therapy of extensive-stage small-cell lung cancer or topotecan in the second-line treatment of recurrent small-cell lung cancer [82–85].

Some protocols indicated for other cancers may also be indicated in the treatment of small-cell lung cancer, such as cisplatin combined with etoposide, which is indicated in the therapy of small-cell lung cancer in a limited stage or an extensive stage [86, 87]. Other protocols will be covered in the next topics [54–56].

9.3.2.1 CAV Protocol (Cyclophosphamide, Doxorubicin, and Vincristine)

The CAV protocol combines cyclophosphamide, doxorubicin, and vincristine in the treatment of extensive small-cell lung cancer. Shepherd et al. [88] tested the CAV protocol in patients with etoposide and cisplatin-resistant small-cell lung cancer. The use of the CAV protocol in these patients promoted a mean survival of 15

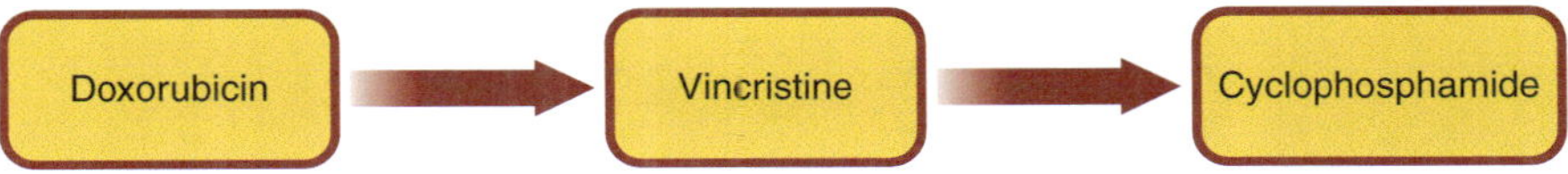

Fig. 9.6 CAV protocol infusion sequence

weeks, with limiting toxicity that included anemia and peripheral neuropathy, proving to be a protocol with limited activity.

Veronesi et al. [89] compared the combination of cisplatin and etoposide with the CAV protocol, showing that the CAV protocol was more tolerated despite not showing superior activity than the combination of cisplatin and etoposide in certain subsets of patients.

Jung et al. [90] looked at the promising effects of the CAV protocol as a third-line treatment in refractory small-cell lung cancer. The CAV protocol appears to improve progression-free survival and the response rate of patients with small-cell lung cancer [90]. Regarding the CAV protocol infusion sequence (Fig. 9.6), it starts with doxorubicin, followed by vincristine, which are the vesicant drugs, and finally the cyclophosphamide infusion [91].

9.3.2.2 PI Protocol (Platinum and Irinotecan)

Second-line treatment of extensive-stage small-cell lung cancer can also be treated with monotherapy with irinotecan or with a combination of irinotecan and platinum (carboplatin or cisplatin) [92]. Georgoulias et al. [93] tested the combination of irinotecan and cisplatin in the treatment of advanced non-small-cell lung cancer. The protocol promoted an overall response rate of 22.5%, a 1-year survival rate of 34.3%, and a median survival of 7.8 months. As for toxicity, cases of febrile neutropenia, neutropenia, and diarrhea have been reported.

Xu et al. [94] report the efficacy of combination therapy of irinotecan with platinum in previously untreated extensive-stage small-cell lung cancer. The authors noted that the protocol improved overall survival, progression-free survival, and overall response rate compared with the combination of etoposide and platinum. These results were also observed by Han et al. [95], which also showed a better overall survival induced by the combination of irinotecan and platinum compared with etoposide combined with platinum.

Hanna et al. [96] showed differences in the toxicity profile between the irinotecan protocol combined with cisplatin and the etoposide protocol combined with cisplatin. Patients who used the etoposide and cisplatin protocol had more cases of anemia, thrombocytopenia, neutropenia, and febrile neutropenia, while patients who used the combination irinotecan and cisplatin had diarrhea and vomiting.

As for the infusion sequence, the IP protocol starts with the infusion of platinum, although irinotecan is cycle specific; when cisplatin is administered first, it promotes synergistic effects [97–99]. Regarding the combination between carboplatin and irinotecan, Sato et al. [100] did not observe pharmacokinetic interactions

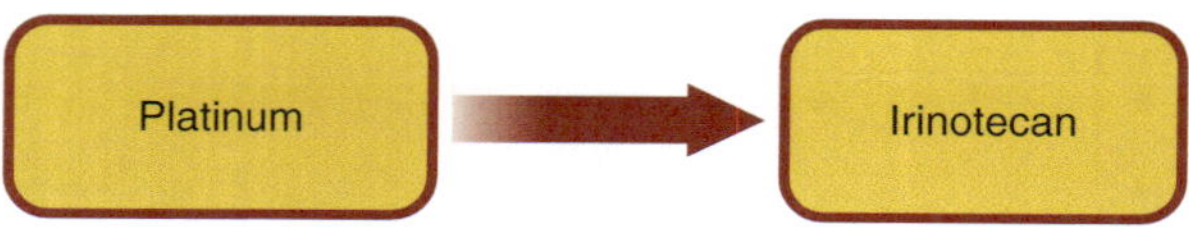

Fig. 9.7 PI protocol infusion sequence

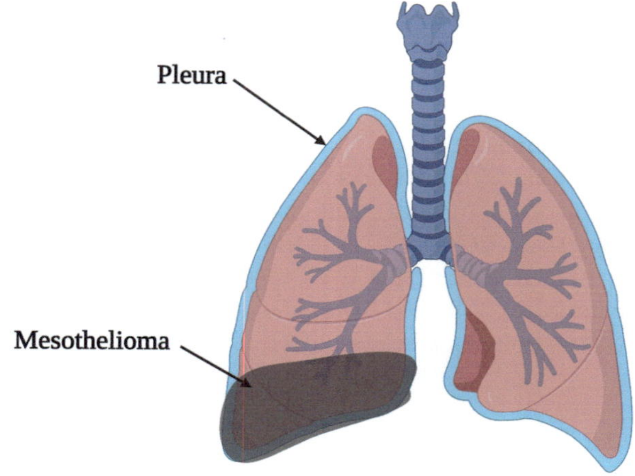

Fig. 9.8 Malignant mesothelioma. Source: Created with BioRender.com

between drugs. Thus, perhaps the infusion sequence is with the infusion initially of platinum followed by the infusion of irinotecan (Fig. 9.7).

9.3.3 Chemotherapy for the Treatment of Malignant Mesothelioma

Mesothelioma (Fig. 9.8) is cancer that originates in cells in the inner lining of the chest, abdomen, and other parts of the body. The treatment of this type of cancer will depend on the stage, in which in stages 1, 2, and 3, when the mesothelioma is resectable, a surgical procedure may be indicated and may be combined with chemotherapy. In cases of unresectable mesothelioma, chemotherapy is the main treatment, and it can be indicated to relieve symptoms and reduce or delay tumor growth [101–106].

Chemotherapy may be indicated as monotherapy, in the case of vinorelbine, which can be used as monotherapy in the treatment of malignant mesothelioma [107, 108]. As for combined therapy, some protocols that have already been mentioned in other cancers may be indicated, in the case of the combination of platinum and gemcitabine that is used in the treatment of head and neck cancers (see Chap. 8, Sect. 8.2.1.3) and the combination between platinum and pemetrexed, which is indicated in the treatment of advanced non-small-cell lung cancer (see Sect. 9.3.1.3) [109–111].

References

1. Alberg AJ, Brock MV, Ford JG, Samet JM, Spivack SD. Epidemiology of lung cancer. Chest. 2013;143(5):1–29. https://doi.org/10.1378/chest.12-2345.
2. Torre LA, Siegel RL, Ward EM, Jemal A. Global cancer incidence and mortality rates and trends-an update. Cancer Epidemiol Biomark Prev. 2016;25(1):16–27. https://doi.org/10.1158/1055-9965.EPI-15-0578.
3. Trufelli DC, Moraes TV, Lima AAPR, Giglio AD. Epidemiological profile and prognostic factors in patients with lung cancer. Rev Assoc Med Bras. 2016;62(5):428–33. https://doi.org/10.1590/1806-9282.62.05.428.
4. WHO – World Health Organization. Estimated number of incident cases from 2018 to 2040. International Agency for Research on Cancer, 2020. Available https://gco.iarc.fr/tomorrow/graphic-isotype?type=0&type_sex=0&mode=population&sex=0&populations=900&cancers=36&age_group=value&apc_male=0&apc_female=0&single_unit=100000&print=0. Accessed Oct 15, 2021.
5. Kligerman S, White C. Epidemiology of lung cancer in women: risk factors, survival, and screening. Am J Roentgenol. 2011;196:287–95. https://doi.org/10.2214/AJR.10.5412.
6. Malhotra J, Malvezzi M, Negri E, Vecchia CL, Boffetta P. Risk factors for lung cancer worldwide. Eur Respir J. 2016;48:889–902. https://doi.org/10.1183/13993003.00359-2016.
7. Kanwal M, Ding XJ, Cao Y. Familial risk for lung cancer. Oncol Lett. 2017;13(2):535–42. https://doi.org/10.3892/ol.2016.5518.
8. Cruz CSD, Tanoue LT, Matthay RA. Lung cancer: epidemiology, etiology, and prevention. Clin Chest Med. 2011;32(4):605–44. https://doi.org/10.1016/j.ccm.2011.09.001.
9. Araujo LH, Baldotto C, Castro G Jr, Katz A, Ferreira CG, Mathias C, Mascarenhas E, Lopes GL, Carvalho H, Tabacof J, Martinez-Mesa J, Viana LS, Cruz MS, Zukin M, Marchi PD, Terra RM, Ribeiro RA, Lima VCC, Werutsky G, Barrios CH. Lung cancer in Brazil. J Bras Pneumol. 2018;44(1):55–64. https://doi.org/10.1590/S1806-37562017000000135.
10. Ridge CA, McErlean AM, Ginsberg MS. Epidemiology of lung cancer. Semin Interv Radiol. 2013;30(2):93–8. https://doi.org/10.1055/s-0033-1342949.
11. Travis WD. Update on small cell carcinoma and its differentiation from squamous cell carcinoma and other non-small cell carcinomas. Mod Pathol. 2012;25:18–30. https://doi.org/10.1038/modpathol.2011.150.
12. Zheng M. Classification and pathology of lung cancer. Surg Oncol Clin N Am. 2016;25:447–68. https://doi.org/10.1016/j.soc.2016.02.003.
13. Molina JR, Yang P, Cassivi SD, Schild SE, Adjei AA. Non-small cell lung cancer: epidemiology, risk factors, treatment, and survivorship. Mayo Clin Proc. 2008;83(5):584–94. https://doi.org/10.4065/83.5.584.
14. Ismael GFV, Coradazzi AL, Neto FAM, Abdalla KC, Milhomem PM, Oliveira JS, Manzoni C, Beato CAM, Segalla JGM. Aspectos clínicos e histopatológicos em câncer de pulmão: análise dos dados de uma instituição no interior paulista entre 1997–2008. Rev Bras Oncol Clín. 2010;7(22):72–8.
15. Pfeifer GP, Denissenko MF, Olivier M, Tretyakova N, Hecht SS, Hainaut P. Tobacco smoke carcinogens, DNA damage and p53 mutations in smoking-associated cancers. Oncogene. 2002;21:7435–51. https://doi.org/10.1038/sj.onc.1205803.
16. Miller YE. Pathogenesis of lung cancer: 100 year report. Am J Respir Cell Mol Biol. 2005;33(3):216–23. https://doi.org/10.1165/rcmb.2005-0158OE.
17. Brambilla E, Gazdar A. Pathogenesis of lung cancer signalling pathways: roadmap for therapies. Eur Respir J. 2009;33:1485–97. https://doi.org/10.1183/09031936.00014009.
18. Dorantes-Heredia R, Ruiz-Morales JM, Cano-García F. Histopathological transformation to small-cell lung carcinoma in non-small cell lung carcinoma tumors. Transl Lung Cancer Res. 2016;5(4):401–12. https://doi.org/10.21037/tlcr.2016.07.10.
19. Siddiqui F, Siddiqui AH. Lung cancer. Treasure Island: StatPearls Publishing; 2021.

20. Sharma A, Fidias P, Hayman LA, Loomis SL, Taber KH, Aquino SL. Patterns of lymph-adenopathy in thoracic malignancies. RadioGraphics. 2004;24(2):419–34. https://doi.org/10.1148/rg.242035075.
21. Terán MD, Brock MV. Staging lymph node metastases from lung cancer in the mediastinum. J Thorac Dis. 2014;6(3):230–6. https://doi.org/10.3978/j.issn.2072-1439.2013.12.18.
22. Purandare NC, Rangarajan V. Imaging of lung cancer: implications on staging and management. Indian J Radiol Imaging. 2015;25(2):109–20. https://doi.org/10.4103/0971-3026.155831.
23. Fernandez A, Jatene FB, Zamboni M. Diagnóstico e estadiamento do câncer de pulmão. J Pneumol. 2002;28(4):219–28. https://doi.org/10.1590/S0102-35862002000400006.
24. Quint LE. Staging non-small cell lung cancer. Cancer Imaging. 2007;7(1):148–59. https://doi.org/10.1102/1470-7330.2007.0026.
25. UyBico SJ, Wu CC, Suh RD, Le NH, Brown K, Krishnam MS. Lung cancer staging essentials: the new TNM staging system and potential imaging pitfalls. RadioGraphics. 2010;30(5):1163–81. https://doi.org/10.1148/rg.305095166.
26. Kay FU, Kandathil A, Batra K, Saboo SS, Abbara S, Rajiah P. Revisions to the tumor, node, metastasis staging of lung cancer (8th edition): rationale, radiologic findings and clinical implications. World J Radiol. 2017;9(6):269–79. https://doi.org/10.4329/wjr.v9.i6.269.
27. Detterbeck FC, Boffa DJ, Tanoue LT, Wilson LD. Details and difficulties regarding the new lung cancer staging system. Chest. 2010;137(5):1172–80. https://doi.org/10.1378/chest.09-2626.
28. Howington JA, Blum MG, Chang AC, Balekian AA, Murthy SC. Treatment of stage I and II non-small cell lung cancer: Diagnosis and management of lung cancer, 3rd ed: American College of Chest Physicians evidence-based clinical practice guidelines. Chest. 2013;143(5):278–313. https://doi.org/10.1378/chest.12-2359.
29. Detterbeck FC, Boffa DJ, Kim AW, Tanoue LT. The eighth edition lung cancer stage classification. Chest. 2017;151(1):193–203. https://doi.org/10.1016/j.chest.2016.10.010.
30. Gensheimer MF, Loo BW Jr. Optimal radiation therapy for small cell lung cancer. Curr Treat Options in Oncol. 2017;18(4):21. https://doi.org/10.1007/s11864-017-0467-z.
31. Benveniste MF, Gomez D, Carter BW, Cuellar SLB, Shroff GS, Benveniste APA, Odisio EG, Marom EM. Recognizing radiation therapy–related complications in the chest. RadioGraphics. 2019;39(2):344–66. https://doi.org/10.1148/rg.2019180061.
32. Majem M, Hernández-Hernández J, Hernando-Trancho F, Dios NR, Sotoca A, Trujillo-Reyes JC, Vollmer I, Delgado-Bolton R, Provencio M. Multidisciplinary consensus statement on the clinical management of patients with stage III non-small cell lung cancer. Clin Transl Oncol. 2019;22(1):21–36. https://doi.org/10.1007/s12094-019-02134-7.
33. Jamil A, Kasi A. Lung metastasis. Treasure Island: StatPearls Publishing; 2021.
34. Mezquita L, Planchard D. Durvalumab in non-small-cell lung cancer patients: current developments. Future Oncol. 2018;14(3):205–22. https://doi.org/10.2217/fon-2017-0373.
35. Witlox WJA, van Asselt AAI, Wolff R, Armstrong N, Worthy G, Chalker A, Buksnys T, Stirk L, Kleijnen J, Joore MA, Grimm SE. Durvalumab for the treatment of locally advanced, unresectable, stage III non-small cell lung cancer: an evidence review group perspective of a NICE single technology appraisal. PharmacoEconomics. 2020;38:317–24. https://doi.org/10.1007/s40273-019-00870-w.
36. Winton T, Livingston R, Johnson D, Rigas J, Johnston M, Butts C, Cormier Y, Goss G, Inculet R, Vallieres E, Fry W, Bethune D, Ayoub J, Ding K, Seymour L, Graham B, Tsao MS, Gandara D, Kesler K, Demmy T, Shepherd F. Vinorelbine plus cisplatin vs. observation in resected non-small-cell lung cancer. N Engl J Med. 2005;352(25):2589–97. https://doi.org/10.1056/NEJMoa043623.
37. Strauss GM, Herndon JE, Maddaus MA, Johnstone DW, Johnson EA, Harpole DH, Gillenwater HH, Watson DM, Sugarbaker DJ, Schilsky RL, Vokes EE, Green MR. Adjuvant paclitaxel plus carboplatin compared with observation in stage IB non–small-cell lung cancer: CALGB 9633 with the cancer and leukemia group B, radiation therapy oncology group,

and north central cancer treatment group study groups. J Clin Oncol. 2008;26(31):5043–51. https://doi.org/10.1200/JCO.2008.16.4855.

38. Palka M, Sanchez A, Córdoba M, Nuevo GD, Ugarte AVD, Cantos B, Méndez M, Calvo V, Maximiano C, Provencio M. Cisplatin plus vinorelbine as induction treatment in stage IIIA non-small cell lung cancer. Oncol Lett. 2017;13(3):1647–54. https://doi.org/10.3892/ol.2017.5620.

39. Cappuzzo F, Ciuleanu T, Stelmakh L, Cicenas S, Szczésna A, Juhász E, Esteban E, Molinier O, Brugger W, Melezínek I, Klingelschmitt G, Klughammer B, Giaccone G. Erlotinib as maintenance treatment in advanced non-small-cell lung cancer: a multicentre, randomised, placebo-controlled phase 3 study. Lancet Oncol. 2010;11(6):521–9. https://doi.org/10.1016/S1470-2045(10)70112-1.

40. Deeks ED. Ceritinib: a review in ALK-positive advanced NSCLC. Target Oncol. 2016;11:693–700. https://doi.org/10.1007/s11523-016-0460-7.

41. Avrillon V, Pérol M. Alectinib for treatment of ALK-positive non-small-cell lung cancer. Future Oncol. 2017;13(4):321–35. https://doi.org/10.2217/fon-2016-0386.

42. Bruckl W, Tufman A, Huber RM. Advanced non-small cell lung cancer (NSCLC) with activating EGFR mutations: first-line treatment with afatinib and other EGFR TKIs. Expert Rev Anticancer Ther. 2017;17(2):143–55. https://doi.org/10.1080/14737140.2017.1266265.

43. Paz-Ares L, Tan EH, O'Byrne K, Zhang L, Hirsh V, Boyer M, Yang JCH, Mok T, Lee KH, Lu S, Shi Y, Lee DH, Laskin J, Kim DW, Laurie SA, Kolbeck K, Fan J, Dodd N, Marten A, Park K. Afatinib versus gefitinib in patients with EGFR mutation-positive advanced non-small-cell lung cancer: overall survival data from the phase IIb LUX-Lung 7 trial. Ann Oncol. 2017;28(2):270–7. https://doi.org/10.1093/annonc/mdw611.

44. Soria JC, Ohe Y, Vansteenkiste J, Reungwetwattana T, Chewaskulyong B, Lee KH, Dechaphunkul A, Imamura F, Nogami N, Kurata T, Okamoto I, Zhou C, Cho BC, Cheng Y, Cho EK, Voon PJ, Planchard D, Su WC, Gray JE, Lee SM, Hodge R, Marotti M, Rukazenkov Y, Ramalingam SS. Osimertinib in untreated EGFR-mutated advanced non-small-cell lung cancer. N Engl J Med. 2018;378:113–25 https://doi.org/10.1056/NEJMoa1713137.

45. Wu YL, Yang JCH, Kim DW, Lu S, Zhou J, Seto T, Yang JJ, Yamamoto N, Ahn MJ, Takahashi T, Yamanaka T, Kemner A, Roychowdhury D, Paolini J, Usari T, Wilner KD, Goto K. Phase II study of crizotinib in East Asian patients with ROS1-positive advanced non-small-cell lung cancer. J Clin Oncol. 2018;36(14):1405–11. https://doi.org/10.1200/JCO.2017.75.5587.

46. Chen R, Tao Y, Xu X, Shan L, Jiang H, Yin Q, Pei L, Cai F, Ma L, Yu Y. The efficacy and safety of nivolumab, pembrolizumab, and atezolizumab in treatment of advanced non-small cell lung cancer. Discov Med. 2018;26(143):155–66.

47. Shields MD, Marin-Acevedo JA, Pellini B. Immunotherapy for advanced non-small cell lung cancer: a decade of progress. Proc Am Soc Clin Oncol. 2021;41:e105–27. https://doi.org/10.1200/EDBK_321483.

48. Friess GG, Baikadi M, Harvey WH. Concurrent cisplatin and etoposide with radiotherapy in locally advanced non-small cell lung cancer. Cancer Treat Rep. 1987;71(7-8):681–4.

49. Zalcberg J, Millward M, Bishop J, McKeage M, Zimet A, Toner G, Friedlander M, Barter C, Rischin D, Loret C, James R, Bougan N, Berille J. Phase II study of docetaxel and cisplatin in advanced non-small-cell lung cancer. J Clin Oncol. 1998;16(5):1948–53. https://doi.org/10.1200/JCO.1998.16.5.1948.

50. Santana-Davila R, Devisetty K, Szabo A, Sparapani R, Arce-Lara C, Gore EM, Moran A, Williams CD, Kelley MJ, Whittle J. Cisplatin and etoposide versus carboplatin and paclitaxel with concurrent radiotherapy for Stage III non-small-cell lung cancer: an analysis of veterans health administration data. J Clin Oncol. 2015;33(6):567–74. https://doi.org/10.1200/JCO.2014.56.2587.

51. Li A, Wei ZJ, Ding H, Tang HS, Zhou HX, Yao X, Feng SQ. Docetaxel versus docetaxel plus cisplatin for non-small-cell lung cancer: a meta-analysis of randomized clinical trials. Oncotarget. 2017;8(34):57365–78. https://doi.org/10.18632/oncotarget.17071.

52. Paz-Ares L, Luft A, Vicente D, Tafreshi A, Gumus M, Mazières J, Hermes B, Senler FÇ, Csoszi T, Fulop A, Rodríguez-Cis J, Wilson J, Sugawara S, Kato T, Lee KH, Cheng Y, Novello S, Halmos B, Li X, Lubiniecki GM, Piperdi B, Kowalski DM. Pembrolizumab plus chemotherapy for squamous non-small-cell lung cancer. N Engl J Med. 2018;379:2040–51. https://doi.org/10.1056/NEJMoa1810865.

53. Scagliotti GV, Parikh P, Pawel JV, Biesma B, Vansteenkiste J, Manegold C, Serwatowski P, Gatzemeier U, Digumarti R, Zukin M, Lee JS, Mellemgaard A, Park K, Patil S, Rolski J, Goksel T, Marinis F, Simms L, Sugarman KP, Gandara D. Phase III study comparing cisplatin plus gemcitabine with cisplatin plus pemetrexed in chemotherapy-naive patients with advanced-stage non-small-cell lung cancer. J Clin Oncol. 2008;26(21):3543–51. https://doi.org/10.1200/JCO.2007.15.0375.

54. Kuehr T, Thaler J, Woell E. Chemotherapy protocols 2017: Current protocols and "targeted therapies". Klinikum Wels-Grieskirchen and Caritas Christi URGET NOS, Austria, 2017. www.chemoprotocols.eu.

55. BC Cancer. Supportive care protocols. BC Cancer. British Columbia, 2021. Available http://www.bccancer.bc.ca/health-professionals/clinical-resources/chemotherapy-protocols/supportive-care. Accessed July 2, 2021.

56. NHS. Chemotherapy protocols. NHS, University Hospital Southampton, NHS Foundation Trust, England, 2021. Available https://www.uhs.nhs.uk/HealthProfessionals/Chemotherapy-protocols/Chemotherapy-protocols.aspx. Accessed July 2, 2021.

57. Konstantinov SM, Berger MR. Antimetabolites. In: Offermanns S, Rosenthal W, editors. Encyclopedia of molecular pharmacology. Berlin: Springer; 2008. https://doi.org/10.1007/978-3-540-38918-7_220.

58. Miller DS, Blessing JA, Krasner CN, Mannel RS, Hanjani P, Pearl ML, Waggoner SE, Boardman CH. Phase II evaluation of pemetrexed in the treatment of recurrent or persistent platinum-resistant ovarian or primary peritoneal carcinoma: a study of the gynecologic oncology group. J Clin Oncol. 2009;27(16):2686–91. https://doi.org/10.1200/JCO.2008.19.2963.

59. Garon EB, Kim JS, Govindan R. Pemetrexed maintenance with or without pembrolizumab in non-squamous non-small cell lung cancer: a cross-trial comparison of keynote-189 versus paramount, pronounce, and JVBL. Lung Cancer. 2021;151:25–9. https://doi.org/10.1016/j.lungcan.2020.11.018.

60. Sun S. BC cancer protocol summary for maintenance therapy of advanced non-squamous non-small cell lung cancer with pemetrexed and pembrolizumab. BC Cancer, British Columbia, 2021. Available http://www.bccancer.bc.ca/chemotherapy-protocols-site/Documents/Lung/LUAVPPMBM_Protocol.pdf. Accessed Oct 16, 2021.

61. Gandhi L, Rodríguez-Abreu D, Gadgeel S, Esteban E, Felip E, Angelis FD, Domine M, Clingan P, Hochmair MJ, Powell SF, Cheng SYS, Bischoff HG, Peled N, Grossi F, Jennens RR, Reck M, Hui R, Garon EB, Boyer M, Rubio-Viqueira B, Novello S, Kurata T, Gray JE, Vida J, Wei Z, Yang J, Raftopoulos H, Pietanza C, Garassino MC. Pembrolizumab plus chemotherapy in metastatic non-small-cell lung cancer. N Engl J Med. 2018;378:2078–92. https://doi.org/10.1056/NEJMoa1801005.

62. Gadgeel S, Rodríguez-Abreu D, Speranza G, Esteban E, Felip E, Dómine M, Hui R, Hochmair MJ, Clingan P, Powell SF, Cheng SYS, Bischoff HG, Peled N, Grossi F, Jennens RR, Reck M, Garon EB, Novello S, Rubio-Viqueira B, Boyer M, Kurata T, Gray JE, Yang J, Bas T, Pietanza MC, Garassino MC. Updated analysis from KEYNOTE-189: pembrolizumab or placebo plus pemetrexed and platinum for previously untreated metastatic nonsquamous non-small-cell lung cancer. J Clin Oncol. 2020;38(14):1505–17. https://doi.org/10.1200/JCO.19.03136.

63. Langer CJ, Gadgeel SM, Borghaei H, Papadimitrakopoulou VA, Patnaik A, Powell SF, Gentzler RD, Martins RG, Stevenson JP, Jalal SI, Panwalkar A, Yang JCH, Gubens M, Sequist LV, Awad MM, Fiore J, Ge Y, Raftopoulos H, Gandhi L. Carboplatin and pemetrexed with or without pembrolizumab for advanced, non-squamous non-small-cell lung cancer: a randomised, phase 2 cohort of the open-label keynote-021 study. Lancet Oncol. 2016;17(11):1497–508. https://doi.org/10.1016/S1470-2045(16)30498-3.

64. Velcheti V, Hu X, Piperdi B, Burke T. Real-world outcomes of first-line pembrolizumab plus pemetrexed-carboplatin for metastatic nonsquamous NSCLC at US oncology practices. Sci Rep. 2021;11:9222. https://doi.org/10.1038/s41598-021-88453-8.

65. NHS. Chemotherapy protocols. Lung cancer-non-small cell (NSCLC). Carboplatin (AUC 5)-pembrolizumab-pemetrexed. NHS, University Hospital Southampton, NHS Foundation Trust, England, 2019. Available https://www.uhs.nhs.uk/Media/SUHTExtranet/Services/Chemotherapy-SOPs/Lung-cancer-non-small-cell(NSCLC)/Carboplatin-Pembrolizumab-Pemetrexed.pdf. Accessed Oct 16, 2021.

66. NHS. Chemotherapy protocols. Lung cancer-non-small cell (NSCLC). Cisplatin-pembrolizumab-pemetrexed. NHS, University Hospital Southampton, NHS Foundation Trust, England, 2019. Available https://www.uhs.nhs.uk/Media/SUHTExtranet/Services/Chemotherapy-SOPs/Lung-cancer-non-small-cell(NSCLC)/Cisplatin-Pembrolizumab-Pemetrexed.pdf. Accessed Oct 16, 2021.

67. NCT00402051. Chemotherapy with pemetrexed in combination with platinum for advanced non-small cell lung cancer (NSCLC). Clinical Trials. 2010. Available https://clinicaltrials.gov/ct2/show/NCT00402051. Accessed Oct 16, 2021.

68. Socinski MA, Weissman C, Hart LL, Beck JT, Choksi JK, Hanson JP, Prager D, Monberg MJ, Ye Z, Obasaju CK. Randomized phase II trial of pemetrexed combined with either cisplatin or carboplatin in untreated extensive-stage small-cell lung cancer. J Clin Oncol. 2006;24(30):4840–7. https://doi.org/10.1200/JCO.2006.07.7016.

69. Xiao H, Tian R, Zhang Z, Du K, Ni Y. Efficacy of pemetrexed plus platinum doublet chemotherapy as first-line treatment for advanced nonsquamous non-small-cell-lung cancer: a systematic review and meta-analysis. Onco Targets Ther. 2016;9:1471–6. https://doi.org/10.2147/OTT.S96160.

70. Fujita T, Kuroki T, Hayama N, Shiraishi Y, Amano H, Nakamura M, Hirano S, Tabeta H, Nakamura S. Pemetrexed plus platinum for patients with advanced non-small cell lung cancer and interstitial lung disease. In Vivo. 2019;33(6):2059–64. https://doi.org/10.21873/invivo.11704.

71. Li M, Zhang Q, Fu P, Li P, Peng A, Zhang G, Song X, Tan M, Li X, Liu Y, Wu Y, Fan S, Wang C. Pemetrexed plus platinum as the first-line treatment option for advanced non-small cell lung cancer: a meta-analysis of randomized controlled trials. PLoS One. 2012;7(5):e37229. https://doi.org/10.1371/journal.pone.0037229.

72. NHS. Chemotherapy protocols. Lung cancer-non-small cell (NSCLC). Carboplatin-pemetrexed. NHS, University Hospital Southampton, NHS Foundation Trust, England, 2014. Available https://www.uhs.nhs.uk/Media/SUHTExtranet/Services/Chemotherapy-SOPs/Lung-cancer-non-small-cell(NSCLC)/CarboplatinandPemetrexedver12.pdf. Accessed Oct 16, 2021.

73. NHS. Chemotherapy protocols. Lung cancer-non-small cell (NSCLC). Cisplatin-pemetrexed. NHS, University Hospital Southampton. NHS Foundation Trust, England, 2014. Available https://www.uhs.nhs.uk/Media/SUHTExtranet/Services/Chemotherapy-SOPs/Lung-cancer-non-small-cell(NSCLC)/CisplatinandPemetrexedver12.pdf. Accessed Oct 16, 2021.

74. Demedts IK, Vermaelen KY, van Meerbeeck JP. Treatment of extensive-stage small cell lung carcinoma: current status and future prospects. Eur Respir J. 2010;35:202–15. https://doi.org/10.1183/09031936.00105009.

75. Carter BW, Glisson BS, Truong MT, Erasmus JJ. Small cell lung carcinoma: staging, imaging, and treatment considerations. RadioGraphics. 2014;34(6):1707–21. https://doi.org/10.1148/rg.346140178.

76. West HJ. Moving beyond limited and extensive staging of small cell lung cancer. JAMA Oncol. 2019;5(3):e185187. https://doi.org/10.1001/jamaoncol.2018.5187.

77. Kalemkerian GP. Staging and imaging of small cell lung cancer. Cancer Imaging. 2011;11(1):253–8. https://doi.org/10.1102/1470-7330.2011.0036.

78. Barnes H, See K, Barnett S, Manser R. Surgery for limited-stage small-cell lung cancer. Cochrane Libr. 2017;4(4):CD011917. https://doi.org/10.1002/14651858.CD011917.pub2.

79. Pezzi TA, Schwartz DL, Mohamed ASR, Welsh JW, Komaki RU, Hahn SM, Sepesi B, Pezzi CM, Fuller CD, Chun SG. JAMA Oncol. 2018;4(8):e174504. https://doi.org/10.1001/jamaoncol.2017.4504.
80. Yang S, Zhang Z, Wang Q. Emerging therapies for small cell lung cancer. J Hematol Oncol. 2019;12:47. https://doi.org/10.1186/s13045-019-0736-3.
81. Zhou T, Zhang Z, Luo F, Zhao Y, Hou X, Liu T, Wang K, Zhao H, Huang Y, Zhang L. Comparison of first-line treatments for patients with extensive-stage small cell lung cancer: a systematic review and network meta-analysis. JAMA Netw Open. 2020;3(10):e2015748. https://doi.org/10.1001/jamanetworkopen.2020.15748.
82. Girling DJ. Comparison of oral etoposide and standard intravenous multidrug chemotherapy for small-cell lung cancer: a stopped multicentre randomised trial. Lancet. 1996;348(9027):563–6. https://doi.org/10.1016/s0140-6736(96)02005-3.
83. Souhami RL, Spiro SG, Rudd RM, Elvira MCR, James LE, Gower NH, Lamont A, Harper PG. Five-day oral etoposide2 treatment for advanced small-cell lung cancer: randomized comparison with intravenous chemotherapy. J Natl Cancer Inst. 1997;89(8):577–80. https://doi.org/10.1093/jnci/89.8.577.
84. Quoix E. Topotecan in the treatment of relapsed small cell lung cancer. Onco Targets Ther. 2008;1:79–86. https://doi.org/10.2147/ott.s3689.
85. Hagmann R, Hess V, Zippelius A, Rothschild SI. Second-line therapy of small-cell lung cancer: topotecan compared to a combination treatment with adriamycin, cyclophosphamide and vincristine (ACO) - a single center experience. J Cancer. 2015;6(11):1148–54. https://doi.org/10.7150/jca.13080.
86. Sundstrom S, Bremnes RM, Kaasa S, Aasebo U, Hatlevoll R, Dahle R, Boye N, Wang M, Vigander T, Vilsvik J, Skovlund E, Hannisdal E, Aamdal S. Cisplatin and etoposide regimen is superior to cyclophosphamide, epirubicin, and vincristine regimen in small-cell lung cancer: results from a randomized phase III trial with 5 years' follow-up. J Clin Oncol. 2002;20(24):4665–72. https://doi.org/10.1200/JCO.2002.12.111.
87. Xenidis N, Kotsakis A, Kalykaki A, Christophyllakis C, Giassas S, Kentepozidis N, Polyzos A, Chelis L, Vardakis N, Vamvakas L, Georgoulias V, Kakolyris S. Etoposide plus cisplatin followed by concurrent chemo-radiotherapy and irinotecan plus cisplatin for patients with limited-stage small cell lung cancer: a multicenter phase II study. Lung Cancer. 2010;68(3):450–4. https://doi.org/10.1016/j.lungcan.2009.08.012.
88. Shepherd FA, Evans WK, MacCormick R, Feld R, Yau JC. Cyclophosphamide, doxorubicin, and vincristine in etoposide- and cisplatin-resistant small cell lung cancer. Cancer Treat Rep. 1987;71(10):941–4.
89. Veronesi A, Cartel G, CriveUari D, Magri MD, Valentina MD, Foladore S, Trovo MG, Nascimben O, Sibau A, Talamini R, Monfardini S. Cisplatin and etoposide versus cyclophosphamide, epirubicin and vincristine in small cell lung cancer: a randomised study. Eur J Cancer. 1994;30(10):1474–8. https://doi.org/10.1016/0959-8049(94)00253-2.
90. Jung SOK, Kim SY, Kim JO, Jung SS, Park HS, Moon JY, Kim SM, Lee JE. Promising effects of 3rd line cyclophosphamide, adriamycin and vincristine (CAV) and 4th line ifosfamide and carboplatin chemotherapy in refractory small cell lung cancer. Thorac Cancer. 2015;6(5):659–63. https://doi.org/10.1111/1759-7714.12198.
91. NHS. Chemotherapy protocols. Lung cancer-small cell (SCLC). Cyclophosphamide-doxorubicin-vincristine. NHS, University Hospital Southampton, NHS Foundation Trust, England, 2013. Available https://www.uhs.nhs.uk/Media/SUHTExtranet/Services/Chemotherapy-SOPs/Lung-cancer-small-cell(SCLC)/Cyclophosphamide,Doxorubicin,Vincristine.pdf. Accessed Oct 16, 2021.
92. Lee C. BC cancer protocol summary for second-line treatment of extensive stage small cell lung cancer (SCLC) with irinotecan with or without platinum. BC Cancer. British Columbia, 2021. Available http://www.bccancer.bc.ca/chemotherapy-protocols-site/Documents/Lung/LUSCPI_Protocol.pdf. Accessed Oct 16, 2021.
93. Georgoulias V, Agelidou A, Syrigos K, Rapti A, Agelidou M, Nikolakopoulos J, Polyzos A, Athanasiadis A, Tselepatiotis E, Androulakis N, Kalbakis K, Samonis G, Mavroudis D. Second-line treatment with irinotecan plus cisplatin vs cisplatin of patients with advanced

non-small-cell lung cancer pretreated with taxanes and gemcitabine: a multicenter randomised phase II study. Br J Cancer. 2005;93:763–9. https://doi.org/10.1038/sj.bjc.6602748.

94. Xu F, Ren X, Chen Y, Li Q, Li R, Chen Y, Xia S. Irinotecan-platinum combination therapy for previously untreated extensive-stage small cell lung cancer patients: a meta-analysis. BMC Cancer. 2018;18(1):808. https://doi.org/10.1186/s12885-018-4715-9.

95. Han D, Wang G, Sun L, Ren X, Shang W, Xu L, Li S. Comparison of irinotecan/platinum versus etoposide/platinum chemotherapy for extensive-stage small cell lung cancer: a meta-analysis. Eur J Cancer Care. 2017;26(6):e12723. https://doi.org/10.1111/ecc.12723.

96. Hanna N, Bunn PA Jr, Langer C, Einhorn L, Guthrie T Jr, Beck T, Ansari R, Ellis P, Byrne M, Morrison M, Hariharan S, Wang B, Sandler A. Randomized phase III Trial comparing irinotecan/cisplatin with etoposide/cisplatin in patients with previously untreated extensive-stage disease small-cell lung cancer. J Clin Oncol. 2006;24(13):2038–43. https://doi.org/10.1200/JCO.2005.04.8595.

97. Jonge MJA, Verweij J, Planting AST, van der Burg ME, Stoter G, Boer-Dennert MM, Bruijn P, Brouwer E, Vernillet L, Sparreboom A. Clin Cancer Res. 1999;5(8):2012–7.

98. Han JY, Lim HS, Lee DH, Ju SY, Lee SY, Kim HY, Park YH, Park CG, Lee JS. Randomized phase II study of two opposite administration sequences of irinotecan and cisplatin in patients with advanced nonsmall cell lung carcinoma. Cancer. 2006;106(4):873–80. https://doi.org/10.1002/cncr.21668.

99. Silva AA, Carlotto J, Rotta I. Padronização da ordem de infusão de medicamentos antineoplásicos utilizados no tratamento dos cânceres de mama e colorretal. Einstein. 2018;16(2):1–9.

100. Sato M, Ando M, Minami H, Ando Y, Ando M, Yamamoto M, Sakai S, Watanabe A, Ikeda T, Sekido Y, Saka H, Shimokata K, Hasegawa Y. Phase I/II and pharmacologic study of irinotecan and carboplatin for patients with lung cancer. Cancer Chemother Pharmacol. 2001;48(6):481–7. https://doi.org/10.1007/s002800100355.

101. Moore AJ, Parker RJ, Wiggins J. Malignant mesothelioma. Orphanet J Rare Dis. 2008;3:34. https://doi.org/10.1186/1750-1172-3-34.

102. Tsao AS, Wistuba I, Roth JA, Kindler HL. Malignant pleural mesothelioma. J Clin Oncol. 2009;27(12):2081–90. https://doi.org/10.1200/JCO.2008.19.8523.

103. Goudreault J, Dagnault A. Mesothelioma: an evidence-based review. London: IntechOpen; 2013.

104. Opitz I. Management of malignant pleural mesothelioma—The European experience. J Thorac Dis. 2014;6(2):238–52. https://doi.org/10.3978/j.issn.2072-1439.2014.05.03.

105. Bibby AC, Tsim S, Kanellakis N, Ball H, Talbot DC, Blyth KG, Maskell NA, Psallidas I. Malignant pleural mesothelioma: an update on investigation, diagnosis and treatment. Eur Respir Rev. 2016;25:472–86. https://doi.org/10.1183/16000617.0063-2016.

106. Kim J, Bhagwandin S, Labow DM. Malignant peritoneal mesothelioma: a review. Ann Transl Med. 2017;5(11):236. https://doi.org/10.21037/atm.2017.03.96.

107. Steele JP, Shamash J, Evans MT, Gower NH, Tischkowitz MD, Rudd RM. Phase II study of vinorelbine in patients with malignant pleural mesothelioma. J Clin Oncol. 2000;18(23):3912–7. https://doi.org/10.1200/JCO.2000.18.23.3912.

108. Petrini I, Lucchesi M, Puppo G, Chella A. Medical treatment of malignant pleural mesothelioma relapses. J Thorac Dis. 2018;10(2):333–41. https://doi.org/10.21037/jtd.2017.10.159.

109. Kindler HL, van Meerbeeck JP. The role of gemcitabine in the treatment of malignant mesothelioma. Semin Oncol. 2002;29(1):70–6. https://doi.org/10.1053/sonc.2002.30232.

110. Kim ST, Park JY, Lee J, Park JO, Park YS, Lim HY, Kang WK, Park SH. The efficacy of the frontline platinum-based combination chemotherapy in malignant peritoneal mesothelioma. Jpn J Clin Oncol. 2010;40(11):1031–6. https://doi.org/10.1093/jjco/hyq083.

111. Ak G, Metintas S, Akarsu M, Metintas M. The effectiveness and safety of platinum-based pemetrexed and platinum-based gemcitabine treatment in patients with malignant pleural mesothelioma. BMC Cancer. 2015;15:510. https://doi.org/10.1186/s12885-015-1519-z.

Chapter 10
Chemotherapeutic Protocols
for the Treatment of Neurological Cancer

10.1 Epidemiological Profile of Neurological Cancers

Neurological tumors represent 1.4–1.8% of all cancers in the world, with the brain being responsible for about 88% of neurological tumors. There are two basic types of brain tumors that are primary and metastatic, in which the primary tumors originate and remain in the brain and the metastatic ones originate in other organs and are spread to the brain [1–3].

According to WHO [4], 308,000 cases of neurological cancers were reported, with 168,000 cases in men and 140,000 in women. Men are at greater risk of developing neurological cancers than women [5, 6]. Due to the location of the tumor, the mortality rate is significant; in the WHO [4] data, 251,000 deaths from neurological cancers were reported. Figure 10.1 shows the estimated incidence and mortality for the year 2040.

The high incidence of neurological cancers occurs in northern Europe, Australia, and North America, while in Africa the incidence is lower [7, 8]. The occurrence of neurological cancers presents a distinct pattern in terms of age, with high incidence rates among adults aged 60 years and over, children aged 0–4 years, and adolescents [7, 9]. As for the histological type, gliomas are the most common in adults, accounting for 70–80% of cases of neurological tumors, but in children, the most common types are pilocytic astrocytomas, medulloblastoma, and germ cell tumors [7, 10, 11].

I. D. Lima Cavalcanti, *Chemotherapy Protocols and Infusion Sequence*,
https://doi.org/10.1007/978-3-031-10839-6_10

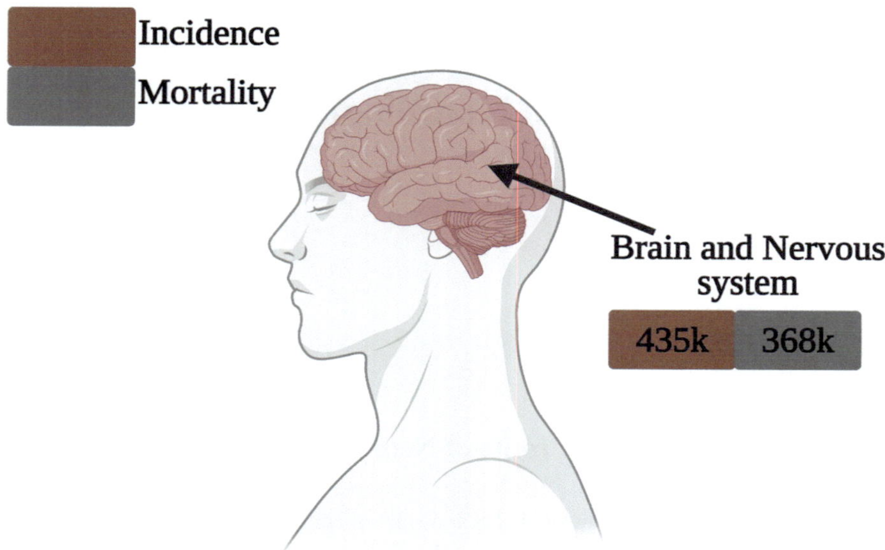

Fig. 10.1 Estimate of incidence and mortality from neurological cancers for the year 2040. (Source: Created with BioRender.com and data were extracted from [4])

10.2 Types of Neurological Cancers

Some risk factors for the development of neurological cancers include high-dose radiation, hereditary syndromes, increasing age, and a family history of brain tumors [12]. Primary brain tumors start in the brain or nearby tissues such as the meninges, cranial nerves, pituitary gland, or pineal gland. As in other tumors, cell DNA mutations induce the development of neurological cancers [13–15]. Some types of neurological tumors are shown in Fig. 10.2.

Glioma is the most common type of neurological cancer, starting in the glial cells that surround the nerve cells and aid their function. Gliomas are classified into three types, which will depend on the type of glial cell that started the tumor development, being classified into astrocytomas, ependymomas, and oligodendrogliomas. Gliomas are characterized by their invasiveness and rapid growth [16–19].

Another type of neurological tumor is the pituitary tumor, which develops in the pituitary gland, thereby disrupting hormone production. Pituitary tumors tend to remain in the pituitary gland or surrounding tissue [20, 21]. The neuroectodermal tumor belongs to the group of small round cell tumors, presenting a neural origin, which can compromise the central or peripheral nervous system. Neuroectodermal tumors are extremely aggressive, with disease-free survival in 2–3 years ranging from 25% to 60% [22–25].

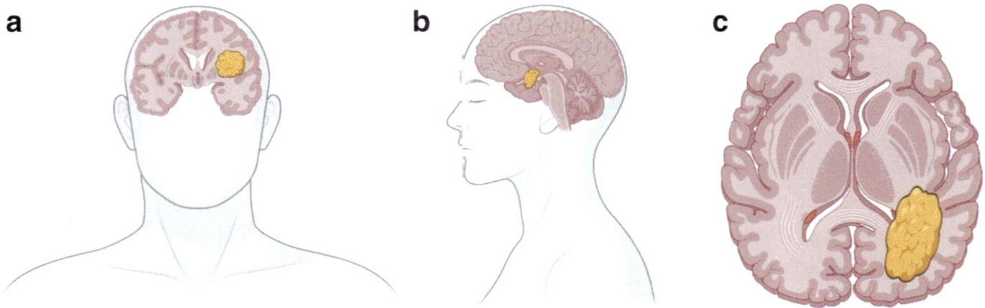

Fig. 10.2 Types of neurological tumors. (**a**) Glioma, (**b**) pituitary tumor, and (**c**) neuroectodermal tumor. (Source: Created with BioRender.com)

Metastatic brain cancer develops from the spread of cancer cells from other organs to the brain, with the most likely cancers that spread to the brain being lung, breast, colon, kidney, and melanoma cancers [2, 26, 27].

10.2.1   Chemotherapy for the Treatment of Glioma

Glioma treatment may include surgery, radiation therapy, chemotherapy, or just medical follow-up. Surgery aims to remove most of the tumor and is usually the first step in treatment. Radiation therapy follows surgery, especially in high-grade gliomas, and chemotherapy may also be indicated and may be combined with radiation therapy [28–31]. Among the drugs used, temozolomide is the most frequent and is indicated for the adjuvant treatment of astrocytomas, oligodendrogliomas, malignant gliomas, and malignant brain tumors with MGMT methylation [32–37].

Another drug indicated as monotherapy is lomustine, which is indicated for the treatment of recurrent malignant brain tumors; etoposide, which is used in the palliative treatment of patients with recurrent malignant gliomas and ependymoma; and procarbazine in the second-line treatment of recurrent brain tumors [38–44]. Some protocols indicated for the treatment of glioma will be covered in the next topics [45–47].

10.2.1.1   BE Protocol (Bevacizumab and Etoposide)

The BE protocol combines bevacizumab with etoposide and has been indicated as palliative therapy for recurrent malignant gliomas [48]. Bevacizumab is the standard treatment for recurrent malignant glioma, but some patients may be resistant to bevacizumab [49, 50]. Fu et al. [49] through a review study evaluated the benefits of the combination of etoposide and bevacizumab in this group of patients. The protocol was observed to promote an 8-month progression-free survival and 28-month overall survival.

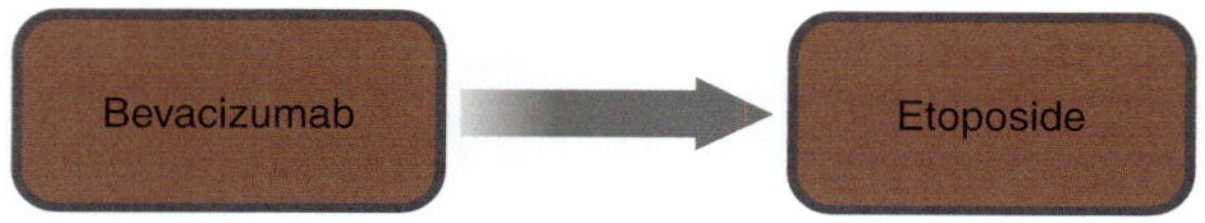

Fig. 10.3 Schedule of administration of the BE protocol with oral administration of etoposide

In a phase 2 study, Reardon et al. [51] and Reardon et al. [52] evaluated the efficacy of bevacizumab combined with etoposide in the treatment of recurrent malignant glioma. The protocol promoted 47-week overall survival and 6-month progression-free survival was 40.6%. As for the toxicity profile, the most common adverse events included neutropenia, thrombosis, hypertension, fatigue, and infection. According to Reardon et al. [52], combining bevacizumab with etoposide increases toxicity compared with monotherapy with bevacizumab.

Regarding the BE protocol administration schedule (Fig. 10.3), bevacizumab is administered by infusion on days 1 and 15 or on days 1 and 22, while etoposide is administered orally from day 1 to day 21, once a day [53].

10.2.1.2   BL Protocol (Bevacizumab and Lomustine)

The combination of bevacizumab with lomustine is also indicated as palliative therapy for recurrent malignant gliomas [54]. Lomustine is a prodrug of the nitrosourea class that undergoes metabolization to its active form; acting from the alkylation and cross-linking of DNA and RNA, it can also inhibit processes such as carbamoylation and modification of cellular proteins [55–57].

The combination of lomustine and bevacizumab has brought benefits for the treatment of glioma. According to Wick et al. [58], the combination promoted an overall survival of 9.1 months and progression-free survival of 2.7 months longer than in the bevacizumab monotherapy group. As for toxicity, 63.6% of patients had grade 3–5 adverse events, but the combination did not affect the patients' quality of life.

Tonder et al. [59] evaluated the benefits of the combination of lomustine and bevacizumab in the treatment of recurrent glioblastoma. The protocol presented leukopenia, neutropenia, thrombocytopenia, and lymphopenia as the most frequent toxicity. As for the benefits of the protocol, a progression-free survival of 2.6 months and overall survival of 5.1 months were observed.

As for the administration schedule, the BL protocol (Fig. 10.4) starts with the infusion of bevacizumab followed by the oral administration of lomustine on day 1 once daily every 6 weeks [53].

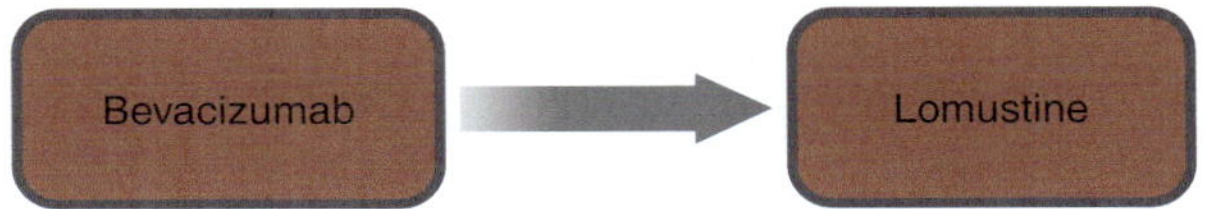

Fig. 10.4 Schedule of administration of the EL protocol with oral administration of lomustine

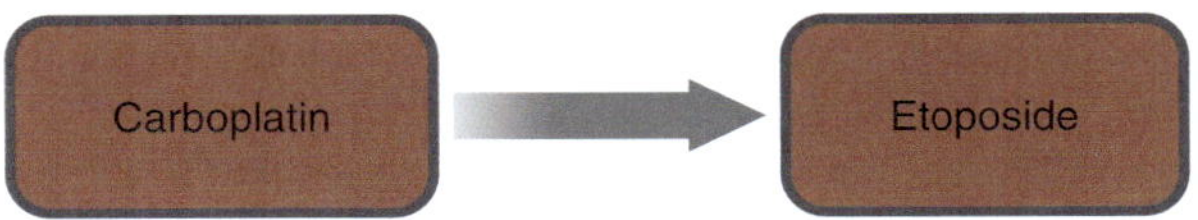

Fig. 10.5 CARV protocol infusion sequence

10.2.1.3   CARV Protocol (Carboplatin and Etoposide)

The CARV protocol combined carboplatin with etoposide in the treatment of recurrent ependymoma [60]. Jeremic et al. [61], in a phase 2 study, verified the efficacy of the combination between carboplatin and etoposide in patients with recurrent malignant glioma. As a result, partial responses were observed in 21% of patients, with a mean time to tumor progression of 42.5 weeks and a mean survival time of 47.5 weeks.

Franceschi et al. [62] treated patients with high-grade recurrent glioma with carboplatin and etoposide. In the study, the authors found that the combination promoted complete response in 20% of patients, the median time to progression of 4 months, 6-month progression-free survival of 33.3%, and median survival time of 10 months.

The combination of carboplatin and etoposide has also been shown to be effective and well tolerated in the treatment of children with brain tumors. According to Castello et al. [63], the protocol promoted a response rate in five of six patients with medulloblastoma and in two of four patients with high-grade astrocytoma. And as for toxicity, the protocol induced anemia, thrombocytopenia, and leukopenia.

In high-grade progressive glioma, Tonder et al. [64] found that the combination of carboplatin and etoposide promoted a progression-free survival of 2.5 months, but at 6 months, the progression-free survival rate was 0%, showing that for heavily pretreated glioma, the combination presented an unfavorable benefit-risk.

The infusion sequence of the CARV protocol (Fig. 10.5) is based on the initial infusion of carboplatin followed by the infusion of etoposide; care must be taken when infusing both drugs, as they may present a risk if extravasated due to their irritating characteristics [65].

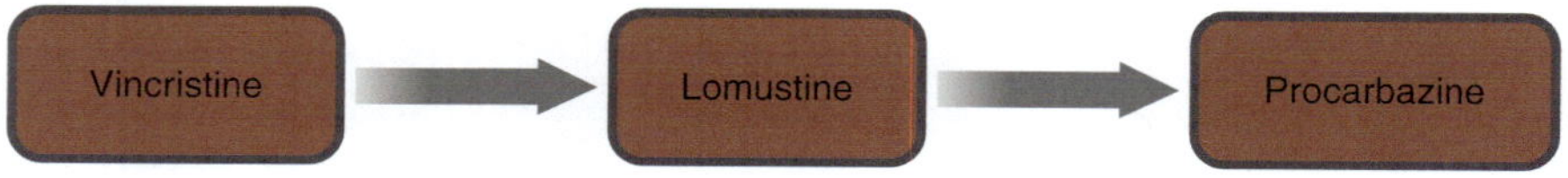

Fig. 10.6 Schedule of administration of the PCV protocol with oral administration of lomustine and procarbazine

10.2.1.4 PCV Protocol (Procarbazine, Lomustine, and Vincristine)

The combination of procarbazine, lomustine, and vincristine is an alternative for the treatment of brain tumors [66]. Cairncross et al. [67] tested the combination in the treatment of oligodendroglial tumors, and as a result, they observed that the protocol associated with radiotherapy in patients with mutant HDI had longer overall survival of 9.4 years. The prolongation of survival by the PCV protocol was also observed by Lassman [68], who compared the protocol with temozolomide monotherapy in the treatment of anaplastic oligodendrogliomas.

Wick and Winkler [69] also compared the PCV protocol with temozolomide in the treatment of gliomas. The authors highlight the importance of balancing the advantages of both therapeutic regimens in terms of the benefits in prolonging survival versus the risks of toxicity and impact on patients' quality of life. In a real-world study, Keogh et al. [70] highlight the frequent toxicities induced by the PCV protocol in clinical practice, with hematological toxicities being the most common, with cases of thrombocytopenia and neutropenia.

As for the PCV protocol infusion schedule (Fig. 10.6), vincristine is administered by infusion followed by oral administration of lomustine once daily and procarbazine once daily for 10 days [71].

10.2.1.5 TMZETO Protocol (Temozolomide and Etoposide)

The association between temozolomide and etoposide may be indicated in the treatment of recurrent malignant brain tumors [72]. In a phase 1 study, Korones et al. [73] evaluated the maximum tolerated dose in the combination of temozolomide and etoposide in the treatment of recurrent malignant glioma. The authors noted that some patients developed thrombocytopenia, neutropenia, fever, herpes zoster infection, and pneumonia, and the maximum tolerated dose of temozolomide was 150 mg/m^2 and that of oral etoposide was 50 mg/m^2.

In children with recurrent malignant brain tumors, Ruggiero et al. [74] evaluated the combination of temozolomide and etoposide through a review study. The advantage of using temozolomide and etoposide in brain tumors is that they both penetrate the blood–brain barrier, thereby acting against malignant brain tumors, and drugs that have distinct cytotoxicity mechanisms can enhance their therapeutic effects [74].

As for the administration schedule, both drugs are administered orally; temozolomide is administered once a day for 5 days, while etoposide is administered once a day for 12 days [72].

10.2.2 Chemotherapy for the Treatment of Primary Neuroectodermal Tumors

The first treatment option for primitive neuroectodermal tumors is surgery to obtain tissue to determine the type of tumor and remove as much of the tumor as possible. Surgery may be followed by radiotherapy and treatment with chemotherapy, targeted therapy, and immunotherapy. Chemotherapy protocols significantly improve outcomes in treating patients with primitive neuroectodermal tumors [75–80].

One of the protocols indicated for the treatment of primitive neuroectodermal tumors is PCV, which is also indicated for the treatment of gliomas (see topic 10.2.1.4) [81, 82]. Another protocol is the CCV, which I will cover in the next topic.

10.2.2.1 CCV Protocol (Lomustine, Cisplatin, and Vincristine)

The CCV protocol combines lomustine, cisplatin, and vincristine for adjuvant treatment in high-risk adult medulloblastoma [83]. Rutkauskiene and Labanauskas [84] evaluated the effectiveness of the CCV protocol in patients with high-risk medulloblastoma. The protocol had a relapse rate of 11.1%, the median time to progression of 47 months, 2-year progression-free survival of 88.9%, and 2-year overall survival of 71.1%.

In the study by Lefkowitz et al. [85], the combination of lomustine, cisplatin, and vincristine promoted a disease-free survival of 18.5 months, and with regard to toxicity, the most frequent adverse events were reversible bone marrow suppression, high-frequency hearing loss, and decreased kidney function.

As for the administration schedule, the CCV protocol (Fig. 10.7) starts with the infusion of vincristine, which is a specific cycle drug with a vesicant characteristic [86, 87], followed by cisplatin infusion, and finally oral administration of lomustine once daily on day 1 [88].

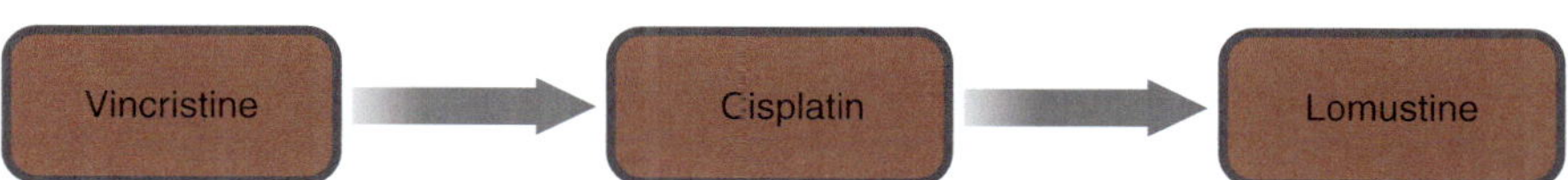

Fig. 10.7 CCV protocol administration schedule

10.2.3   Treatment of Pituitary Tumor

Some pituitary tumors do not require treatment; the choice of treatment depends on the type of tumor and the size of the tumor. Among the therapeutic modalities, surgery is indicated in cases where the tumor is pressing on the optic nerves or if it is overproducing some hormones. After surgery, radiotherapy or isolated therapy may be indicated in cases where surgery is not indicated [89–92].

Concerning drug treatment, drugs that block excessive hormone secretion may be indicated, for example, bromocriptine and cabergoline, which act by decreasing prolactin secretion, and are indicated in the treatment of pituitary adenomas [93–95]. Lanreotide and octreotide are octapeptide analogs of the endogenous somatostatin that act by decreasing the production of growth hormone and are indicated in the treatment of growth hormone-secreting pituitary adenoma [96, 97]. Quinagolide is another drug used in the treatment of pituitary adenomas; it acts as a selective dopamine D2 receptor agonist and reduces elevated levels of prolactin [98–100].

References

1. Araújo DS, Soares EA, Freitas WLS, Araújo MS. Analysis of the mortality rate for tumors in the central nervous system between 1979 to 2018 in the State of Piauí, Brazil. Res Soc Develop. 2021;10(1):e2510111269. https://doi.org/10.33448/rsd-v10i1.11269.
2. Eichler AF, Chung E, Kodack DP, Loeffler JS, Fukumura D, Jain RK. The biology of brain metastases—translation to new therapies. Nat Rev Clin Oncol. 2011;8(6):344–56. https://doi.org/10.1038/nrclinonc.2011.58.
3. Motah M, Massi DG, Bekolo FF, Nju NA, Ndoumbe A, Moumi M, Sango A, Shu P, Eyenga V. Epidemiological profile of brain tumors in Cameroon: a retrospective study. Egypt J Neurol Psychiatr Neurosurg. 2021;57:126. https://doi.org/10.1186/s41983-021-00381-6.
4. WHO – World Health Organization. Estimated number of incident cases from 2018 to 2040. International Agency for Research on Cancer; 2020. Available in: https://gco.iarc.fr/tomorrow/graphic-isotype?type=0&type_sex=0&mode=population&sex=0&populations=900&cancers=36&age_group=value&apc_male=0&apc_female=0&single_unit=100000&print=0. Accessed 17 Oct 2021.
5. Fisher JL, Schwartzbaum JA, Wrensch M, Wiemels JL. Epidemiology of brain tumors. Neurol Clin. 2007;25(4):867–90. https://doi.org/10.1016/j.ncl.2007.07.002.
6. Darefsky AS, Dubrow R. International variation in the incidence of adult primary malignant neoplasms of the brain and central nervous system. Cancer Causes Control. 2009;20:1593–604. https://doi.org/10.1007/s10552-009-9404-1.
7. Piñeros M, Sierra MS, Izarzugaza MI, Forman D. Descriptive epidemiology of brain and central nervous system cancers in central and South America. Cancer Epidemiol. 2016;44(Suppl 1):S141–9. https://doi.org/10.1016/j.canep.2016.04.007.
8. Farmanfarma KHK, Mohammadian M, Shahabinia Z, Hassanipour S, Salehiniya H. Brain cancer in the world: an epidemiological review. World Cancer Res J. 2019;6:e1356. https://doi.org/10.32113/wcrj_20197_1356.
9. Arora RS, Alston RD, Eden TOB, Estlin EJ, Moran A, Birch JM. Age–incidence patterns of primary CNS tumors in children, adolescents, and adults in England. Neuro-Oncology. 2009;11(4):403–13. https://doi.org/10.1215/15228517-2008-097.

10. Rodríguez JL. Pilocytic astrocytoma, another way to reach your diagnosis. Rev Bras Oftalmol. 2020;79(4):276–7. https://doi.org/10.5935/0034-7280.20200060.

11. Tan AC, Ashley DM, López GY, Malinzak M, Friedman HS, Khasraw M. Management of glioblastoma: state of the art and future directions. CA Cancer J Clin. 2020;70(4):299–312. https://doi.org/10.3322/caac.21613.

12. Bondy ML, Scheurer ME, Malmer B, Barnholtz-Sloan JS, Davis FG, Il'yasova D, Kruchko C, McCarthy BJ, Rajaraman P, Schwartzbaum JA, Sadetzki S, Schlehofer B, Tihan T, Wiemels JL, Wrensch M, Buffler PA. Brain tumor epidemiology: consensus from the brain tumor epidemiology consortium (BTEC). Cancer. 2008;113(7 Suppl):1953–68. https://doi.org/10.1002/cncr.23741.

13. Reilly KM. Brain tumor susceptibility: the role of genetic factors and uses of mouse models to unravel risk. Brain Pathol. 2009;19(1):121–31. https://doi.org/10.1111/j.1750-3639.2008.00236.x.

14. Miller KD, Ostrom QT, Kruchko C, Patil N, Tihan T, Cioffi G, Fuchs HE, Waite KA, Jemal A, Siegel RL, Barnholtz-Sloan JS. Brain and other central nervous system tumor statistics, 2021. CA Cancer J Clin. 2021;71(5):381–406. https://doi.org/10.3322/caac.21693.

15. Perkins A, Liu G. Primary brain tumors in adults: diagnosis and treatment. Am Fam Physician. 2016;93(3):211–7.

16. Louis DN, Holland EC, Cairncross JG. Glioma classification: a molecular reappraisal. Am J Pathol. 2001;159(3):779–86. https://doi.org/10.1016/S0002-9440(10)61750-6.

17. Gladson CL, Prayson RA, Liu WM. The pathobiology of glioma tumors. Ann Rev Pathol Mechan Dis. 2010;5:33–50. https://doi.org/10.1146/annurev-pathol-121808-102109.

18. Honasoge A, Sontheimer H. Involvement of tumor acidification in brain cancer pathophysiology. Front Physiol. 2013;4:316. https://doi.org/10.3389/fphys.2013.00316.

19. Mesfin FB, Al-Dhahir MA. Gliomas. Treasure Island: StatPearls Publishing; 2021.

20. Melmed S. Mechanisms for pituitary tumorigenesis: the plastic pituitary. J Clin Invest. 2003;112(11):1603–18. https://doi.org/10.1172/JCI20401.

21. Chang M, Yang C, Bao X, Wang R. Genetic and epigenetic causes of pituitary adenomas. Front Endocrinol. 2021;11:596554. https://doi.org/10.3389/fendo.2020.596554.

22. Costa CML, Rondinelli P, Camargo B. Tumor neuroectodérmico primitivo na infância: relato de 13 casos e revisão da literatura. Revista Brasileira de Cancerologia. 2000;46(3):293–8.

23. Mattos JP, Bonilha L, Ferreira D, Borges W, Fernandes YB, Borges G. Multiple systemic metastases of posterior fossa - primitive neuroectodermal tumor (PF-PNET) in adult: case report. Arq Neuropsiquiatr. 2003;61(1):100–3. https://doi.org/10.1590/S0004-282X2003000100019.

24. He X, Chen Z, Dong Y, Tong D. A primitive neuroectodermal tumor in an adult: case report of a unique location and MRI characteristics. Medicine. 2018;97(7):e9933. https://doi.org/10.1097/MD.0000000000009933.

25. Rios CI, Jesus OD. Primitive neuroectodermal tumor. Treasure Island: StatPearls Publishing; 2021.

26. Riva M, Landonio G, Arena O, Citterio A, Galli C, Ferrante E, Brioschi A, Collice M, Gambacorta M, Scialfa G, Defanti CA, Siena S. Pathophysiology, clinical manifestations and supportive care of metastatic brain cancer. Forum (Genova). 2001;11(1):4–26.

27. Witzel I, Oliveira-Ferrer L, Pantel K, Müller V, Wikman H. Breast cancer brain metastases: biology and new clinical perspectives. Breast Cancer Res. 2016;18:8. https://doi.org/10.1186/s13058-015-0665-1.

28. Croteau D, Mikkelsen T. Adults with newly diagnosed high-grade gliomas. Curr Treat Options in Oncol. 2001;2(6):507–15. https://doi.org/10.1007/s11864-001-0072-y.

29. Stupp R, Mason WP, van den Bent MJ, Weller M, Fisher B, Taphoorn MJB, Belanger K, Brandes AA, Marosi C, Bogdahn U, Curschmann J, Janzer RC, Ludwin SK, Gorlia T, Allgeier A, Lacombe D, Cairncross JG, Eisenhauer E, Mirimanoff RO. Radiotherapy plus concomitant and adjuvant temozolomide for glioblastoma. N Engl J Med. 2005;352:987–96. https://doi.org/10.1056/NEJMoa043330.

30. Bush NAO, Chang S. Treatment strategies for low-grade glioma in adults. J Oncol Pract. 2016;12(12):1235–41. https://doi.org/10.1200/JOP.2016.018622.

31. Weller M, van den Bent M, Preusser M, Rhun EL, Tonn JC, Minniti G, Bendszus M, Balana C, Chinot O, Dirven L, French P, Hegi ME, Jakola AS, Platten M, Roth P, Rudà R, Short S, Smits M, Taphoorn MJB, von Deimling A, Westphal M, Soffietti R, Reifenberger G, Wick W. EANO guidelines on the diagnosis and treatment of diffuse gliomas of adulthood. Nat Rev Clin Oncol. 2021;18:170–86. https://doi.org/10.1038/s41571-020-00447-z.

32. Yung WK. Temozolomide in malignant gliomas. Semin Oncol. 2000;27(3 Suppl 6):27–34.

33. Hegi ME, Diserens AC, Gorlia T, Hamou MF, Tribolet N, Weller M, Kros JM, Hainfellner JÁ, Mason W, Mariani L, Bromberg JEC, Hau P, Mirimanoff RO, Cairncross G, Janzer RC, Stupp R. MGMT gene silencing and benefit from temozolomide in glioblastoma. N Engl J Med. 2005;352:997–1003. https://doi.org/10.1056/NEJMoa043331.

34. Villano JL, Seery TE, Bressler LR. Temozolomide in malignant gliomas: current use and future targets. Cancer Chemother Pharmacol. 2009;64(4):647–55. https://doi.org/10.1007/s00280-009-1050-5.

35. Cohen KJ, Pollack IF, Zhou T, Buxton A, Holmes EJ, Burger PC, Brat DJ, Rosenblum MK, Hamilton RL, Lavey RS, Heideman RL. Temozolomide in the treatment of high-grade gliomas in children: a report from the Children's Oncology Group. Neuro-Oncology. 2011;13(3):317–23. https://doi.org/10.1093/neuonc/noq191.

36. Thon N, Kreth S, Kreth FW. Personalized treatment strategies in glioblastoma: MGMT promoter methylation status. Onco Targets Ther. 2013;6:1363–72. https://doi.org/10.2147/OTT.S50208.

37. NCT03633552. Efficacy of two temozolomide regimens in adjuvant treatment of patients with brain high grade glioma. Clinical Trials. 2018. Available in: https://clinicaltrials.gov/ct2/show/NCT03633552. Accessed 17 Oct 2021.

38. Fulton D, Urtasun R, Forsyth P. Phase II study of prolonged oral therapy with etoposide (VP16) for patients with recurrent malignant glioma. J Neuro-Oncol. 1996;27(2):149–55. https://doi.org/10.1007/BF00177478.

39. Brandes AA, Ermani M, Turazzi S, Scelzi E, Berti F, Amistà P, Rotilio A, Licata C, Fiorentino MV. Procarbazine and high-dose tamoxifen as a second-line regimen in recurrent high-grade gliomas: a phase II study. J Clin Oncol. 1999;17(2):645. https://doi.org/10.1200/JCO.1999.17.2.645.

40. Sandri A, Massimino M, Mastrodicasa L, Sardi N, Bertin D, Basso ME, Todisco L, Paglino A, Perilongo G, Genitori L, Valentini L, Ricardi U, Gandola L, Giangaspero F, Madon E. Treatment with oral etoposide for childhood recurrent ependymomas. J Pediatr Hematol Oncol. 2005;27(9):486–90. https://doi.org/10.1097/01.mph.0000181430.71176.b7.

41. Kesari S, Schiff D, Doherty L, Gigas DC, Batchelor TT, Muzikansky A, O'Neill A, Drappatz J, Chen-Plotkin AS, Ramakrishna N, Weiss SE, Levy B, Bradshaw J, Kracher J, Laforme A, Black PM, Folkman J, Kieran M, Wen PY. Phase II study of metronomic chemotherapy for recurrent malignant gliomas in adults. Neuro-Oncology. 2007;9(3):354–63. https://doi.org/10.1215/15228517-2007-006.

42. Leonard A, Wolff JE. Etoposide improves survival in high-grade glioma: a meta-analysis. Anticancer Res. 2013;33(8):3307–15.

43. NCT00004004. Procarbazine in treating patients with recurrent brain tumor. Clinical Trials. 2013. Available in: https://clinicaltrials.gov/ct2/show/NCT00004004. Accessed 17 Oct 2021.

44. Weller M, Rhun EL. How did lomustine become standard of care in recurrent glioblastoma? Cancer Treat Rev. 2020;87:102029. https://doi.org/10.1016/j.ctrv.2020.102029.

45. Kuehr T, Thaler J, Woell E. Chemotherapy protocols 2017: current protocols and "Targeted therapies". Klinikum Wels-Grieskirchen and Caritas Christi URGET NOS. Austria. 2017. www.chemoprotocols.eu.

46. BC Cancer. Supportive care protocols. BC Cancer. British Columbia. 2021. Available in: http://www.bccancer.bc.ca/health-professionals/clinical-resources/chemotherapy-protocols/supportive-care. Accessed 2 July 2021.

47. NHS. Chemotherapy protocols. NHS. University Hospital Southampton. NHS Foundation Trust. England. 2021. Available in: https://www.uhs.nhs.uk/HealthProfessionals/Chemotherapy-protocols/Chemotherapy-protocols.aspx. Accessed 2 July 2021.

48. NCT00612430. Ph II bevacizumab + etoposide for Pts w recurrent MG. Clinical Trials. 2013. Available in: https://clinicaltrials.gov/ct2/show/NCT00612430. Accessed 19 Oct 2021.

49. Fu BD, Linskey ME, Bota DA. Bevacizumab and etoposide combination chemotherapy in patients with recurrent malignant gliomas who failed bevacizumab. Drug Therapy Stud. 2012;2(1):e6. https://doi.org/10.4081/dts.2012.e6.

50. Carrillo JA, Hsu FPK, Delashaw J, Bota DA. Efficacy and safety of bevacizumab and etoposide combination in patients with recurrent malignant gliomas who have failed bevacizumab. Rev Health Care. 2014;5(1):23–32.

51. Reardon D, Desjardins A, Vredenburgh JJ. Gururangan S, Peters KB, Norfleet JA. Bevacizumab plus etoposide among recurrent malignant glioma patients: Phase II study final results. J Clin Oncol. 2009;27(15_suppl):2046. https://doi.org/10.1200/jco.2009.27.15_suppl.2046.

52. Reardon DA, Desjardins A, Vredenburgh JJ, Gururangan S, Sampson JH, Sathornsumetee S, McLendon RE, Herndon JE, Marcello JE, Norfleet J, Friedman AH, Bigner DD, Friedman HS. Metronomic chemotherapy with daily, oral etoposide plus bevacizumab for recurrent malignant glioma: a phase II study. Br J Cancer. 2009;101(12):1986–94. https://doi.org/10.1038/sj.bjc.6605412.

53. Thiessen B. BC cancer protocol summary for palliative therapy for recurrent malignant gliomas using bevacizumab with or without concurrent etoposide or lomustine. BC Cancer. British Columbia. 2021. Available in: http://www.bccancer.bc.ca/chemotherapy-protocols-site/Documents/Neuro-Oncology/CNBEV_Protocol.pdf. Accessed 19 Oct 2021.

54. NCT01290939. Bevacizumab and lomustine for recurrent GBM. Clinical Trials. 2021. Available in: https://clinicaltrials.gov/ct2/show/NCT01290939. Accessed 19 Oct 2021.

55. Liang XJ, Choi Y, Sackett DL, Park JK. Nitrosoureas inhibit the stathmin mediated migration and invasion of malignant glioma cells. Cancer Res. 2008;68(13):5267–72. https://doi.org/10.1158/0008-5472.CAN-07-6482.

56. Weber GF. DNA damaging drugs. Mol Therap Cancer. 2014;8:9–112. https://doi.org/10.1007/978-3-319-13278-5_2.

57. Nassar AEF, Wisnewski AV, King I. Biotransformation and rearrangement of laromustine. Drug Metab Dispos. 2016;44:1349–63. https://doi.org/10.1124/dmd.116.069823.

58. Wick W, Gorlia T, Bendszus M, Taphoorn M, Sahm F, Harting I, Brandes AA, Taal W, Domont J, Idbaih A, Campone M, Clement PM, Stupp R, Fabbro M, Rhun EL, Dubois F, Weller M, von Deimling A, Golfinopoulos V, Bromberg JC, Platten M, Klein M, van der Bent MJ. Lomustine and bevacizumab in progressive glioblastoma. N Engl J Med. 2017;377:1954–63. https://doi.org/10.1056/NEJMoa1707358.

59. Tonder M, Eisele G, Weiss T, Hofer S, Seystahl K, Valavanis A, Stupp R, Weller M, Roth P. Addition of lomustine for bevacizumab-refractory recurrent glioblastoma. Acta Oncol. 2014;53(10):1436–40. https://doi.org/10.3109/0284186X.2014.920960.

60. Thiessen B. BC cancer protocol summary for CARBOplatin and etoposide in the treatment of recurrent ependymoma and oligodendroglioma. BC Cancer. British Columbia. 2021. Available in: http://www.bccancer.bc.ca/chemotherapy-protocols-site/Documents/Neuro-Oncology/CNCARV_Protocol.pdf. Accessed 20 Oct 2021.

61. Jeremic B, Grujicic D, Jevremovic S, Stanisavljevic B, Milojevic L, Djuric L, Mijatovic L. Carboplatin and etoposide chemotherapy regimen for recurrent malignant glioma: a phase II study. J Clin Oncol. 1992;10(7):1074–7.

62. Franceschi E, Cavallo G, Scopece L, Paioli A, Pession A, Magrini E, Conforti R, Palmerini E, Bartolini S, Rimondini S, Degli Esposti R, Crinò L. Phase II trial of carboplatin and etoposide for patients with recurrent high-grade glioma. Br J Cancer. 2004;91(6):1038–44. https://doi.org/10.1038/sj.bjc.6602105.

63. Castello MA, Clerico A, Deb G, Dominici C, Fidani P, Donfrancesco A. High-dose carboplatin in combination with etoposide (JET regimen) for childhood brain tumors. Am J Pediatr Hematol Oncol. 1990;13(3):297–300. https://doi.org/10.1097/00043426-199023000-00008.

64. Tonder M, Weller M, Eisele G, Roth P. Carboplatin and etoposide in heavily pretreated patients with progressive high-grade glioma. Chemotherapy. 2014;60:375–8. https://doi.org/10.1159/000440678.

65. NHS. Chemotherapy protocols. Brain tumours. Carboplatin (AUC5)-etoposide. NHS. University Hospital Southampton. NHS Foundation Trust. England. 2019. Available in: https://www.uhs.nhs.uk/Media/SUHTExtranet/Services/Chemotherapy-SOPs/CNS/CarboplatinAUC5Etoposide.pdf. Accessed 20 Oct 2021.

66. Thiessen B. BC cancer protocol summary for modified PCV chemotherapy of brain tumours using procarbazine, lomustine (CCNU) and vincristine. BC Cancer. British Columbia. 2021. Available in: http://www.bccancer.bc.ca/chemotherapy-protocols-site/Documents/Neuro-Oncology/CNMODPCV_Protocol.pdf. Accessed 20 Oct 2021.

67. Cairncross JG, Wang M, Jenkins RB, Shaw EG, Giannini C, Brachman DG, Buckner JC, Fink KL, Souhami L, Laperriere NJ, Huse JT, Mehta MP, Curran WJ Jr. Benefit from procarbazine, lomustine, and vincristine in oligodendroglial tumors is associated with mutation of IDH. J Clin Oncol. 2014;32(8):783–90. https://doi.org/10.1200/JCO.2013.49.3726.

68. Lassman AB. Procarbazine, lomustine and vincristine or temozolomide: which is the better regimen? CNS Oncol. 2015;4(5):341–6. https://doi.org/10.2217/cns.15.36.

69. Wick W, Winkler F. Regimen of procarbazine, lomustine, and vincristine versus temozolomide for gliomas. Cancer. 2018;124(13):2674–6. https://doi.org/10.1002/cncr.31371.

70. Keogh RJ, Aslam R, Hennessy MA, Coyne Z, Hennessy BT, Breathnach OS, Grogan L, Morris PG. One year of procarbazine lomustine and vincristine is poorly tolerated in low grade glioma: a real world experience in a national neuro-oncology Centre. BMC Cancer. 2021;21:140. https://doi.org/10.1186/s12885-021-07809-5.

71. NHS. Chemotherapy protocols. Central Nervous System. Lomustine-Procarbazine-Vincristine (PCV). NHS. University Hospital Southampton. NHS Foundation Trust. England. 2015. Available in: https://www.uhs.nhs.uk/Media/SUHTExtranet/Services/Chemotherapy-SOPs/CNS/Lomustine-Procarbazine-Vincristine%20(PCV)%20ver%201.1.pdf. Accessed 20 Oct 2021.

72. Thiessen B. BC cancer protocol summary for therapy for recurrent malignant brain tumours using temozolomide and etoposide. BC Cancer. British Columbia. 2021. Available in: http://www.bccancer.bc.ca/chemotherapy-protocols-site/Documents/Neuro-Oncology/CNTMZETO_Protocol.pdf. Accessed 20 Oct 2021.

73. Korones DN, Benita-Weiss M, Coyle TE, Mechtler L, Bushunow P, Evans B, Reardon DA, Quinn JA, Friedman H. Phase I study of temozolomide and escalating doses of oral etoposide for adults with recurrent malignant glioma. Cancer. 2003;97(8):1963–8. https://doi.org/10.1002/cncr.11260.

74. Ruggiero A, Ariano A, Triarico S, Capozza MA, Romano A, Maurizi P, Mastrangelo S, Attinà G. Temozolomide and oral etoposide in children with recurrent malignant brain tumors. Drugs Context. 2020;9:2020-3-1. https://doi.org/10.7573/dic.2020-3-1.

75. Grier HE, Krailo MD, Tarbell NJ, Link MP, Fryer CJH, Pritchard DJ, Gebhardt MC, Dickman PS, Perlman EJ, Meyers PA, Donaldson SS, Moore S, Rausen AR, Vietti TJ, Miser JS. Addition of ifosfamide and etoposide to standard chemotherapy for Ewing's sarcoma and primitive neuroectodermal tumor of bone. N Engl J Med. 2003;348(8):694–701. https://doi.org/10.1056/NEJMoa020890.

76. NCT00003859. Surgery plus radiation therapy with or without chemotherapy in treating children with primitive neuroectodermal tumors of the CNS. Clinical Trials. 2013. Available in: https://clinicaltrials.gov/ct2/show/NCT00003859. Accessed 20 Oct 2021.

77. Friedrich C, Warmuth-Metz M, von Bueren AO, Nowak J, Bison B, von Hoff K, Pietsch T, Kortmann RD, Rutkowski S. Primitive neuroectodermal tumors of the brainstem in children treated according to the HIT trials: clinical findings of a rare disease. J Neurosurg Pediatr. 2015;15(3):227–35. https://doi.org/10.3171/2014.9.PEDS14213.

78. Aridgides PD, Kang G, Mazewski C, Merchant TE. Outcomes after radiation therapy for very young children with high-risk medulloblastoma or supratentorial primitive neuroectodermal

tumor treated on COG ACNS0334. Int J Radiat Oncol Biol Phys. 2019;105(1):S109. https://doi.org/10.1016/j.ijrobp.2019.06.602.

79. Bruschi M, Petretto A, Cama A, Pavanello M, Bartolucci M, Morana G, Ramenghi LA, Garré ML, Ghiggeri GM, Panfoli I, Candiano G. Potential biomarkers of childhood brain tumor identified by proteomics of cerebrospinal fluid from extraventricular drainage (EVD). Sci Rep. 2021;11:1818. https://doi.org/10.1038/s41598-020-80647-w.

80. Maier H, Dalianis T, Kostopoulou ON. New approaches in targeted therapy for medulloblastoma in children. Anticancer Res. 2021;41(4):1715–26. https://doi.org/10.21873/anticanres.14936.

81. van den Bent MJ, Chinot O, Boogerd W, Marques JB, Taphoorn MJB, Kros JM, van der Rijt CCD, Vecht CJ, Beule ND, Baron B. Second-line chemotherapy with temozolomide in recurrent oligodendroglioma after PCV (procarbazine, lomustine and vincristine) chemotherapy: EORTC Brain Tumor Group phase II study 26972. Ann Oncol. 2003;14(4):599–602. https://doi.org/10.1093/annonc/mdg157.

82. Cakar M, Aksoy S, Kilickap S, Harputluoglu H, Erman M. Procarbazine, lomustine, vincristine combination may be effective in adult medulloblastoma patients with systemic metastases. J Neuro-Oncol. 2005;75:233–4. https://doi.org/10.1007/s11060-005-4177-1.

83. Thiessen B. BC cancer protocol summary for adjuvant lomustine, CISplatin and vincristine in adult high-risk medulloblastoma or other primitive neuro-ectodermal tumour (PNET). BC Cancer. British Columbia. 2021. Available in: http://www.bccancer.bc.ca/chemotherapy-protocols-site/Documents/Neuro-Oncology/CNCCV_Protocol.pdf. Accessed 20 Oct 2021.

84. Rutkauskiene G, Labanauskas L. Treatment of patients of high-risk group of medulloblastoma with the adjuvant lomustine, cisplatin, and vincristine chemotherapy. Medicina (Kaunas). 2005;41(12):1026–34.

85. Lefkowitz IB, Packer RJ, Siegel KR, Sutton LN, Schut L, Evans AE. Results of treatment of children with recurrent medulloblastoma/primitive neuroectodermal tumors with lomustine, cisplatin, and vincristine. Cancer. 1990;65:412–7.

86. Almeida VL, Leitão A, Reina LCB, Montanari CA, Donnici CL, Lopes MTP. Câncer e agentes antineoplásicos ciclo-celular específicos e ciclo-celular não específicos que interagem com o DNA: uma introdução. Química Nova. 2005;28(1):118–29. https://doi.org/10.1590/S0100-40422005000100021.

87. Gama CS, Nobre SMPC, Neusquen LPDG. Extravasamento de medicamentos antineoplásicos. Eurofarma. São Paulo. Brazil. 2016. Available in: https://cdn.eurofarma.com.br//wp-content/uploads/2019/11/530382..pdf. Accessed 18 July 2021.

88. NHS. Chemotherapy protocols. Central Nervous System. Cisplatin-Lomustine-Vincristine (Packer LCV3). NHS. University Hospital Southampton. NHS Foundation Trust. England. 2015. Available in: https://www.uhs.nhs.uk/Media/SUHTExtranet/Services/Chemotherapy-SOPs/CNS/Cisplatin-Lomustine-Vincristine-Packer-LCV3.pdf. Accessed 20 Oct 2021.

89. Chanson P, Salenave S. Diagnosis and treatment of pituitary adenomas. Minerva Endocrinol. 2004;29(4):241–75.

90. Dekkers OM, Pereira AM, Romijn JA. Treatment and follow-up of clinically nonfunctioning pituitary macroadenomas. J Clin Endocrinol Metabol. 2008;93(10):3717–26. https://doi.org/10.1210/jc.2008-0643.

91. Lake MG, Krook LS, Cruz SV. Pituitary adenomas: an overview. Am Fam Physician. 2013;88(5):319–27.

92. Neto LV, Boguszewski CL, Araújo LA, Bronstein MD, Miranda PAC, Musolino NRC, Naves LA, Vilar L, Oliveira Júnior AR, Gadelha MR. A review on the diagnosis and treatment of patients with clinically nonfunctioning pituitary adenoma by the Neuroendocrinology Department of the Brazilian Society of Endocrinology and Metabolism. Arch Endocrinol Metabol. 2016;60(4):374–90. https://doi.org/10.1590/2359-3997000000179.

93. Ribeiro MF, Spritzer PM, Barbosa-Coutinho LM, Oliveira MC, Pavanato MA, Silva ISB, Reis FM. Effects of bromocriptine on serum prolactin levels, pituitary weight and immunoreactive prolactin cells in estradiol-treated ovariectomized rats: an experimental model of estrogendependent hyperprolactinemia. Braz J Med Biol Res. 1997;30(1):113–7.

94. Cannavò S, Curtò L, Squadrito S, Almoto B, Vieni A, Trimarchi F. Cabergoline: a first-choice treatment in patients with previously untreated prolactin-secreting pituitary adenoma. J Endocrinol Investig. 1999;22(5):354–9. https://doi.org/10.1007/BF03343573.

95. Banskota S, Adamson DC. Pituitary adenomas: from diagnosis to therapeutics. Biomedicine. 2021;9(5):494. https://doi.org/10.3390/biomedicines9050494.

96. Heaney AP, Melmed S. Molecular targets in pituitary tumours. Nat Rev Cancer. 2004;4:285–95. https://doi.org/10.1038/nrc1320.

97. Ferraz-Filho JRL, Torres US, Teixeira ACV, Castro MLS, Dias MAF. Ectopic growth hormone-secreting pituitary adenoma involving the clivus treated with octreotide: role of magnetic resonance imaging in the diagnosis and clinical follow-up. Arq Neuropsiquiatr. 2012;70(9):741–5. https://doi.org/10.1590/S0004-282X2012000900019.

98. Barlier A, Jaquet P. Quinagolide – a valuable treatment option for hyperprolactinaemia. Eur J Endocrinol. 2006;154(2):187–95. https://doi.org/10.1530/eje.1.02075.

99. Nobels FR, Herder WW, van den Brink WM, Kwekkeboom DJ, Hofland LJ, Zuyderwijk J, Jong FH, Lamberts SW. Long-term treatment with the dopamine agonist quinagolide of patients with clinically non-functioning pituitary adenoma. Eur J Endocrinol. 2000;143(5):615–21. https://doi.org/10.1530/eje.0.1430615.

100. Sarno AD, Landi ML, Marzullo P, Somma CD, Pivonello R, Cerbone G, Lombardi G, Colao A. The effect of quinagolide and cabergoline, two selective dopamine receptor type 2 agonists, in the treatment of prolactinomas. Clin Endocrinol. 2000;53(1):53–60. https://doi.org/10.1046/j.1365-2265.2000.01016.x.

Index